Veterinary epidemiology

SECOND EDITION

Michael Thrusfield

Department of Veterinary Clinical Studies
Royal (Dick) School of Veterinary Studies
University of Edinburgh

b

Blackwell
Science

First edition © 1986 by Butterworth & Co.
   (Publishers) Ltd
Second edition © 1995 by
   Blackwell Science Ltd
Editorial Offices:
Osney Mead, Oxford OX2 0EL
25 John Street, London WC1N 2BL
23 Ainslie Place, Edinburgh EH3 6AJ
350 Main Street, Malden
   MA 02148 5018, USA
54 University Street, Carlton
   Victoria 3053, Australia
10, rue Casimir Delavigne
   75006 Paris, France

Other Editorial Offices:

Blackwell Wissenschafts-Verlag GmbH
Kurfürstendamm 57
10707 Berlin, Germany

Blackwell Science KK
MG Kodenmacho Building
7–10 Kodenmacho Nihombashi
Chuo-ku, Tokyo 104, Japan

First published 1986 by
   Butterworth & Co. (Publishers) Ltd
Second edition published 1995 by
   Blackwell Science Ltd
Reissued in paperback with updates 1997
Reprinted 1999, 2000

Set in 9/11 Times
by MHL Typesetting Ltd, Coventry
Printed and bound in the United Kingdom
at the University Press, Cambridge

DISTRIBUTORS

Marston Book Services Ltd
PO Box 269
Abingdon, Oxon OX14 4YN
(*Orders*: Tel: 01235 465500
          Fax: 01235 465555)

USA
   Blackwell Science, Inc.
   Commerce Place
   350 Main Street
   Malden, MA 02148 5018
   (*Orders*: Tel: 800 759 6102
                781 388 8250
          Fax: 781 388 8255)

Canada
   Login Brothers Book Company
   324 Saulteaux Crescent
   Winnipeg, Manitoba R3J 3T2
   (*Orders*: Tel: 204 837-2987
          Fax: 204 837 3116)

Australia
   Blackwell Science Pty Ltd
   54 University Street
   Carlton, Victoria 3053
   (*Orders*: Tel: 03 9347 0300
          Fax: 03 9347 5001)

A catalogue record for this title
is available from the British Library

ISBN 0-632-04851-4

For further information on
Blackwell Science, visit our website:
www.blackwell-science.com

To Marjory and Harriet

Contents

From the preface to the first edition

The common aim of the many disciplines that comprise veterinary medicine is an increase in the health of animal populations, notably of domestic livestock and companion animals. This goal has traditionally been achieved by individual diagnosis and treatment: procedures that evolved contemporaneously in veterinary and human medicine, when infectious diseases, which had predominantly single causes and clearly identifiable signs, were commonplace.

Four major changes in the veterinarian's appreciation of and approach to disease problems have occurred over the past 20 years. First, despite traditional control techniques, for example slaughter and vaccination, some diseases remain at refractory levels and now require continuous scrutiny to detect changing levels of occurrence associated with ecological and management factors. An example is the detection of 'pockets' of bovine tuberculosis in England in areas where infection of badgers is recorded. Secondly, the control of infectious disease has freed animals from major causes of death, thereby facilitating the emergence of non-infectious diseases as major problems: examples are the cardiac, dermal and renal diseases of dogs. Many of these diseases have a poorly understood, often complex (i.e., multifactorial) cause. Thirdly, the intensification of animal industries has highlighted new 'diseases of production', often manifested as poor performance, rather than clinical disease, and frequently with multifactorial causes. Fourthly, economic evaluation has become important: the economic advantages of disease control, which are obvious with the major animal plagues such as rinderpest, can be difficult to identify when overt disease and dramatic changes in levels of performance are not involved. These four changes in the approach to, and appreciation of, disease have added momentum to the emergence of veterinary epidemiology as a discipline concerned with the measurement of the amount of disease and its economic effects, the identification and quantification of the effects of factors associated with disease, and the assessment of the effects of prevention and treatment of disease in groups of animals.

A knowledge of elementary statistics is essential for an understanding of the full range of epidemiological techniques. Hitherto, most epidemiology books either have assumed a knowledge of statistics or have avoided a description of the mathematical manipulations that are commonly used in epidemiology. However, the extent of statistical teaching varies widely between veterinary schools. Two chapters therefore are included as an introduction to basic statistics, and are intended to make this book statistically self-sufficient (though not comprehensive). Similarly, a chapter includes an introduction to computers, which are now used widely in the recording and analysis of epidemiological data.

Preface to the second edition

Since publication of the first edition, veterinary medicine has faced several new problems, and has been forced to evaluate established ones more critically. Bovine spongiform encephalopathy emerged as a serious problem in the United Kingdom. Rinderpest is still the subject of a global eradication campaign. There is an increasing demand for comprehensive, high-quality technical and economic information on animal disease and productivity at the national and international level; and information systems, such as the United States' National Animal Health Monitoring System, have been designed to suit these requirements. The moves towards an open market, both in the European Union and internationally following the Uruguay round of the General Agreement on Tariffs and Trade, highlight the need for information on animal disease status in trading nations. Multifactorial diseases continue to predominate in intensive production systems, and many companion animal diseases are similarly complex. The solving of these problems and fulfilling of these tasks rely heavily on epidemiological principles and techniques.

All chapters of the first edition have been revised. Chapter 11 has been modified to take account of the increasing popularity of microcomputers, and the rapid development of veterinary information systems. New chapters on clinical trials and comparative epidemiology have been added in response to suggestions from colleagues. More statistical methods are included in Chapters 13–15 and 17. The goal of this edition nevertheless remains the same as that of the first: to provide an introduction to veterinary epidemiology for veterinary undergraduates, postgraduates who have received limited or no training in epidemiology, and practising veterinarians and members of other disciplines with an interest in the subject.

I am again indebted to the colleagues who gave advice during the writing of the second edition. Colin Aitken, Martin Hugh-Jones, Stuart MacDiarmid, Alex Russell, Gordon Scott, Jill Thomson and Andrew Wyllie criticized various parts of the text. George Gettinby again provided considerable indispensable information relating to statistics and modelling, and Keith Howe gave me further insight into animal health economics. A valuable discussion on cluster sampling was also held with Helen Brown, and Ronald Smith's comments on multiple testing were also useful. Helen London, librarian at the University of Edinburgh's Veterinary Field Station, acquired many of the publications cited in the text. Kath Tracey typed several tables, and Rhona Muirhead produced numerous figures. I am also grateful to John Wilesmith of the Central Veterinary Laboratory for permission to reproduce, in *Table 14.9*, details of BSE-affected herds in Northern Ireland. Finally, I am grateful to the Literary Executor of the late Sir Ronald A. Fisher, FRS, to Dr Frank Yates, FRS, and to the Longman Group Limited, London, for permission to reprint Tables III, IV, V and VII from their book, *Statistical Tables for Biological, Agricultural and Medical Research* (6th edition, 1974).

Author's note on the paperback reissue

The publication of this paperback edition has provided the opportunity to correct several errors, particularly in the *t*-test for independent samples with unequal variances (page 272), and in the risk analysis presented in *Table 22.4*. The author is indebted to colleagues who identified these, and other, faults.

Chapter 16 has also been expanded by the inclusion of an appendix on meta-analysis of clinical trials (Appendix XXI, p. 413).

Michael Thrusfield
Edinburgh
1997

1 The development of veterinary medicine

Veterinary epidemiology is concerned with disease in animal **populations**. Its evolution has spanned several centuries and has been central to the successful control of animal disease. This introductory chapter traces the development of veterinary medicine in general, showing that it has been inseparably linked to that of veterinary epidemiology.

Although man's association with animals began in prehistoric times, the development of scientific veterinary medicine is comparatively recent. A milestone in this growth was the establishment of the first permanent veterinary school at Lyons, France, in 1762. Early developments were governed largely by economic rather than humanitarian motives, associated with the importance of domestic stock as a source of food and as working animals; and there are still important economic reasons for concern about disease in animal populations. Later, with the advent of the industrial revolution and the invention of the internal combustion engine, the importance of draft animals declined in the developed countries. Although dogs and cats have been companion animals for several thousand years, it is only recently that they and other pets have increased in importance as components of human society.

Until recently, the emphasis of veterinary medicine has been on the treatment of individual animals with clearly identifiable diseases or defects. Apart from routine immunization and prophylactic treatment of internal parasites, restricted attention has been given to herd health and comprehensive preventive medicine which give proper consideration to both infectious and non-infectious diseases.

Currently, the nature of traditional clinical practice is changing in all developed countries. The stock owner is better educated, and the value of individual animals relative to veterinary fees has decreased. Therefore, contemporary large animal practitioners, if they are to meet modern requirements, must improve their knowledge of herd health programmes, designed to increase production by preventing disease, rather than just dispensing traditional treatment to clinically sick animals.

In the developing countries, the infectious diseases still cause considerable loss of animal life and production. Traditional control techniques, based on identification of recognizable signs and pathological changes, cannot reduce the level of some diseases to an acceptable degree. Different techniques, based on the study of patterns of disease in groups of animals, are needed.

Similarly, contemporary companion animal practitioners, like their medical counterparts, are becoming increasingly involved with chronic and refractory diseases which can be understood better by an investigation of the diseases' characteristics in populations.

This chapter outlines the changing techniques of veterinary medicine by tracing man's attempts at controlling disease in animals, and introduces some current animal disease problems that can be solved by an epidemiological approach.

Historical perspective

Domestication of animals and early methods of healing

The importance of animal healers has been acknowledged since animals were initially domesticated. The dog, naturally a hunter, was probably the first animal to be domesticated over 14 000 years ago when it became the companion of early hunters. Sheep and goats were domesticated by 9000 BC in the fertile Nile valley and were the basis of early pastoral cultures. A few of these societies have lasted, for example the Jews, but many were superseded by cattle cultures; in some the pig

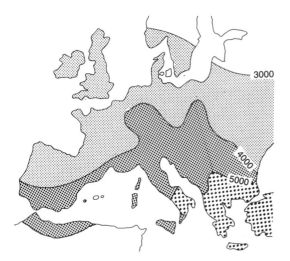

Fig. 1.1 A generalized map to show the spread of farming from the Near East to Europe in years BC. (From Dyer, 1990.)

increased in importance (Murray, 1968). An Egyptian cattle culture evolved from 4000 BC, and farming spread from the Near East into Europe (*Figure 1.1*). There is archaeological evidence of cattle shrines in Anatolia dating back to 6000 BC (Mellaart, 1967). This record illustrates that animals had a religious as well as an economic significance in early civilizations. The aurochs was central to the religion of the Sumerians, who migrated throughout Asia, North Africa and Europe in the third millennium BC taking their animals and beliefs with them. India is the largest cattle culture that remains. Cattle cultures also persist in north-east Africa, the result of interaction between the Ancient Egyptians and early Nilotic tribes. Cattle still play important roles in these cultures: they are food, companionship, and status and religious symbols to the Suk (Beech, 1911) and Dinka tribes (Lienhardt, 1961) of the Sudan.

The first extensive colonization of the Eurasian steppe and semi-arid areas occurred in the third millenium BC. The horse provided the key to successful exploitation of the area north of the Black Sea, the Caucasus, and the Taurus and Zagros mountains (Barraclough, 1984), and a Eurasian horse culture, associated with warrior tribes, emerged. Some of these tribes overran the older cattle cultures. The horse is represented in Iranian, Greek and Celtic pantheons. It has become a symbol of veterinary medicine in the form of a centaur, one of which, Chiron, was considered to be the mythological founder of Greek medicine.

There have been several movements of animals with concomitant social and agricultural modifications since the early changes. The camel was introduced into Saharan Africa in the first century BC. The Spanish introduced cattle, sheep, pigs and goats to North America in the 16th century. Haired sheep were introduced to Africa by European slave traders. The Spanish brought turkeys to Europe from North America.

The early Egyptian healers combined religious and medical roles by being priest-healers, often associated with temples. Their therapeutic techniques are recorded in the veterinary *Papyrus of Kahun* (*c.* 1900 BC). Literary records of similar age, describing veterinary activities, are extant from other parts of the world, such as Indian Sanskrit texts from the Vedic period (1800 – 1200 BC).

Changing concepts of the cause of disease

A method of treatment used by early Egyptians was incantation. This was partly ritual, but also reflected their belief in supernatural spirits as a possible cause of disease. Approaches to treatment and prevention are the direct result of theories of cause. There have been five main theories up to the middle of this century. One theory was often superseded by another, but traces of each can still be seen in different parts of the world.

Demons

Early man attributed disease to supernatural powers, the product of animism which imbued all moving things with a spirit. In this 'spirit-world' disease could be produced by witches, superhuman entities and spirits of the dead (Valensin, 1972). Treatment therefore included: placation, for example by sacrifice; exorcism (forcible expulsion); evasion, for instance scattering millet seeds to avoid vampires (Summers, 1961); and transference, the best known example of which is the Gadarene swine (the *Bible*: Mark 5, i – xiii). The techniques included: ritual ceremonies; material objects that could be suspended (amulets and periapts), carried (talismans), hung in a building (fetishes and icons) or displayed in the community (totems); the use of special people such as witch doctors; and incantations. The meaning of the Indian word 'brahmin' originally was 'healer' because the brahmin were a class of healers. In the neolithic period (4200 – 2100 BC), trepanning (the removal of a bone disc from the skull) may have been practised to release demons from sick people.

During the 19th century, many European peasants still believed that diseases of cattle were caused by evil spirits which could be kept at bay by fire (Frazer, 1890), and the

African Nuer tribe still uses incantations during ritual sacrifice when cattle epidemics occur (Evans-Pritchard, 1956). Moreover, sacrifice was practised in England as late as the 19th century (Baker, 1974).

Divine wrath

The demonic theory involved many spirits; the next development, monotheistic in origin, argued that disease was the product of a displeased supreme being: disease was punishment. This belief is prominent in the Old Testament, for example the animal plague of Egypt (the *Bible*: Exodus 9, iii) and is also evident in Persian and Aztec writings. The only effective treatment of disease induced in this way was placation because exorcism and evasion would not be effective against a supreme being. Traces of this belief have persisted until recent times. The English veterinary surgeon, William Youatt, writing in 1835, supported the practice of burning crosses on the heads of cattle to cure and prevent disease. In 1865, Queen Victoria, recognizing that the current British rinderpest outbreak was the result of divine displeasure, ordered that a prayer should be used in each church in England while the epidemic continued.

Metaphysical medicine

The next development did not assume the existence of a supreme being, either demonic or divine, but assumed the presence of occult forces beyond the physical universe. This 'metaphysical' medicine embodied a theory of natural laws but excluded scientific principles such as observation and the repeatability of phenomena. The moon, stars and planets were considered to affect health (Whittaker, 1960), these concepts being obvious predecessors of astrology. Several outbreaks of rinderpest in Dark Age Europe were ascribed to earthquakes, floods and comets.

Treatment frequently included particularly foul medicines and practices that persisted for many centuries. A recommended 17th century cure for broken wind in horses comprised toads, swallows and moles roasted alive and mixed with shoe soles. Divination, practised by the Babylonians using sheep livers, and the 'Doctrine of Signatures' which suggested a similarity between the disease and its cure — for example, using toads to treat warts — were notable metaphysical developments.

The universe of natural law

A major intellectual revolution began in Greece in the sixth century BC in which the universe was rationalized without either demonic or metaphysical influences. The Greeks thought that disease was the result of derangement

CHARACTERISTIC		Moisture	Dryness
CHARACTERISTIC	Heat	Humour = Blood Associated element = Air Source = Heart Excess → Sanguine temperament	Humour = Yellow bile Associated element = Fire Source = Liver Excess → Choleric (bilious) temperament
	Cold	Humour = Phlegm Associated element = Water Source = Pituitary gland Excess → Phlegmatic temperament	Humour = Black bile Associated element = Earth Source = Spleen Excess → Melancholic temperament

Fig. 1.2 Components of humoral pathology.

of four humours of the body, which were associated with four properties (heat, moisture, dryness and cold) and with four elements (air, earth, water and fire) (*Figure 1.2*). Diseases were considered to be caused by external forces, including climatic and geological changes that affected the population. Local outbreaks of disease were thought to be the result of local eruptions of noxious air: **miasmata (miasmas)**. The word 'malaria' literally means 'bad air' and hints at the 19th century belief that the disease was caused by stale air around swamps.

The concept of humoral derangement was reimported into medieval Europe, via Sicily, during the Crusades, and food was imbued with the same properties as the humours (Tannahill, 1968). The concept persists in several cultures. In indigenous Indian Ayurvedic human and veterinary medicine, based on the Hindu scriptures (Vedas), there are three humours (tridosa): vata (wind), pitta (bile) and kapha (phlegm); derangement of vata, for example, causing asthma and diarrhoea. This concept is also central to modern Mahayana Buddhist medicine. However, in Europe, the popularity of the miasmatic theory declined at the beginning of the 20th century, by which time the microbial theory of infectious disease was adequately supported.

The Greek idea of disease was susceptible to scientific investigation. Careful observation and the identification of specific causes became the hallmarks of the fifth century BC school of medicine at Cos, and were refined by Hippocrates whose text *Discourse on Airs, Waters and Places* (Jones, 1923) dominated medicine for many centuries. Therapy was consistent with causal concepts, and included alterations in diet and purges.

Contagion

The idea that some diseases can be transmitted from one animal to another has its ubiquitous origins in antiquity. The Romans, Galen and Lucretius, believed that disease could be spread by airborne **seeds** or **animacula** (not necessarily living) which were taken in through the nose and mouth. The Jewish Talmud describes demons as hiding 'everywhere' — in water, crumbs and air — implying transmissibility. The primitive Hindus associated sick rats with human plague, the first suggestion of a zoonosis. The Veronan, Fracastorius, writing in the early 16th century, argued that diseases were transmitted by minute, invisible particles; and Lancisi, physician to Pope Clement XI, freed Rome from rinderpest by using a slaughter policy to prevent infection of unaffected animals. Thomas Lobb, writing in London in the 18th century, considered that human plague and rinderpest were caused by particles that multiplied in infected individuals and then infected others by contact or through the air (Lobb, 1745).

The main advances in the identification of microbes as causes of infectious diseases occurred in the 19th century, although the concept of a living contagious agent, **contagium animatum**, was founded in the 17th century. Edward Jenner's development of a smallpox vaccine using cowpox-infective material, and early biological warfare conducted by American settlers who gave blankets belonging to smallpox victims to Indians as presents, implicitly recognized contagion.

Louis Pasteur's investigation of anthrax and rabies, and Robert Koch's discovery of the bacteria causing tuberculosis and cholera, firmly established microbiology and marked the downfall of the miasmatic theory. The set of postulates formulated by Koch to define causal agents has been used to identify many microbial diseases since those early days of bacteriology (see Chapter 3).

Viruses were also discovered in the late 19th century, although not actually 'seen' until the invention of the electron microscope in the 1930s. In 1892, Iwanowsky demonstrated that tobacco mosaic disease could be transmitted by sap that had been filtered through bacteria-proof filters. Beijerinck serially transmitted the disease using bacteria-free filtrates, and coined the term **contagium vivum fluidum** to describe the infectious 'living' agent. In 1898−99 Loeffler and Frosch discovered the first animal virus, foot-and-mouth disease virus, and in 1911 Rous reported the first virus-induced transmissible tumour.

Towards the end of the 19th century, the first arthropod carrier (a tick) of an infectious disease was identified by Kilborne, Smith and Curtis, investigating Texas fever of cattle in the US.

Impetus for change

Changing attitudes towards the cause of disease and the concomitant alterations in techniques of treatment and prevention are a small part of shifts in overall scientific thought. These changes have not taken place gradually, but have occurred as distinct 'revolutions', which terminate periods of stable science (Kuhn, 1970). Each period has its paradigm (model) which serves to guide research. As time passes, anomalies accumulate. Initially, scientists accommodate these by modifying the paradigm, but a time comes when the pressures on the old framework become so great that a crisis occurs, and there is a revolutionary shift in paradigms. For example, in astronomy the old Ptolemaic model of the universe had to be modified and remodified by adding new planetary epicycles to account for the observed motion of the heavenly bodies, but eventually the critical point was reached when the old model was falling apart under the strain and was ceasing to be credible. Thus, the time was ripe for the dramatic shift in models called the Copernican revolution. Kuhn's thesis has also been applied to political, social and theological 'revolutions' (Macquarrie, 1978) and to the applied sciences (Nordenstam and Tornebohm, 1979) of which veterinary medicine is a part.*

Veterinary medicine has experienced five stable periods and revolutions up to the middle of the 20th century relating to disease control (Schwabe, 1982), which stimulated the changes in the causal concepts already described. The major problem that persisted during these periods, precipitating crises, was large-scale outbreaks of infectious disease: the classical animal plagues† (*Table*

---

*The concept of dramatic paradigm shifts, however, may not be applicable to all areas of thought and progress. The 17th century German philosopher, Leibnitz, argued that change (e.g., in ethics and aesthetics) is gradual.

†A plague (Greek: *plege* = a stroke, a blow; Latin: *plangere* = to strike) traditionally is any widespread infectious disease with a high fatality rate among clinically affected individuals. In veterinary medicine, the term is extended to any widespread infectious disease causing major economic disruption, although the fatality rate may not be high (e.g., foot-and-mouth disease). In human medicine, the term is now commonly restricted to infection with the bacterium, *Pasteurella pestis*.

1.1). Military campaigns frequently assisted the spread of these infections (*Table 1.2*).

The first period: until the first century AD

The initial domestication of animals brought man into close contact with animals and therefore with their diseases. The demonic theory was prevalent. However, despite the use of control techniques consistent with the theory, draft animals continued to die, and a crisis arose when urbanization increased the importance of animals as food resources. This resulted in the development of the first stable phase of veterinary medicine. This was characterized by the emergence of veterinary specialists such as the early Egyptian priest-healers and the Vedic *Salihotriya* who founded the first veterinary hospitals. Humoral pathology developed and the miasmatic theory of cause evolved. Techniques of treatment required careful recognition of clinical signs following the Greek Coan tradition. Quarantine (derived from the Italian word meaning 'forty' — the traditional length, in days, of isolation in the Middle Ages) and slaughter became preventive strategies. These local actions, which lasted until the first century AD, were incapable of solving major problems in the horse, which was becoming an important military animal. This crisis resulted in the second phase: that of military healers.

The second period: the first century AD until 1762

Veterinarians specialized in equine medicine and surgery, reflecting the importance and value of horses (e.g., Richards, 1954). A major veterinary text, the *Hippiatrika*, comprising letters between veterinarians, cavalry officers and castrators, dates from early Byzantine times. The major contributor to this work was Apsyrtus, chief *hippiatros* to the army of Constantine the Great. This phase lasted until the mid-18th century and was marked by a continuing interest in equine matters. Several important texts were written, including Ruini's *Anatomy of the Horse* (published in 1598). Some interest was taken in other animals. John Fitzherbert's *Boke of Husbandrie* (published in 1523) included diseases of cattle and sheep. The horse, however, was pre-eminent. This bias survived in Europe until early this century when equine veterinary medicine was still considered to be a more respectable occupation than the care of other species.

Varying emphasis was placed on the miasmatic and metaphysical theories of cause and on humoral pathology. The Arabians, for example, based their medicine largely on the metaphysical theory.

The third period: 1762–1884

The animal plagues, especially those of cattle, became particularly common in Europe in the mid-18th century with the introduction of rinderpest from Asia. They provided the next major crisis involving civilian animals. The miasmatic theory persisted but the miasmata were thought to originate from filth generated by man, rather than from natural sources. A third stable phase developed, characterized by improvement of farm hygiene, slaughter and treatment as control techniques. When rinderpest entered England from Holland in 1714, Thomas Bates, surgeon to George I, advocated fumigation of buildings, slaughter and burning of affected animals, and resting of contaminated pasture as typical tactics. Cattle owners were also compensated for loss.

Half of the cattle in France were destroyed by rinderpest between 1710 and 1714. The disease occurred irregularly until 1750 when it again became a serious problem. Little was known about the disease. This provided impetus for the establishment of the first permanent veterinary school at Lyons in 1762, and others were subsequently founded to combat the disease (*Table 1.3*).

The lifting of animal importation restrictions in England in 1842 increased the risk of disease occurring in Britain. Sheep pox entered Britain in 1847 from Germany, and pleuropneumonia became a serious problem. Public concern, highlighted by the rinderpest outbreak of 1865, was responsible for the establishment of the British State Veterinary Service in the same year. Similar services were founded in other countries. The legislature continued to strengthen the power of the veterinary services by passing Acts relating to the control of animal diseases.

The fourth period: 1884–1960

The animal plagues continued despite sanitary campaigns. This crisis coincided with the inception and acceptance of the microbial theory which, epitomized by Koch's postulates, defined a specific, single cause of an infectious disease and therefore implied a suitable control strategy directed against the causal agent.

This fourth stable phase of campaigns or mass actions began in the 1880s. Treatment of disease was based on laboratory diagnosis involving isolation of agents and identification of lesions followed by therapy. Control of disease by prevention and, subsequently, eradication involved mass testing of animals and immunization when an increasing number of vaccines became available. The discovery of disease vectors facilitated prevention by vector control. An improved understanding of infectious agents' life histories enabled their life-cycles to be broken

Table 1.1 Some dates of occurrence of animal plagues. (Most dates before 1960 extracted from Smithcors, 1957.)

Date	Animal plagues						
	Rinderpest	Pleuropneumonia	Canine distemper	Anthrax	Foot-and-mouth disease	Equine influenza	Ill-defined diseases
500 BC							Egypt 500 BC – time of Christ; Egypt 278 BC abortion
AD				Rome AD 500			Rome 4th century AD (cattle); France 6th century AD (cattle); Ireland 8th century AD; France 820, 850, 940–43 (cattle); England 1314 (cattle)
AD 1400					Italy 1514	England 1688	
AD 1700	France 1710–14, Rome 1713, England 1714, 1745–46, France 1750	Europe 18th century	US 1760, Spain 1761, England 1763			England 1727, Ireland 1728, England 1733, 1737, 1750, 1760, 1771, 1788	
AD 1800	England 1865	England 1841–98			England 1839; England 1870–72, 1877–85	England 1837; North America 1872; England 1889–90	
AD 1900	Africa 1890–1900; Belgium 1920; Middle East 1969–70, Africa 1979–84, India 1983–85, Turkey 1991–92				England 1922–25, 1942, 1952, 1967–68; Italy 1987, 1993; Greece 1994	Czechoslovakia 1957, Britain 1963, US 1963, Europe 1965, Poland 1969, USSR 1976, France, the Netherlands, Sweden 1978–79, England 1989	

Table 1.2 Military campaigns that disseminated rinderpest.

Century	Campaign
5th	Fall of Rome
8 – 9th	Charlemagne's conquest of Europe
12th	Genghis Khan's invasion of Europe
13th	Kublai Khan's invasion of Europe
15 – 16th	Spanish-Hapsburg conquest of Italy
17th	War of the League of Augsberg
18th	War of the Spanish Succession
18th	War of the Austrian Succession
18th	Seven Years' War
18 – 19th	Napoleonic Wars
19 – 20th	Italian conquest of Eritrea
20th	World War I
20th	World War II
20th	Vietnam War
20th	Lebanese War
20th	Azerbaijan conflict
20th	Gulf War

by manipulating the environment; the draining of land to prevent fascioliasis is a good example. Bacterial diseases remained as major clinical problems until the discovery and synthesis of antibiotics in the 20th century, which increased the therapeutic power of the veterinarian.

Many infectious diseases were either effectively controlled or eradicated between the latter part of the 19th century and the middle of the 20th century in the developed countries using the new techniques of the microbial revolution and older techniques including quarantine, importation restrictions, slaughter and

Table 1.3 Veterinary schools founded to combat rinderpest.

Year of foundation	City	Country
1762	Lyon	France
1766	Alfort	France
1767	Vienna	Austria
1769	Turin	Piedmont
1773	Copenhagen	Denmark
1777	Giessen	Hesse
1778	Hannover	Hannover

hygiene. In 1892, pleuropneumonia in the US was the first disease to be regionally eradicated after a campaign lasting only five years. Notable British successes included rinderpest, eradicated in 1877, pleuropneumonia in 1898, and glanders and equine parasitic mange in 1928.

Contemporary veterinary medicine

Current perspectives

The animal plagues

The mass infectious diseases still pose problems in both developed and developing countries. Some have emerged as major problems this century, although there is circumstantial evidence that the infectious agents have existed for some time (*Table 1.4*). Others are apparently novel (*Table 1.5*). Military conflict continues to be responsible for spreading these diseases (*Table 1.2*); for example, at the end of the Second World War, retreating Japanese soldiers brought rinderpest from Myanmar (Burma) to north-eastern Thailand.

The infectious diseases are particularly disruptive in the developing countries. There have been some successes, for example, the JP15 campaign against rinderpest in Africa (Lepissier and MacFarlane, 1966), although the benefits of this campaign have subsequently been negated by civil strife. Several vector-transmitted diseases with complex life-cycles, including haemoprotozoan infections such as trypanosomiasis, have not been controlled satisfactorily. More than half of the world's livestock are located in developing countries (*Table 1.6*), where they still provide over 80% of power and traction (Pritchard, 1986), and are exposed to these disease problems. The techniques of the microbial revolution have enabled these diseases to be identified. However, accurate means of assessing the extent and distribution of the diseases also are necessary in order to plan control programmes (e.g., the Pan-African Rinderpest Campaign: IAEE, 1991).

Some infectious diseases, for example brucellosis and tuberculosis, persist at low levels in developed countries, despite the application of traditional control methods. This problem can result from inadequate survey techniques and insensitive diagnostic tests (Martin, 1977). In some cases, an infectious agent may have a more complex natural history than initially suspected. For example, continued outbreaks of bovine tuberculosis in problem herds in England (Wilesmith *et al.*, 1982) have been shown to be associated with pockets of infection in wild badgers (Little *et al.*, 1982).

Table 1.4 Some emergent infectious diseases and plagues of animals in the 20th century.

Year	Country	Infection	Source
1907	Kenya	African swine fever	Montgomery (1921)
1910	Kenya	Nairobi sheep disease	Montgomery (1917)
1918	US	Swine influenza	Shope (1931)
1929	South Africa	Lumpy skin disease	Thomas and Maré (1945)
1939	Colombia	Venezuelan equine encephalomyelitis	Kubes and Rios (1939)
1946	Canada	Mink enteritis	Schofield (1949)
1947	US	Transmissible mink encephalopathy	Hartsough and Burger (1965)
1953	US	Bovine mucosal disease	Ramsey and Chivers (1953)
1972	US	Lyme disease	Steere *et al.* (1977)
1977	Worldwide	Canine parvovirus	Eugster *et al.* (1978)
1986	UK	Bovine spongiform encephalopathy	Wells *et al.* (1987)
1987	US	Porcine reproductive and respiratory syndrome	Keffaber (1989)

Table 1.5 Some novel infectious diseases and plagues of animals in the 20th century.

Year	Country	Infection	Source
1912	Kenya	Rift Valley fever	Daubney *et al.* (1931)
1923	The Netherlands	Duck plague	Baudet (1923)
1926	Java	Newcastle disease	Doyle (1927)
1945	US	Duck virus hepatitis-1	Levine and Fabricant (1950)
1946	US	Aleutian disease of mink	Hartsough and Gorham (1956)
1954	Japan	Akabane disease	Miura *et al.* (1974)
1956	China	Goose plague	Fang and Wang (1981)
1962	US	Avian infectious bursitis-1	Cosgrove (1962)
1974	Japan	Kunitachi virus	Yoshida *et al.* (1977)
1978	Iraq	Pigeon paramyxovirus-1	Kaleta *et al.* (1985)
1979	Japan	Chick anaemia agent	Yuasa *et al.* (1979)
1984	China	Rabbit haemorrhagic disease	Liu *et al.* (1984)
1985	UK	Rhinotracheitis of turkeys	Anon. (1985)
1987	USSR	Phocid distemper-2 (Baikal)	Grachev *et al.* (1989)
1988	The Netherlands	Phocid distemper-1 (North Sea)	Osterhaus and Vedder (1988)

The effective control of the animal plagues has allowed an increase in both animal numbers (*Table 1.7*) and productivity (*Table 1.8*) in the developed countries (mechanization making draft horses the exception). There has been an increase in the size of herds and flocks, notably in dairy, pig (*Table 1.9*) and poultry enterprises. Intensification of animal industries is accompanied by changes in animal health problems.

Complex infectious diseases

The animal plagues are caused by 'simple' agents, that is, their predominant causes can be identified as single infectious agents. Diseases caused by single agents still constitute problems in developed countries. Examples include salmonellosis, leptospirosis, babesiosis and coccidiosis. However, diseases have been identified that are produced by simultaneous infection with more than one agent (mixed infections), and by interaction between infectious agents and non-infectious factors. These are common in intensive production enterprises. Diseases of the internal body surfaces — enteric and respiratory diseases — are particular problems. Single agents alone cannot account for the pathogenesis of these complex diseases.

Table 1.6 World livestock populations, 1990 (1000s of animals). (From FAO, 1991.)

	Cattle	Sheep	Goats	Pigs	Horses	Chickens	Buffaloes
USA and Canada	110 449	121 23	1 927	64 384	5 630	1 570 000	—
Central America	49 638	7 109	11 928	24 415	8 499	371 796	9
South America	263 864	112 622	23 374	55 645	14 329	932 892	1 200
Europe	124 002	152 215	15 448	181 897	4 198	1 270 767	375
Africa	187 771	205 094	173 944	13 585	4 987	860 701	29 047
Asia	393 869	338 215	321 973	432 598	16 859	4 447 274	136 254
Oceania	31 264	226 122	1 956	5 339	498	83 592	25
USSR	118 400	137 000	6 480	78 900	5 920	1 200 000	420
All developed countries	400 556	560 479	31 675	341 612	16 417	4 511 267	795
All developing countries	878 701	630 021	525 355	515 150	44 503	6 228 757	139 963
World	1 279 257	1 190 500	567 030	856 762	60 920	10 740 024	140 758

Table 1.7 The livestock population of Great Britain, 1866–1989 (1000s of animals). (From HMSO, 1968, 1982, 1991.)

Year	Cattle	Sheep	Pigs	Horses (agricultural use)	Fowls	Turkeys
1866	4 786	22 048	2 478	—	—	—
1900	6 805	26 592	2 382	1 078	—	—
1925	7 368	23 094	2 799	910	39 036	730
1950	9 630	19 714	2 463	347	71 176	855
1965	10 826	28 837	6 731	21	101 956	4 323
1980	11 919	30 385	7 124	—	115 895	6 335
1989	10 510	38 869	7 391	—	121 279	—

—, Data not available.

Table 1.8 World cattle productivity, 1990. (From FAO, 1991.)

	Number of animals slaughtered (1000s of animals)	Carcass weight (kg/animal)	Milk yield (kg/animal)	Milk production (1000s tonnes)
World	241 283	212	2 129	475 507
US	35 256	297	6 711	67 383
South America	36 698	212	1 073	30 797
Asia	31 948	123	987	54 318
Africa	23 024	156	487	14 149
Europe	44 220	251	3 771	170 889
USSR	44 000	198	2 549	106 275
Oceania	10 015	217	3 633	14 317
Developed countries	141 408	244	3 605	378 458
Developing countries	99 874	166	820	97 048

Table 1.9 Pig herd structure in England and Wales (June). (Data supplied by the Meat and Livestock Commission.)

	1965	1971	1975	1980	1991
Number of farms with pigs	94 639	56 900	32 291	22 973	13 738
Total sows (1000s)	756.3	791.0	686.0	701.1	672.4
Average herd size (sows)	10.4	18.5	27.6	41.4	70.4
Number of herds by herd size (sows):					
1–49	56 560 (75.4%)	39 000 (90.9%)	20 873 (84.0%)	12 900 (76.3%)	6 471 (67.8%)
50–99	10 445 (13.9%)	2 700 (6.3%)	2 401 (9.7%)	2 000 (11.8%)	1 050 (11.0%)
100–199	8 034 (10.7%)	1 000 (2.3%)	1 141 (4.6%)	1 300 (7.7%)	1 115 (11.7%)
200 and over	—	200 (0.5%)	426 (1.7%)	700 (4.1%)	914 (9.5%)
Total number of herds with sows	75 039	42 900	24 841	16 900	9 500

Subclinical diseases

Some diseases do not produce overt clinical signs although they often affect production. These are called **subclinical** diseases. Helminthiasis and marginal mineral deficiencies, for example, decrease rates of liveweight gain. Porcine adenomatosis decreases growth in piglets, although there may be no clinical signs (Roberts *et al.*, 1979). Infection of pregnant sows with porcine parvovirus in early pregnancy destroys fetuses, the only sign being small numbers of piglets in litters. These diseases are major causes of production loss; their identification often requires laboratory investigations.

Non-infectious diseases

Non-infectious diseases have increased in importance following control of the major infectious ones. They can be predominantly genetic (e.g., canine hip dysplasia), metabolic (e.g., bovine ketosis) and neoplastic (e.g., canine mammary cancer). Their cause may be associated with several factors; for example, feline urolithiasis is associated with breed, sex, age and diet (Willeberg, 1977). Moreover, the role of genes in the pathogenesis of a wide variety of diseases is gradually being discovered (*Figure 1.3*).

Some conditions, such as ketosis, are particularly related to increased levels of production; ketosis is more likely in cows with high milk yields than in those with low yields. Intensive production systems may also be directly responsible for some conditions, for example foot lesions in individually caged broilers (Pearson, 1983).

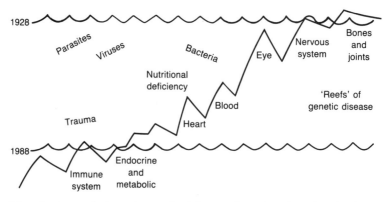

Fig. 1.3 The discovery of the role of genes in the pathogenesis of disease. An analogy is made using the sea and reefs. The sea represents environmental factors (infectious and non-infectious); the reefs represent genetic factors. Only the reefs above the water level are known. As time passes, the water level falls, and more genetic factors are identified. (From Thrusfield, 1993.)

Diseases of unknown cause

The cause of some diseases has not been identified, despite intensive investigation. Some of these diseases, such as feline dysautonomia (Edney *et al.*, 1987), have emerged and apparently declined without their causes being elucidated. Others, such as equine grass sickness (Pinsent, 1989), persist.

In some situations, infectious agents have been isolated from cases of a disease but cannot be unequivocally associated with the disease. An example is *Pasteurella haemolytica* in relation to 'shipping fever' (Martin *et al.*, 1982c). This syndrome occurs in cattle soon after their arrival at feedlots. Post-mortem examination of fatal cases has revealed that fibrinous pneumonia is a common cause of death. Although *P. haemolytica* is frequently isolated from lungs, it is not invariably present. Attempts to reproduce the disease experimentally using the bacterium alone have failed (Jericho, 1979). Other factors also seem to be involved. These include mixing animals and then penning them in large groups, the feeding of corn silage, dehorning, and, paradoxically, vaccination against agents that cause pneumonia, including *P. haemolytica* — factors associated with adrenal stress (see *Figure 3.5b* and Chapter 5).

Management and environment also appear to play significant, although often not clearly defined, roles in other diseases. Examples include enzootic pneumonia and enteritis in calves (Roy, 1980), enteric disease in suckling pigs, porcine pneumonia, bovine mastitis associated with *Escherichia coli* and *Streptococcus uberis* (Francis *et al.*, 1979), and mastitis in intensively housed sows (Muirhead, 1976).

In some instances, the infectious agents that are isolated are ubiquitous and can also be isolated from healthy animals, for example, enteric organisms (Isaacson *et al.*, 1978). These are 'opportunistic' pathogens, which cause disease only when other detrimental factors are also present.

In all of these cases, attempts to identify a causal agent fulfilling Koch's postulates frequently fail, unless unnatural techniques, such as abnormal routes of infection and the use of gnotobiotic animals, are applied.

The fifth period

These 20th century animal health problems and anomalies stimulated a change, which began in the 1960s, in attitude towards disease causality and control.

Causality

The inappropriateness of Koch's postulates as criteria for defining the cause of some syndromes suggested that more than one factor may sometimes operate in producing disease. A **multifactorial** theory of disease has developed, equally applicable to non-infectious and infectious diseases. Interest in human diseases of complex and poorly understood cause grew in the early years of the 20th century (Lane-Claypon, 1926) and was responsible for the development of new methods for analysing risk factors, for example smoking in relation to lung cancer (Doll, 1959). These epidemiological techniques are also being applied in veterinary medicine.

New control strategies

Two major strategies have been added to the earlier techniques (Schwabe, 1980a, b):

1. the structured recording of information on disease;
2. the analysis of disease in populations.

The collecting of disease information is not new; the ancient Japanese reported outbreaks of animal disease and in the 17th century John Graunt collected human mortality data in England (Graunt, 1662). The newer methods, however, involve two complementary approaches: the continuous collection of data on disease — termed **surveillance** and **monitoring** — and the intensive investigation of particular diseases. A further technique, used at the individual farm level, is the recording of information on both the health and productivity of each animal in a herd, as a means of improving production by improving herd health.

Emerging trends

Several trends are emerging in relation to the services that the veterinarian supplies to his clients, and to national and international disease reporting.

Veterinary services

Veterinarians practising in the livestock sector continue to control and treat disease in individual animals. Developments in molecular biology are improving diagnostic procedures (Goldspink and Gerlach, 1990), and offer new opportunities for vaccine production (Report, 1990). Additionally, in intensive production systems, the multifactorial nature of many diseases necessitates modification of the environment of the animal and management practices, rather than concentrating exclusively on infectious agents.

Diseases of food animals are also being considered directly in relation to their effect on **production**. Reduced

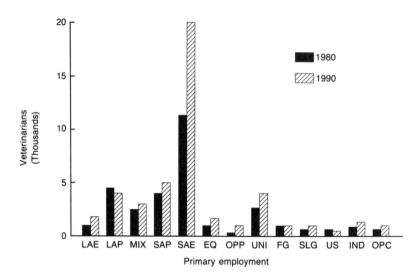

Fig. 1.4 Areas of employment of veterinarians in the US, 1980 and 1990. LAE: exclusively large animal; LAP: predominantly large animal; MIX: mixed practice; SAP: predominantly small animal; SAE: exclusively small animal; EQ: equine; OPP: other private practice; UNI: university; FG: federal government; SLG: state or local government; US: uniformed services; IND: industry; OPC: other public and corporate. (From Wise and Yang, 1992.)

levels of production can be used as 'diagnostic indicators'; for example, small litter size as an indicator of infection with porcine parvovirus. More significantly, veterinary emphasis has shifted from disease as a clinical entity in the individual animal to disease assessed in terms of suboptimal health, manifested by decreased herd performance: disease is being defined as the unacceptable performance of **groups** of animals. There is thus a need to identify all factors that contribute to the occurrence of disease, to select suitable 'performance indicators' (e.g., 'calving to conception interval'), and to define targets for these indicators in herds under a particular system of husbandry. It is then possible to identify those herds that miss the targets. This is called **performance-related diagnosis** (Morris, 1982), and includes not only the measurement of overt indicators, such as liveweight gain, but also estimation of covert biochemical values, such as metabolite levels in serum. Thus, clinical disease, subclinical disease and production need to be monitored in the context of anticipated ('normal') levels for a particular production system (Dohoo, 1993).

The veterinarian therefore is becoming more involved in husbandry, management and nutrition than previously, and less involved in traditional 'fire brigade' treatment of clinically sick animals. However, the livestock owner frequently still regards the veterinarian solely as a dispenser of treatment (Goodger and Ruppanner, 1982),

relying on feed representatives, dairy experts and nutritionists for advice on breeding, nutrition and management. The extent of this problem varies from one country to another, but indicates that the veterinarian's evolving role in animal production requires a change not only in veterinary attitudes but also sometimes in those of animal owners.

Government veterinary services, too, are becoming increasingly concerned with investigations of specific animal health problems of complex cause, such as mastitis, thereby extending their role beyond the traditional control of mass infectious diseases.

As the mass infectious diseases are controlled, and animal production becomes more intensive, other diseases become relatively more important. They are currently major problems in developed countries, and in some developing countries which have intensive enterprises, such as poultry and pig units in Malaysia, the Philippines and Taiwan. These diseases will become increasingly significant in the developing countries when the mass infectious diseases are controlled.

Attention is being focused on the health of companion animals, particularly in the developed countries. This is reflected in the employment trends in the veterinary profession (*Figure 1.4*). Many health problems of companion animals are complex too, and a full understanding of their cause and control is possible only when the contribution of genetic and environmental factors is appreciated. Examples include urinary tract infections in bitches, in which concurrent disease and recent chemotherapy are important factors (Freshman *et al.*, 1989), and equine colic which is related to age and breed (Morris *et al.*, 1989; Reeves *et al.*, 1989).

Animal welfare

The attitude of the public to animals (notably in developed countries) is reflected in contemporary concern for animal welfare (Seamer and Quimby, 1992; Moss, 1994). This encompasses health and 'well-being' (Ewbank, 1986). The latter term is difficult to define, and is also included in the World Health Organization's definition of human health (Old English: *hal* = whole) as 'a state of complete physical, mental and social well-being and not merely the absence of disease or infirmity' (WHO, 1983). Although this definition was not designed to be a framework for formulating goals of health policy (Noack, 1987), it illustrates that health is more than just absence of disease. An obvious aspect of animal welfare is deliberate abuse and neglect which may cause suffering; contentious topics are surgical mutilation such as tail docking in dogs (Morton, 1992) and horses (Cregier, 1990) and velvet antler removal from deer (Pollard *et al.*, 1992). There are wider and less tangible issues, though (Ewbank, 1986). These include behavioural deprivation which is associated with some intensive husbandry systems (e.g., the tethering of sows in stalls). The veterinarian therefore is concerned with disease, productivity and well-being, all of which can be interrelated (Ewbank, 1988).

National and international disease reporting

There is a requirement for improved disease reporting systems at the national and international level to identify problems, define research and control priorities and assist in the prevention of spread of infectious agents from one country to another. Additionally, residues need to be identified and eliminated (WHO, 1993). This includes contamination of meat by pesticides (Corrigan and Seneviratna, 1989) and hormones (McCaughey, 1992), as well as the more long-standing issue of antibiotic residues.

The move towards a free internal market in the European Union (Anon., 1992), and global goals to liberalize international trade through the Uruguay Round of the General Agreement on Tariffs and Trade (GATT) are highlighting the need for comprehensive disease reporting. If liberalization is achieved, it will have advantageous effects on world trade, including that in livestock commodities (Page *et al.*, 1991). An important

component of free trade therefore is assessment of the **risk** of disease and related events (e.g., carcass contamination) associated with the importation of animals and animal products (Morley, 1993). Established organizations, such as the Office International des Epizooties (OIE), are modifying their goals and reporting techniques, taking account of these new requirements (Blajan and Chillaud, 1991).

The advent of low-cost computing following the microelectronic revolution offers powerful means of storing, analysing and distributing data. Information can be transported rapidly using modern communications systems. These developments increase the scope for efficient disease reporting and analysis of the many factors that contribute to clinical disease and suboptimal production, both of which require increased statistical acumen among veterinarians. Epidemiology has developed to supply these contemporary veterinary requirements.

Further reading

British Veterinary Association Trust Project (1982) *Future of Animal Health Control — The Control of Infectious Diseases in Farm Animals*. Report of a symposium, University of Reading, 14–16 December 1982. British Veterinary Association, London

Davies, G. (1985) Art, science and mathematics: new approaches to animal health problems in the agricultural industry. *Veterinary Record*, **117**, 263–267

Dorn, C.R. (1992) Veterinary epidemiology and its economic importance in AD 2000. *Preventive Veterinary Medicine*, **13**, 129–136

Faber, K. (1930) *Nosography: The Evolution of Clinical Medicine in Modern Times*, 2nd edn. Paul B. Hoeber, New York. Reprinted by AMS Press, New York, 1978. (*A history of concepts of pathogenesis*)

Melby, E.C. (1985) The veterinary profession: changes and challenges. *Cornell Veterinarian*, **75**, 16–26

Michell, A.R. (Ed.) (1993) *The Advancement of Veterinary Science. The Bicentenary Symposium Series. Volume 1: Veterinary Medicine Beyond 2000.* CAB International, Wallingford

Michell, A.R. (Ed.) (1993) *The Advancement of Veterinary Science. The Bicentenary Symposium Series. Volume 3: History of the Healing Professions, Parallels between Veterinary and Medical History.* CAB International, Wallingford

Ministry of Agriculture, Fisheries and Food (1965) *Animal Health: A Centenary 1865–1965.* Her Majesty's Stationery Office, London. (*A history of the government veterinary service in the UK*)

Morris, R.S. (1988) The veterinarian and the livestock industries — fire in the heart or smoke in the eyes? *New Zealand*

Veterinary Journal, **36**, 161–166. (*Mainly a discussion of current requirements in the livestock sector*)

OIE (1994) Early methods of animal disease control. *Revue Scientifique et Technique, Office International des Epizooties*, **13**, 332–614

Pritchard, W.R. (1986) Veterinary education for the 21st century. *Journal of the American Veterinary Medical Association*, **189**, 172–177. (*A general review of contemporary veterinary requirements in developed countries*)

Rollinson, D.H.K. and Callear, J.F.F. (Eds) (1973) *A history of the overseas Veterinary Services. Part 2*. British Veterinary Association, London. (*Second part of an account of the British Colonial Veterinary Services*)

Schwabe, C.W. (1978) *Cattle, Priests, and Progress in Medicine*. The Wesley W. Spink lectures on comparative medicine, Vol. 4. University of Minnesota Press, Minneapolis. (*A comparative history of veterinary and human medicine*)

Schwabe, C.W. (1993) The current epidemiological revolution in veterinary medicine. Part II. *Preventive Veterinary Medicine*, **18**, 3–16

Smithcors, J.F. (1957) *Evolution of the Veterinary Art*. Veterinary Medicine Publishing Company, Kansas City. (*A general history of veterinary medicine to the 1950s*)

Thrusfield, M. (1988) The application of epidemiological techniques to contemporary veterinary problems. *British Veterinary Journal*, **144**, 455–469

Thrusfield, M. (1990) Trends in epidemiology. *Society for General Microbiology Quarterly*, **17**, 82–84

West, G.P. (Ed.) (1961) *A history of the overseas Veterinary Services. Part 1*. British Veterinary Association, London. (*First part of an account of the British Colonial Veterinary Services*)

Winslow, C.E.A. (1944) *The Conquest of Epidemic Disease*. Princeton University Press, Princeton. (*An historical account of the control of infectious diseases*)

2 The scope of epidemiology

Many contemporary disease problems can be solved by an investigation of animal populations rather than the individual. The natural history of infectious diseases can be understood by studying their distribution in different populations. The measurement of the amount of infectious and non-infectious disease in a population assists in determining their importance and the efficacy of control campaigns. Complex and unknown causes of diseases can be elucidated by studying the diseases in various groups of animals. The effects of diseases on production can be realistically estimated only in relation to decreased production in the herd or flock rather than in a single animal. The economic impact of disease and of attempts at its control similarly are evaluated best in groups of animals, ranging from the individual farm to the national level. The investigation of disease in **populations** is the basis of epidemiology.

Definition of epidemiology

Epidemiology is the **study of disease in populations and of factors that determine its occurrence**; the key word being **populations**. Veterinary epidemiology additionally includes investigation and assessment of other health-related events, notably **productivity**. All of these investigations involve **observing** animal populations and making **inferences** from the observations.

A literal translation of the word 'epidemiology', based on its Greek roots $\epsilon\pi\iota$- (*epi-*) = upon, $\delta\eta\mu o$- (*demo-*) = people, and $\lambda o\gamma o$- (*logo-*) = discoursing, is 'the study of that which is upon the people' or, in modern parlance, 'the study of disease in populations'. Traditionally, 'epidemiology' related to studies of human populations, and 'epizootiology', from the Greek $\zeta\omega o$- (*zoo-*) = animal, to the studies of animal (excluding human)

populations (e.g., Karstad, 1962). Outbreaks of disease in human populations were called 'epidemics', in animal populations were called 'epizootics', and in avian populations were called 'epornitics', from the Greek $o\rho\nu\iota\theta$- (*ornith-*) = bird (e.g., Montgomery *et al.*, 1979). Other derivatives, such as 'epidemein' ('to visit a community'), give hints of the early association between epidemiology and infections that periodically entered a community, in contrast to other diseases which were usually present in the population.

The various derivatives can be used in different contexts. A study of a disease that is present only in an animal population, such as *Brucella ovis* infection of sheep, would not involve a simultaneous study of disease in humans; the term 'epizootiology' might then be used by some to indicate that the study was confined to animals other than man. Many diseases, called **zoonoses**, may be shared by man and lower animals. Thus, when studying diseases such as bovine brucellosis and leptospirosis, both of which are zoonoses, mechanisms of transfer of disease between human and non-human populations have to be considered. An important factor that determines the occurrence of such occupationally acquired zoonoses (in veterinarians, abattoir workers and farmers in these examples) is the amount of disease in domestic animals. The 'epidemiology' of brucellosis and leptospirosis in dairy farmers is therefore closely associated with the 'epizootiology' of these diseases in cattle. The semantic differentiation between studies involving human diseases and those concerned with animal diseases therefore is considered neither warranted nor logical (Dohoo *et al.*, 1994). Throughout this book, the word 'epidemiological' is therefore used to describe any investigation relating to disease in a population, whether or not the population consists of humans, domestic animals, or wildlife.

The uses of epidemiology

There are five objectives of epidemiology:

1. determination of the origin of a disease whose cause is known;
2. investigation and control of a disease whose cause is either unknown or poorly understood;
3. acquisition of information on the ecology and natural history of a disease;
4. planning and monitoring of disease control programmes;
5. assessment of the economic effects of a disease and analysis of the costs and economic benefits of alternative control programmes.

Determination of the origin of a disease whose cause is known

Many diseases with a known cause can be diagnosed precisely by the signs exhibited by the affected animals, by appropriate laboratory tests and by other clinical procedures such as radiological investigation. For instance, the diagnosis of salmonellosis in a group of calves is relatively straightforward (the infection frequently produces distinct clinical signs). However, determining why an outbreak occurred and using the correct procedures to prevent recurrence can be difficult. For example, the outbreak may have been caused either by the purchase of infected animals or by contaminated food. Further investigations are required to identify the source of infection. When the food is suspected, the ration may consist of several components. Even if a sample of each component is still available, it would be expensive and possibly uneconomic to submit all of the samples for laboratory examination. Consideration of the risk associated with the consumption of each component of the ration may narrow the field of investigation to only one or two items.

There are many examples of the investigation of diseases with known causes that involve answering the questions 'Why has an outbreak occurred?' or 'Why has the number of cases increased?'. For instance, an increased number of actinobacillosis cases in a group of cattle might be associated with grazing a particular pasture of 'burnt off' stubble. Such an occurrence could be associated with an increase in abrasions of the buccal mucosae which could increase the animals' susceptibility to infection with *Actinobacillus lignieresi*. An increased number of cases of bone defects in puppies might be due to local publicity given to the use of vitamin supplements, resulting in their administration to animals that were already fed a balanced diet, with consequent hypervitaminosis D and osteodystrophy (Jubb and Kennedy, 1971). An increase in the number of lamb carcasses with high ultimate pH values could be associated with excessive washing of the animals prior to slaughter (Petersen, 1983). These possible explanations can be verified only by epidemiological investigations.

Investigation and control of a disease whose cause is either unknown or poorly understood

There are many instances of disease control based on epidemiological observations before a cause was identified. Contagious bovine pleuropneumonia was eradicated from the US by an appreciation of the infectious nature of the disease before the causal agent, *Mycoplasma mycoides*, was isolated (Schwabe, 1984). Lancisi's slaughter policy to control rinderpest, mentioned in Chapter 1, was based on the assumption that the disease was infectious, even though the causal agent had not been discovered. Edward Jenner's classical observations on the protective effects of cowpox virus against human smallpox infection in the 18th century (Fisk, 1959), before viruses were isolated, laid the foundations for the global eradication of smallpox.

More recently, epidemiological studies in the UK suggested that cattle develop bovine spongiform encephalopathy (BSE) following consumption of feedstuffs containing meat and bone meal contaminated with a scrapie-like agent (Wilesmith *et al.*, 1988). This was sufficient to introduce legislation prohibiting the feeding of ruminant-derived protein, although the causal agent had not been identified.

Although the exact cause of 'blood splashing' (eccymoses in muscle) in carcasses is still not known, observations have shown that there is a correlation between this defect and electrical stunning by a 'head only' method (Blackmore, 1983); and the occurrence of this condition can be reduced by adopting a short 'stun-to-stick' interval, stunning animals with a captive bolt, or using a method of electrical stunning that causes concurrent cardiac dysfunction (Gracey, 1986). Similarly, there is a strong correlation between grass sickness and grazing, and the disease can be almost totally prevented by stabling horses continuously during spring and summer, although the cause of the disease is unknown (Gilmour, 1989).

The cause of squamous cell carcinoma of the eye in Hereford cattle ('cancer eye') is not known. Epidemiological studies have shown that animals with unpigmented eyelids are much more likely to develop the condition than those with pigment (Anderson *et al.*, 1957). This information can be utilized by cattle breeders to select animals with a low susceptibility to this neoplasm.

Epidemiological studies are also used to identify causes of disease (many of which are multifactorial and initially poorly understood) so that the most appropriate disease control techniques can be applied. Thus, the identification of low levels of water intake as an important component of the cause of feline urolithiasis (Willeberg, 1981) facilitated control of this syndrome by dietary modification. Investigations can also be used to identify characteristics of animals that increase the risk of disease. For example, entire bitches with a history of oestrus irregularity and pseudopregnancy are particularly at risk of developing pyometra (Fidler *et al.*, 1966); this information is of diagnostic value to the clinician, and is of assistance when advising owners on breeding policy.

Acquisition of information on the ecology and natural history of a disease

An animal that can become infected with an infectious agent is a **host** of that agent. Hosts and agents exist in communities that include other organisms, all of which live in particular environments. The aggregate of all facts relating to animals and plants is their **natural history**. Related communities and their environments are termed **ecosystems**. The study of ecosystems is **ecology**.

A comprehensive understanding of the natural history of infectious agents is possible only when they are studied in the context of their hosts' ecosystems. Similarly, an improved knowledge of non-infectious diseases can be obtained by studying the ecosystems and the associated physical features with which affected animals are related. The geological structure of an ecosystem, for example, can affect the mineral content of plants and therefore can be an important factor in the occurrence of mineral deficiencies and excesses in animals.

The environment of an ecosystem affects the survival rate of infectious agents and of their hosts. Thus, infection with the helminth *Fasciola hepatica* is a serious problem only in poorly drained areas, because the parasite spends part of its life-cycle in a snail which requires moist surroundings.

Each of the 200 antigenic types (serovars) of *Leptospira interrogans* is maintained in one or more species of hosts. Serovar *copenhageni*, for instance, is maintained primarily in rats (Babudieri, 1958). Thus, if this serovar is associated with leptospirosis in either man or domestic stock, then part of a disease control programme must involve an ecological study of rat populations and control of infected rats. Similarly, in Africa, a herpesvirus that

produces infections without signs in wildebeeste is responsible for malignant catarrhal fever of cattle (Plowright *et al.*, 1960). Wildebeeste populations, therefore, must be investigated when attempting to control the disease in cattle.

An ecosystem's climate also is important because it limits the geographical distribution of infectious agents that are transmitted by arthropods by limiting the distribution of the arthropods. For example, the tsetse fly, which transmits trypanosomiasis, is restricted to the humid parts of Sub-Saharan Africa (Ford, 1971).

Infectious agents may extend beyond the ecosystems of their traditional hosts. This has occurred in bovine tuberculosis in the UK, where the badger population appears to be an alternative host for *Mycobacterium tuberculosis* (Little *et al.*, 1982; Wilesmith *et al.*, 1982). Similarly, in certain areas of New Zealand, wild opossums are infected with this bacterium and can therefore be a source of infection to cattle (Thorns and Morris, 1983). Purposeful routine observation of such infections provides valuable information on changes in the amount of disease and relevant ecological factors and may therefore indicate necessary changes in control strategies.

Infectious diseases that are transmitted by insects, ticks and other arthropods, and which may be maintained in wildlife, present complex ecological relationships and even more complex problems relating to their control. Comprehensive epidemiological studies of these diseases help to unravel their life-cycles, and can indicate suitable methods of control.

Planning and monitoring of disease control programmes

The institution of a programme to either control or eradicate a disease in an animal population must be based on a knowledge of the amount of the disease in that population, the factors associated with its occurrence, the facilities required to control the disease, and the costs and benefits involved. This information is equally important for a mastitis control programme on a single dairy farm and for a national brucellosis eradication scheme involving all the herds in a country. The epidemiological techniques that are employed include the routine collection of data on disease in populations (**monitoring** and **surveillance**) to decide if the various strategies are being successful.

Surveillance is also required to determine whether the occurrence of a disease is being affected by new factors. For example, during the eradication scheme for bovine tuberculosis in New Zealand, opossums became infected in certain areas. New strategies had to be introduced to control this problem (Julian, 1981). During the foot-and-mouth disease epidemic in the UK in 1967 and 1968, surveillance programmes indicated the importance of wind-borne virus particles in the transmission of the disease (Smith and Hugh-Jones, 1969). This additional knowledge was relevant to the establishment of areas within which there was a restriction of animal movement, thus facilitating eradication of the disease.

Assessing the economic effects of a disease and of its control

The cost of the control of disease in the livestock industry must be balanced against the economic loss attributable to the disease. Economic analysis therefore is required. This is an essential part of most modern planned animal health programmes. Although it may be economic to reduce a high level of disease in a herd or flock, it may be uneconomic to reduce even further the level of a disease that is present at only a very low level. If 15% of the cows in a herd were affected by mastitis, productivity would be severely affected and a control programme would be likely to reap financial benefit. On the other hand, if less than 1% of the herd were affected, the cost of further reduction of the disease might not result in a sufficient increase in productivity to pay for the control programme.

This introduction to the uses of epidemiology indicates that the subject is relevant to many areas of veterinary science. The general agricultural practitioner is becoming increasingly concerned with herd health. The companion animal practitioner is faced with chronic refractory diseases, such as the idiopathic dermatoses, which may be understood better by an investigation of the factors that are common to all cases. The state veterinarian cannot perform his routine duties without reference to disease in the national animal population. The diagnostic pathologist investigates the associations between causes and effects (i.e., lesions); this approach is epidemiological when inferences are made from groups of animals. The veterinarian in abattoirs and meat-processing plants attempts to reduce the occurrence of defects and contamination by understanding and eliminating their causes. Similarly, industrial veterinarians, concerned with the design of clinical trials, compare disease rates and response to treatment in groups of animals to which different prophylactic and therapeutic compounds are administered.

Types of epidemiological investigation

There are four approaches to epidemiological investigation that traditionally have been called 'types' of epidemiology. These types are **descriptive**, **analytical**, **experimental** and **theoretical** epidemiology.

Descriptive epidemiology

Descriptive epidemiology involves observing and recording diseases and possible causal factors. It is usually the first part of an investigation. The observations are sometimes partially subjective, but, in common with observations in other scientific disciplines, may generate hypotheses that can be tested more rigorously later. Darwin's theory of evolution, for example, was derived mainly from subjective observations, but with slight modification it has withstood rigorous testing by plant and animal scientists.

Analytical epidemiology

Analytical epidemiology is the analysis of observations using suitable diagnostic and statistical tests.

Experimental epidemiology

The experimental epidemiologist observes and analyses data from groups of animals from which he can select, and in which he can alter, the factors associated with the groups. An important component of the experimental approach is the control of the groups. Experimental epidemiology developed in the 1920s and 1930s, and utilized laboratory animals whose short lifespans enabled events to be observed more rapidly than in humans (see Chapter 18). A notable example is the work of Topley (1942) who infected colonies of mice with ectromelia virus and *Pasteurella* spp. The effects of varying the rate of exposure of mice maintained in groups of various sizes provided insights into the behaviour of human epidemic diseases such as measles, scarlet fever, whooping cough and diptheria which followed similar patterns to the experimental infections (MRC, 1938). This work demonstrated the importance of the proportion of susceptible individuals in the population in determining the progress of epidemics (see Chapter 8); hitherto, changes in the virulence of a microorganism were thought to be the most important factor affecting epidemic patterns.

Rarely, a 'natural' experiment can be conducted when the naturally occurring disease or other fortuitous circumstance approximates closely to the ideally designed experiment. For instance, when BSE occurred in the UK, outbreaks of the disease on the Channel Islands (Jersey and Guernsey), which maintain isolated populations of cattle, provided an ideal situation in which to study the disease, uncomplicated by the possibility of transmission by contact with infected animals (Wilesmith, 1993). This added credence to the hypothesis that the disease was transmitted in contaminated feedstuffs.

Theoretical epidemiology

Theoretical epidemiology consists of the representation of disease using mathematical 'models' that attempt to simulate natural patterns of disease occurrence.

Epidemiological subdisciplines

Various epidemiological subdisciplines are now recognized. These reflect different areas of interest, rather than fundamentally different techniques. They all apply the four types of epidemiology described above, and can overlap, but their separate identities are considered by some to be justifiable.

Clinical epidemiology

Clinical epidemiology is the use of epidemiological principles, methods and findings in the care of individuals, with particular reference to diagnosis and prognosis (Last, 1988), and therefore brings a numerate approach to traditional clinical medicine, which has tended to be anecdotal and subjective (Grufferman and Kimm, 1984). It is concerned with the frequency and cause of disease, the factors that affect prognosis, the validity of diagnostic tests, and the effectiveness of therapeutic and preventive techniques (Fletcher *et al.*, 1988).

Computational epidemiology

Computational epidemiology involves the application of computer science to epidemiological studies (Habtemariam *et al.*, 1988). This includes the representation of disease by **mathematical models** (see 'Quantitative investigations', below) and the use of **expert systems**. These systems are commonly applied to disease diagnosis where they incorporate a set of rules for solving problems, details of clinical signs, lesions, laboratory results, and the opinions of experts; examples are the identification of the cause of coughing in dogs (Roudebush, 1984), and the diagnosis of bovine mastitis (Hogeveen *et al.*, 1993). Expert systems are also employed in formulating disease control strategies (e.g., for East coast fever: Gettinby and Byrom, 1989), predicting animal productivity (e.g., reproductive performance in dairy herds: McKay *et al.*, 1988), and

supporting management decisions (e.g., decisions on replacing sows: Huirne *et al.*, 1991).

Genetic epidemiology

Genetic epidemiology is the study of the cause, distribution and control of disease in related individuals, and of inherited defects in populations (Morton, 1982; Roberts, 1985). It indicates that the disciplinary boundary between genetics and epidemiology is blurred. Many diseases involve both genetic and non-genetic factors (see Chapter 5), and genes are increasingly incriminated in diseases of all organ systems (*Figure 1.3*). Thus, the geneticist and epidemiologist are both concerned with interactions between genetic and non-genetic factors — only the frequently indistinct time of interaction may be used to classify an investigation as genetic or epidemiological.

Molecular epidemiology

New biochemical techniques now enable microbiologists and molecular biologists to study small genetic and antigenic differences between viruses and other microorganisms at a higher level of discrimination than has been possible using conventional serological techniques. The methods include peptide mapping, nucleic acid 'fingerprinting' and hybridization (Keller and Manak, 1989; Kricka, 1992), restriction enzyme analysis, monoclonal antibodies (Oxford, 1985; Goldspink and Gerlach, 1990; Goldspink, 1993) and the polymerase chain reaction (Belák and Ballagi-Pordány, 1993). For example, nucleotide sequencing of European foot-and-mouth disease virus has indicated that recent outbreaks of the disease involved vaccinal strains, suggesting that improper inactivation or escape of virus from vaccine production plants may have been responsible for the outbreaks (Beck and Strohmaier, 1987). Similarly, infections that hitherto have been difficult to identify are now readily distinguished using these new molecular techniques; examples are infection with *Mycobacterium paratuberculosis* (the cause of Johne's disease) (Murray *et al.*, 1989) and latent infection with Aujeszky's disease virus (Belák *et al.*, 1989). The application of these new diagnostic techniques constitutes **molecular epidemiology**. A general description of the methods is given by Persing *et al.* (1993).

Molecular epidemiology is part of the wider use of **biological markers** (Hulka *et al.*, 1990). These are cellular, biochemical or molecular alterations that are measurable in biological media such as tissues, cells or fluids. They may indicate susceptibility to a causal factor, or a biological response, suggesting a sequence of events from exposure to disease (Perera and Weinstein, 1982). Some have been used by veterinarians for many years, for instance, serum magnesium levels as indicators of susceptibility to clinical hypocalcaemia (Whitaker and Kelly, 1982; Van de Braak *et al.*, 1987), serum transaminase levels as markers for liver disease, and antibodies as indicators of exposure to infectious agents (see Chapter 17).

Other subdisciplines

Several other epidemiological subdisciplines have also been defined. **Chronic disease epidemiology** is involved with diseases of long duration (e.g., cancers), many of which are non-infectious. **Environmental epidemiology** is concerned with the relationship between disease and environmental factors such as industrial pollution and, in human medicine, occupational hazards. Domestic animals can act as monitors of environmental hazards and can provide early warning of disease in man (see Chapter 18). **Micro-epidemiology** is the study of disease in a small group of individuals with respect to factors that influence its occurrence in larger segments of the population. For example, studies of feline acquired immunodeficiency syndrome (FAIDS) in groups of kittens have provided insights into the widespread human disease, AIDS (Torres-Anjel and Tshikuka, 1988). Micro-epidemiology, which frequently uses animal biological models of disease, therefore is closely related to **comparative epidemiology** (see Chapter 18). In contrast, **macro-epidemiology** is the study of national patterns of disease, and the social, economic and political factors that influence them (Hueston and Walker, 1993). Other subdisciplines, such as **nutritional epidemiology** (Willett, 1990) and **subclinical epidemiology** (Evans, 1987), can also be identified to reflect particular areas of interest.

Components of epidemiology

The components of epidemiology are summarized in *Figure 2.1*. The first stage in any investigation is the collection of relevant data. The main sources of information are outlined in Chapter 10. Methods of storing, retrieving and disseminating information are discussed in Chapter 11. Investigations can be either **qualitative** or **quantitative** or a combination of these two approaches.

Qualitative investigations

The natural history of disease

The ecology of diseases, including the distribution, mode of transmission and maintenance of infectious diseases, is investigated by field observation. Ecological principles are outlined in Chapter 7. Methods of transmission and maintenance are described in Chapter 6, and patterns of disease occurrence are described in Chapter 8. Field observations also may reveal information about factors that may directly or indirectly cause disease. The various factors that act to produce disease are described in Chapter 5.

Causal hypothesis testing

If field observations suggest that certain factors may be causally associated with a disease, then the association must be assessed by formulating a causal hypothesis. Causality (the relating of causes to effects) and hypothesis formulation are described in Chapter 3.

Qualitative investigations were the mainstay of epidemiologists before the Second World War. These epidemiologists were concerned largely with the identification of unknown causes of infectious disease and sources of infection. Some interesting examples of the epidemiologist acting as a medical 'detective' are described by Roueché (1991).

Quantitative investigations

Quantitative investigations involve measurement (e.g., the number of cases of disease), and therefore expression and analysis of numerical values. Basic methods of expressing these values are outlined in Chapters 4 and 12. The types of measurement that are encountered in veterinary medicine are described in Chapter 9. Quantitative investigations include **surveys**, **monitoring** and **surveillance**, **studies**, **modelling**, and the biological and economic **evaluation of disease control**.

Surveys

A survey is an examination of an aggregate of units (Kendall and Buckland, 1982). A group of animals is an example of an aggregate. The examination usually involves counting members of the aggregate and characteristics of the members. In epidemiological surveys, characteristics might include the presence of particular diseases, weight, and milk yield. Surveys can be undertaken on a **sample** of the population. Less commonly, a **census**, which examines the total animal population, can be undertaken (e.g., tuberculin testing). A **cross-sectional** survey records events occurring at a particular point in time. A **longitudinal** survey records events over a period of time. These latter events may be recorded **prospectively** from the present into the future; or may be a **retrospective** record of past events.

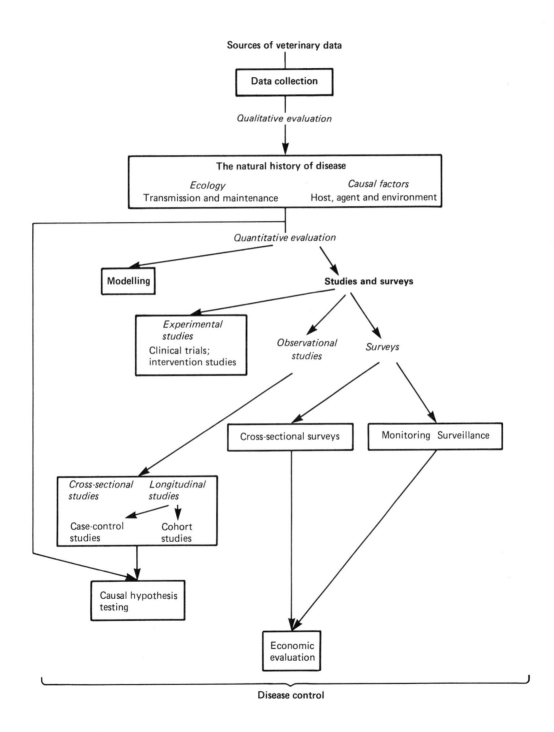

Fig. 2.1 Components of veterinary epidemiology. (Adapted from Thrusfield, 1985a.)

A particular type of diagnostic survey is **screening**. This is the identification of undiagnosed cases of disease using rapid tests or examinations. The aim is to separate individuals that probably have a disease from those that probably do not. Screening tests are not intended to be definitive; individuals with positive test results (i.e., that are classified as diseased by the screening test) require further investigation for definite diagnosis.

Diagnostic tests, including serological surveys and screening, are considered in Chapter 17. The design of surveys in general is described in Chapter 13.

Monitoring and surveillance

Monitoring is the making of routine observations on health, productivity and environmental factors and the recording and transmission of these observations. Thus, the regular recording of milk yields is monitoring, as is the routine recording of meat inspection findings at abattoirs. The identity of individual diseased animals usually is not recorded.

Surveillance is a more intensive form of data recording than monitoring. Originally, surveillance was used to describe the tracing and observation of people who were in contact with cases of infectious disease. It is now used in a much wider sense (Langmuir, 1965) to include all types of disease — infectious and non-infectious — and involves the collation and interpretation of data collected during monitoring programmes, usually with the recording of the identity of diseased individuals, with a view to detecting changes in a population's health. It is normally part of control programmes for specific diseases. The recording of tuberculosis lesions at an abattoir, followed by tracing of infected animals from the abattoir back to their farms of origin, is an example of surveillance. The terms 'monitoring' and 'surveillance' have previously been used synonymously, but the distinction between them is now generally accepted. The national and international aspects of surveillance are reviewed by Blajan (1979), Davies (1980, 1993), Ellis (1980) and Blajan and Welte (1988), and some animal disease information systems are described in Chapter 11.

Monitoring and surveillance can include all of the national herd. Alternatively, a few farms, abattoirs, veterinary practices or laboratories may be selected; these are then referred to as 'sentinel' units, because they are designed to 'keep watch' on a disease. Similarly, horses can be used as sentinels for Venezuelan equine encephalitis virus infection (Dickerman and Scherer, 1983), and stray dogs as sentinels for canine parvovirus infection (Gordon and Angrick, 1985), the infections being identified serologically. Other species of animals that also are susceptible to an infectious agent can be used as sentinels for the infection in the main animal population. For example, wild birds can be used to monitor the activity of St Louis encephalitis virus, providing early information on the activity of the virus at a time when avian infection rates are still too low to pose an immediate threat to man (Lord *et al.*, 1974). Domestic animals can also be used as sentinels of human environmental health hazards such as carcinogens and insecticides; this topic is discussed in detail in Chapter 18.

Studies

'Study' is a general term that refers to any type of investigation. However, in epidemiology, a study usually involves **comparison** of groups of animals, for example, a comparison of the weights of animals that are fed different diets. Thus, although a survey generally could be classified as a study, it is excluded from epidemiological studies because it involves only **description** rather than comparison and the analysis that the comparison requires. There are four main types of epidemiological study:

1. experimental studies;
2. cross-sectional studies;
3. case—control studies;
4. cohort studies.

In an **experimental study** the investigator has the ability to allocate animals to various groups, according to factors which the investigator can randomly assign to animals (e.g., treatment regimen, preventive technique); such studies are therefore part of experimental epidemiology. An important example is the **clinical trial**. In a clinical trial, the investigator assigns animals either to a group to which a prophylactic or therapeutic procedure is applied, or to a control group. It is then possible to evaluate the efficacy of the procedure by comparing the two groups. Clinical trials are discussed in Chapter 16.

The other types of study — cross-sectional, case—control and cohort — are **observational**. An observational study is similar to an experimental study: animals are allocated to groups with respect to certain characteristics that they possess (trait, disease, etc.). However, in observational studies, it is not possible to assign animals to groups randomly because the investigator has little control over the factors that are being studied; the characteristics are **inherent** (e.g., sex, weight or normal diet).

A **cross-sectional study** investigates relationships between disease (or other health-related factors) and hypothesized causal factors in a specified population. Animals are categorized according to presence and absence of disease and hypothesized causal factors; inferences can then be made about associations between disease and the hypothesized causal factors, for example, between heart valve incompetence (the disease) and breed (the hypothesized causal factor).

A **case–control study** compares a group of diseased animals with a group of healthy animals with respect to exposure to hypothesized causal factors. For example, a group of cats with urolithiasis (the disease) can be compared with a group of cats without urolithiasis with respect to consumption of dry cat food (the factor) to determine whether that type of food has an effect on the pathogenesis of the disease.

In a **cohort study**, a group exposed to factors is compared with a group not exposed to the factors with respect to the development of a disease. It is then possible to calculate a level of risk of developing the disease in relation to exposure to the hypothesized causal factors.

Case–control and cohort studies have often been applied in human medicine in which experimental investigations of cause are usually unethical. For example, it would not be possible to investigate the suspected toxicity of a drug by intentionally administering the drug to a group of people in order to study possible side-effects. However, if symptoms of toxicity have occurred, then a case–control study could be used to evaluate the association between the symptoms and the drug suspected of causing the toxicity. There are fewer ethical restraints on experimental investigation in veterinary medicine than in human medicine and so experimental investigation of serious conditions is more tenable. However, observational studies have a role in veterinary epidemiology; for example, when investigating diseases in farm and companion animal populations. The increasing concern for animal welfare is making these techniques even more useful than previously.

Basic methods of assessing association between disease and hypothesized causal factors in observational studies are described in Chapters 14 and 15.

Observational studies form the majority of epidemiological studies. Observational and experimental science have their own strengths and weaknesses which are discussed in detail by Trotter (1930). A major advantage of an observational investigation is that it studies the natural occurrence of disease. Experimentation may separate factors associated with disease from other factors that may have important interactions with them in natural outbreaks.

Modelling

Disease dynamics and the effects of different control strategies can be represented using mathematical equations. This representation is 'modelling'. Many modern methods rely heavily on computers. Another type of modelling is biological simulation using experimental animals (frequently laboratory animals) to simulate the pathogenesis of diseases that occur naturally in animals and man. Additionally, the spontaneous occurrence of disease in animals can be studied in the field (e.g., using observational studies) to increase understanding of human diseases. Mathematical modelling is outlined in Chapter 19, and spontaneous disease models are described in Chapter 18.

Disease control

The goal of epidemiology is to improve the veterinarian's knowledge so that diseases can be controlled effectively, and productivity thereby optimized. This can be fulfilled by treatment, prevention or eradication. The economic evaluation of disease and its control is discussed in Chapter 20. Health schemes are described in Chapter 21. Finally, the principles of disease control are outlined in Chapter 22.

The different components of epidemiology apply the four epidemiological approaches to varying degrees. Surveys and studies, for example, consist of a descriptive and an analytical part. Modelling additionally may include a theoretical approach.

Is epidemiology a science?

The interplay between epidemiology and other sciences

During the first half of the 20th century most epidemiologists were trained initially as bacteriologists, reflecting epidemiologists' early involvement in the investigation of outbreaks of infectious disease. The epidemiological approach is now practised by veterinarians from many disciplines: the parasitologist studying the life-cycles and dynamics of helminth, arthropod and protozoan infections, the geneticist concerned with an hereditary defect in a population, and the nutritionalist investigating a deficiency or toxicity.

Today, members of a variety of other sciences also take part in epidemiological studies: statisticans analysing data from groups of animals, mathematicians modelling diseases, economists assessing the economic impact of disease, and ecologists studing the natural history of disease. Each of these sciences is concerned with different facets of epidemiology, ranging from the purely descriptive, qualitative approach to the quantitative analytical approach. There have been many definitions of epidemiology (Lilienfeld, 1978), which reflect these facets. These definitions vary from the ecological relating only to infectious diseases ('the study of the ecology of infectious diseases': Cockburn, 1963), to the mathematical, referring only to human populations ('the study of the distribution and dynamics of diseases in human populations': Sartwell, 1973). However, they all have the study of populations in common, and so are encompassed by the broad definition that was given at the beginning of this chapter.

Many of the techniques used in epidemiological investigations have been developed in sciences other than epidemiology; statistical tests for assessing association and methods of sampling populations are examples. This raises the question: is epidemiology a separate science or merely a way of thinking that applies a variety of methods borrowed from other sciences? (Terris, 1962). When undertaking a field survey, is the bacteriologist practising a distinct science called epidemiology, or using statistical sampling methods merely to add credence to a bacteriological hypothesis, formulated from experimental results derived in the laboratory? The difference between a science and a method is more than a semantic one: 'If epidemiology is seen merely as an adjunct to experimental research, it will be shackled with the same limitations and subject to the same narrow perspectives. It will either continue to be an amateur sport — that of making subjective observations in the field in order to raise an hypothesis that can be examined at the laboratory bench — or exist simply to add some respectablity to experimental findings that on their own are unconvincing' (Davies, 1983). If epidemiology is a science then it has a separate identity and is free to develop its own methods.

The differentiation between science and method may not be easy (Himsworth, 1970). There will be those who hold the opinion that a proposed new science is merely a variation of their own, and there will be those who feel, with equal conviction, that the concepts and methods of traditional subjects are inadequate, and that an allegedly new field can be approached only on its own merits.

Trotter (1932) has suggested two considerations when judging the individuality of a science: **quality** and **distinction**. The quality of data relating to the science must be such that they can be analysed scientifically, and methods of analysis must be available. The field of natural experience that is to be investigated by the science must

also be distinct from those investigated by other sciences, to the extent that only the methods of the new science will extend knowledge in that field.

Since the 1960s, veterinary epidemiology has fulfilled these two criteria (Davies, 1983). An example is the field investigation of foot-and-mouth disease by Smith and Hugh-Jones (1969), mentioned earlier in this chapter. They plotted the spread of the disease during the 1967—68 epidemic in the UK and concluded that virus particles could be disseminated by wind. The epidemiological data have been refined by laboratory investigation of virus excretion and, with meteorological data, have been used to formulate a model to predict dispersion of the virus that is of direct value in the planning of disease control campaigns (Gloster *et al.*, 1981). This work fulfils the two criteria of quality and distinction; the quality of the data is such that they can be analysed, and the field of natural experience — spread of disease in this case — provides distinctive knowledge. The results of these investigations and the concomitant increased understanding of disease are possible only because of the amalgamation of the techniques of the different sciences that constitute epidemiology.

The relationship between epidemiology and other diagnostic disciplines

The biological sciences form a hierarchy, ranging from the study of non-replicating molecules to nucleic acids, organelles, cells, tissues, organs, systems, individuals, groups and, finally, whole communities and ecosystems (Wright, 1959). The various disciplines in veterinary medicine operate at different levels in this hierarchy. The histologist and physiologist study the structure and dynamics of the individual. The clinician and pathologist are concerned with disease processes in the individual: the clinician diagnoses disease using the signs displayed by the patient; the pathologist interprets lesions to produce a diagnosis. The epidemiologist investigates populations, using the frequency and distribution of disease to produce a diagnosis. These three diagnostic disciplines, operating at different levels in the hierarchy, are complementary (Schwabe *et al.*, 1977). Epidemiologists, dealing with the higher level, must have a knowledge of those disciplines 'lower' in the hierarchy — they must be able to see both the 'wood' and the 'trees'. This means that they must adopt a broad rather than a specialist approach, avoiding the dangers of the specialist; dangers that have been described (somewhat cynically) by Konrad Lorenz (1977) in his book on the natural history of human knowledge:

'The specialist comes to know more and more about less and less, until finally he knows everything about a mere nothing. There is a serious danger that the specialist, forced to compete with his colleagues in acquiring more and more specialised knowledge, will become more and more ignorant about other branches of knowledge, until he is utterly incapable of forming any judgement on the role and importance of his own sphere within the context of human knowledge as a whole.'

Thus, the major attributes required to become a competent veterinary epidemiologist are a natural curiosity, a logical approach, a general interest in and knowledge of veterinary medicine, and a capability for lateral thinking. In spite of the preceding remarks on specialists, a special interest and expertise in a particular sphere of veterinary science may, however, be useful in some investigations; for example, a knowledge of economics when undertaking an evaluation of the economic effects of disease.

Epidemiology is becoming more quantitative than previously. A basic knowledge of statistics is therefore required. However, many problems can be solved without the use of complex statistical methods, and statisticians can be consulted if necessary; the epidemiologist should know when to seek their advice.

The ensuing chapters describe epidemiological concepts, principles and techniques. They also include material from other sciences, such as statistics, immunology, economics and computer science, that is relevant to the practice of contemporary veterinary epidemiology.

Further reading

Davies, G. (1983) Development of veterinary epidemiology. *Veterinary Record*, **112**, 51−53

Ferris, D.H. (1967) Epizootiology. *Advances in Veterinary Science*, **11**, 261−320. (*An early description of veterinary epidemiology*)

Riemann, H. (1982) Launching the new international journal 'Preventive Veterinary Medicine'. *Preventive Veterinary Medicine*, **1**, 1−4

Thrusfield, M. (1992) Quantitative approaches to veterinary epidemiology. In: *The Royal Veterinary College Bicentenary Symposium Series: The Advancement of Veterinary Science, London 1991. Volume 1: Veterinary Medicine Beyond 2000.* Ed. Michell, A.R., pp. 121−142. Commonwealth Agricultural Bureaux, Farnham Royal

3 Some general epidemiological concepts and principles

Chapters 1 and 2 have outlined the development and scope of veterinary epidemiology. This chapter introduces some specific epidemiological concepts and principles that will be applied in succeeding chapters.

Endemic, epidemic, pandemic and sporadic occurrence of disease

Endemic occurrence

'Endemic' is used in two senses to describe:

1. the **usual frequency of occurrence** of a disease in a population;
2. the **constant presence** of a disease in a population.

Thus the term implies a stable state; if a disease is well understood, then its endemic level is often **predictable**. The term endemic can be applied not only to overt disease but also to disease in the absence of clinical signs and to levels of circulating antibodies. Therefore, the exact context in which the term is used should always be defined. For example, laboratory mice kept under conventional systems of 'non-barrier maintenance' (i.e., with no special precautions being taken to prevent entry and spread of infection into the population) are invariably infected with the nematode *Syphacia obvelata*. Infection of 100% of the mice would be considered the usual level of occurrence, that is, the endemic level of infection. When a disease is continuously present to a high level, affecting all age groups equally, it is **hyperendemic**. In contrast, the endemic level of actinobacillosis in a dairy herd is likely to be less than 1%.

'Endemic' is applied not only to infectious diseases but also to non-infectious ones: the veterinary meat hygienist is just as concerned with the endemic level of carcass bruising as is the veterinary practitioner with the endemic level of pneumonia in pigs.

When endemic disease is described, the affected population and its location should be specified. Thus, although bovine tuberculosis is endemic in badgers in south-west England, the infection apparently is not endemic in all badger populations in the UK (Little *et al.*, 1982).

Epidemic occurrence

'Epidemic' originally was used only to describe a sudden, usually unpredictable, increase in the number of cases of an infectious disease in a population. In modern epidemiology, an epidemic is an occurrence of an infectious or non-infectious disease to a level **in excess of the expected (i.e., endemic) level**. Thus, infection with *S. obvelata* should be absent from specific-pathogen-free (SPF) mice kept under strict barrier conditions where precautions are taken to prevent entry and spread of infectious agents in the colony. If an infected mouse gained entry to the colony the infection would be transmitted throughout the resident population and an epidemic of the nematode infection would occur. Such an infection in SPF mice colonies would be **unusually frequent**, that is, epidemic. Similarly, if cattle grazed on rough pasture which could abrade their mouths there might be an increase in the number of cases of actinobacillosis. Although only 2% of the animals might become infected, this would be an unusually high (epidemic) level compared with the endemic level of 1% in the herd. Thus, an epidemic need not involve a large number of individuals.

When an epidemic occurs, the population must have been subjected to one or more factors that were not present previously. In the example of the SPF mouse colony that became infected with *S. obvelata*, the factor was a breakdown in barrier maintenance and the entry of an infected mouse. In the case of the herd with actinobacillosis, the new factor was an increased consumption of vegetation that could cause buccal abrasions.

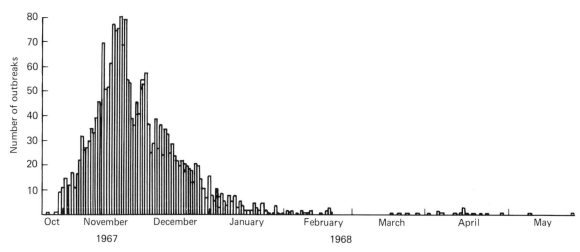

Fig. 3.1 The British 1967–68 foot-and-mouth disease epidemic: number of outbreaks per day. (From HMSO, 1969.)

The popular conception of an epidemic frequently is an outbreak of disease that is noticed immediately. However, some epidemics may go undetected for some time after their occurrence. Thus, in London, in 1952, the deaths of 4000 people were associated with a particularly severe smog (fog intensified by smoke). The deaths occurred at the same time as the Smithfield fat stock show (HMSO, 1954). Although an epidemic of severe respiratory disease in the cattle was recognized immediately and was associated with the air pollution caused by the smog, the epidemic of human respiratory disease was not appreciated until statistics recording human deaths were published more than a year later.

In contrast, some epidemics may be exaggerated. An increased number of deaths in foxes occurred in the UK in the late 1950s. This apparent epidemic of a 'new' fatal disease received considerable publicity and every dead fox was assumed to have died from the disease. Subsequent laboratory analyses identified chlorinated hydrocarbon poisoning as the cause of the increased fox fatality, but only 40% of foxes submitted for post-mortem examination had died from the poisoning. The other 60% had died of endemic diseases that had not previously stimulated general interest (Blackmore, 1964). This example illustrates that the endemic level of disease in a population has to be known before an epidemic can be recognized.

Pandemic occurrence

A pandemic is a widespread epidemic that usually affects a large proportion of the population. Many countries may be affected. Pandemics of rinderpest (see *Table 1.1*),

foot-and-mouth disease, and African swine fever have been the cause of considerable financial loss. By the 1970s, rinderpest was found only in north-west Africa and the Indian subcontinent, but the disease became pandemic in Africa and the Middle East during the early 1980s (Sasaki, 1991), and is now the target of a global eradication campaign (Wojciechowski, 1991). In the late 1970s, a pandemic of parvovirus infection occurred in dogs in many parts of the world (Carmichael and Binn, 1981). Serious human pandemics have included plague (the Black Death) in the Middle Ages, cholera in the 19th century, and influenza soon after the First World War.

Sporadic occurrence

A sporadic outbreak of disease is one that occurs **irregularly and haphazardly**. This implies that appropriate circumstances have occurred **locally**, producing small, localized outbreaks.

Foot-and-mouth disease is not endemic in the UK. A sporadic outbreak, thought to be associated with the importation of infected meat from South America, occurred in Oswestry in October 1967 (Hugh-Jones, 1972). Unfortunately, this incident resulted in an epidemic that was not eliminated until the middle of 1968 (*Figure 3.1*). However, the disease did not become endemic, because of veterinary intervention. Conversely, in 1969, a single sporadic case of rabies occurred in a dog in the UK after it had completed the statutory six-month quarantine period (Haig, 1977). No other animal was infected and so this sporadic outbreak was confined to the original case.

Thus, 'sporadic' can indicate either a single case or a cluster of cases of a disease or infection (without obvious disease) that is not normally present in an area.

Infection with *Leptospira interrogans*, serovar *pomona*, is endemic in domestic pigs in New Zealand. The bacterium is also frequently the cause of sporadic epidemics of abortion in cattle. Infected cattle excrete the bacterium in their urine only for approximately three months. The bacterium therefore cannot usually be maintained, and so becomes endemic, in the herd. If a cow becomes infected with the bacterium by direct or indirect contact with pigs, this constitutes sporadic infection. This animal may now become a short-term source of infection to other pregnant cattle in the herd, and a sporadic epidemic of abortion, of three or four months duration, is likely to occur. Post-infection leptospiral antibodies persist for many years in cattle, and sporadic infection with the bacterium is not uncommon; 18% of New Zealand cattle have been reported to have detectable antibodies to this organism. Thus, although infection and the abortion that may ensue are **sporadic**, there is an **endemic** level of antibody in the bovine population (Hathaway, 1981).

The cause of disease

The cause of events is of relevance to all branches of science. It is discussed in general by Taylor (1967), and in the epidemiological context by Buck (1975) and Evans (1993). In epidemiology, studies are generally undertaken to identify causes of disease so that preventive measures can be developed and implemented, and their subsequent effectiveness identified (Wynder, 1985). Chapter 1 indicated that there has been a transition from the idea that disease has a predominantly single cause to one of multiple causes.* The former idea is epitomized by Koch's postulates.

Koch's postulates

The increased understanding of microbial diseases in the late 19th century led Robert Koch to formulate his

---

*Complexity, however, should not be sought when it is not justified. This guideline is encapsulated in the 'principle of parsimony', whose frequent and thorough use by the medieval English philosopher, William of Ockham, gained it the name of 'Ockham's razor': *'Pluralitas non est ponenda sine necessitate'*: ('multiplicity ought not to be posited without necessity'). More generally, one should choose the simplest hypothesis that will fit the facts (Edwards, 1967).

postulates to determine the cause of infectious disease. These postulates state that an organism is causal if:

1. it is present in all cases of the disease;
2. it does not occur in another disease as a fortuitous and non-pathogenic parasite;
3. it is isolated in pure culture from an animal, is repeatedly passaged, and induces the same disease in other animals.

Koch's postulates brought a necessary degree of order and discipline to the study of infectious disease. Few would argue that an organism fulfilling the above criteria does not cause the disease in question; but is it the **sole** and **complete** cause? Koch provided a rigid framework for testing the causal importance of a microorganism but ignored the influence of environmental factors that were relatively unimportant in relation to the lesions that were being studied. Microbiologists found it difficult enough to satisfy the postulates without concerning themselves with interactions between complex environmental factors. Therefore, the microorganisms were assumed to be the sole causes of the diseases that the microbiologists were investigating.

Dissatisfaction became evident in two groups (Stewart, 1968). Some microbiologists thought that the postulates were too difficult to satisfy because there can be obstacles to fulfilling Koch's postulates with some infectious agents that are causes of disease (e.g., some pathogens can be isolated in pure culture from cases, but do not readily induce disease in other animals; e.g., see 'Diseases caused by mixed agents' in Chapter 5). Others thought that the postulates were insufficient because they did not specify the environmental conditions that turned vague associations into specific causes of disease. Furthermore, the postulates were not applicable to non-infectious diseases. A more cosmopolitan theory of cause was needed.

Evans' postulates

Evans (1976) has produced a set of postulates that are consistent with modern concepts of causation:

1. the proportion of individuals with the disease should be significantly higher in those exposed to the supposed cause than in those who are not;
2. exposure to the supposed cause should be present more commonly in those with than those without the disease, when all other risk factors are held constant;
3. the number of new cases of disease should be significantly higher in those exposed to the supposed

cause than in those not so exposed, as shown in prospective studies;

4. temporally, the disease should follow exposure to the supposed cause with a distribution of incubation periods on a bell-shaped curve;*

5. a spectrum of host responses, from mild to severe, should follow exposure to the supposed cause along a logical biological gradient;

6. a measurable host response (e.g., antibody, cancer cells) should appear regularly following exposure to the supposed cause in those lacking this response before exposure, or should increase in magnitude if present before exposure; this pattern should not occur in individuals not so exposed;

7. experimental reproduction of the disease should occur with greater frequency in animals or man appropriately exposed to the supposed cause than in those not so exposed; this exposure may be deliberate in volunteers, experimentally induced in the laboratory, or demonstrated in a controlled regulation of natural exposure;

8. elimination (e.g., removal of a specific infectious agent) or modification (e.g., alteration of a deficient diet) of the supposed cause should decrease the frequency of occurrence of the disease;

9. prevention or modification of the host's response (e.g., by immunization or use of specific lymphocyte transfer factor in cancer) should decrease or eliminate the disease that normally occurs on exposure to the supposed cause;

10. all relationships and associations should be biologically and epidemiologically credible.

An important characteristic of Evans' postulates is that they require the association between an hypothesized causal factor and the disease in question to be **statistically significant**. This involves comparing **groups** of animals, rather than investigating associations in the individual.

Demonstration of a statistically significant association, however, **does not prove** that a factor is causal. The logical reduction of proof requires that the mechanism of induction of a disease by a cause needs to be explained by describing the chain of events, from cause to effect, at the

molecular level. However, in the absence of experimental evidence, epidemiological identification of an association can be of considerable preventive value because it can indicate factors, the reduction or removal of which reduce the occurrence of disease, although a specific cause has not been identified (see Chapter 2). Some of the statistical techniques of demonstrating association are described in Chapters 14 and 15.

Variables

The object of detailed statistical analysis is to identify those factors that cause disease. Disease and causal factors are examples of **variables**.

Variable

A variable is any observable event that can vary. Examples of variables are the weight and age of an animal and the number of cases of disease.

Study variable

A study variable is any variable that is being considered in an investigation.

Response and explanatory variables

A **response** variable is one that is affected by another (**explanatory**) variable. In epidemiological investigations, disease is often the response variable. For example, when studying the effects of dry cat food on the occurrence of urolithiasis, cat food is the explanatory variable and urolithiasis is the response variable.

Types of association

Association is the degree of dependence or independence between two variables. There are two main types of association (*Figure 3.2*):

1. non-statistical association;
2. statistical association.

Non-statistical association

A non-statistical association between a disease and an hypothesized causal factor is an association that arises by chance; that is, the frequency of joint occurrence of the disease and factor is no greater than would be expected by chance. For example, *Mycoplasma felis* has been isolated from the eyes of some cats with conjunctivitis. This represents an association between the mycoplasma and conjunctivitis in these cats. However, surveys have shown that *M. felis* also can be recovered from the

---

*The bell shape is often obtained only when the horizontal 'time' axis is mathematically transformed (Sartwell, 1950, 1966; Armenian and Lilienfeld, 1974; Armenian, 1987); if a linear time-scale is used then the curve is usually positively skewed, that is, there are few long incubation periods relative to the number of short incubation periods. Mathematical transformation is described in Chapter 12.

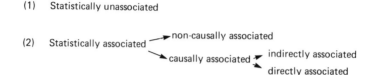

(1)   Statistically unassociated

(2)   Statistically associated — non-causally associated
                                 causally associated — indirectly associated
                                                        directly associated

Fig. 3.2 Types of association between disease and hypothesized causal factors.

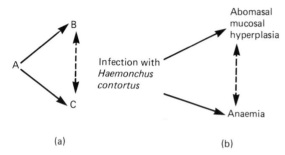

(a)   (b)

Fig. 3.3 Path diagrams indicating the paradigm (**a**) and an example (**b**) of causal and non-causal statistical associations. A = cause of disease (explanatory variable); B and C = manifestations of disease (response variables); ——►causal association;◄–►non-causal association.

conjunctivae of 80% of apparently normal cats (Blackmore *et al.*, 1971). Analysis of these findings revealed that the association between conjunctivitis and the presence of *M. felis* arose by chance: the mycoplasma could be present in healthy cats as well as in those with conjunctivitis. In such circumstances, where a chance, non-statistical association occurs, a factor cannot be inferred to be causal.

Statistical association

Variables are positively statistically associated when they occur together more frequently than would be expected by chance. They are negatively statistically associated when they occur together less frequently than would be expected by chance.

Positive statistical associations may therefore indicate a causal relationship. However, not all factors that are positively statistically associated with a disease are necessarily causal. This can be understood with the aid of a simple path diagram (*Figure 3.3a*). The explanatory variable, A, is the cause of a disease. The response variables, B and C, are two manifestations of the disease. In these circumstances, there is a statistical causal association between A and B, and between A and C. There is also a positive statistical association between the two response variables, B and C, arising from their

separate associations with A, but this is a non-causal association.

An example of these associations is given in *Figure 3.3b*. If infection of cattle with *Haemonchus contortus* were being investigated, then the following positive statistical associations could be found:

1. between the presence of the parasite and abomasal mucosal hyperplasia;
2. between the presence of the parasite and anaemia;
3. between abomasal mucosal hyperplasia and anaemia.

The first two associations are causal and the third non-causal.

Abomasal mucosal hyperplasia and infection with *H. contortus* are **risk factors** for anaemia, that is, their presence increases the risk of anaemia. Similarly, in cats, lack of skin pigmentation results in white fur and also increased ultraviolet irradiation of the skin. The latter is associated with cutaneous squamous cell carcinoma (Dorn *et al.*, 1971), and white fur is a risk factor for this condition.

Risk factors therefore may be either causal or non-causal. (Some authors reserve 'risk factor' exclusively for causal factors, and use 'risk indicator' or 'risk marker' to describe both causally and non-causally associated factors: Last, 1988.) A knowledge of risk factors is useful in identifying populations at which veterinary attention should be directed. Thus, high milk yield is a risk factor for ketosis in dairy cattle. When developing preventive measures it is important to identify those risk factors that are causal, against which control should be directed, and those that are non-causal and will not therefore affect the development of disease.

Explanatory and response variables can be causally associated either **directly** or **indirectly** (*Figure 3.4*). Path diagrams 1 and 2 illustrate direct causal associations. Indirect associations are characterized by an intervening variable. Path diagram 3 illustrates an indirect causal association between A and C where the effect of A is entirely through the intervening variable B, whose effect is direct. This is equivalent to saying that A and B operate at different levels, therefore either A or B can be described as the cause of C. Leptospirosis, for example,

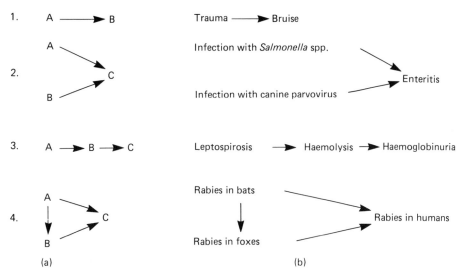

Fig. 3.4 Path diagrams indicating paradigms (**a**), and examples (**b**) of direct and indirect causal associations: 1 and 2 = direct causal associations; 3 = indirect causal association (A with C), direct causal association (B with C); 4 = direct and indirect causal association (A with C).

causes haemoglobinuria by haemolysing red blood cells; a clinician would say that leptospirosis causes the haemoglobinuria, whereas a pathologist might attribute it to intravascular haemolysis.

Path diagram 4 in *Figure 3.4* illustrates the situation where one explanatory variable, A, has not only a direct causal association with a response variable, C, but also an indirect effect on C by influencing another variable, B. For example, in the US people have contracted rabies by inhalation on entering caves where rabies-infected bats roost. They can also contract rabies from foxes that are infected by living in bat-infested caves.

Causal models

The associations and interactions between direct and indirect causes can be viewed in two ways, producing two causal 'models'.

Causal model 1

The relationship of causes to their effects allows classification of causes into two types: 'sufficient' and 'necessary' (Rothman, 1976).

A cause is **sufficient** if it inevitably produces an effect (assuming that nothing happens that interrupts the development of the effect, such as death or prophylaxis). A sufficient cause virtually always comprises a range of component causes; disease therefore is **multifactorial**. Frequently, however, one component is commonly

described, in general parlance, as **the** cause. For example, distemper virus is referred to as the cause of distemper, although the sufficient cause actually involves exposure to the virus, lack of immunity and, possibly, other components. It is not necessary to identify all components of a sufficient cause to prevent disease because removal of one component may render the cause insufficient. For example, an improvement in floor design can prevent foot abscesses in pigs even though the main pyogenic bacteria are not identified.

A particular disease may be produced by different sufficient causes. The different sufficient causes may have certain component causes in common, or they may not. If a cause is a component of every sufficient cause then it is **necessary**. Therefore, a necessary cause must always be present to produce an effect.

In *Figure 3.5a*, A is the only necessary cause, because it is the only component appearing in all of the sufficient causes. The remaining causes (B−J) are not necessary because there are some sufficient causes without them. This concept is exemplified in *Figure 3.5b* which depicts hypothesized sufficient causes of pneumonic pasteurellosis in cattle. Infection with *Pasteurella* spp. is the necessary cause, but other component causes, including lack of immunity, are required for induction of the disease.

Another example of a cause that is necessary but not sufficient is infection with *Actinobacillus ligneresi*, which must occur before actinobacillosis ('wooden tongue') can

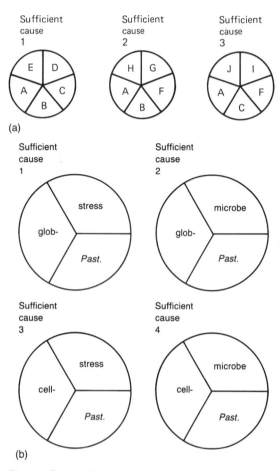

(a)

(b)

Fig. 3.5 Scheme for the causes of disease (causal model 1). (**a**) Paradigm. (**b**) Hypothetical example for bovine pneumonic pasteurellosis. glob-: lack of specific globulins; stress: adrenal stress of environmental origin (e.g., weather); *Past.*: presence of *Pasteurella* spp.; microbe: presence of viruses or mycoplasmata; cell-: lack of cellular immunity. ((**a**) From Rothman, 1976; (**b**) modified from Martin *et al.*, 1987.)

develop. However, other factors that damage the buccal mucosae (e.g., sharp, abrasive vegetation) must be present before the disease develops. In the absence of these factors the bacterium can be present without disease developing.

It is obvious that necessary causes are frequently related to the definition of a disease; for example, lead is a necessary cause of lead poisoning, and *P. multocida* is a necessary cause of pneumonic pasteurellosis.

A cause may be necessary, sufficient, neither, or both, but it is unusual for a single component cause to be both necessary and sufficient. One example is exposure to

large doses of gamma radiation with the subsequent development of radiation sickness.

Component causes therefore include factors that can be classified as:

1. **predisposing factors**, which increase the level of susceptibility in the host (e.g., age and immune status);
2. **enabling factors**, which facilitate manifestation of a disease (e.g., housing and nutrition);
3. **precipitating factors**, which are associated with the definitive onset of disease (e.g., many toxic and infectious agents);
4. **reinforcing factors**, which tend to aggravate the presence of a disease (e.g., repeated exposure to an infectious agent in the absence of an immune response).

Pneumonia is an example of a disease that has sufficient causes, none of which has a necessary component. Pneumonia may have been produced in one case by heat stress where a dry, dusty environment allowed microscopic particulate matter to reach the alveoli. Cold stress could produce a clinically similar result.

Multifactorial syndromes such as pneumonia can have many sufficient causes, although no single component cause is necessary. Part of the reason is taxonomic: pneumonia is a loosely connected group of diseases whose classification (see Chapter 9) is based on lesions (inflammation of the lungs), rather than specific causes; the lesions can be produced by many different causes. When a disease is classified according to aetiology there is, by definition, usually only one major cause, which therefore is likely to be necessary. Examples include lead poisoning, actinobacillosis and pasteurellosis, mentioned above, and many 'simple' infectious diseases, such as tuberculosis and brucellosis.

The object of epidemiological investigations of cause is the identification of sufficient causes and their component causes. Removal of one or more components from a sufficient cause will then prevent disease produced by that sufficient cause.

Causal model 2

Direct and indirect causes represent a chain of actions, with the indirect causes activating the direct causes (e.g., *Figure 3.4*, path diagram 3). When many such relationships occur, a number of factors can act at the same level (but not necessarily at the same intensity), and there may be several levels, producing a 'web of causation'. Again, disease is **multifactorial**. *Figure 3.6* illustrates the causal web of bovine hypomagnesaemia.

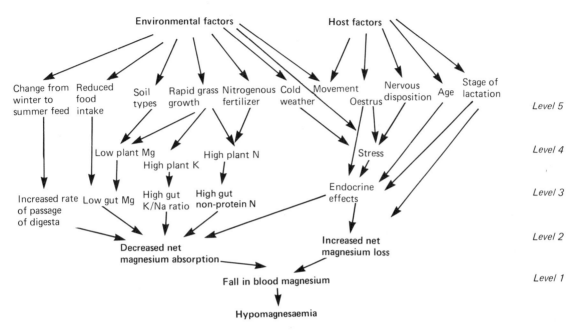

Fig. 3.6 Causal web of bovine hypomagnesaemia (causal model 2).

Confounding

Confounding (Latin: *confundere* = to mix together) is the effect of an extraneous variable that can wholly or partly account for an apparent association between variables. Confounding can produce a spurious association between study variables, or can mask a real association. A variable that confounds is called a **confounding variable** or **confounder**.

A confounding variable is distributed non-randomly (i.e., is positively or negatively correlated with the explanatory and response variables that are being studied). A confounding variable must:*

1. be a risk factor for the disease that is being studied; and
2. be associated with the explanatory variable, but not be a consequence of exposure to it.

Examples to illustrate the concept

An investigation of leptospirosis in dairy farmers in New Zealand (Mackintosh *et al.*, 1980) revealed that wearing

an apron during milking was associated with an increased risk of contracting leptospirosis. Further work showed that the larger the herd being milked, the greater the chance of contracting leptospirosis. It also was found that farmers with large herds tended to wear aprons more frequently for milking than farmers with small herds. The association between the wearing of aprons and leptospirosis was not causal but was produced spuriously by the confounding effect of large herd size (*Figure 3.7a*), because large herd size was associated with leptospirosis, and also with the wearing of aprons. *Figure 3.7b* illustrates a similar confounding effect in relation to respiratory disease in pigs (Willeberg, 1980b). A statistical association was demonstrated between fan ventilation and respiratory disease. This was not because fan ventilation caused respiratory disease. The association resulted from the confounding effect of herd size: large herds are more likely to develop respiratory disease than small herds, and are also more likely to have fan ventilation rather than natural ventilation.

These two examples have been selected to illustrate confounding in situations where the spurious association is obviously rather implausible. In most situations, confounding is less obvious but must be considered; for example, age, breed and sex can be common confounders in observational studies that test causal hypotheses (see Chapter 15).

*Criteria for confounding are given in standard texts (e.g., Schlesselman, 1982), but there is controversy over conflicting definitions of confounding, and therefore over the conditions required (Kass and Greenland, 1991).

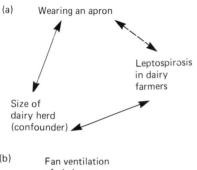

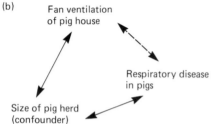

Fig. 3.7   Examples of confounding: (**a**) large dairy herds in relation to leptospirosis in dairy farmers and the wearing of milking aprons; (**b**) large pig herds in relation to respiratory disease in pigs and fan ventilation. ←→ 'Real' association; ←- -→ spurious association.

Formulating a causal hypothesis

The first step in any epidemiological investigation of cause is descriptive. A description of **time**, **place** and **population** is useful initially.

Time

Associations with year, season, month, day or even hour in the case of food poisoning investigations, should be considered. Such details may provide information on climatic influences, incubation periods and sources of infection. For example, an outbreak of salmonellosis in a group of cattle may be associated with the introduction of infected cattle feed.

Place

The geographical distribution of a disease may indicate an association with local geological, management or ecological factors, for example nutritionally deficient soil or arthropod transmitters of infection. Epidemiological maps (see Chapter 4) are a valuable aid to identifying geographical associations.

Population

The type of animal that is affected often is of considerable importance. Hereford cattle are more susceptible to squamous cell carcinoma of the eye than other breeds, suggesting that the cause may be partly genetic. In many parts of the world, meat workers are affected more often by Q Fever than are other people, implying a source of infection in meat-processing plants.

When the major facts have been established, alternative causal hypotheses can be formulated. An epidemiological investigation is similar to any detective novel that unfolds a list of 'suspects' (possible causal factors), some of which may be non-statistically associated with a disease, and some statistically associated with the disease, either causally or non-causally.

There are four major methods of arriving at an hypothesis:

1. method of difference;
2. method of agreement;
3. method of concomitant variation;
4. method of analogy.

Method of difference

If the frequency of a disease is different in two different circumstances, and a factor is present in one circumstance but is absent from the other, then the factor may be suspected of being causal. For instance, Wood (1978) noted an increased occurrence of stillbirths in pigs in one of three farrowing houses. The only difference between this house and the other two was a different type of burner on its gas heaters. An hypothesis was formulated: that the different type of burner caused the stillbirths. Subsequently, the burners were shown to be defective and producing large amounts of carbon monoxide; the carbon monoxide was assumed to cause the stillbirths. The occurrence of stillbirths decreased when the faulty burners were removed, thus supporting the hypothesis.

Similarly, BSE occurred to a different extent on the Channel Islands (Jersey and Guernsey), and meat and bone meal was used more frequently in feedstuffs on the island with the greater frequency of BSE (Wilesmith, 1993). This added credence to the hypothesis that the causal agent was transmitted in meat and bone meal in concentrate rations.

A defect of an hypothesis based on the method of difference is that several different factors may usually be incriminated as possible causes. The value of an hypothesis generated by this method is reduced if many alternative hypotheses can be formulated. For example, a comparison of the different disease patterns of pigs in Africa and Denmark would involve a large number of variables, many of which could be hypothesized as

Table 3.1 The relationship between frequency of milking and serological evidence of exposure to leptospirosis in dairy farm personnel in the Manawatu region of New Zealand.

Frequency of milking of cows by personnel	Serological leptospirosis		Total number of personnel	Percentage of personnel with serological leptospirosis
	Present	Absent		
9 times/week	61	116	177	34.5
1−8 times/week	4	11	15	26.7
Rarely or never	8	20	20	0.0

causal. In contrast, the marked occurrence of mannosidosis in Angus cattle (Jolly and Townsley, 1980), compared with the absence of this disease in other breeds, strongly suggests that a genetic factor is the cause.

Method of agreement

If a factor is common to a number of different circumstances in which a disease is present then the factor may be the cause of the disease. Thus, if a batch of meat and bone meal was associated with salmonellosis on widely different types of pig farms, and this was the only circumstance in common, then the causal hypothesis — that disease was caused by contamination of that batch — is strengthened.

A second example relates to bovine hyperkeratosis which was identified in cattle in the US (Schwabe *et al.*, 1977). The disease was called 'X disease' because initially the cause was unknown. It occurred in different circumstances:

1. in cattle that were fed sliced bread;
2. in calves that had been licking lubricating oil;
3. in cattle that were in contact with wood preservative.

The bread-slicing machine was lubricated with a similar oil to that which had been licked by the calves. The lubricating oil and the wood preservative both contained chlorinated naphthalene. This chemical was common to the different circumstances and subsequently was shown to cause hyperkeratosis.

Method of concomitant variation

This method involves a search for a factor, the frequency or strength of which varies continuously with the frequency of the disease in different situations. Thus, the distance over which cattle are transported before slaughter appears to be related to the occurrence of bruises in their carcasses (Meischke *et al.*, 1974).

Similarly, there appear to be relationships between the occurrence of squamous cell carcinoma of the skin of animals and the intensity of ultraviolet radiation, between the occurrence of bovine hypomagnesaemia and pasture levels of magnesium, and between infection of dairy personnel with leptospires and the frequency with which the personnel milk cows (*Table 3.1*). The classical medical epidemiological investigation of the association between smoking and lung cancer (Doll and Hill, 1964a, b) also illustrates this method of reasoning (*Table 3.2*): the number of deaths due to lung cancer is proportional to the number of cigarettes smoked per day.

Method of analogy

This method of reasoning involves comparison of the pattern of the disease under study with that of a disease that is already understood, because the cause of a disease that is understood may also be the cause of another poorly understood disease with a similar pattern. For example, some mammary tumours of mice are known to be caused by a virus, therefore some mammary tumours of dogs may have a viral cause. The climatic conditions associated with outbreaks of Kikuyu grass poisoning of cattle may suggest a mycotoxin as the cause because the circumstance is similar to those circumstances present in other

Table 3.2 The relationship between number of cigarettes smoked per day and deaths by lung cancer in British doctors, 1951−61. (From Doll and Hill, 1964a.)

Cigarettes/day in 1951	Annual lung cancer death rate/1000 (1951−61)
None	0.07
1−14	0.54
15−24	1.39
≥25	2.27

mycotoxicoses (Bryson, 1982). Bovine petechial fever, caused by *Cytoecetes ondiri*, is present in a limited area of Kenya (Snodgrass, 1974). The mode of transmission of this infectious agent is unknown. However, other members of the genus *Cytoecetes* are known to be transmitted by arthropods, and geographic limitation is a feature of arthropod-transmitted diseases. Therefore, using the method of analogy, it has been suggested that *C. ondiri* may be transmitted by arthropods.

Evidence by analogy is not, in the strictest sense, evidence of fact. It can point to probabilities, and can confirm conclusions that may be reached by other means; but it can be dangerously misleading. A classical example is the inference made by the 19th century medical epidemiologist, John Snow, that yellow fever was transmitted by sewage (Snow, 1855). He had already demonstrated that cholera was transmitted by sewage, and then observed that cholera and yellow fever were both associated with overcrowding. He then inferred that cholera and yellow fever had similar modes of transmission, whereas the latter is actually transmitted by an arthropod rather than by contaminated sewage.

When attempting to establish a causal association, five principles should be considered:

1. the time sequence of the events;
2. the strength of the association;
3. biological gradient;
4. consistency;
5. compatibility with existing knowledge.

Time sequence

Cause must precede effect. In a bacteriological survey, Millar and Francis (1974) found an increased occurrence of various infections in barren mares compared with others whose reproductive function was normal. However, unless the bacterial infections were present **before** the mares became infertile, it would be incorrect to infer that the bacterial infections caused infertility. The causal pathway may have been in the other direction: absence of normal reproductive cyclic activity may allow previously harmless infections to flourish.

Strength of association

If a factor is causal then there will be a strong positive statistical association between the factor and the disease.

Biological gradient

If a dose–response relationship can be found between a factor and a disease, the plausibility of a factor being causal is increased. This is the basis of reasoning by the method of concomitant variation. Examples have already been cited: frequency of milking in relation to leptospirosis (see *Table 3.1*) and smoking in relation to lung cancer (see *Table 3.2*).

Consistency

If an association exists in a number of different circumstances, then a causal relationship is probable. This is the basis of reasoning by the method of agreement. An example is bovine hyperkeratosis, mentioned above.

Compatibility with existing knowledge

It is more reasonable to infer that a factor causes a disease if a plausible biological mechanism has been identified than if such a mechanism is not known. Thus, smoking can be suggested as a likely cause of lung cancer because other chemical and environmental pollutants are known to have a carcinogenic effect on laboratory animals. Similarly, if a mycotoxin were present in animal foodstuffs, then it might be expected to produce characteristic liver damage. On the other hand, the survey of leptospirosis of dairy farmers, mentioned earlier, showed a positive association between wearing an apron and having a leptospiral titre. This finding was not compatible with either existing knowledge or common sense and a factor that might have confounded the result was sought and found.

This chapter has discussed hypothesis formulation. The testing of hypotheses using observational studies is described in Chapter 16.

A fuller discussion of reasoning and causal inference in epidemiological studies is presented by Maclure (1985) and Weed (1986).

Further reading

Evans, A.S. (1993) *Causation and Disease: A Chronological Journey.* Plenum Publishing Corporation, New York

Last, A.M. (1988) *A Dictionary of Epidemiology*, 2nd edn. Oxford University Press, New York

Susser, M. (1973) *Causal Thinking in the Health Sciences. Concepts and Strategies of Epidemiology.* Oxford University Press, New York, London and Toronto

Taylor, R. (1967) Causation. In: *The Encyclopedia of Philosophy*, Vol. 2. Ed. Edwards, P., pp. 56–66. The Macmillan Company and The Free Press, New York

4 Describing disease occurrence

A necessary part of the investigation of disease in a population is the counting of affected animals so that the **amount** of disease can be described. Furthermore, it is usually desirable to describe **when** and **where** disease occurs, and to relate the number of diseased animals to the size of the **population at risk** of developing disease so that a disease's importance can be assessed. A report of 10 cases of infectious enteritis in a cattery, for example, does not indicate the true extent of the problem unless the report is considered in terms of the number of cats in the cattery: there may be only 10 cats present, in which case all of the cats are affected, or there may be 100 cats, in which case only a small proportion of the cats is affected.

The amount of disease is the **morbidity** (Latin: *morbus* = disease); the number of deaths is the **mortality**. The times of occurrence of cases of a disease are its **temporal** distribution; the places of occurrence are its **spatial** distribution. The measurement and description of the size of populations and their characteristics is **demography*** (Greek: *demo-* = people; *-graphia* = writing, description).

This chapter discusses the types of animal population that are encountered in veterinary medicine, and describes the methods of expressing the amount of, and temporal and spatial distribution of, disease and associated demographic data.

The structure of animal populations

The structure of populations influences the extent to which population sizes can be assessed, as well as

*A distinction between zoography and demography is not made in this book, for the reasons given in Chapter 2 in relation to epizootiology and epidemiology.

affecting the ways in which disease occurs and persists in animals. The organization of animal populations can usually be described as either **contiguous** or **separated**.

Contiguous populations

A contiguous population is one in which there is much contact between individuals in the population and members of other populations. Contiguous populations therefore predispose to transfer and persistence of infectious diseases over large areas because of the inherent mixing and movement of animals.

Most human populations are contiguous because there is mixing of individuals by travel. Populations of small domestic animals also are usually contiguous. Dogs and cats move freely within cities, coming into contact with other urban, suburban and rural animals of their own and different species. African nomadic tribes similarly own animals that comprise contiguous groups. Many wild animals belong to this category, too.

Assessing the size of contiguous populations

It is often difficult to assess the size of contiguous animal populations. Only limited demographic data about small domestic animals are available; for example, from Kennel Club registers (Tedor and Reif, 1978; Wong and Lee, 1985). In some developed countries, dogs must be legally registered, but this is a difficult law to enforce and so many dogs may not be recorded. There are pet registries that record and identify animals, for example, by ear or leg tattooing (Anon., 1984), but these records are voluntary and so exclude the majority of animals.

Some surveys have been undertaken to establish the size and other characteristics of small animal populations (*Table 4.1*). However, such animals are kept in small numbers — often only one animal per household. It is therefore necessary to contact many owners to gain

Table 4.1 Some demographic surveys of pet dog and cat populations.

Country/region	Characteristics recorded	Source
Canada: Ontario	Breed, age, owner characteristics*	Leslie *et al.* (1994)
Cyprus	Population size	Pappaioanou *et al.* (1984)
Europe	Population size (by country) For UK: regional distribution, owner characteristics	Anderson (1983)
Malaysia	Breed, sex, litter size, seasonal distribution of whelping	Wong and Lee (1985)
UK	Sex, age, diet Breed Breed, sex, age	Fennell (1975) Edney and Smith (1986) Thrusfield (1989)
US: California	Breed, sex, age, owner characteristics	Dorn *et al.* (1967); Franti and Kraus (1974)†
	Breed, sex, age Owner characteristics	Schneider and Vaida (1975) Franti *et al.* (1974)
	Breed, sex, age, owner characteristics	Franti *et al.* (1980)
US: Illinois	Sex, age, reproductive history, owner characteristics	Griffiths and Brenner (1977)
US: Indiana	Population size Sex, age, owner characteristics	Lengerich *et al.* (1992) Teclaw *et al.* (1992)
US: Kansas	Age, population dynamics	Nasser and Mosier (1980, 1982)
US: Nevada	Age, population dynamics	Nasser *et al.* (1984)
US: New Jersey	Breed, sex, age	Cohen *et al.* (1959)
US: Ohio	Breed, sex, age, owner characteristics	Schnurrenberger *et al.* (1961)

*Owner characteristics vary between studies, and include age, occupation, location (urban versus rural), number and age of children, and type of dwelling.
†Also reports horse ownership.

information about relatively few animals (i.e., the animal:owner ratio is low). This can be a difficult and costly exercise. The results may also be distorted by the lack of information on undetectable segments of the population such as stray, semi-domesticated and feral animals.

Non-thoroughbred horses and ponies kept as leisure animals similarly are difficult to count, and their enumeration is frequently indirect. In the UK, for example, estimation of population size has been based on the number of farriers (McClintock, 1988), the amount of shoeing steel produced (*Horse and Hound*, 1992), aerial counts (Barr *et al.*, 1986), and surveys of private households (McClintock, 1988; *Horse and Hound*, 1992).

These methods have shortcomings. The first counted farriers, assuming that each shod 250 horses, and ignored unshod horses; the second assumed an average of four new sets of shoes per horse per year, again ignoring unshod horses; the aerial survey omitted horses indoors; and the household surveys excluded some categories of animals such as those in riding centres. However, each produced similar figures (for thoroughbred and non-thoroughbred horses, combined), ranging from 500 000 to 560 000 animals, suggesting valid, but conservative, estimates.

Populations of wild animals can be enumerated by aerial and ground counts (Norton-Griffiths, 1978; Southwood, 1978). A common method is **capture–release–**

recapture in which animals are caught, marked and released. A second sample is then captured. The numbers of marked animals recaptured in the second sample is then related to the number initally marked. The simplest index for estimating the number of individuals (Lincoln, 1930) is:

$$\hat{N} = \frac{an}{r}$$

where:

$\hat{N}$ = estimated population size;
a = number of individuals initially marked;
n = number of individuals in the second sample;
r = number of marked individuals recaptured in the second sample.

The validity of this method depends on several assumptions such as complete mixing of marked animals in the population (Southwood, 1978).

Capture – release – recapture and other marking techniques can also provide information on the movement, home range and territories of wild animals, which can be relevant to disease transmission (see Chapter 7). The marking of bait, for example, has facilitated identification of badgers' territories which overlap with dairy farms in the south-west of England on which tuberculosis is present, indicating that infected badgers could be the source of infection on these farms (Cheeseman *et al.*, 1981).

Separated populations

Separated populations occur as discrete units such as herds and flocks. They are particularly common in countries that practise intensive animal production, with many animals on one farm (e.g., many of the developed countries). *Table 4.2* illustrates the various sizes of these units in the UK; most animals of all species are kept in larger units.

A separated population can be **closed**, with no movement of animals into or out of the unit (except to slaughter). An example is a dairy herd that raises its own replacements, or is under statutory control of movement. Two extreme examples of closed populations are the specific-pathogen-free (SPF) and gnotobiotic colonies of laboratory animals.

A separated population can also be **open**, with limited movement of individuals in and out. Examples include

beef herds where animals are brought in from other farms and markets for fattening, and dairy herds that receive replacements from other farms.

Separated populations, especially of the closed type, are less likely to be infected with agents from other areas than contiguous populations. However, if infection enters separated populations, it may spread rapidly because the animal density is frequently high.

Assessing the size of separated populations

It is often easier to obtain information on the size of a separated population than a contiguous one. The large numbers of animals kept under conditions of intensive husbandry in a single separated unit usually have only one owner (i.e., the animal:owner ratio is high). Many demographic data about food animals are available as a result of regular censuses and estimations. The most extensive sources are the *Animal Health Yearbook* of the Food and Agriculture Organization of the United Nations and Office International des Epizooties; animal population sizes in *Tables 1.6* and *1.8* were obtained from the first source.

Thoroughbred horses are members of separated (usually open) populations. They are concentrated in stables in major training areas and can be counted easily. Published figures, however, may not be comprehensive. Thoroughbred horses in training in the UK, for example, are recorded annually, but they comprise only a small and variable age group. Stud books provide information on stallions, mares and foals, but may be incomplete.

Measures of disease occurrence

Prevalence

Prevalence, P, is the number of instances of disease or related attributes (e.g., infection or presence of antibodies) in a known population, at a designated time, without distinction between old and new cases. When the time is not specified, prevalence usually refers to **point prevalence**, that is, the amount of disease in a population at a particular point in time.

Period prevalence refers to the number of cases that are known to have occurred during a specified period of time; for example, a year (**annual prevalence**). It is the sum of the point prevalence at the beginning of the period and the number of new cases that occur during the period, and can therefore be used when the exact time of onset of

Table 4.2 Holdings by size of herd or flock; UK, June 1989. (From HMSO, 1991.)

Dairy herds

	1–2	3–4	5–9	10–15	15–19	20–29	30–39	40–49	50–59	60–69	70–79	100–199	200+	Total
No. of holdings	1 944	627	1 345	1 810	1 985	4 524	5 194	5 164	4 250	3 667	7 845	6 855	974	46 184
No. of cattle	2 625	2 167	9 359	21 596	33 741	110 617	178 437	227 218	229 460	647 621	647 902	891 032	272 622	2 861 397

Beef herds

	1–2	3–4	5–9	10–14	15–19	20–29	30–39	40–49	50–59	60–69	70–99	100–199	200+	Total
No. of holdings	12 834	8 933	13 554	8 644	5 637	7 688	4 751	3 085	2 004	1 384	2 263	1 696	238	72 711
No. of cattle	19 166	30 991	90 872	101 480	94 375	182 561	160 071	134 762	107 283	88 066	185 629	219 310	64 923	1 479 489

Pig herds

	1–2	3–9	10–19	20–29	30–49	50–69	70–99	100–199	200–399	400–999	1000–4999	5000+	Total
No. of holdings		4 731	1 784		2 233		1 706	1 589	1 552	2 120	2 082		17 797
No. of pigs		16 148	24 464		71 377		120 648	229 719	444 046	1 371 908	5 200 441		7 478 751

Sheep flocks

	1–24	25–49	50–99	100–199	200–299	300–399	400–499	500–699	700–999	1000–1499	1500–1999	2000+	Total
No. of holdings	10 364	7 761	11 504	14 957	10 111	7 168	5 366	7 622	7 799	5 720	2 848	3 277	93 497
No. of sheep	118 164	280 244	834 552	2 169 033	2 492 644	2 484 483	2 395 234	4 506 176	5 683 008	6 972 055	4 890 022	9 736 621	42 562 236

Laying fowls

	1–25	26–49	50–99	100–199	200–499	500–999	1000–2499	2500–4999	5000–9999	10 000–19 999	20 000–49 999	50 000+	Total
No. of holdings	32 712		2 303	1 952		320	471	435	364	254	185	130	39 126
No. of fowls	493 400		143 800	374 644		214 004	752 532	1 535 560	2 530 624	3 424 193	5 484 716	18 717 853	33 671 326

Broiler flocks

	1–999	1000–1999	2000–4999	5000–9999	10 000–19 999	20 000–49 999	50 000–99 999	100 000–249 999	250 000–499 999	500 000–999 999	1 000 000+	Total
No. of holdings	603		220	203		349		392				1 767
No. of fowls	58 381		1 080 688	1 961 293		10 972 945		53 926 405				69 233 812

a condition is not known (e.g. some behavioural conditions). **Lifetime prevalence** is the number of individuals known to have had disease for at least part of their life..

Although prevalence can be defined simply as the number of affected animals, it is most meaningful when expressed in terms of the number of diseased animals in relation to the number of animals in the population at risk of developing the disease:

$$P = \frac{\text{number of individuals having a disease at a particular point in time}}{\text{number of individuals in the population at risk at that point in time}}$$

For example, if 20 cows in a herd of 200 cows were lame on a particular day, then the prevalence of lameness in the herd on that day would be 20/200, that is, 0.1. This is a **proportion** that represents the **probability** of an animal having a specified disease at a given time. Prevalence can take values between 0 and 1 and is dimensionless. Sometimes, it is expressed as a percentage. Thus, a prevalence of 0.1 = 10%. Additionally, if a disease is rare, its prevalence may be expressed as:

$$\frac{\text{number of cases of disease}}{\text{population at risk}} \times 10^n$$

where n is an integer depending on the rarity of the disease. Thus, prevalence may be expressed per 10 000 population at risk ($n = 4$) or per 1 000 000 population at risk ($n = 6$).

Incidence

Incidence is the number of new cases that occur in a known population over a specified period of time. The two essential components of an incidence value are:

1. the number of new cases;
2. the period of time over which the new cases occur.

Incidence, like prevalence, can be defined simply in terms of the number of affected animals, but again is usually expressed in relation to the population at risk.

Cumulative incidence

The **cumulative incidence**, *CI* (also termed **risk**), is the proportion of non-diseased individuals at the beginning of a period of study that become diseased during the period:

$$CI = \frac{\text{number of individuals that become diseased during a particular period}}{\text{number of healthy individuals in the population at the beginning of that period}}$$

It is therefore a proportion that can take values between 0 and 1 (or 0–100%) and is dimensionless.

Thus, if 20 animals in a cattery develop feline viral rhinotracheitis during a week, and there are 100 healthy cats in the cattery at the beginning of the week, then, for the week:

$$CI = \frac{20}{100}$$

$$= 0.2.$$

The longer the period of observation, the greater the risk. Thus, if 10 more cats developed the disease during a second week of observation, the cumulative incidence would be 0.3 for the two-week period. If the cumulative incidence has been estimated for one time period, x, it can be extrapolated to other periods, y:

$$CI_y = 1 - (1 - CI_x)^{y/x},$$

assuming that the risk is constant (Martin *et al.*, 1987). For example, if the cumulative incidence in one year is 0.30, for three years:

$$\begin{aligned} CI &= 1 - (1 - 0.30)^{3/1} \\ &= 1 - 0.7^3 \\ &= 1 - 0.34 \\ &= 0.66. \end{aligned}$$

Cumulative incidence is an indication of the average risk of developing disease during a particular period, in both the individual and the population. It is calculated only for the first occurrence of a disease (rather than for multiple occurrences). When calculating cumulative incidence, additional animals at risk cannot be added to the initial number at risk during the period of observation; it is therefore appropriate when populations are relatively static (e.g. 'all in/all out' production systems). If non-diseased animals are removed from the population during this period, the denominator is modified by subtraction of *half* the value of the number removed (Kleinbaum *et al.*, 1982). Cumulative incidence is also used in dynamic populations if the period of risk is short and related to a specific event (e.g. dystokia at calving in dairy herds), because all relevant animals can then be observed for the entire risk period.

Table 4.3 Example of calculation of incidence rate: enzootic bovine leucosis (EBL) (hypothetical data).

Cow number	Period of observation	Time of development of EBL after beginning of observation	Contribution to animal-years at risk
1	7 years	No disease	7 years
2	7 years	No disease	7 years
3	4 years	4 years	4 years
4	5 years	No disease	5 years
5	6 years	No disease	6 years
6	8 years	No disease	8 years
7	5 years	5 years	5 years
8	2 years	No disease	2 years
9	9 years	No disease	9 years
10	5 years	No disease	5 years
Total			58 years

Calculation:
Total number of cases = 2.
Incidence rate   = 2 per 58 animal-years at risk
          = 3.5 per 100 animal-years at risk, i.e. 0.035 per animal-year at risk.

Incidence rate

Incidence rate, I, measures the rapidity with which new cases of disease develop over time:

$$I = \frac{\text{number of new cases of disease that occur in a population during a particular period of time}}{\text{the sum, over all individuals, of the length of time at risk of developing disease}}$$

The denominator is often measured as 'animal-years at risk' (other observed time units, such as days, weeks and months, can also be used). This is the sum of the periods of observation for each animal during which the latter is free from the disease (i.e., is at risk). As soon as an animal becomes diseased, it no longer contributes to this value. For example, six cows, free from disease, observed for one year would constitute 'six animal-years at risk'; equally, one cow observed for six years would constitute 'six animal-years at risk'. An example of calculation of incidence rate is given in *Table 4.3*. Note that incidence rate has a dimension, **time**$^{-1}$; incidence rate is calculated **per animal-week**, **per animal-year**, and so on. If the incidence rate has been estimated for one time period, x, it can be extrapolated to other periods, y:

$$I_y = I_x(y/x),$$

assuming that the rate is constant (Martin *et al.*, 1987). For example, if the incidence rate has been estimated as two cases per animal-year at risk, and the rate per animal-

month is required, then $y = 1$ and $x = 12$ (one year = 12 months), and:

$$I_y = 2(1/12)$$
$$= 0.17 \text{ per animal-month at risk.}$$

Similarly, an incidence rate of two cases per animal-month at risk is equivalent to 24 cases per animal-year at risk.

The technique is based on the idea that the movement to the diseased state depends on:

1. the size of the population;
2. the period of observation;
3. the 'force of morbidity'.

The force of morbidity (also termed the 'hazard rate' and 'instantaneous incidence rate') is a theoretical measure of the risk of occurrence of disease at a point in time, and it is this that is estimated by the incidence rate. It relates to the population, and cannot be interpreted at the level of the individual. The measure accommodates movement into and out of the population (e.g., heifers being brought into, and cows leaving, a dairy herd) during an observed time period and is calculated when the population is relatively dynamic and disease is not restricted to a particular period of time.

Frequently, the exact period of observation of individual animals cannot be recorded. An approximate calculation is then:

$$I = \frac{\begin{array}{c}\text{number of new cases of disease that occur in a}\\\text{population during a particular period of time}\end{array}}{\begin{array}{c}\text{(number at risk at the start of the time period}\\\text{+ number at risk at the end of the time period)}/2\end{array}}$$

using a denominator that represents the average number at risk (Martin *et al.*, 1987).

Thus, if a herd with an average size of 70 cows was observed for a year, and pneumonia was reported in 7 cows, the incidence rate is approximated by:

7/70 per animal-year at risk
= 0.10 per animal-year at risk.

When calculating an incidence rate, the time unit that is used should be short enough to allow only one bout of illness in each animal (after which time the animal ceases to be at risk). Thus, when measuring the incidence rate for bovine mastitis, an appropriate time unit could be one month, in which circumstance the rate would be expressed in terms of animal-months at risk. However, in practice, some diseases may recur within the specified time unit (e.g. injuries). If the disease is of short duration, and subsequent recovery (and immunity) is brief, affected individuals can continue to be included in the population at risk, without interruption (Kleinbaum *et al.*, 1982). Alternatively, recovery periods can be defined, in which circumstance animals re-enter the population at risk after expiry of the periods (Bendixen, 1987).

The incidence rate is sometimes called, more fully, the **true incidence rate**, the **person-time incidence rate** (from human epidemiology), or the **incidence density** (Miettinen, 1976).

Cumulative incidence can be estimated from the incidence rate thus:

$$CI = 1 - e^{-I}$$

where *e* is the base of natural logarithms, 2.718 (see Appendix II). For example, if the incidence rate is 0.03 per year, for one year:

$$
\begin{aligned}
CI &= 1 - 2.718^{-0.03}\\
&= 1 - (1/2.718^{0.03})\\
&= 1 - 0.97\\
&= 0.03.
\end{aligned}
$$

Note that, in this example, the cumulative incidence and incidence rate are equal; this equality is roughly maintained when $I < 0.10$ (Kleinbaum *et al.*, 1982). (Recall that cumulative incidence relates disease to the number at risk at the beginning of the period of observation, whereas an incidence rate relates disease to the average population at risk during the period — two different denominators.)

The rate is higher because the number under observation at the start of the period is reduced as cases occur and are therefore removed from the population at risk.)

Incidence is discussed in detail by Kleinbaum *et al.* (1982) and Bendixen (1987).

Attack rate

Sometimes a population may be at risk for only a limited period of time, either because exposure to a causal agent is brief, or because the risk of developing the disease is limited to a narrow age range such as the neonatal period. Examples of the first reason would be the feeding of a batch of food contaminated with a mycotoxin to a herd of cattle (e.g., Griffiths and Done, 1991), and exposure to radiation during nuclear accidents. Even if observations were made on the animals for a long time, the incidence would not change. In these circumstances, when the period of risk is brief, the term **attack rate** is used to describe the proportion of animals that develop the disease.

A **secondary attack rate** can also be defined (Lilienfeld and Lilienfeld, 1980). This is the proportion of cases of a transmissible disease that develop as a result of contact with the primary case:

Secondary attack rate =
$$\frac{\begin{array}{c}\text{number of individuals exposed to the primary}\\\text{case that develop the disease within the range}\\\text{of the incubation period}\end{array}}{\begin{array}{c}\text{total number of individuals exposed to}\\\text{the primary case}\end{array}}$$

(Cases occurring outside the range of the incubation period are usually the result of contact with secondary cases, and are therefore called tertiary cases.) If the incubation period of the disease is not known, the numerator can be expressed in terms of a specified time period. The secondary attack rate is usually applied to closed aggregates of individuals such as pens and stables (and, in human populations, families and households) and is a useful measure of contagiousness (see Chapter 6).

The relationship between prevalence and incidence rate

A disease with a long duration is more likely to be detected during a cross-sectional survey than is a disease of short duration. For example, chronic arthritis, lasting for several months, could be detected by a cross-sectional abattoir survey that was undertaken any time during the several months that the arthritis was present. However, clinical louping ill, lasting for a few days, could be detected by a cross-sectional survey only if the survey was conducted during the short period that the disease was apparent.

Prevalence, P, therefore depends on the duration, D, and the incidence rate, I, of a disease:

$$P \propto I \times D.$$

This means that a change in prevalence can be due to:

1. a change in incidence rate;
2. a change in the average duration of the disease;
3. a change in both incidence rate and duration.

A decrease in the incidence rate of a disease such as Johne's disease in cattle eventually will decrease the overall prevalence of the disease. Improvements in the therapy of diseases that are frequently fatal may decrease mortality, but could increase prevalence by prolonging the life of diseased animals that otherwise would have died quickly. For example, antibiotic treatment of acute bacterial pneumonia could decrease the fatality of the disease but could increase the number of convalescent animals with chronic pneumonia.

The prevalence of a disease also can be decreased if the duration of the disease is reduced. Improvements in therapy, for instance, may accelerate recovery.

Calculation of incidence rate from prevalence

The exact relationship between prevalence and incidence rate is complex (Kleinbaum et al., 1982), but a simple mathematical relationship can be derived under **steady-state** conditions (i.e., assuming a stable population and a constant incidence rate and prevalence):

$$P/(1 - P) = I \times D$$

When P is small, this simplifies to:

$$P = I \times D$$

and:

$$I = P/D.$$

Therefore, if two components of the equation are known, the third can be calculated. For example, the annual incidence rate of occupationally-acquired leptospirosis in New Zealand dairy farmers has been estimated (Blackmore and Schollum, 1982). Surveys had shown that 34% of farmers had serological reactions to leptospirosis (i.e., the prevalence of seropositive farmers was 0.34). Other work indicated that leptospiral titres of 1/24 or greater persist, on average, for 10 years (i.e., the duration of the infection, expressed as persistence of antibody at that titre, was 10 years). The number of notified cases of human leptospirosis had remained at approximately the same level for more than ten years. Therefore, it could be assumed that a stable endemic level of disease existed in the human population. Thus:

$$P = 0.34,$$
$$D \text{ (years)} = 10.$$

Therefore:

$$I = 0.34/10$$
$$= 0.034 \ (3.4\%) \text{ per year.}$$

This estimated annual incidence rate compares favourably with an annual notification value of 2.1% in dairy farmers in a large dairy region of New Zealand because official notifications are generally an underestimate of the true incidence of a disease. (See Chapter 17 for a further discussion of seroconversion rates.)

Application of prevalence and incidence values

Prevalence and incidence have different applications. Prevalence is useful if interest is focused on existing cases; for example, in identifying disease problems for administrative purposes, for defining research priorities and long-term disease control strategies and in evaluating diagnostic tests (see Chapter 17). Cumulative incidence is used to predict an individual's change in health status because it indicates the probability of an individual becoming ill over a specified period of time. In contrast, an incidence rate cannot be directly interpreted at the individual level, but is appropriate when the speed of development of new cases in a population needs to be known.

Causal studies

Investigations of causal factors ideally require a knowledge of incidence. This is because incidence values directly estimate the risk or rate of developing disease during a specified period of time, and therefore permit the epidemiologist to determine whether the probability of developing disease differs in different populations or time periods in relation to suspected causal factors (Lilienfeld and Lilienfeld, 1980). The choice of the appropriate incidence measure (cumulative incidence versus incidence rate) in causal studies is discussed briefly in Chapter 15 and in detail by Kleinbaum et al. (1982).

When attempting to identify causal associations, disease occurrence in the presence of an hypothesized causal factor is compared with disease occurrence in the absence of the factor. This can be conducted either by:

1. comparing the **absolute** difference between values (e.g., the absolute difference between a cumulative incidence of 0.0010 over 10 years in a group 'exposed' to a factor, and of 0.0001 in an 'unexposed' group, is 0.0009); or
2. comparing the **relative** difference between the two groups (0.0010/0.0001 = 10 in the above example).

A relative measure gives a clear indication of the **magnitude** of the difference, and is often applied in causal studies. This topic is discussed in detail in Chapter 15.

Mortality

Mortality measures are analogous to incidence measures where the relevant outcome is death associated with, rather than new cases of, a specific disease.

Cumulative mortality

Cumulative mortality, CM, can be estimated in a similar way to cumulative incidence, but with the numerator comprising the number of deaths due to a particular disease over a specified period of time, and the denominator comprising the number of individuals at risk of dying during that period. Diseased animals present at the beginning of the period of observation are included in the denominator.

$$CM = \frac{\text{number of individuals that die during a particular period}}{\text{number of individuals in the population at the beginning of that period}}$$

Mortality rate

Mortality rate (**mortality density**), M, is calculated similarly to incidence rate. The numerator comprises the number of deaths. However, since an animal is at risk of dying **after** onset of disease, animals that develop disease continue to be included in the denominator until they die.

$$M = \frac{\text{number of deaths due to a disease that occur in a population during a particular period of time}}{\text{the sum, over all individuals, of the length of time at risk of dying}}$$

Death rate

The **death rate** is the total mortality rate for **all** diseases — rather than one specific disease — in a population. (Some authors do not distinguish between mortality rate and death rate. Thus, a disease-specific death rate may be encountered. Similarly, a crude mortality rate, referring to deaths from all causes, may be described.)

Case fatality

The tendency for a condition to cause the death of **affected** animals in a specified time is the **case fatality**, CF. This is the proportion of diseased animals that die:

$$CF = \frac{\text{number of deaths}}{\text{number of diseased animals}}$$

It measures the probability of death in diseased animals, is dimensionless, and can take values between 0 and 1 (or $0 - 100\%$).

The value of the case fatality depends on the time of observation which can range from a brief period of hospitalization to several years. If the period of observation is long (e.g., in cases of chronic diseases such as cancer), it is more appropriate to quote **survival**.

Survival

Survival, S, is the probability of individuals with a specific disease remaining alive for a specified length of time:

$$S = \frac{N - D}{N},$$

where:

$D =$ the number of deaths observed in a specified period of time,

$N =$ the number of newly diagnosed cases under observation during the same period of time.

Survival is the complement of case fatality. Thus, for a given period of observation, the sum of the case fatality and survival should equal 1 (100%).

During observation, an animal may die, survive, or be 'censored'. An animal is censored when follow-up ends before death or completion of the full period of observation (e.g., if an animal cannot be traced or the study is terminated).

One- or two-year (and in humans, five- or ten-year) survival times are often quoted for cancer cases. These times also provide a useful way of summarizing prognosis with or without treatment.

In domestic animals, survival depends not only on the characteristics of the disease but also on subjective factors, such as humane and economic reasons for euthanasia in pet animals and farm livestock, respectively. The effects of these factors can be removed when

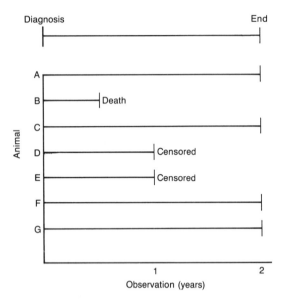

Fig. 4.1 Survival of seven diseased animals (hypothetical data).

evaluating the nett effect of therapeutic procedures by including only animals that died from the disease or that were killed in its terminal stage.

Using the data in *Figure 4.1*, survival for at least one year can be estimated:

$$S = \frac{6}{7}$$

$$= 0.86 \ (86\%).$$

However, two-year survival is more difficult to calculate because of the two censored observations (animals D and E). If these animals survived for at least two years, the two-year survival would again be 6/7 (0.86). However, if these two animals died within two years, the survival would be 4/7 = 0.57. Statistical techniques, termed **survival analyses**, have been devised to deal with such incomplete data. Two common methods are **life table analysis** and **Kaplan–Meier analysis**. A detailed description of these methods is beyond the scope of this book and may be found elsewhere (Lee, 1992).

Table 4.4 lists the one-year survival of cats with mammary carcinoma, after surgical removal of the tumour, estimated by the Kaplan–Meier technique, in relation to some prognostic factors (indicators). The results of survival analyses can also be presented graphically; an example is given in *Figure 4.2*.

Other measures of survival are also used in cancer studies (Misdorp, 1987). Thus, **tumour-free (disease-free)** survival can be estimated; however, this requires careful periodic examination for local recurrence or metastases. The success of local treatment can be expressed in terms of the **percentage recurrence** or **non-recurrence**. Systemic treatment (e.g., chemotherapy) can be assessed by the **percentage of complete or partial remission**.

Example of calculation of prevalence, incidence, mortality, case fatality and survival

Suppose a veterinarian investigates a disease that runs a clinical course ending in either recovery or death, in a herd of cattle. On 1 July 1993 the herd is investigated when the disease is already present. The herd is then observed for the following year, during which period there are no additions and all animals are followed up (i.e., there are no censored observations).

Total herd size on 1 July 1993:	600
Total number clinically ill on 1 July 1993:	20
Total number developing clinical disease between 1 July 1993 and 1 July 1994:	80
Total number dying from the disease from 1 July 1993 to 1 July 1994:	30

Prevalence on 1 July 1993 = 20/600 = 0.03
Cumulative incidence 1 July 1993 – 1 July 1994
   = 80/580 = 0.14
Incidence rate = 80/{(580 + 500)/2}
   = 0.15 per animal-year at risk
Cumulative mortality 1 July 1993 – 1 July 1994
   = 30/600 = 0.05
Mortality rate = 30/{(600 + 570/2)}
   = 0.05 per animal-year at risk
Case fatality 1 July 1993 – 1 July 1994
   = 30/100 = 0.30
Survival 1 July 1993 – 1 July 1994
   = 70/100 = 0.70

(Note that in this calculation approximate incidence and mortality rates are calculated using the average population at risk as the denominator. Calculation of a true incidence and mortality rate would require observation of each animal so that the time of onset of disease, and occurrence of death, respectively, in each could be noted, and the number of animal-months at risk therefore recorded, as in *Table 4.3*.)

Table 4.4 One-year survival of cats with mammary carcinoma according to some prognostic factors. (Based on Weijer and Hart, 1983.)

Prognostic factor	Number of cats	Survival
No tumour +ve lymph nodes	107	0.58
Tumour +ve lymph nodes	43	0.22
Diameter of primary tumour:		
1 cm	27	0.72
2 cm	31	0.41
3−5 cm	98	0.40
≥6 cm	44	0.23

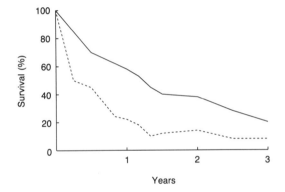

Fig. 4.2 Survival curve of cats with mammary carcinoma in relation to the presence of tumours in lymph nodes at initial diagnosis. The survival of cats was calculated at three-monthly intervals, and the points joined by straight lines. ———— no tumour-positive lymph nodes; ------- tumour-positive lymph nodes. (Redrawn from Weijer and Hart, 1983.)

Ratios, proportions and rates

The preceding parts of this chapter have introduced some descriptive measures of disease occurrence as proportions and rates. These two terms, and a third — ratios — have been widely and sometimes improperly used in veterinary and human medicine, and therefore require further discussion.

A ratio is a value obtained by dividing one quantity by another. For example, a male:female sex ratio might be 3:2, the upper figure being the **numerator** and the lower figure the **denominator**. A proportion is a special case of a ratio in which the numerator consists of some of (i.e., is a subset of) the individuals in the denominator. Thus, prevalence, cumulative incidence, case fatality and survival are proportions. In epidemiology, the term ratio is usually confined to measures where the numerator is **not** drawn from the denominator. For example:

$$\text{foetal death ratio} = \frac{\text{number of foetal deaths}}{\text{number of live births}}$$

A rate is a ratio that expresses a change in one quantity (the numerator) with respect to another quantity (the denominator). 'Time' is usually included in the denominator. Velocity (e.g., 10 m per second) is a rate. True epidemiological rates have time as part of the denominator. Incidence rate is the commonest epidemiological rate.

However, 'rate' has sometimes been suffixed incorrectly to epidemiological ratios in which the numerator is a subset of the denominator (i.e., proportions). Thus, 'prevalence rate', 'cumulative incidence rate', 'case fatality rate' and 'survival rate' are sometimes used as synonyms for prevalence, cumulative incidence, case fatality and survival, respectively, although they are not true rates.

Table 4.5 lists some common epidemiological ratios and rates. In most instances, the rates are proportions, rather than true rates, but the terms are so well-established that they are retained in this table.

Proportions and rates are expressed in three main forms: **crude**, **specific** and **adjusted**.

Crude measures

Crude prevalence, incidence and mortality values are an expression of the amount of disease and deaths in a population as a whole; they take no account of the structure of the population affected. For instance, the crude death rate of two laboratory colonies of mice could be 10/1000/day and 20/1000/day respectively. Initially, this might suggest that the second colony has twice the

Table 4.5 Some commonly used rates and ratios (indices usually refer to a defined population of animals observed for one year).* (Modified and expanded from Schwabe *et al.*, 1977.)

Name	Definition
Rates	
No-return rate at n days:	$\dfrac{\text{No. animals bred that have not come back in heat in } n \text{ days after breeding}}{\text{No. animals bred}} \times 10^{a\dagger}$
Pregnancy rate at n days:	$\dfrac{\text{No. animals pregnant at } n \text{ days after breeding}}{\text{No. animals bred}} \times 10^{a}$
Crude live birth rate:	$\dfrac{\text{No. live births occurring}}{\text{Average population}} \times 10^{a}$
General fertility rate:	$\dfrac{\text{No. live births occurring}}{\text{Average no. female animals of reproductive age}} \times 10^{a}$
Crude death rate:	$\dfrac{\text{No. deaths occurring}}{\text{Average population}} \times 10^{a}$
Age-specific death rate:	$\dfrac{\text{No. deaths among animals in a specified age-group}}{\text{Average no. in the specified age-group}} \times 10^{a}$
Calf (lamb, piglet, puppy, etc.) mortality rate:	$\dfrac{\text{No. deaths under a specified age**}}{\text{No. live births}} \times 10^{a}$
Neonatal (calf, lamb, etc.) mortality rate:	$\dfrac{\text{No. deaths under a specified age**}}{\text{No. live births}} \times 10^{a}$
Foetal death rate (also called stillbirth rate):	$\dfrac{\text{No. foetal deaths}}{\text{No. live births plus foetal deaths}} \times 10^{a}$
Cause-specific death rate:	$\dfrac{\text{No. deaths from a specified cause}}{\text{Average population}} \times 10^{a}$
Proportional morbidity rate:	$\dfrac{\text{No. of animals with a specified disease}}{\text{Total no. of diseased animals}} \times 10^{a}$
Proportional mortality rate:	$\dfrac{\text{No. deaths from a specified cause}}{\text{Total no. deaths}} \times 10^{a}$
Ratios	
Foetal death ratio (also called stillbirth ratio):	$\dfrac{\text{No. foetal deaths}}{\text{No. live births}} \times 10^{a}$
Maternal mortality ratio:	$\dfrac{\text{No. deaths in dams from puerperal causes}}{\text{No. live births}} \times 10^{a}$
Zoonosis incidence ratio (ZIR):	$\dfrac{\text{No. new cases of a zoonotic disease in an animal species in a given geographic area in a stated time period}}{\text{Average human population in the same are during the same period} \times \text{time}} \times 10^{a}$
Area incidence ratio (AIR):	$\dfrac{\text{No. new cases of a disease in a given time period}}{\text{Unit geographic area in which the observations are made} \times \text{time}} \times 10^{a}$

*All rates could use other specified time periods.

**There is not a universal agreement on the age at which animals cease to be neonates in veterinary medicine.

†a = a whole number, usually between 2 and 6; for example, if $a = 3$, then $10^a = 10^3 = 1000$.

disease problem of the first, but this difference in crude rates might be due only to a difference in age structure. Mice have a lifespan of about two years, and so if the second colony consisted of much older animals than the first, greater mortality would be expected in the second than the first colony, even without concurrent disease. Although crude rates may express the prevalence or incidence of a particular disease, they take no account of specific host characteristics, such as age, which can have a profound effect on the occurrence of disease in a population.

Specific measures

Specific measures of disease are those that describe disease occurrence in specific categories of the population related to host attributes such as age, sex, breed and method of husbandry, and, in man, also race, occupation and socio-economic group. They convey more information than crude measures on the pattern of disease. They can indicate categories of animal that are particularly at risk of disease, and can provide evidence of its cause.

Specific measures are calculated in a similar manner to crude ones, except that the numerator and denominator apply to one or more categories of a population with specific host attributes. For instance, a whole series of different age-specific incidence rates could be calculated that would cover the entire lifespan of a particular population.

Age-specific incidence rates of many enteric diseases, such as salmonellosis and colibacillosis, can be higher in young than old animals. Sex-specific incidence rates of diabetes mellitus are higher in females than in males. The breed-specific prevalence of squamous cell carcinoma of the eye in cattle reveals that Herefords have the highest prevalence: although there is a crude prevalence of 93/100 000 for all breeds of cattle, the specific prevalence for Herefords and Hereford crosses is 403/100 000. The prevalence of goitre in budgerigars is higher in pet birds than in breeders' birds (Blackmore, 1963). Similarly, the occupation-specific prevalence values of human Q fever in Australia indicate that meat workers are the group at greatest risk (Scott, 1981).

Table 4.6a illustrates that the crude incidence rate of testicular neoplasia in castrated dogs (12.67 per 1000 dog-years at risk) reveals much less about the period at risk in a dog's life than the age-specific values. Likewise, the rates specific to location (*Table 4.6b*) indicate at which sites the lesion is most likely to occur.

Calculation of age-specific incidence values has given further clues to the cause of BSE (see Chapters 2 and 3).

The mode (most frequent value) of the disease's incubation period is 4–5 years, and very few cases occur in two-year-old animals. A statutory ban on ruminant-derived protein (meat and bone meal), the suspected source of the infection, was introduced in July 1988. Its impact therefore would be detected initially in two-year-old animals two years later. None of the two-year-old animals affected then had been born after the ban (Wilesmith and Ryan, 1992). This finding added credence to the hypothesis that meat and bone meal were the source of the infection.

Adjusted (standardized) measures

Crude values can only be used to make **comparisons** between two different populations if the populations are similar with respect to characteristics that might affect disease occurrence. If the populations are dissimilar with respect to such characteristics, erroneous conclusions might be drawn because these characteristics may act as confounders (see Chapter 3).

For example, *Table 4.7a* presents the results of a survey of the prevalence of leptospiral antibodies (sero-prevalence) in samples of unvaccinated dogs taken in two

Table 4.6 Specific incidence rates of testicular neoplasia in cryptorchid dogs. (From Reif *et al.*, 1979.)

(a) Age-specific rates				
Age (years)	No. of dogs	Dog-years at risk	No. of neoplasms	Age-specific rate/1000 dog-years
≤2	262	411.3	0	0.00
2–3	153	288.8	0	0.00
4–5	93	199.4	0	0.00
6–7	49	103.0	7	67.96
8–9	31	59.2	4	67.57
≥10	21	43.3	3	69.28
Total	609	1 105.0	14	12.67

(b) Rates specific to location				
Location of testicles	No. of dogs	Dog-years at risk	No. of neoplasms	Incidence/1000 dog-years
Bilateral scrotal (controls)	329	680.0	0	0.00
Abdominal-scrotal	210	392.8	5	12.73
Inguinal-scrotal	188	372.2	9	24.18
Bilateral abdominal	54	96.8	0	0.00
Bilateral inguinal	27	52.5	0	0.00
Inguinal-abdominal	16	30.5	0	0.00
Cryptorchid unknown	114	160.2	0	0.00

Table 4.7 Numbers and proportions (seroprevalence) of urban dogs with microscopic agglutination test antibody titres ≥ 1:10 to leptospires, Edinburgh and Glasgow, 1986−88. (Based on van den Broek *et al.*, 1991.)

| | (a) Crude seroprevalence | | |
	No. of dogs with positive titres	No. of dogs sampled	Seroprevalence
Edinburgh	61	260	0.24
Glasgow	69	251	0.27
Total	130	511	

| | (b) Sex-specific seroprevalence | | | | | | | |
| | No. of dogs with positive titres | | | No. of dogs sampled | | | Seroprevalence | |
	Male	Female	Total	Male	Female	Total	Male	Female
Edinburgh	15	46	61	48	212	260	0.31	0.22
Glasgow	53	16	69	180	71	251	0.29	0.23
Total	68	60	130	228	283	511		

cities, Glasgow and Edinburgh. The crude seroprevalence in Glasgow is 3% higher than in Edinburgh (0.27 compared with 0.24). Assuming that the rate of antibody decline (i.e., the duration of seropositivity) is constant, this might suggest that the incidence of leptospiral infection is greater in Glasgow than in Edinburgh (reasons might include a larger population of infected feral animals in the former than the latter city).

However, factors other than location might also affect seroprevalence. Male dogs, for instance, may run a higher risk of infection because of sexual behaviour, particularly the licking of the vulva of females (Dunbar, 1979) which is likely to bring them into contact with infected urine. Other studies have already shown that leptospiral seroprevalence is higher in male dogs than in bitches (Stuart, 1946; Cunningham *et al.*, 1957; Arimitsu *et al.*, 1989).

The confounding effect of sex can be removed by **adjustment** (**standardization**) by direct and indirect methods. This involves adjusting the crude values to reflect the values that would be expected if the potentially confounding characteristics were similarly distributed in the two study populations.

Direct adjustment: In direct adjustment, the specific values in each population are required. The sex-specific seroprevalence values for the data in *Table 4.7a* are listed in *Table 4.7b*. Note that the seroprevalence in males is higher than that in females. Note, too, that the crude values are the **weighted** average of the specific values,

with the number of males and females used as the weights:

Edinburgh:

$$\text{Crude seroprevalence} = \frac{(0.31 \times 48) + (0.22 \times 212)}{(48 + 212)}$$

$$= 0.24.$$

Glasgow:

$$\text{Crude seroprevalence} = \frac{(0.29 \times 180) + (0.23 \times 71)}{(180 + 71)}$$

$$= 0.27.$$

To adjust these values directly, a **standard** population is selected, in which the frequency of the characteric (sex, in this example) is known. Its choice is somewhat arbitrary, but it should be realistic and relevant. Thus, it may be a large population obtained from published demographic data, one of the two groups being compared, or the totals of the two groups. In this example, the totals of the two groups are used, that is, 228 males and 283 females.

The specific values in each group are now weighted by the frequency of the characteristic in the standard population:

$$\text{direct adjusted value} = sr_1 \times \frac{S_1}{N} + sr_2 \times \frac{S_2}{N}$$

where:

sr = specific value in study population,
S = frequency of characteristic in the standard population,
N = total number in the standard population ($S_1 + S_2 = N$).

For Edinburgh:

sr_1 (male)   = 0.31
S_1 = 228
sr_2 (female)   = 0.22
S_2 = 283
N = 511
Adjusted value = $\{0.31 \times (228/511)\}$ +
$\{0.22 \times (283/511)\}$
 = 0.138 + 0.122
 = 0.26.

For Glasgow:

sr_1 (male)   = 0.29
S_1 = 228
sr_2 (female)   = 0.23
S_2 = 283
N = 511

Adjusted value = $\{0.29 \times (228/511)\}$ +
$\{0.23 \times (283/511)\}$
 = 0.129 + 0.127
 = 0.26.

The adjusted values are similar. This suggests that sex is the factor responsible for the difference in seroprevalence between Edinburgh and Glasgow. If other characteristics (e.g., location or age) were responsible for the difference, the sex-adjusted values would be different.

In veterinary medicine, direct adjustment is indicated for age, sex, breed and other factors which may be confounders. However, the specific data are the 'facts'; the combination of specific values into a weighted average is merely a useful way of combining the values into a single index for the purpose of comparison of groups.

Indirect adjustment: If specific values for one or both populations are not available, or the numbers with each characteristic are so small that large fluctuations in morbidity or mortality occur through the presence or absence of a few cases, the indirect method of adjustment can be used.

In indirect adjustment, only crude values are required for the two study populations, but the frequencies of the adjusting characteristic in these populations must be known. Additionally, specific values are required for the

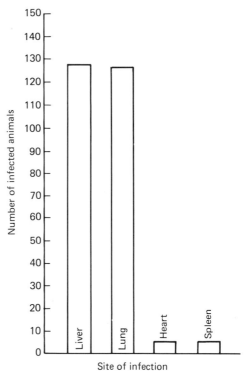

Fig. 4.3 The distribution of hydatid cysts in organs of 765 Somalian cattle in Kuwait: an example of a bar chart. (Modified from Behbehani and Hassounah, 1976.)

standard population. First, calculate the overall value *expected* in each population if the standard population's specific values applied:

$$\text{expected value} = Sr_1 \times \frac{s_1}{n} + Sr_2 \times \frac{s_2}{n}$$

where:

Sr = specific value in standard population
s = frequency of characteristic in the study population
n = total number in the study population ($s_1 + s_2 = n$).

In each population being compared, the ratio of the *observed* crude value to the *expected* value is termed the **standardized morbidity ratio** (or **standardized mortality ratio, SMR**, when mortality is being indirectly adjusted). These standardized ratios provide *relative* comparisons between two populations. They are multiplied by the crude value in the standard population to give the indirectly adjusted values for each population.

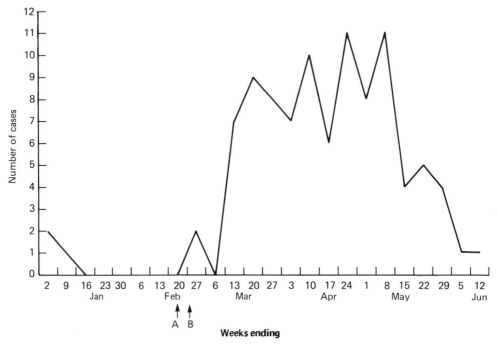

Fig. 4.4 An anthrax outbreak in cattle in England, 1 January – 12 June 1977, associated with a batch of feedstuff: an example of a time trend graph. A = feedstuff unloaded at docks; B = feedstuff arrived at mills. (Modified from MAFF, 1977.)

Age-adjusted SMRs, expressed as percentages, are commonly used in human medicine to relate mortality in particular occupations to the mortality experience of the general population (HMSO, 1958). The adjustment is made in five-year blocks for adults between 20 and 64 years of age.

The advantages, disadvantages and pitfalls associated with adjustment are discussed in detail by Fleiss (1981) and Kahn and Sempos (1989).

Displaying morbidity and mortality values and demographic data

Morbidity and mortality values and demographic data should be recorded in a way that immediately conveys their salient features such as fluctuations in values. The methods of presentation include **tables**, **bar charts** and **time trend graphs**.

Tables

Tabulation is one of the commoner techniques of displaying numerical data. It involves listing numerical values in rows and columns. An example is *Table 4.1*.

Bar charts

Bar charts display variables by vertical bars that have heights proportional to the number of occurrences of the variable (*Figure 4.3*). The bar chart is used to display categories in which counts are **discrete**, that is, they comprise whole numbers, such as numbers of cases of disease. (The frequency distribution of **continuous** data — defined in Chapter 9 — can be displayed in a similar fashion, in which case adjacent bars touch, and the chart is called a **histogram**; an example is given in *Figure 12.1*.) The bar chart strikingly demonstrates differences that would not be noted as easily in tables.

Time trend graphs

In a time trend graph the vertical position of each point represents the number of cases; the horizontal position corresponds to the midpoint of the time interval in which the cases were recorded. In *Figure 4.4*, for instance, the vertical coordinate of each point is the number of new cases of anthrax and the horizontal coordinate is the midpoint of the weekly intervals for which cases of anthrax were reported. The plotting of epidemics in this way produces **epidemic curves** (see Chapter 8).

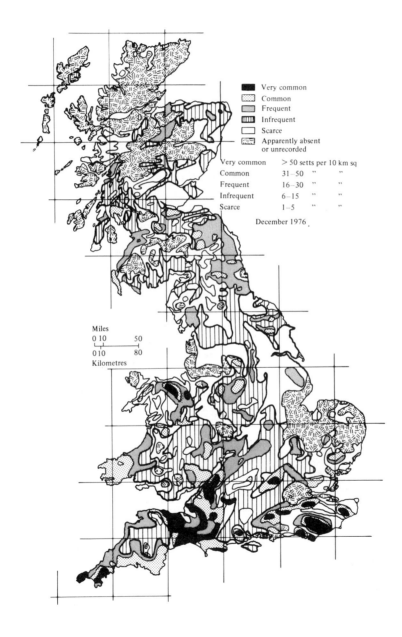

Fig. 4.5 Density of badger setts in Great Britain: an example of an isoplethic map (geographic base). (From Zuckerman, 1980.)

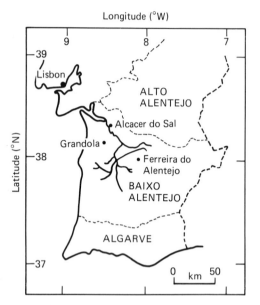

Fig. 4.6 Outbreaks of bluetongue in Portugal, July 1956: an example of a point map. (From Sellers *et al.*, 1978.)

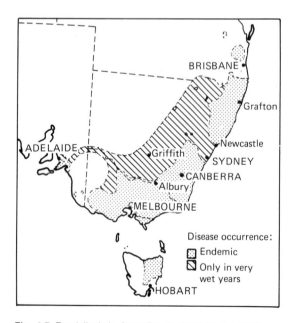

Fig. 4.7 Fascioliasis in Australia: an example of a distribution map. (Modified from Barger *et al.*, 1978.)

Mapping

A common method of displaying the geographical (spatial) distribution of disease and related factors is by drawing maps (cartography). This is of value not only in the recording of areas where diseases exist but also in investigating the mode and direction of transmission of infectious diseases. For example, the spatial distribution of cases of foot-and-mouth disease during the British outbreak in 1967 suggested that the infection may have been disseminated by wind (Smith and Hugh-Jones, 1969). Subsequent investigations have supported this idea (Hugh-Jones and Wright, 1970; Sellers and Gloster, 1980).

Maps can also suggest possible causes of diseases of unknown aetiology. Mapping indicated that tumours (notably of the jaw) in sheep in Yorkshire clustered in areas where bracken was common (McCrea and Head, 1978). This led to the hypothesis that bracken causes tumours. Subsequently, the hypothesis was supported by experimental investigation (McCrea and Head, 1981). Similarly, comparison of the maps of hypocupraemia in cattle (Leech *et al.*, 1982) with a geochemical atlas (Webb *et al.*, 1978) has indicated areas in England and Wales where bovine copper deficiency may be caused by excess dietary molybdenum.

At their simplest, maps may be qualitative, indicating location without specifying the amount of disease. They can also be quantitative, displaying the number of cases of disease (the numerator in proportions, rates and ratios), the population at risk (the denominator), and prevalence and incidence (i.e., including both numerator and denominator).

Map bases

Maps can be constructed according to the shape of a country or region, in which case they are drawn to a **geographic base**. Alternatively, they can be drawn to represent the size of the population concerned, that is, to a **demographic (isodemographic) base** (Forster, 1966), in which morbidity and mortality information is presented in relation to population size. Demographic maps require accurate information on both the numerators and denominators in morbidity and mortality values and are not common in veterinary medicine because this information is often missing.

Geographic base maps

Figure 4.5 is an example of a geographic base map. It is a 'conventional' map of Great Britain, showing the shape of

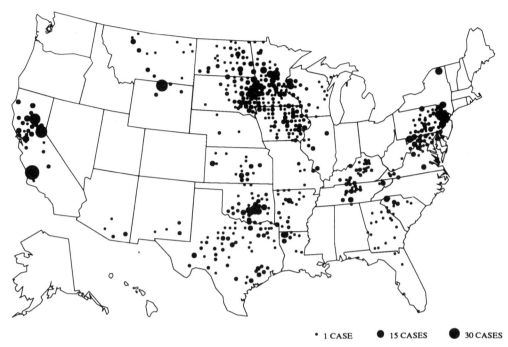

Fig. 4.8 Reported cases of rabies in skunks in the US, by county, 1990: an example of a proportional circle map. The area of each circle is proportional to the number of cases in each county. (From Uhaa *et al.*, 1992.)

the country. Most atlases consist of geographic base maps. There are several types of geographic base map, each with a different purpose, and displaying information in varying detail.

Point (dot or location) maps

These maps illustrate outbreaks of disease in discrete locations, by circles, squares, dots or other symbols. An example is *Figure 4.6*, where the solid circles with adjacent names indicate the sites of outbreaks of bluetongue in Portugal. Point maps are qualitative; they do not indicate the extent of the outbreaks which could each involve any number of animals. Point maps can be refined by using arrows to indicate direction of spread of disease. A series of point maps, displaying occurrence at different times, can indicate the direction of spread of an outbreak of disease.

Distribution maps

A distribution map is constructed to show the area over which disease occurs. An example is given in *Figure 4.7*, illustrating areas in south-east Australia in which fascioliasis is continually present (endemic areas) and those that only experience the disease in wet years. Further

examples, showing the world distribution of the major animal virus diseases, are presented by Odend'hal (1983).

Proportional circle maps

Morbidity and mortality can be depicted using circles whose area is proportional to the amount of disease or deaths (*Figure 4.8*). If the large values are substantially greater than the small values, the values can be represented by proportional spheres whose volume is proportional to the magnitude of the depicted characteristic. (Shading is used to give the impression of spheres on a two-dimensional map.)

Choroplethic maps

It is also possible to display quantitative information as discrete shaded units of area, graded in intensity to represent the variability of the mapped data. The units can be formed from grid lines, but are commonly administrative areas such as parishes, shires, counties or states. Maps that portray information in this way are **choroplethic** (Greek: *choros* = an area, a region; *plethos* = a

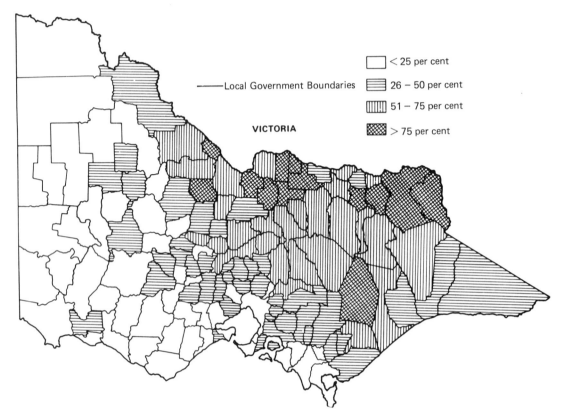

Fig. 4.9 Prevalence of fluke-affected livers by shire, Victoria, Australia, 1977 – 78: an example of a choroplethic map. (From Watt, 1980.)

throng, a crowd, the population). *Figure 4.9* is an example.

Choroplethic maps display quantitative data, but the boundaries between different recorded values are artificial. They are not the actual boundaries between, for example, high and low prevalence; they are merely the administrative boundaries of the areas over which the displayed values are averaged.

Isoplethic maps

True boundaries between different values can be depicted by joining all points of equal value by a line, such as joining points of equal height to produce the familiar contour map. Maps produced this way are **isoplethic** (Greek: *iso* = equal). Lines joining points of equal morbidity are **isomorbs**, and those joining points of equal mortality are **isomorts**. If these lines are to be constructed, accurate estimates of both the number of cases of

disease (numerator) and the size of the population at risk (denominator) over an area must be known.

Figure 4.5 is an isoplethic map showing badger density in Great Britain, also drawn in relation to bovine tuberculosis. In this example, the 'contours' are the boundaries between different ranges of badger density.

Medical mapping is discussed in detail by Cliff and Haggett (1988).

Geographical information systems

Disease distribution can be mapped and analysed using **geographical information systems** (GIS) (Maguire, 1991). These are computerized systems for collecting, storing, managing, interrogating and displaying spatial data. They have a range of powerful functions in addition

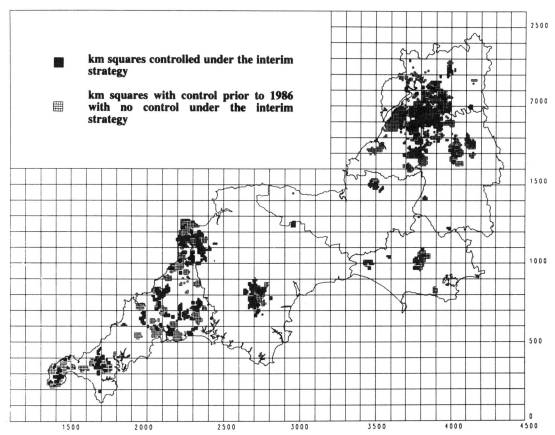

km squares controlled under the interim strategy

km squares with control prior to 1986 with no control under the interim strategy

Fig. 4.10 Areas of statutory badger control in south-west England: an example of a grid-based map generated by a geographical information system. Badgers are reservoirs of infection with *Mycobacterium tuberculosis* in this region. Statutory badger removal to control bovine tuberculosis started in 1975 and was based on areas delineated by physical barriers such as roads, so that the instigating herd of cattle and nearby herds were included. This strategy was costly and, in 1986, was replaced by an 'interim' strategy in which badgers were removed only from land used by infected herds in which infection had been unequivocally associated with badgers. Further analysis with the GIS identified areas where pre-emptive badger control could be applied. (From Clifton-Hadley, 1993.)

to simple mapping; these include graphical analysis based on spatial location, statistical analysis, and modelling.

Structure of GIS

Data that are input may be **cartographic data**, describing the location of features; and textual **attribute data**, describing characteristics of the features. These types of data may be **primary** or **secondary**. Primary data may be **directly sensed** from field sketching, interviews and measurements. Alternatively, they may be **remotely sensed**, that is, collected by a device not in direct contact with the object that is being sensed (e.g., a photographic camera). Meteorological satellites have also been used to

detect habitats of ticks, mosquitoes, trematodes (Hugh-Jones, 1989) and tsetse flies (Rogers, 1991).

The GIS then store these **geographically referenced data** in a database management system (see Chapter 11) in a form that can be graphically queried and summarized.

Cartographic data must be stored in **digital form** on computers (see Chapter 11). The digital maps are stored in two basic formats: **grid-based (raster-based)** and **vector-based**. In grid-based systems, information is stored uniformly in relation to each cell that forms the grid (*Figure 4.10*). In vector-based systems, points and lines (arcs) are used to represent geographical features, the lines being composed of their respective straight-line

Table 4.8 Some applications of geographical information systems and remote sensing in veterinary and related fields.

Area of application	Country/continent	Source
Aujeszky's disease	US	Marsh et al. (1991)
Bovine tuberculosis	Ireland New Zealand UK	Hammond and Lynch (1992) Sanson et al. (1991a) Clifton-Hadley (1993)
Dracunculiasis	West Africa	Clarke et al. (1991)
Foot-and-mouth disease control	Brazil New Zealand	Arámbulo and Astudillo (1991) Sanson et al. (1991b)
Gastric cancer	UK	Matthews (1989)
Habitat of the snail *Fossaria bulimoides* (intermediate host of *Fasciola hepatica*)	US	Zukowski et al. (1991)
Handling epidemiological data	US	Campbell (1989)
Mosquito population dynamics	US	Wood et al. (1991)
Site selection for fish farming	Ghana	Kapetsky et al. (1991)
Theileriosis	Africa	Lessard et al. (1988, 1990)
Tick habitats *Amblyomma variegatum* Lyme disease tick distribution *Rhipicephalus appendiculatus*	St Lucia Guadeloupe US Czechoslovakia Africa	Hugh-Jones (1991c) Hugh-Jones and O'Neil (1988) Hugh-Jones et al. (1992) Kitron et al. (1991) Daniel and Kolár (1990) Lessard et al. (1990) Perry et al. (1990)

segments. Areas enclosed by lines (e.g., farms) are termed polygons. A **digitizing tablet** is used to convert maps to a digital format for vector-based storage. This is an electronic board and pointer that accurately transcribes a map to digital format. A **scanner** is used for raster-based storage.

Grid-based systems store and manipulate regional and remotely sensed data conveniently, but data-processing is relatively slow if high resolution is required. In contrast, vector-based systems have inherently high resolution but are complex to implement. Many current systems can analyse both vector and raster data.

Applications of GIS

Applications of GIS (Sanson et al., 1991b) include:

1. **cartography**, with the advantage over traditional techniques that thematic maps can be produced and updated rapidly;

2. **neighbourhood analysis**, which allows an investigator to list all features that meet specified criteria (e.g., identification of livestock units adjacent to an infected farm);

3. **buffer generation** around or along certain features (e.g., definition of all properties at risk of infection within a given distance of an infected farm, or along a road that has been used by infected animals);

4. **overlay analysis** in which two or more data sets are superimposed on top of one another and areas of intersection (overlay) of features identified (e.g., overlaying land-form, vegetation and watering-point locations to identify areas where animals are difficult to muster for tuberculin testing: Laut, 1986);

5. **network analysis** permitting optimal routing along networks of linear features;

6. **three-dimensional surface modelling** (e.g., construction of isoplethic maps with height proportional to

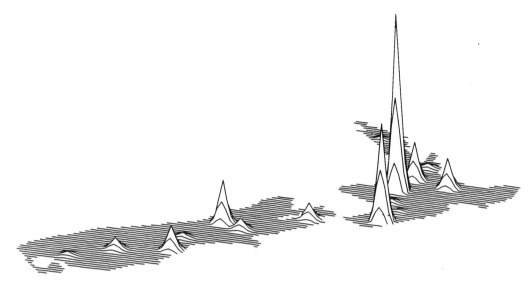

Fig. 4.11 Spatial distribution of the number of tuberculin test reactors in cattle in New Zealand, 1988–89: an example of an isoplethic map generated by a geographical information system. The heights of the peaks represent numbers of tuberculin test reactors; the bases represent geographical areas of the country. (From *OIE Scientific and Technical Review*, **10**(1), March 1991.)

disease incidence or other characteristics: *Figure 4.11*).

The ability of GIS to link graphic and non-graphic data facilitates powerful analysis of the spatial distribution of disease and related factors. These systems are being increasingly applied to animal disease control as integral parts of veterinary decision support systems (see Chapter 11). Some GIS applications are listed in *Table 4.8*, and the value of GIS and remote sensing are discussed by Hugh-Jones (1991a, b).

Further reading

Dawson-Saunders, B. and Trapp, R.G. (1990) *Basic and Clinical Biostatistics*. Appleton and Lange, East Norwalk

Hugh-Jones, M. (Ed.) (1991) Applications of remote sensing to epidemiology and parasitology. *Preventive Veterinary Medicine*, **11**, 159–366. (*A collection of papers on remote sensing and geographical information systems*)

Last, J.M. (1988) *A Dictionary of Epidemiology*, 2nd edn. Oxford University Press, New York

Roht, L.H., Selwyn, B.J., Holguin, A.H. and Christensen, B. (1982) *Principles of Epidemiology. A Self-teaching Guide*. Academic Press, New York

5 Determinants of disease

Chapter 3 introduced the concept that disease is caused by multiple factors. The factors are **determinants** of disease. A determinant is any characteristic that affects the health of a population. Diet, for example, is a determinant of bovine hypomagnesaemia: reduced food intake and low levels of plant magnesium, related to rapid grass growth, are associated with an increased incidence of the disease (*Figure 3.6*). A knowledge of determinants facilitates identification of categories of animal that are at particular risk of developing disease. It therefore is a prerequisite for disease prevention and is an aid to differential diagnosis. This chapter discusses the types of determinant and the interactions that occur between them.

Classification of determinants

Determinants can be classified in three ways, as:

1. **primary** and **secondary**;
2. **intrinsic** and **extrinsic**;
3. associated with **host**, **agent** or **environment**.

Primary and secondary determinants

Primary determinants are factors whose variations exert a major effect in inducing disease. Frequently, primary determinants are necessary causes (see Chapter 3). Thus, exposure to distemper virus is a primary determinant of canine distemper.

Secondary determinants correspond to predisposing, enabling and reinforcing factors. For example, sex is a secondary determinant of canine heart valve incompetence: male dogs are more likely to develop incompetence than females (Buchanan, 1977; Thrusfield *et al.*, 1985). The primary determinants may include other genetically determined factors such as the rate of ageing of the valves, which may be associated with breed. Primary and secondary determinants are listed in *Table 5.1*.

Intrinsic and extrinsic determinants

Table 5.1 also illustrates that some determinants (both primary and secondary) are internal to the host; for example, genetic constitution, including aberrant genes (which are the primary causes of genetic disorders), species, breed and sex. These determinants are **intrinsic**, also termed **endogenous** (Greek: *endon* = 'within'). In contrast, some determinants are external to the host; for instance, transportation, which may result in physical trauma, producing bruising of carcasses (Meischke *et al.*, 1974). Such determinants are **extrinsic**, also termed **exogenous** (Greek: *exo* = outside). *Table 5.2* exemplifies this scheme of classification in relation to canine pruritus (tendency to itch), a common problem in small animal practice. Internal disease, such as hepatitis and nephritis, may act as an intrinsic predisposing factor by increasing the sensitivity of the skin (Kral, 1966). Mastocytomas contain an excess of histamine and proteolytic enzymes which induce itching. Conditions that are not usually associated with pruritus, such as hypothyroidism, may become pruritic when bacterial infections are superimposed. Dietary factors, such as a high potassium:calcium ratio, also increase skin sensitivity.

Determinants associated with host, agent and environment

Many diseases include infectious agents in their sufficient causes. Most infectious agents enter the host as challenges from the environment (see *Figure 1.3*), and, when foetal infection occurs, the dam can be the 'environment' too. However, during the microbial revolution, the early emphasis on microbes as the primary causes of disease resulted in their being considered separately from other environmental factors such as husbandry, trauma and toxic agents. Thus, determinants commonly are classified into those associated with the **host**, the **agent** and the

Table 5.1 Primary and secondary determinants.

PRIMARY DETERMINANTS

Intrinsic determinants	*Extrinsic determinants*				
	Animate		*Inanimate*		
	Endoparasitic	*Ectoparasitic*	*Physical*	*Chemical*	*Allergic*
Genetic constitution	Viruses	Arthropods	Trauma	Excess	Allergens
Metabolism	Bacteria		Climate	Deficiency	
Behaviour	Fungi		Radiation	Imbalance	
	Protozoa		Stressors	Poisons	
	Metazoa			Photosensitizers	

SECONDARY DETERMINANTS

Intrinsic determinants	*Extrinsic determinants*
Genetic constitution (including sex, species and breed)	Location
	Climate
Age	Husbandry (housing, diet, general management, animal use)
Size and conformation	Trauma
Hormonal status	Concurrent disease
Nutritional status	Vaccination status
Immunological status	Stressors
Functional status (e.g. pregnant, lactating)	
Behaviour	

environment. These three groups of factors are sometimes called the **triad** (*Figure 5.1*). Some authors (e.g., Schwabe, 1984) consider that management and husbandry are important enough in intensive animal enterprises to be classified separately from the environment, as a fourth major group.

In some diseases, an infectious agent is the main determinant, and host and environmental factors are of relatively minor importance. Such diseases are 'simple'; examples are major animal plagues such as foot-and-mouth disease and rinderpest occurring in susceptible populations. A multifactorial nature is not obvious. In other diseases, termed 'complex', their multifactorial nature predominates and a clear **interaction** between

host, agent and environment can be identified. Thus, 'environmental' mastitis involves an interaction between *Escherichia coli* or *Streptococcus uberis* (the agent), milking machine faults, and poor hygiene resulting from inadequate bedding, drainage and cleaning of passageways (the environment) (Francis *et al.*, 1979). In addition, cows (the hosts) are most susceptible in early lactation.

The complexity of a multifactorial disease depends upon how the disease is defined. Most 'diseases' with which the veterinarian is initially concerned are actually clinical signs presented by animals' owners. Thus, pruritus in a dog is a clinical sign which can be caused by several different lesions each with their own sufficient causes. Further examples of signs and lesions with

Table 5.2 Some determinants of canine pruritus. (Modified from Thoday, 1980.)

Intrinsic determinants		*Extrinsic determinants*				
Internal disease	*Temperament*	*Trauma*	*Chemicals*	*Diet*	*Parasites*	*Bacteria*
Renal disease	Lick granuloma	Abrasion	Relative	Fat deficiency	Fleas	Causing:
Hepatic disease		Aural and	primary	Carbohydrate	Lice	Juvenile impetigo
Diabetes mellitus		nasal	irritants	excess	Mites:	Anal sacculitis
Maldigestion or		foreign		High potassium:	*Otodectes* spp.	Impetigo
malabsorption		bodies		calcium ratio	*Sarcoptes* spp.	Short-haired dog
Tumours					*Trombicula* spp.	folliculitis
					Demodex	Acute moist
					(pustular)	dermatitis

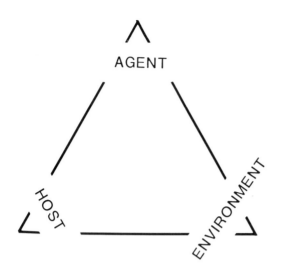

Fig. 5.1 The 'triad': three main headings under which determinants can be classified.

different causes are given in *Figures 9.3b* and *9.3c*. The causal web can become very complex when the 'disease' is defined in terms of a production shortfall in a herd or flock. Thus, 'reproductive failure' in a pig herd, reflected in unacceptably low numbers of piglets being born in a herd in a defined period of time, can be produced by decreased male or female fertility, or infection or metabolic derangement of the sow or foetus during pregnancy. *Figure 5.2* divides the causes of reproductive failure in pigs into six main areas relating to genetic constitution, nutrition, infections, toxic agents, environment and management. It therefore represents a subdivision of agent, host and environmental determinants. These six areas are discussed in detail by Wrathall (1975).

Genetic factors include genetic defects affecting the parents (e.g., abnormal genitalia or gametes) and the offspring (e.g., malformations and inherited predisposition to disease).

Failure to supply nutritional requirements for specific micronutrients (vitamins, minor minerals and trace elements) can result in reduced litter sizes, embryonic death and delayed puberty. The plane of nutrition can also affect performance. Restriction of diet can delay puberty. In contrast, 'flushing' (increasing the amount fed) a few days before ovulation is due can increase the number of ova released in gilts.

Infections are classified into three groups:

1. opportunistic pathogens;
2. common viruses;

3. specific infectious diseases.

Group 1 pathogens are ubiquitous and frequently endogenous. They cause disease sporadically when host resistance is lowered. Examples include *Staphylococcus* and *Listeria* spp. — infections causing prenatal deaths and abortions. Notable in group 2 are the porcine parvoviruses, also termed SMEDI viruses, an acronym for stillbirth, mummification, embryonic death and infertility, which effects they produce. Group 3 infections include brucellosis, leptospirosis, toxoplasmosis and swine fever — infections caused by exogenous pathogens, which can produce low conception rates and induce abortion.

Toxic substances include those ingested in the food (e.g., mycotoxins which can induce vulvovaginitis and abnormal oestrus), and environmental pollutants such as wood preservatives which can cause abortion.

The environment affects reproduction through its climatic, social and structural components. High environmental temperatures, for example, can induce infertility in males.

Important management factors include herd age (young females may have a low ovulation rate and therefore small litter size), the boar:sow ratio, boar management, efficiency of heat detection and pregnancy diagnosis, breeding policy and record keeping.

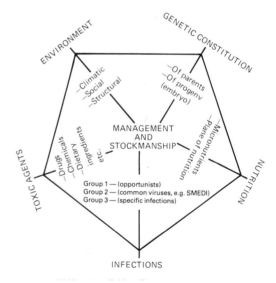

Fig. 5.2 Diagrammatic representation of causes of reproductive failure in a pig herd. (Modified from Pritchard *et al.*, 1985.)

The three schemes of determinant classification are not mutually exclusive. They are just three different ways of viewing the multifactorial nature of disease. Determinants are described below using the third system of classification: into those associated with host, agent or environment. This system is also followed by Schwabe *et al.* (1977), Martin *et al.* (1987) and Smith (1991) in their discussion of determinants of animal diseases, and by Reif (1983) in his consideration of determinants of diseases of dogs and cats.

Host determinants

Genotype

The genetic constitution of a host is its **genotype**. Some diseases appear to have an almost totally genetic cause, that is, alterations in gene structure are considered to have a marked effect on their pathogenesis, and they may be inherited by succeeding generations; an example is haemophilia A and B in dogs. Such diseases, in which aberrant genes are primary determinants, are traditionally termed **genetic diseases**. Other diseases, such as the simple infectious diseases, appear to have little or no genetic component. Many diseases, however, occupy positions intermediate to these two extremes; examples are bovine foot lameness (Peterse and Antonisse, 1981) and mastitis (Wilton *et al.*, 1972).

Genetic diseases generally belong to one of three categories (Nicholas, 1987):

1. chromosomal disorders;
2. Mendelian (simply inherited) disorders;
3. multifactorial disorders.

The first two categories represent diseases that are almost totally genetic. The third category represents diseases that have a variable, complex genetic component. Such diseases have been reported to occur more commonly than those belonging to the first two categories and their mode of inheritance will therefore be discussed in more detail.

Multifactorial inheritance

Many of the simply inherited disorders are qualitative, 'all-or-none' characteristics. In contrast, other characteristics, such as muscle mass and the severity of some diseases (e.g., hip dysplasia), are quantitative, displaying continuous variation. The genetic component of this variation is explained by the cumulative (usually additive) effects of many genes at several sites (loci) on the

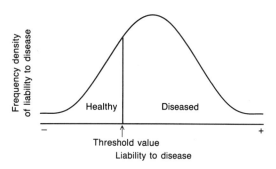

Fig. 5.3 Genetic model for manifestation of a multifactorial disease. The disease occurs when the number and combination of genes, in association with environmental factors, exceeds a threshold value.

chromosomes. This is **polygenic** inheritance. The polygenic component additionally interacts with environmental factors; thus there is a **multifactorial** cause to such traits. For example, canine hip dysplasia requires both a genetic weakness of the muscles supporting the hip joint, and conditions in early life that favour separation of the joint, resulting in the osseous changes that characterize the disease. These changes can be prevented by confining to cages pups that have genetically weak muscles, with their hindlimbs flexed and abducted. There is clearly a non-genetic component relating to management early in life. The relative (but not exclusive) occurrence of hip dysplasia in different giant breeds, between which there is no genetic movement, supports the hypothesis that large, poorly muscled breeds (whose conformation is genetically determined) are particularly at risk. Furthermore, litter mates can be affected to different degrees, suggesting a polygenic cause.

Some disorders, such as congenital heart defects, do not show continuous variation, but liability to the condition nevertheless can be interpreted as having a polygenic component. An individual can inherit the 'right' number and combination of genes, and be exposed to environmental determinants, to pass beyond a **threshold value**, beyond which the disease occurs (Falconer, 1989). *Figure 5.3* illustrates this concept. The horizontal axis is the 'liability to disease', with '+' indicating the presence of many, and '−' of few, of the right genes and environmental factors. The vertical axis is the relative frequency of values of liability to disease in the population. The congenital heart defect, patent ductus arteriosus, for example, is inherited multifactorially, and is discussed in more detail in Chapter 18 in the context of comparative epidemiology.

The likelihood of a relative inheriting the right combination of causal genes becomes less as a relationship becomes more distant. The likelihood of the right number and combination of genes being inherited also decreases as the number of genes required for manifestation of the disorder increases.

Initially, simple and polygenic modes of inheritance appeared to be mutually exclusive. However, it is now clear that the additive effects of many genes, inherited in a Mendelian manner, can be applied to the polygenic model for continuous traits. Conversely, a single-gene model can be applied to quantitative traits by converting the trait to a dichotomy, with an animal characterized as to whether its trait value is above or below a threshold value. Moreover, liability to disease can be applied to simple, single-gene traits where environmental factors have an effect (e.g., human phenylketonuria).

Although it is currently believed that many common diseases have a genetic component, it is unclear whether this amounts to a multifactorial (polygenic) predisposition or to the involvement of a single major chromosomal locus interacting with environmental factors. It is also difficult to infer a genetic component to the cause of a disease in the absence of data relating to genetically distinct groups (breeds, families, and sire and dam lines).

Foley *et al.* (1979) describe heritable diseases of companion animals and livestock in detail.

Age

The occurrence of many diseases shows a distinct association with age. Many bacterial and virus diseases, for instance, are more likely to occur, and to be fatal, in young than in old animals, either because of an absence of acquired immunity or because of a low non-immunological host resistance. Many protozoan and rickettsial infections, in contrast, induce milder responses in the young than in the old.

The absolute number of cases of a disease clearly is not an indication of the impact of disease in a particular age range because the ranges are present in different proportions in the total population. This is illustrated in *Figure 5.4* which depicts **population pyramids** for dogs and cats. These show the age distribution of animals (male and female indicated separately). Thus, age-specific rates (see Chapter 4) provide the most valuable information about disease in particular age groups, because they relate morbidity and mortality to a uniform size of population at risk. *Figure 5.5* displays age-specific rates for canine neoplasia and shows that tumours are more common in old than in young animals. (There are some notable

exceptions, such as canine osteosarcoma and lymphosarcoma, which show peak incidences between 7 and 10 years of age: Reif, 1983.)

Sex

Sexual differences in disease occurrence may be attributed to hormonal, occupational, social and ethological, and genetic determinants.

Hormonal determinants

The effects of sex hormones may predispose animals to disease. Bitches are more likely to develop diabetes mellitus than dogs (Marmor *et al.*, 1982) and signs often develop after oestrus, possibly related to the increased insulin requirements of diabetic bitches during oestrus. Similarly, the neutering of bitches decreases the likelihood of mammary carcinoma developing (Schneider *et al.*, 1969), perhaps from the effect of oestrogens on this tumour (see Chapter 18).

Occupational determinants

Sex-associated occupational hazards, although more relevant to human than animal disease, can be identified occasionally in animals, where animal use is equated with occupation. Thus, the increased risk of contracting heartworm infection by male dogs relative to bitches (Selby *et al.*, 1980) may result from increased 'occupational' exposure of male dogs during hunting to the mosquito that transmits the infection.

Social and ethological determinants

Behavioural patterns may account for bite wound abscesses being more common in male than in female cats. Behaviour can also affect the likelihood of transmission of infection from one species to another. Thus, in New Zealand, opossums stand their ground when confronted by cattle, thereby increasing the chance of aerosol transmission (see Chapter 6) of tuberculosis from infected opossums to cattle by inhalation. In contrast, in the UK, badgers' immediate response to threatening behaviour is to retreat, and so aerosol transmission of tuberculosis from infected badgers is less likely (Benham and Broom, 1989).

Genetic determinants

Genetic differences in disease incidence may be inherited either by being **sex-linked**, **sex-limited** or **sex-influenced**. Sex-linked inheritance is commonly associated with Mendelian inheritance, and occurs when the DNA responsible for a disease is carried on either the X

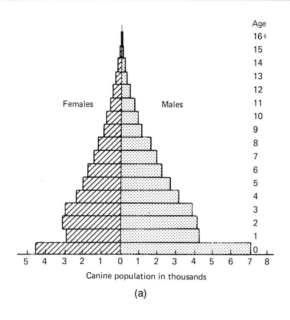

(a)

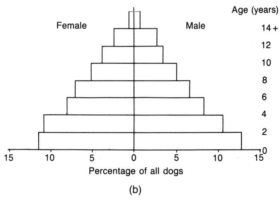

(b)

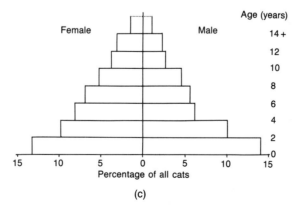

(c)

Fig. 5.4 Canine and feline population pyramids. (a) Canine: New Jersey, USA, 1957; (b) canine: UK, 1986; (c) feline: UK, 1986. ((a) From Cohen *et al.*, 1959; (b) and (c) from Thrusfield, 1989.)

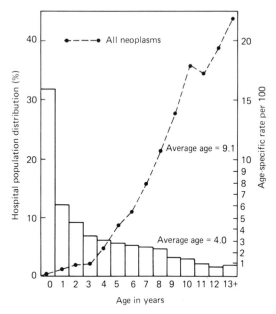

Fig. 5.5 Age distribution of a total canine hospital population (bars) and age-specific rates (graph) for canine neoplasia: University of Pennsylvania, 1952–64. (From Reif, 1983.)

or Y sex chromosomes. Canine haemophilia A and B, for example, are associated with the X chromosome and are inherited recessively, the defects being predominant in males (Patterson and Medway, 1966). Sex-limited inheritance occurs when the DNA responsible for the disease is not in the sex chromosomes, but the disease is expressed only in one sex; for example, cryptorchidism in dogs. In sex-influenced inheritance, the threshold for the overt expression of a characteristic (based on the multifactorial genetic model: *Figure 5.3*) is lower in one sex than the other; therefore, there is an excess incidence in one sex over the other. Canine patent ductus arteriosus (see Chapter 18) may be an example.

In many diseases, there may be excess disease occurrence in one sex over the other, but either a genetic component has not been identified clearly or the method of inheritance has not been established. Examples that are reported to occur predominantly in male dogs include epilepsy (Bielfelt *et al.*, 1971), melanoma and pharyngeal fibrosarcoma (Cohen *et al.*, 1964).

Some diseases may be apparently sex-associated, but are actually associated with other determinants that are related to gender. For instance (Schwabe *et al.*, 1977), the increased mortality rate in male dairy calves may

appear to be sex-associated. However, the real association is with husbandry: male dairy calves may not be given as much attention as females because they are worth less (in this instance husbandry, therefore, is a confounder).

Species and breed

Species and breeds vary in their susceptibility and responses to different infectious agents. Thus, dogs do not develop heartwater. Rottweilers and Doberman pinschers react more severely to canine parvovirus enteritis than other breeds (Glickman *et al.*, 1985), and boxers appear to be more susceptible than other breeds to mycotic diseases, such as coccidioidomycosis (Maddy, 1958) (see *Figure 7.2* for a distribution map of the fungus).

The reasons for species susceptibility are many and not fully understood. The efficacy of the immune mechanism against an infectious agent may be important. Thus, humans are not usually susceptible to infection with *Babesia* spp. but splenectomized individuals can develop the disease. Different species have been shown to have different receptors for infectious agents on the cell surface. This is particularly important with viruses, which must enter the host cell. Monkeys are not susceptible to poliovirus because they do not have the 'right' cell receptors. Removal of the virus capsid allows the virus to divide lytically in monkey cells if it is first made to enter them. Susceptibility can vary within a species, too. Thus, only certain pigs are susceptible to the strain of *Escherichia coli* possessing the K88 antigen because susceptibility is determined by the presence of an intestinal receptor which is specified by one or more genes (Vögeli *et al.*, 1992).

Phylogenetically closely related animals are likely to be susceptible to infection by the same agent, albeit with different signs. Herpesvirus B causes labial vesicular lesions in non-human primates, and a fatal encephalitis in man. The rider to this — that phylogenetically closely related agents infect the same species of animal — is not, however, generally true. Measles, distemper and rinderpest are closely related paramyxoviruses, yet usually infect quite different species: man, dogs and cattle, respectively.

Apparently new diseases can develop when a species or breed is placed in a new ecosystem (see Chapter 7) that contains a pathogen that has a well-balanced relationship with local species or breeds. In such circumstances, inapparent infection (discussed later in this chapter) is common in the local animals but clinical disease occurs in the exotic ones. This happened in South Africa, when European breeds of sheep were exposed to bluetongue virus. The agent did not produce clinical signs in the indigenous sheep, but caused severe disease in imported Merino sheep. Similarly, malaria developed as a clinical disease in early European visitors to West Africa, whereas the local population was tolerant of the parasite. The importation of European cattle to West Africa also accentuated the problem of dermatophilosis.

There is also species and breed variation in the occurrence of non-infectious diseases. Thus, British breeds of sheep develop intestinal carcinoma more frequently than fine wool breeds, and Hereford cattle develop ocular squamous cell carcinoma more commonly than other breeds (see Chapter 4).

Many diseases having distinct associations with a particular familial line or breed are considered to be primarily genetic. Patterson (1980) has described over 100 such diseases in the dog. A genetic causal component is more likely when disease incidence is higher in pedigree animals than in crossbreds. Examples include congenital cardiovascular defects (Patterson, 1968) and valvular heart disease (Thrusfield *et al.*, 1985) in dogs.

Diseases may be present in a range of breeds because the breeds are genetically related. Boston terriers and bull terriers show a high risk of developing mastocytoma, which may be related to their common origin (Peters, 1969). In contrast, the risk of a particular breed developing a disease may vary between countries, indicating different genetic 'pools' (or a different environment or method of management). Thus, Das and Tashjian (1965) found an increased risk of developing valvular heart disease in cocker spaniels in North America, whereas, in Scotland, Thrusfield *et al.* (1985) did not detect an increased risk in that breed. Similarly valvular heart disease is commoner in Cavalier King Charles spaniels in Scotland (Thrusfield *et al.*, 1985) than in Australia (Malik *et al.*, 1992).

Other host determinants

Size and conformation

Size, independent of particular breed associations, has been identified as a disease determinant. Hip dysplasia and osteosarcoma are more common in large breeds than in small breeds of dog (Tjalma, 1966). Interestingly, the latter disease is also more common in large than small children (Fraumeni, 1967). The conformation of animals may similarly increase the risk of some diseases. For instance, cows with a small pelvic outlet relative to their size (e.g., Chianina and Belgian blue) are predisposed to dystocia. Conformation may also have less direct effects. Thus, some calves cannot suckle their dams because the latter have large, bulbous teats (Logan *et al.*, 1974). This can result in the calves being hypogammaglobulinaemic, with the increased risk of fatal colibacillosis.

Coat colour

Predisposition to some diseases is associated with coat colour, which is heritable and a risk indicator. For example, white cats have a high risk of developing cutaneous squamous cell carcinoma (Dorn *et al.*, 1971) related to the lack of pigment which protects the skin from the carcinogenic effects of the sun's ultraviolet radiation. In contrast, canine melanomas occur mainly in deeply pigmented animals (Brodey, 1970). White cats often have a genetic defect associated with deafness (Bergsma and Brown, 1971). White hair colour is also associated with congenital deafness in Dalmatians (Anderson *et al.*, 1968).

Agent determinants

Virulence and pathogenicity

Infectious agents vary in their ability to infect and to induce disease in animals. The ability to infect is related to the inherent susceptibility of a host and whether or not the host is immune. The ability to induce disease is expressed in terms of **virulence** and **pathogenicity**. Virulence is the ability of an infectious agent to cause disease, in a **particular** host, in terms of **severity**. Highly virulent organisms therefore are often associated with high case fatality rates. Pathogenicity is sometimes incorrectly used as a synonym for virulence, with virulence reserved for variations in the disease-inducing potential of different strains of the same organism. However, 'pathogenicity' refers to the quality of disease induction (Stedman, 1982). Thus, the protozoan parasite *Naegleria fowleri* is pathogenic to man in warm water but not in cold water, the pathogenicity being governed in this instance by environment. Additionally, some authorities quantify pathogenicity as the ratio of the number of individuals developing clinical illness to the number exposed to infection (Last, 1988). A highly pathogenic organism thus induces clinical disease in a large proportion of infected animals.

Pathogenicity and virulence are commonly intrinsic characteristics of an infectious agent and are either **phenotypically** or **genotypically** conditioned. Phenotypic changes are transient, and are lost in succeeding gene-rations. For example, Newcastle disease virus cultivated in the chorioallantois of hens' eggs is more virulent to chicks than virus that is cultivated in calf kidney cells. Genotypic changes result from a change in the DNA (and RNA, in RNA viruses) of the microbial genome (the agent's total genetic complement).

Pathogenicity and virulence are determined by a variety of host and agent characteristics. The infectious agent must be able to multiply in, and resist the clearance and defence mechanisms of, the host. Multiplication and spread of bacteria are assisted by their release of toxins. An agent may achieve pathogenicity, or increase viru-lence, by a change in antigenic composition to a type to which the host is not genetically or immunologically resistant. However, antigenic changes are not always the cause of changes in pathogenicity. They may simply be indicators of such changes, the determinants being associated with the production of inhibitory, toxic or other substances by the agent. Genotypic changes also can alter the sensitivity of bacteria to antibiotics.

Types of genotypic change

Genotypic changes in infectious agents can result from **mutation**, **recombination**, **conjugation**, **transduction** and **transformation**. Mutation is an alteration in the sequence of nucleic acids in the genome of a cell or virus particle. There may be either **point mutation** of one base, resulting in misreading of succeeding codon triplets, or **deletion mutation**, where whole segments of genome are removed. Deletion mutants are more likely to occur because they result in changes without redundant genetic material. Frequent mutation may produce antigenic diversity, which may induce recurrent outbreaks of disease in a population that is not immune to the new antigen. Within the same organism, mutation rates can vary for different genetic markers by a factor of 1000. Sites within the genome that frequently mutate are termed 'hot spots'. If these spots code for virulence determinants and antigens in the infectious agent then the agent can change virulence and antigens frequently. If mutation occurs at sites that are not associated with either virulence or antigenic type, then changes in these two characteris-tics are rare.

Recombination is the reassortment of segments of a genome that occurs when two microbes exchange genetic material. Thus, influenza A viruses have a genome that is packaged in each virion (virus particle) as eight strands of RNA. Influenza viruses are divided into groups based on the structure of two major antigens: the haemagglutinin and neuraminidase (see also *Table 17.6*). Reassortment

between current human and avian strains of the virus (possibly in pigs) is likely to produce recombinants with novel haemagglutinin and neuraminidase combinations (Webster *et al.*, 1992). Major changes are referred to as 'shift' and minor changes as 'drift'. The major changes are responsible for the periodic — approximately decadal — pandemics of influenza in man (Kaplan, 1982). (Note that antigenic drift also occurs in trypanosomes, but by a totally different mechanism. The superficial cell mem-brane is shed to reveal new antigens. The epidemiological result, though, is similar: new antigens, therefore a partially or totally susceptible population.) Recombina-tion may also occur in the orbiviruses (e.g., African horse sickness and bluetongue) where the precise mechanism is not known, and the term 'genetic reassortment' has been applied (Gorman *et al.*, 1979).

Conjugation (Finnegan, 1976) involves transmission of genetic material from one bacterium to another, by a conjugal mechanism (i.e., they touch) through a sex pilus. Not only can surface antigens change by this means but also drug resistance, especially to antibiotics. This is common in *E. coli*, and *Salmonella*, *Proteus*, *Shigella* and *Pasteurella* spp.

Transduction (Primrose, 1976) is the transfer of a small portion of genome from one bacterium to another by a bacterial virus (bacteriophage). Again, resistance factors, as well as surface antigens, may be transferred in this way. It occurs in *Shigella*, *Pseudomonas* and *Proteus* spp.

Transformation is transmission of naked nucleic acid between bacteria, without contact. It occurs sponta-neously in *Neisseria* spp. but, to occur in other bacterial species, DNA has to be extracted in the laboratory. (This type of transformation should not be confused with the *in vitro* production of malignant cells, which is also called transformation.)

In addition to these five methods of genetic alteration, infection by more than one type of virus particle may be necessary to produce disease. Such infections do not strictly involve a change in a virus genome, rather a complementation of it, which may render a non-pathoge-nic virus particle pathogenic. This occurs in some plant virus infections because several plant viruses have split genomes that are packaged in separate particles. Each particle carries a portion of the total genome which is, itself, non-infectious, but which contributes to the whole infectious unit. For example, tobacco rattle virus has two virions: one containing a promoting gene, and the other containing replication and maturation genes. All three genes, and therefore both types of virion, are necessary to instigate the successful infection of a tobacco plant. In animals, Rous sarcoma virus has capsid proteins that are

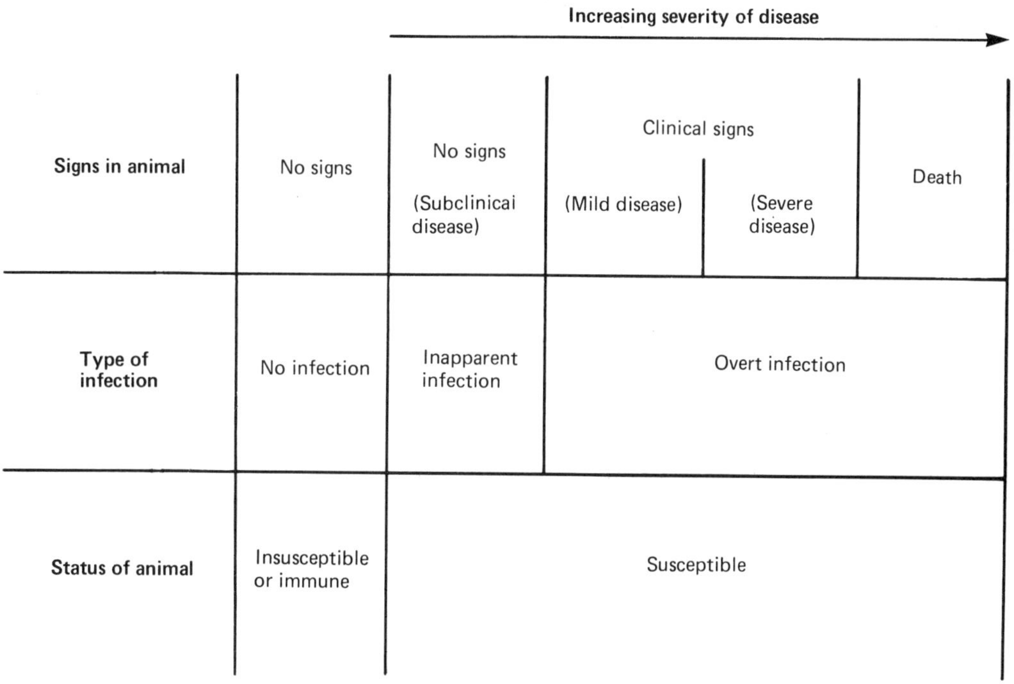

Increasing severity of disease

Signs in animal	No signs	No signs (Subclinical disease)	Clinical signs (Mild disease)	(Severe disease)	Death
Type of infection	No infection	Inapparent infection	Overt infection		
Status of animal	Insusceptible or immune	Susceptible			

Fig. 5.6 Gradient of infection: the various responses of an animal to challenge by an infectious agent.

genetically determined by a separate helper virus. Similarly, some adeno-associated viruses require an adenovirus for infectivity. The different particles present in human hepatitis B fall into this double infection group too.

Infection with immunosuppressive viruses can exacerbate other infections (e.g., rinderpest infection aggravates haemoprotozoan infections). Conversely, infection by one virus may prevent infection by, or lessen the virulence of, a second virus. This occurs when the first virus induces the host's cells to release an inhibitory substance now known as interferon.

The ways in which virulence and pathogenicity affect the transmission and maintenance of infection are discussed in Chapter 6.

Gradient of infection

'Gradient of infection' refers to the variety of responses of an animal to challenge by an infectious agent (*Figure 5.6*) and therefore represents the combined effect of an agent's pathogenicity and virulence, and host characteristics such as susceptibility and pathological and clinical reactions. These responses affect the further availability of the agent to other susceptible animals, and the ability of the veterinarian to detect, and therefore to treat and control, the infection. If an animal is either insusceptible or immune then infection and significant replication and shedding of an agent do not usually occur, and the animal is not important in the transmission of infection to others.

Inapparent (silent) infection

This is infection of a susceptible host without clinical signs. The infection usually runs a similar course to that which produces a clinical case, with replication and shedding of agent. The inapparently infected animal poses a considerable problem to the disease controller because it is impossible to detect without auxiliary diagnostic aids such as antigen detection or serology.

Subclinical infection occurs without overt clinical signs. Some authors use this term and inapparent infection synonymously. Others ascribe a loss of productivity to subclinical infection, which is absent from inapparent infection. 'Subclinical' can also be applied to noninfectious conditions, such as hypomagnesaemia, where there may be no clinical signs.

Clinical infection

Clinical infection produces clinical signs. Disease may be **mild**. If the disease is very mild with an illness too indefinite to permit a clinical diagnosis then it is termed an **abortive reaction**. There is a gradation to severe disease, which is called a **frank clinical reaction**, when the intensity is sufficient to allow a clinical diagnosis. The severest reaction results in death. Paradoxically, death is the logical climax of some infections since it is the only means by which the agent can be released to infect other animals. An example is infection with *Trichinella spiralis* which is transmitted exclusively by flesh eating.

Inapparent and mild clinical infections commonly indicate an adaptation of some antiquity between host and parasite; the relationship between bluetongue virus and indigenous South African sheep has already been cited.

Outcome of infection

Clinical disease may result in the development of a long-standing chronic clinical infection, recovery or death. Chronically infected cases are potential sources of an infectious agent. Death usually removes an animal as a source of infection, although there are important exceptions such as infection with *T. spiralis*, and anthrax infection where carcasses contaminate the soil. Recovery may result in **sterile immunity** following an effective host response, which removes all of the infectious agent from the body. Animals that have sterile immunity no longer constitute a threat to the susceptible population.

Two states, however, are important determinants:

1. the carrier state;
2. latent infection.

The carrier state

'Carrier' is used loosely to describe several situations. In a broad sense, a carrier is any animal that sheds an infectious agent without demonstrating clinical signs. Thus, an inapparently or subclinically infected animal may be a carrier, and may shed agent, either continuously or intermittently. The periods for which animals are carriers vary. They are rarely lifelong, but carriers may be important sources of infection to susceptible animals during these periods.

Incubatory carriers are animals that excrete agent during the disease's incubation period. For instance, dogs usually shed rabies virus in their saliva for up to 5 days before clinical signs of rabies develop (Fox, 1958), and periods as long as 14 days have been reported (Fekadu

and Baer, 1980). Thus, in countries in which rabies is endemic, the World Health Organization recommends that dogs and cats that have bitten a person should be confined for 10 days; this protocol is designed to determine if the bitten person was exposed to rabies virus.

Convalescent carriers are animals that shed agent when they are recovering from a disease, and the agent may then persist for prolonged periods. An example is infection with foot-and-mouth disease virus, where there is circumstantial evidence that carriers can establish further outbreaks (Salt, 1994).

Latent infection

A latent infection is one that persists in an animal, and in which there are no overt clinical signs. Thus, the distinction between latency, chronic infection and the carrier state is blurred. Latency may or may not be accompanied by transmission to other susceptible animals. In persistent bacterial infections (e.g., tuberculosis) a balance occurs between host and agent such that the agent replicates, but the disease may not progress for a long time. In virus and rickettsial infections, persistence is not usually associated with demonstrable replication of the agent, unless the latter is reactivated. Many examples of virus and rickettsial latency are known, but the role of latency in perpetuating infection in a population, except in a minority of infections, such as infection with the virus causing bovine virus diarrhoea (Harkness, 1987), is still unclear.

The likelihood of persistence can depend not only on the particular infectious agent and host species but also on the host's age at the time of infection. For instance, all kittens transplacentally infected with feline leukaemia virus become permanently infected (Jarrett, 1985). However, from 8 weeks of age, an increasing proportion of cats resist infection: by 4−6 months of age only about 15% of naturally infected cats become permanently infected. Latently infected cats do not appear to transmit infection (except possibly female cats to their kittens, in milk).

Unidentified latent infections can be obstacles to the control of disease. For example, the bacterium *Serpulina* (*Treponema*) *hyodysenteriae*, the cause of swine dysentery, can latently infect pigs. Attempts to control swine dysentery in the Thuringia region of Germany in the 1960s and 1970s were unsuccessful because only pigs in clinically affected herds were treated, and the infection was maintained in latently infected animals. However, when latently infected herds were identified by examining faecal samples for presence of the bacterium, and control measures were instituted in these herds, the disease

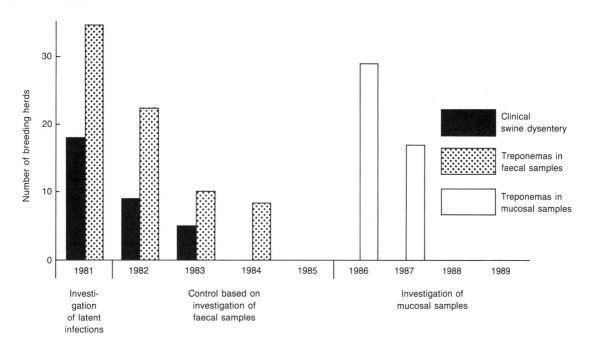

Fig. 5.7 Control and eradication of swine dysentery: Thuringia, Germany, 1981–89. (Modified from Blaha, 1992.)

declined (*Figure 5.7*). Pathogen-free status was subsequently monitored by examination of mucosal scrapings from the colon.

Microbial colonization of hosts

Infectious agents enter a host at varying times during its life. Some — the vertically transmitted ones (see Chapter 6) — infect the host before birth. Initial infection may or may not be followed by the immediate development of disease.

Exogenous and endogenous pathogens

The previous description of microbes involved with reproductive failure in pigs illustrates that pathogenic infectious agents can be classified into two groups: **exogenous** and **endogenous** (Dubos, 1965).

The exogenous pathogens are not usually present in the host. They cannot normally survive for a long time in the external environment (soil, water, etc.). They do not usually form persistent relationships with the host. They are generally acquired by exposure to an infected animal, and usually produce disease with clearly identifiable clinical signs and pathological lesions. Examples include

canine distemper, rinderpest, and the other traditional animal plagues.

The endogenous pathogens are often found in healthy animals, commonly in the gastrointestinal and respiratory tracts, and usually do not cause disease unless the host is stressed. An example is *E. coli*, which is commonly found in the intestinal tract of calves, and which may cause disease only when a calf is immunodeficient, for example, due to deprivation of colostrum (Isaacson *et al.*, 1978).

This twofold classification is somewhat simplistic. Some pathogens possess characteristics of both groups. For example, *Salmonella* spp. usually produce distinct clinical signs when they infect animals. However, some animals can permanently carry and intermittently excrete the agent without showing signs, as carriers. The bacterium can also be transmitted by methods other than direct contact with infected animals, for example, in contaminated food.

Opportunistic pathogens

Some organisms cause disease only in a host whose resistance is lowered; for example, by drug therapy and other diseases. Such organisms are **opportunistic**, may colonize the host at any time during life, and may be endogenous or exogenous. Examples described earlier are the group 1 pathogens that can cause prenatal deaths and abortions in pigs.

Environmental determinants

The environment includes location, climate and husbandry. Particular attention has been paid to environmental determinants of disease in livestock enterprises, where intensive production systems expose animals to unnatural environments (e.g., chicken battery houses), and in human medicine, where social and occupational exposure to possible causal factors (e.g., to smoke in relation to lung cancer: *Table 3.2*) can occur.

Location

Local geological formations, vegetation and climate affect the spatial distribution of both animals and disease. Thus, the incidence of jaw tumours in sheep, mentioned in Chapter 4, is associated with the distribution of bracken, and illustrates the value of maps in identifying causes of disease. Non-specific chronic canine pulmonary disease in middle-aged and old dogs has been shown to be associated with urban residence in the US (Reif and Cohen, 1970); urban residence being defined in relation to atmospheric pollution (see Chapter 18). This investigation has been refined by demonstrating an urban/rural gradient in the occurrence of canine pulmonary disease (Reif and Cohen, 1979): an example of the application of the method of concomitant variation (see Chapter 3) in inferring cause.

Noise is associated with location and may also be considered as being related to 'occupation' and husbandry. The effect of noise on animal health has not been studied in detail. Most investigations have been conducted on man and laboratory animals where, apart from the obvious induction of temporary or permanent deafness, noise has been shown to cause a general stress reaction (discussed later in this chapter) with altered secretion of adrenocortical hormones. In a review of the effects of noise on animal health, Algers *et al.* (1978) describe leucopenia (which could be associated with immunosuppression), decreased milk production in dairy cows, and oligospermia and an increased incidence of abortion in rats. Studies in horses, however, suggest that impulse noises (sonic booms) have no effect on animal health or behaviour (Ewbank and Cullinan, 1984).

The temporal distribution of disease is also affected by location because of the seasonal effects of climate. These effects, and methods of identifying them, are discussed in Chapter 8.

Climate

Two types of climate can be identified: **macroclimate** and **microclimate**.

Macroclimate

The macroclimate comprises the normal components of weather to which animals are exposed: rainfall, temperature, solar radiation, humidity and wind, all of which can affect health (Webster, 1981). Temperature may be a primary determinant; for example, low temperatures in the induction of hypothermia, to which newborn animals are particularly prone. Wind and rain increase heat loss from animals. Cold stress predisposes animals to disease; for example, by reducing efficiency of digestion, which may predispose to infectious enteritis. Wind can also carry infectious agents (e.g., foot-and-mouth disease virus) and arthropod vectors (e.g., *Culicoides* spp. infected with bluetongue virus) over long distances (see Chapter 6).

Solar radiation can act as a primary determinant: the carcinogenic effect of solar ultraviolet radiation has already been mentioned in relation to cutaneous squamous cell carcinoma. It is also an important component of the sufficient cause of infectious bovine keratoconjunctivitis, in which the primary determinant is infection with *Moraxella bovis* (Hughes *et al.*, 1965). The bacterium alone only produces mild clinical signs; the classical disease only occurs when high levels of ultraviolet radiation are present. The disease therefore tends to be seasonal, occurring most frequently during summer, and occasionally in winter, when ultraviolet radiation is reflected from fresh snow (Hubbert and Hermann, 1970). Current stratospheric ozone depletion, with the associated increase in ultraviolet radiation, may therefore cause an increase in the incidence of this and other diseases, including Uberreiter's syndrome (chronic superficial keratoconjunctivitis) in dogs, and cataracts and skin lesions in farmed fish (Mayer, 1992).

The macroclimate can also affect the stability of infectious agents, in which circumstance it is a secondary determinant. Bovine rhinotracheitis virus survives well when humidity is low, whereas rhinoviruses survive when it is high. Porcine transmissible gastroenteritis virus is sensitive to solar ultraviolet radiation, and therefore is more likely to be inactivated in summer than in winter. The statistical association between respiratory disease and cool damp weather conditions is probably due to a build-up of pathogens, rather than a reduction in host resistance by climatic stress (Webster, 1981).

Climatic impact can be measured in several ways. A common method is to calculate the **wind-chill index**. This combines the effects of temperature and wind-speed, and is especially important at temperatures below freezing, where convective heat losses are magnified by wind. The **standard environmental temperature** (McArthur, 1991) relates the effects of temperature, wind-speed and humidity, and can take values considerably below or above actual air temperature.

The macroclimate, in conjunction with geological features, determines vegetation and affects the spatial distribution of disease because of the resultant distribution of hosts and vectors; this is discussed in Chapter 7. Macroclimatic changes may therefore alter the frequency and distribution of many diseases, and it has been speculated that global warming, resulting from an increase in the 'greenhouse effect' caused by industrial carbon dioxide and other emissions, may be an important determinant during the next century (Aitken, 1993). For example, if there is a mean rise in temperature of $2-4$ °C in Europe over that period, the growing season in the UK would be extended and the rainfall pattern would alter. Extension of the grazing season could increase the incidence of bovine hypomagnesaemia (see Figure 3.6) and selenium and cobalt deficiency in lambs. A concomitant change to 'softer' grazing with more lush pasture could also lead to an increase in dental problems in sheep. The distribution of biological vectors may also alter, resulting in changes in vector-transmitted diseases; for example, louping ill, Lyme disease and tick-borne fever could become more common as the pattern of activity of the agents' vector, the tick *Ixodes ricinus*, shifted. Moreover, the patterns of parasitic diseases such as fascioliasis, nematodiriasis and haemonchosis could also be modified because of the importance of temperature in the development of the parasites' stages in the environment and cold-blooded intermediate hosts.

Microclimate

A microclimate is a climate that occurs in a small defined space. This may be as small as within a few millimetres of a plant's or an animal's surface or as large as a piggery or calf house. In the former, microclimate may be **terrestrial** (e.g., over the surface of leaves) or **biological** (e.g., over the surface of a host's body). The terrestrial microclimate affects the development of arthropods and helminths. The biological microclimate can change during the course of a disease, assisting in its spread. For instance, sweating during the parasitaemic phase of human malaria increases the humidity of the body's surface and attracts more mosquitoes to the humid skin surface at a time when the protozoon is readily available.

The microclimate in intensive animal production units is an important determinant of disease. Stable dust is associated with respiratory hypersensitivity and non-allergic pulmonary disease, and can act as a vehicle for microorganisms (Collins and Algers, 1986). Poor ventilation is associated with chronic equine respiratory disease (Clarke, 1987). Therefore, adequate ventilation is recommended to remove stale air, microbial aerosols and dust, and to reduce humidity (Wathes *et al.*, 1983; Wathes, 1989). Although the effects of high concentrations of non-pathogenic airborne bacteria on livestock are unclear, there is evidence (Pritchard *et al.*, 1981) that reduced levels of airborne bacteria are associated with a reduced incidence of clinical and subclinical respiratory disease.

Husbandry

Housing

The importance of well-designed ventilation in an animal house has already been mentioned. The structure of bedding materials and surfaces is also a determinant. Thus, claw lesions are more common and severe in pigs reared on aluminium slats than in pigs reared on steel or concrete slabs, or on soil (Fritschen, 1979). Limb lesions are more common in pigs reared on concrete than on asphalt-based floors (Kovacs and Beer, 1979); and hoof lesions and vulva biting (associated with aggression) are common problems in group-housed sows (Kroneman *et al.*, 1993). Smith (1981) suggests that excessive floor slope may predispose to rectal prolapse in pigs because of the increased effect of gravity.

Diet

Diet has obvious effects in diseases caused by energy, protein, vitamin and mineral deficiencies. Sometimes the effects are less clearly defined. There is evidence, for example, that increased dietary levels of biotin reduce the incidence of foot lesions in sows (Penny *et al.*, 1980). However, there is no evidence of an association between a deficiency of the vitamin and an increased incidence of the lesions.

Feeding regimes may be a determinant. Thus, gastric torsion in sows kept in sow stalls has been associated with once-a-day, rather than twice-a-day feeding, which may indicate that the ingestion of a relatively large amount of food is a causal factor (Crossman, 1978).

Management (including animal use)

Management determines stocking density and production policy. Increased densities increase the challenge of microbial pathogens. An internal replacement policy (i.e., maintaining a 'closed' population) is less likely to introduce pathogens into an enterprise than a policy involving buying in animals from outside the herd.

The use to which an animal is put (its 'occupation') can affect disease occurrence. Equine limb injuries are relatively common in hunters. 'Hump-sore' ('yoke gall') occurs more frequently in draught zebus than in non-working cattle. Apparently sex-related differences in disease occurrence, which actually are related to animal use, have been described earlier.

Stress

No general theory of stress has been universally accepted (Moberg, 1985), and there has been conflict and confusion over interpretation of the related physiological responses (Becker, 1987). Stress is generally associated with adverse conditions. In human medicine, it is used to describe emotional conflicts and displeasure. In veterinary medicine, it is often considered as arising from factors such as weaning, overcrowding, transportation, changes in diet and other environmental factors. However, in such circumstances, stress may just be a convenient term to describe an area of interest or particular conditions of management, and may mask understanding of underlying principles and mechanisms (Rushen, 1986). Stress can be considered to be the normal and complex summation of a wide variety of responses to any environmental change (Coffey, 1988). If the responses are inappropriate or inadequate then stress may contribute to the development of pathological lesions (Moberg, 1985).

Stress was initially considered in relation to the physiological 'flight or fight' reaction (Cannon, 1914). Factors such as physical exertion and fear stimulate secretion of catechol amines by the adrenal medulla. These in turn assist muscular exercise by redistributing blood to the muscles, enabling animals to respond by either 'flight' or 'fight'.

A more comprehensive theory of stress was formulated by Selye (1946) who described the effects of noxious stimuli (e.g., cold, heat, immobilization and severe infections) in laboratory animals. These stimuli were called **stressors**, and their effects were later collectively

termed the **general adaptation syndrome**. This was divided into three parts:

1. general alarm reaction;
2. phase of resistance (phase of adaptation);
3. phase of reaction.

The general alarm reaction occurred 6 – 48 hours after exposure to a stressor and comprised a decrease in the size of the liver, lymph nodes, spleen and thymus, disappearance of adipose tissue, loss of muscular tone, hypothermia, the development of erosions in the digestive tract, and increased lacrimation and salivation. The phase of resistance began after approximately 48 hours and included adrenal enlargement associated with increased release of adrenotropic hormones mediated by the hypothalamus, reappearance of lipoid granules, hyperplasia of the thyroid associated with increased production of thyrotropic hormones, cessation of body growth and milk secretion, and atrophy of the gonads. The various organs became almost normal, even when the stressor was still applied. The phase of reaction resulted in death with signs similar to those of the first part.

Selye argued that there was a similar, that is, **non-specific**, response to all stressors, which always involved adrenal activity. This resulted in an adrenal response being used as proof of stress. However, later studies (Mason *et al.*, 1968) demonstrated that the adrenal response is closely related to psychological stimuli, and that it does not occur when some stressors (e.g., fasting) are applied in the absence of psychological stressors. This resulted in the rejection of a non-specific stress response (Mason, 1971). Consequently, the particular stimulus responsible for an observed reaction should be identified; this is particularly important in practical situations (e.g., transportation) where several stimuli are involved. Moreover, the response may include a number of hormones, either with or without adrenal involvement, and several may therefore need to be monitored.

Stress theory is still contentious, and evidence for the role of stress as a determinant of disease has usually been in the context of particular conditions of management, rather than in relation to a well-understood, unequivocal physiological response. It is in the former context that stress is now discussed.

Stress can be a primary determinant. A notable example is when stress results from the capture of animals, where it can produce a **postcapture myopathy syndrome**. This syndrome is reported in wild animals in South Africa (Basson and Hofmeyer, 1973). It is characterized by ataxia, paresis or paralysis, the production of brown urine, and asymmetric muscular and myocardial lesions.

A similar disease occurs in red deer following capture (McAllum, 1985).

Stress is also a primary determinant of the **porcine stress syndrome**. This is the inability of susceptible pigs to tolerate the usual environmental stressors (e.g., castration, vaccination, movement and high ambient temperatures) that are associated with normal management. The syndrome occurs rapidly — often within minutes — after exposure to a stressor. The disease, which is considered to be identical to malignant (fulminant) hyperthermia in humans, dogs, cats, horses and pigs, is characterized initially by muscle and tail tremors. Further stress can produce dyspnoea, cyanosis, increased body temperature and acidosis. The final stage is marked by total collapse, muscle rigidity, hyperthermia and death. The condition is a genetically determined error of metabolism which induces a switch of energy utilization in muscles of affected pigs from aerobic to anaerobic metabolism. It is inherited through an autosomal recessive gene with high or complete penetrance. Susceptible pigs can be detected by the rapid development of malignant hyperthermia under halothane anaesthesia, and by certain blood group linked genes (Archibald and Imlah, 1985).

Stress may be a secondary determinant of several diseases. The immune system can be suppressed by stressors (Dohms and Metz, 1991). Although the significance of such immunosuppression in predisposing animals to infectious disease is unclear, epidemiological studies have provided evidence that it is functionally relevant. Thus, shipping fever (see Chapter 1) is associated with transportation, dehorning, castration and winter weather, and the increased incidence of malignant catarrhal fever and yersiniosis in deer in winter may be due to prolonged exposure to cold and a low plane of nutrition.

Interaction

Determinants associated with host, agent or environment do not exert their effects in isolation, but **interact** to induce disease. 'Interaction' refers to the interdependent operation of factors to produce an effect. Thus, factors that result in net decreased magnesium intake interact with those that induce net increased loss to produce hypomagnesaemia (see *Figure 3.6*). Bovine alimentary papillomas, caused by a papilloma virus (the agent), can transform to carcinomas in areas where bracken fern (the environment) is common, indicating an interaction between agent and environment (Jarrett, 1980). There is an interaction between a gene (the host) and stressors (the environment) which induces the porcine stress syndrome.

Diseases caused by mixed agents

An important example of interaction between agents is the **mixed infection**, that is, an infection with more than one type of agent. The main infectious disease problems in intensive production systems relate to the body surfaces. Common problems are enteric and respiratory diseases and mastitis. These diseases are frequently caused by mixed infections. Two categories of diseases can be identified (Rutter, 1982):

1. those diseases in which clinical signs can be reproduced by single agents independently, although mixed infections usually occur in animals;
2. those diseases in which two or more microbial components are necessary to induce disease.

Some examples are listed in *Table 5.3*. Category I agents include *E. coli*, rotaviruses, caliciviruses, and *Cryptosporidium* spp., all of which can induce diarrhoea. Category II agents are exemplified by those that cause calf pneumonia, which include 5 viruses, 4 mycoplasmata and 19 bacterial species. The precise mechanism of the interaction is unclear, but investigations in mice (Jakab, 1977) suggest that pulmonary phagocytosis of bacteria may be reduced by virus inhibition of intracellular killing mechanisms in macrophages, and that increased bacterial adherence to virus-infected cells may increase.

Foot rot in sheep also demonstrates interaction. There are four component organisms: *Corynebacterium pyogenes*, *Fusobacterium necrophorum*, *Dichelobacter nodosus* and non-pathogenic motile fusobacteria. Each of these four alone is only poorly virulent but supplies growth factors or substances that overcome the host's defence mechanisms in the complete infection (Roberts, 1969).

Other examples of interactions demonstrated experimentally include intestinal coccidiosis in chickens which may predispose to necrotic enteritis with the associated proliferation of *Clostridium perfringens* (Shane *et al.*, 1985), and haemorrhagic enteritis virus infection of turkey poults which increases their susceptibilty to colibacillosis (Larsen *et al.*, 1985). A full discussion of microbial interactions is presented by Woolcock (1991).

In addition to this general concept of interaction, two specific meanings are attached to interaction, defining **biological** and **statistical interaction**.

Biological interaction

Biological interaction involves a dependence between two factors based on an underlying physical or chemical

Table 5.3 Examples of diseases caused by mixed infections. (Modified from Rutter, 1982.)

Disease	Classification*	Agents
Enteric disease (most species)	I (?II)	Enterotoxigenic *Escherichia coli*
		Rotavirus Coronavirus Calicivirus *Cryptosporidium* spp.
Atrophic rhinitis (pigs)	I	*Bordetella bronchiseptica* *Pasteurella multocida*
Foot rot (sheep)	II	*Corynebacterium pyogenes* *Fusobacterium necrophorum* *Dichelobacter nodosus* Motile fusobacteria
Pneumonia (sheep)	II	Parainfluenza 3 *Pasteurella haemolytica*
Swine dysentery (pigs)	II	*Treponema hyodysenteriae* Gut anaerobes
'Coli septicaemia' (chickens)	II	*Escherichia coli* Infectious bronchitis virus
Respiratory disease (bovine)	?II	*Mycoplasma bovis* *Mycoplasma dispar* Parainfluenza 3 Respiratory syncytial virus Infectious bovine rhinotracheitis virus *Pasteurella* spp. Other bacteria
Summer mastitis (bovine)	?II	*Corynebacterium pyogenes* *Peptococcus indolicus* *Streptococcus dysgalactiae* Micro-aerophilic cocci

*I = Single agents can reproduce clinical signs but mixed infections frequently occur.
II = Mixed infections are essential with cooperative or synergistic interactions.
? = Insufficient evidence for definitive classification.

association. For instance, there is a chemical interaction between the K88 antigen of *E. coli* (the agent) and receptors in the intestines of some pigs (the host), described earlier in this chapter, which results in the bacteria that possess the antigen being pathogenic to pigs with the receptors. There appears to be a physical interaction, also mentioned earlier, between the presence of bacteria and poor ventilation in the induction of calf respiratory disease, associated with the density of airborne bacteria. Biological interaction similarly is demonstated by category II mixed agents. Biological interactions

therefore relate to identifiable stages in a causal pathway, and represent many of the known general qualitative interactions.

Two or more factors also can interact biologically to produce an effect that is greater than that expected of either factor alone; this is **synergism**. An example would be the potentiating effect of combinations of antibiotics. Similarly, there is synergism between the four component organisms of ovine foot rot, described above.

'Synergism' should be reserved to describe **biological** mechanisms. In the epidemiological literature, however, synergism has also been used to describe certain types of statistical, rather than biological, interactions, and this has led to some confusion (Kleinbaum *et al.*, 1982). The use of 'synergism' in a statistical context is discussed in the following section.

Statistical interaction

Statistical interaction is a quantitative effect involving two or more factors. Often disease occurrence does not depend simply on the presence or absence of a factor; there may be continuous variation in the frequency of occurrence of disease associated with both the strength of a factor (e.g., the frequency with which dairy farm personnel milk cows and infection with *Leptospira* spp.: see *Table 3.1*) and the number of factors involved. There is often a 'background' frequency of occurrence associated with none of the factors under consideration. When two or more factors are associated with disease, the frequency of disease may be proportional to the occurrence of disease resulting from the **separate** frequencies attributable to each factor (i.e., the frequency when each factor is present singly, minus the 'background' frequency). Alternatively, the frequency may be either in excess of or less than that expected from the combined effects of each factor, in which case **statistical interaction** occurs. For example, Willeberg (1976), in his study of the feline urological syndrome (FUS), showed that castration and high levels of dry cat food intake, when present simultaneously, resulted in a frequency of the FUS in excess of that expected from the combined effects of each factor, indicating positive statistical interaction between the two factors.

When several component causes are present simultaneously, their joint effect can be explained quantitatively in terms of two causal models: **additive** and **non-additive** (Kupper and Hogan, 1978). The additive model interprets disease occurrence, when two or more factors are present, as the **sum** of the amount of disease attributable to each factor. If no interaction exists, then, for example:

when X and Y are both absent, suppose 'background' disease occurrence = γ;
when cause X is present alone, disease occurrence = $2 + \gamma$;
when cause Y is present alone, disease occurrence = $5 + \gamma$;
when X and Y are both present, disease occurrence = $7 + \gamma$.

If positive interaction occurs, then the level of disease occurrence, when X and Y are present, will be greater than $7 + \gamma$.

The commonest non-additive model is the multiplicative. This interprets disease occurrence, when two or more factors are present, as the **product** of the amount of disease attributable to each factor. If no interaction exists, then, for example:

when X and Y are both absent, suppose 'background' disease occurrence = δ;
when cause X is present alone, disease occurrence = 2δ;
when cause Y is present alone, disease occurrence = 5δ;
when X and Y are both present, disease occurrence = 10δ.

If positive interaction occurs, then the level of disease occurrence, when X and Y are present, will be greater than 10δ.

Disease occurrence can be measured in terms of incidence or other measures of the risk of disease developing (see Chapter 15). The type of model depends on the means of expressing disease occurrence; for example, a multiplicative model may become additive if log transformation of the measure of occurrence is conducted.

In epidemiology the additive model is of particular relevance to assessing the impact of a factor on disease occurrence in a population, whereas the multiplicative model has a role in elucidation of causes (Kleinbaum *et al.*, 1982). When there is evidence of positive interaction based on the additive model, the model has sometimes been described as **synergistic**. However, there are arguable differences between interaction and synergism (Blot and Day, 1979). Evidence of a positive statistical interaction does not necessarily imply a causal relationship. However, if it can be inferred that the factors are part of an aggregate of causes with a common causal pathway then synergism is said to have occurred (MacMahon, 1972). Synergism, in a statistical context, therefore may be thought of as a positive statistical interaction where a causal pathway may be inferred. Thus, castration and high levels of dry cat food intake (usually associated with overfeeding and sometimes related to insufficient water intake) are synergistically associated in the FUS: both may result in inactivity, thereby reducing blood flow to the kidneys, impairing renal function, and therefore promoting changes in the urine that are conducive to the formation of uroliths.

The value of assessing statistical interaction lies in its ability to identify the **degree** to which various determinants interact. It then may be possible to predict the extent to which disease incidence may be reduced by modification of the determinants. Thus, the value often lies in its ability to **predict** outcome, rather than to explain **biological** interaction (Kupper and Hogan, 1978). The quantification of statistical interaction is described in Chapter 15.

The cause of cancer

The cause of cancer exemplifies interaction between host, agent and environment. The abnormal, unrestricted multiplication of cells produces a tumour. Tumours may be benign, in which growth is restricted and spread to other parts of the body does not occur; or malignant, in which growth is unrestricted and spread (metastasis) may occur. Malignant tumours are commonly termed cancers, the word taking its meaning from the zodiacal constellation of the crab, because malignant tumours 'put out' extensions like the limbs of a crab.

The induction of cancer

The mass of cancerous cells that constitutes a malignant tumour originates from a single 'founder' cell which once was normal, but which has undergone a fundamental change. This change is manifested in several abnormal characteristics such as excessive dependence on anaerobic metabolism and the presence of unusual tumour antigens, in addition to the disregard for normal territorial boundaries which is a cancer's most obvious characteristic. These complex alterations in cell behaviour appear to originate from a surprisingly restricted set of genetic changes (Weinberg, 1983). Thus, cancer can be induced in laboratory animals by the introduction of cells that have been transformed to the cancerous state, *in vitro*, by infection with polyoma virus.

Epidemiological investigations had previously revealed that chemical and physical agents can induce cancer. Hydrocarbons in soot were the first chemicals to be incriminated. In 1775, Percival Pott, a London surgeon, recorded an increased incidence of scrotal epithelioma in chimney sweeps. Since then, a range of chemical carcinogens have been identified (Coombs, 1980), including hydrocarbons, aromatic amines (associated with bladder cancer in dyestuff workers), *N*-nitroso compounds (associated with liver cancer in fish, birds and mammals), steroids (e.g., oestrone, inducing mammary

cancer in mice), inorganic products such as asbestos (associated with mesothelioma in man; see Chapter 18) and some natural products (e.g., the fungal aflatoxins, which are contaminants of peanut oil, implicated in liver cancer in humans and in fish exposed to contaminated foodstuffs).

Evidence suggests that tumour-inducing (oncogenic) viruses, chemical and physical carcinogens, and spontaneous mutations alter cellular DNA and, therefore, that cancer results from alterations to genetic material. The critical genes that are the targets of these alterations fall into two families: proto-oncogenes and oncosuppressor genes. **Proto-oncogenes** code for the products that directly support cell proliferation or, sometimes, inhibit cell death. These products form a group of cell regulatory molecules, including growth factors, membrane-associated growth factor receptors, GTP-binding proteins, tyrosine and serine kinases, and transcription factors. These molecules are vital for the normal modulation of cell behaviour. When modified, for example by mutation, through interaction with chemical carcinogens or ionizing radiation, they acquire the potential to transform cells directly towards the cancerous state. Such modified forms of the proto-oncogenes are called **oncogenes**. Many transforming animal retroviruses contain versions of such oncogenes, presumably acquired during the sojourn of the virus within host cells.

Oncosuppressor genes have the property of restraining growth. In association with proto-oncogenes, such genes exert extremely important roles in physiological cell regulation. One such gene (the retinoblastoma susceptibility gene, Rb-1) regulates cell movement into and around the replication cycle. Another (p53) initiates cell cycle arrest in response to genotoxic injury, so permitting DNA repair. Others may modulate the passage of signals from cell to cell or from substratum to cell, via adhesion molecules, and so adjust cell behaviour and proliferation in response to prevailing cell density within a tissue. In carcinogenesis, these genes are silenced, usually by mutation or by acquired loss of part of the chromosome containing the gene. Normal diploid cells contain two copies of each oncosuppressor gene, and in general both must be inactivated to achieve the full change of phenotype that is recognized as cancer. However, these paired events do not necessarily occur at the same time. They may be acquired one after the other through continuous exposure to a carcinogen, or only one may be acquired, the other being inherited in the germ line. Animals that inherit such defective oncosuppressor genes are clearly at higher risk of acquiring cancer through subsequent exposure to environmental carcinogens, and several well-known inherited cancer-susceptibility syndromes in man (e.g., familial retinoblastoma and familial polyposis coli) are the result of this type of inherited gene defect. Interestingly, the transforming genes of several animal DNA viruses (e.g., in the papova-, papilloma-, adeno- virus groups) appear to act through binding to the products of endogenous oncosuppressor genes.

Many tumours show a steeply rising age–incidence relationship (Armitage and Doll, 1954; Peto, 1977; and see *Figure 5.5*). This can be accurately modelled by assuming that carcinogenesis requires multiple independent events. Laboratory reconstructions, in which different oncogenes are inserted, in active form, into previously normal cells, also confirm the view that multiple changes are required to achieve full transformation from normality to the cancer cell. Hence, it is not surprising that the majority of known cancers can be shown to contain multiple oncogene and oncosuppressor gene alterations. The concept of **multistage carcinogenesis**, however, also includes interactions between agents which may not effect permanent changes in DNA structure in the manner outlined above for oncogenes and oncosuppressor genes. Early experiments with chemical carcinogens delineated two main processes in carcinogenesis (Becker, 1981): **initiation** and **promotion**.

Initiation, either by oncogenic viruses, ionizing radiation, chemical carcinogens, or inherited or spontaneous changes in the genome, is assumed to involve an irreversible alteration in cellular DNA.

Initiation alone is not sufficient to induce a cancer, but it produces a cell with a high risk of becoming malignant. Malignancy results when promotion occurs. This step was considered to be reversible, although there is evidence that, when cells have reached a certain stage of change, they progress irreversibly to cancer (e.g., Peraino *et al.*, 1977). Several chemical promoters have been identified, such as croton oil, which promotes skin tumours. The active ingredient in croton oil is an ester which is an analogue of an endogenous cellular regulatory molecule, but the biochemical basis of promotion is generally still poorly understood. Many chemical carcinogens are both initiators and promoters (**complete carcinogens**).

'Co-carcinogen' is a general term for a factor that furthers the action of a carcinogen, such as chronic inflammation or a chemical promoter. Squamous cell carcinoma of sheep in northern Australia occurs predominantly on the ears, the prevalence increasing with decreasing latitude. Solar ultraviolet radiation has been incriminated as a physical carcinogen. An infectious agent, transmitted on ear marking instruments, may be a co-carcinogen, and would explain why the lesions are commoner on the ear than on other parts of the head.

Investigating the cause of cancer

Biochemists, virologists and molecular biologists have identified inducers and promoters, using animals and tissue cultures. At the top of the biological hierarchy, epidemiologists have identified risk factors using observational studies. Two groups of factors are defined (Gopal, 1977):

1. specific causal agents;
2. modifying factors.

Specific physical causal agents that have been incriminated include ultraviolet and ionizing radiation (the latter experimentally inducing thyroid tumours and leukaemia in dogs), chronic irritation (associated with some horn cancers in Indian cattle: Somvanshi, 1991) and parasites (e.g., *Spiroceria lupi* associated with canine oesophageal osteosarcoma and fibrosarcoma). Specific chemical and biological initiators, such as viruses, have already been described. Modifying factors are not incriminated as initiators, but in some way affect the incidence of cancer, and include co-carcinogens. The genetic composition of the host is the most important modifying factor and may be related to the presence of suitable proto-oncogenes. Some cancers can be hereditary; for example, porcine lymphosarcoma (McTaggart *et al.*, 1979).

Interactions have been demonstrated in which chemical carcinogens enhance the production of tumours *in vitro* by oncogenic viruses. One outstanding example is the interaction between bracken fern and infection with bovine papilloma virus, described above. Some non-oncogenic viruses are also reported to interact with chemical carcinogens (Martin, 1964). Thus, chickens infected with pox viruses, and mice infected with influenza virus, are more susceptible to chemical carcinogenesis than non-infected animals. Doll (1977) has contended that most cancers have environmental causes either as initiators or promoters.

Investigation of the cause of cancer therefore involves cooperation between several disciplines: biochemistry, pathology, molecular biology and epidemiology. Tumours of domestic animals and some of their causes are reviewed by Cotchin (1984). Cancers of domestic animals can also be useful biological models of human cancer (Pierrepoint, 1985); this topic is discussed further in Chapter 18.

Further reading

Clarke, A. (1987) Air hygiene and equine respiratory disease. *In Practice*, **9**, 196–204

Darcel, C. (1994) Reflections on viruses and cancer. *Veterinary Research Communications*, **18**, 43 – 61

Dennis, M.J. (1986) The effects of temperature and humidity on some animal diseases — a review. *British Veterinary Journal*, **142**, 472 – 485

Doll, R. and Peto, R. (1983) Epidemiology of cancer. In: *Oxford Textbook of Medicine*, Vol. 1. Eds Weatherall, D.J., Ledingham, J.G.G. and Warrell, A., pp. 4.51 – 4.79. Oxford University Press, Oxford

Ekesbo, I. (1988) *Environment and Animal Health*. Proceedings of the 6th International Congress on Animal Hygiene, Skara, Sweden, 2 vols. Swedish University of Agricultural Sciences, Report No. 21

MacMahon, B. (1972) Concepts of multiple factors. In: *Multiple Factors in the Causation of Environmentally Induced Disease*. Fogarty International Center Proceedings No. 12. Eds Lee, D.H.K. and Kotkin, P., pp. 1 – 12. Academic Press, New York and London

Madwell, B.R. and Theilen, G.H. (1987) Etiology of cancer in animals. In: *Veterinary Cancer Medicine*, 2nd edn. Eds Theilen, G.H. and Madewell, B.R., pp. 13 – 26. Lea and Febiger, Philadelphia

Mims, C.A. (1987) *The Pathogenesis of Infectious Disease*, 3rd edn. Academic Press, London and New York

Phillips, C. and Piggins, D. (Eds) (1992) *Farm Animals and the Environment*. CAB International, Wallingford. (*Includes discussions of environment-dependent diseases, stress, and the effects of ventilation on health and performance*)

Reif, J.S. (1983) Ecologic factors and disease. In: *Textbook of Veterinary Internal Medicine. Vol. 1: Diseases of the Dog and Cat*, 2nd edn. Ed. Ettinger, S.Y., pp. 147 – 173. W.B. Saunders Company, Philadelphia

Sainsbury, D.W.B. (1981) Health problems in intensive animal production. In: *Environmental Aspects of Housing for Animal Production*. Ed. Clark, J.A., pp. 439 – 454. Butterworths, London

Sainsbury, D.W.B. (1991) Environmental factors affecting susceptibility to disease. In: *Microbiology of Animals and Animal Products*. World Animal Science, A6. Ed. Woolcock, J.B., pp. 77 – 94. Elsevier, Amsterdam

Smith, H., Skehel, J.J. and Turner, M.J. (Eds) (1980) *The Molecular Basis of Pathogenicity*. Report of the Dahlem workshop on the molecular basis of the infective process, Berlin, 22 – 26 October 1979. Verlag Chemie, Weinheim

Wyllie, A.H. (1992) Growth and neoplasia. In: *Muir's Textbook of Pathology*, 13th edn. Eds MacSween, R.N.M. and Whaley, K., pp. 355 – 410. Edward Arnold, London

6 The transmission and maintenance of infection

Infectious disease is the result of the invasion of a host by a pathogenic organism. The continued survival of infectious agents, with or without the induction of disease, depends on their successful transmission to a susceptible host, the instigation of an infection therein and replication of the agent to maintain the cycle of infection. The complete cycle of an infectious agent is its **life history (life-cycle)**. A knowledge of the life history of an infectious agent is essential when selecting the most applicable control technique (see Chapter 22). This involves knowledge of:

1. the modes of transmission and maintenance of infection;
2. the ecological conditions that favour the survival and transmission of infectious agents.

This chapter is concerned with the first topic; the second is considered in Chapter 7 with reference to basic ecology.

Transmission may be either **horizontal (lateral)** or **vertical**. Horizontally transmitted infections are those transmitted from any segment of a population to another; for example, influenza virus from one horse to a stable-mate. Vertically transmitted infections are transmitted from one generation to the next by infection of the embryo or foetus while in *utero* (in mammals) or *in ovo* (in birds, reptiles, amphibians, fish and arthropods). Transmission by milk to offspring is also considered, by some, to be vertical.

Horizontal transmission

Infections can be transmitted horizontally either **directly** or **indirectly** (*Figure 6.1*).

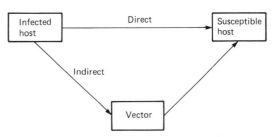

Fig. 6.1 Basic mechanisms of transmission of infectious agents.

Direct transmission occurs when a susceptible host contracts an infection, either by physical contact with an infected host or by contact with the latter's infected discharges (e.g., the transmission of canine distemper in infected urine and faeces).

Indirect transmission involves an intermediate vehicle, living or inanimate, that transmits infection between infected and susceptible hosts. This vehicle generally may be termed a **vector**, although the term is usually restricted, by common usage, to living carriers (see 'vector' below). Indirect transmission can involve a vector of a different species from that of the initially infected host. The life-cycle of infectious agents therefore may be complex with several different hosts. Details of specific life-cycles are not presented in this chapter, but a basic knowledge of veterinary microbiology and parasitology is assumed.

Airborne transmission of infectious agents, sometimes over long distances, is often defined as indirect, although it is more correctly classified as direct because no intermediate vehicle is involved.

Types of host and vector

A variety of terms describe the range of host/parasite relationships, and are used by the epidemiologist, proto-zoologist, entomologist, helminthologist and microbiologist. Each of these may use terms specific to his discipline, that have the same general meaning, from the point of view of the life-cycle of the disease, as different words from other disciplines; for example, **intermediate host** in helminthology and **biological vector** in entomology (see below).

Hosts

Host: a plant, animal or arthropod that is capable of being infected with, and therefore giving sustenance to, an infectious agent. Replication or development of the agent usually occurs in the host.

Definitive host: a parasitological term describing a host in which an organism undergoes its sexual phase of reproduction (e.g., *Taenia pisiformis* in dogs; *Plasmodium* spp. in mosquitoes).

Final host: a term used in a more general sense (i.e., in connection with all types of infectious agent) as a synonym for **definitive host**. Both 'final' and 'definitive' imply the 'end of the line', in other words the termination of a dynamic process. They are, in most cases, therefore, improperly used.

Primary (natural) host: an animal that maintains an infection in the latter's endemic area (e.g., dogs infected with distemper virus). Since an infectious agent frequently depends upon a primary host for its long-term existence, the host is also called a **maintenance host**.

Secondary host: a species that additionally is involved in the life-cycle of an agent, especially outside typical endemic areas (e.g., cattle infected with strains of foot-and-mouth virus that usually cycle in buffaloes). A secondary host sometimes can act as a maintenance host.

Paratenic host: a host in which an agent is transferred **mechanically**, without further development (e.g., fish, containing *Diphyllobothrium* spp. larvae, which are preyed upon by larger fish). This term is exclusive to helminthology, and could be considered to have its entomological analogue in the term **mechanical vector**.

Intermediate host: an animal in which an infectious agent undergoes some development, frequently with **asexual reproduction** (e.g., *Cysticercus pisiformis* in rabbits and hares). This term is parasitological in origin.

Amplifier host: an animal which, because of temporally associated changes in population dynamics that produce a sudden increase in the host population size, may suddenly increase the amount of infectious agent. Multiplication of the agent occurs in this type of host. This term is most commonly used in relation to virus diseases. An example is litters of baby pigs infected with Japanese encephalitis virus (*Figure 6.2*).

Hibernating host: an animal in which an agent is held, probably without replication, in a state of 'suspended animation' (e.g., hibernating snakes infected with either western, eastern or Japanese encephalitis virus).

Incidental (dead-end or **accidental) host:** one that does not usually transmit an infectious agent to other animals (e.g., bulls infected with *Brucella abortus*). 'Final' and 'definitive' can be applied validly to this type of host.

Link host: a host that forms a link between other host species (e.g., pigs linking infected herons to man in Japanese encephalitis: *Figure 6.2*).

Reservoir: a term commonly used as a synonym for, or prefix to, 'host'; (**reservoir host**). A reservoir host is one in which an infectious agent normally lives and multiplies, and therefore is a common source of infection to other animals. Thus, in Kenya, buffalo and waterbuck are reservoirs of bovine ephemeral fever virus, acting as a source of infection for cattle (Davies *et al.*, 1975). Similarly, in the tropics, cattle are reservoirs of bluetongue virus, and therefore can be sources of infection for sheep (Hourrigan and Klingsporn, 1975). Animals may

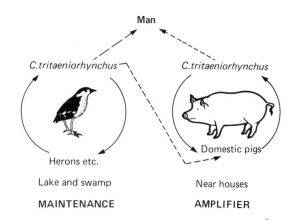

Fig. 6.2 The maintenance and amplifier hosts of Japanese encephalitis virus in Japan. The vector is the mosquito, *Culex tritaeniorhynchus*. (From Gordon Smith, 1976, based on Buescher *et al.*, 1959, and Scherer *et al.*, 1959.)

be important reservoirs of infection for humans. In Sierra Leone, the multimammate mouse, *Mastomys natalensis*, is the primary host and reservoir of Lassa fever, a virus disease with a high case fatality rate in man (Monath *et al.*, 1974). The mouse is adapted to life both within houses and in fields, and comes into contact with man in rural areas, particularly during the wet season, when it may seek shelter in houses, and thus may transmit the infection to man. Reservoirs may be primary or secondary hosts.

'Reservoir' is also used to refer to any substance that is a common source of infection (e.g., soil as a source of anthrax spores).

Vector: an animate transmitter of infectious agents. By common usage, vectors are defined as invertebrate animals — usually arthropods — that transmit infectious agents to vertebrates. The dictionary definition of the term implies independent movement, that is, a living vehicle. Inanimate carriers of agents (e.g., feed concentrates contaminated with *Salmonella* spp.) usually are called 'fomites' (singular: fomes, from the Greek meaning 'tinder'; because fomites were thought metaphorically to be the 'tinder' by which the 'fire' of an epidemic was ignited).

Mechanical vector: an animal (usually an arthropod) that physically carries an infectious agent to its primary or secondary host (e.g., mosquitoes and fleas transmitting myxomatosis virus between rabbits). The infectious agent neither multiplies nor develops in the mechanical vector.

Biological vector: a vector (usually an arthropod) in which an infectious agent undergoes either a necessary part of its life-cycle, or multiplication, before transmission to the natural or secondary host.

Three types of biological transmission occur:

1. **developmental transmission:** with an essential phase of development occurring in the vector (e.g., *Dirofilaria immitis* in mosquitoes);
2. **propagative transmission:** when the agent multiplies in the vector (e.g., louping ill virus in ixodid ticks);
3. **cyclopropagative transmission:** a combination of 1 and 2 (e.g., *Babesia* spp. in ticks).

Development in the vector involves migration of the infectious agent. Thus, two types of transmission are identified in the life-cycles of members of the protozoan genus *Trypanosoma*. The African trypanosomes that parasitize the blood and tissues of infected animals are ingested by insects of the genus *Glossina*, in which they undergo a developmental cycle that involves migration from their initial focus of infection in the midgut and back to the salivary glands, from which infective forms are released; this is **salivarian** transmission. In contrast, members of the species *Trypanosoma cruzi* (the cause of Chagas' disease in man in South America, with dogs, cats and some wild animals implicated as reservoirs) are ingested by bugs of the family *Reduviidae*, from which infective forms are shed in the faeces, human infection occurring by contamination of wounds and the eyes; this is **stercorarian** transmission.

Biological vectors are frequently either definitive or intermediate hosts; for example, mosquitoes are biological vectors and the definitive hosts of *Plasmodium* spp. (the cause of malaria).

Factors associated with the spread of infection

Three factors are important in the transmission of infection (Gordon Smith, 1982):

1. characteristics of hosts;
2. characteristics of pathogens;
3. effective contact.

Characteristics of hosts

A host's **susceptibility** and **infectiousness** determine its ability to transmit infection. Susceptibility to infection may be limited to a single species or group of species. For example, only equids are naturally susceptible to equine rhinopneumonitis virus infection. Alternatively, several widely different species may be susceptible to an infection; for example, all mammals are susceptible to rabies.

Susceptibility within a species may vary markedly and may be associated with selection of genetically resistant animals following exposure to an infectious agent. For example, the mortality in rabbits exposed experimentally to a standard dose of myxomatosis fell from 90% to 25% over a seven-year period (Fenner and Ratcliffe, 1965).

'Infectiousness' refers to:

1. the duration of the period when an animal is infective;
2. the relative amount of an infectious agent that an animal can transmit.

An animal is not infectious as soon as it is infected — a period of time elapses between infection and the shedding of the agent; this is a parasite's **prepatent** period, a virus'

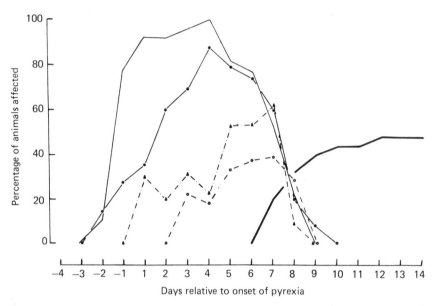

Fig. 6.3 Correlation of viraemia and virus excretion in cattle infected experimentally with virulent rinderpest virus (strain RGK/1): ———— viraemia; ●———● nasal excretion of virus; ▲······▲ urinary excretion of virus; ●---● faecal excretion of virus: ———— mortality. (From Liess and Plowright, 1964).

eclipse phase and a bacterium's **latent period**.* In contrast, the **incubation period** is the period of time between infection and the development of clinical signs. Thus, inapparent infections have a prepatent period, but do not have an incubation period. The **generation time** is the period between infection and maximum infectiousness. These periods, for a given agent and host species, are not the same for all animals but show natural variation. The frequency distribution of incubation periods, for example, follows a lognormal statistical distribution (see *Figure 12.4* and Sartwell, 1950, 1966).

Figure 6.3 plots the excretion of rinderpest virus in a group of experimentally infected cattle. It illustrates that nasal excretion is the most common form of shedding of the virus, that virus is shed **before** the appearance of clinical signs, and that, for **the group**, the period of maximum infectiousness is four days after the onset of clinical signs (i.e., pyrexia).

Diseases with short incubation periods run a clinical course, terminating in either recovery or death, relatively quickly. Thus, a high host density is required to ensure

that the agent's life-cycle can be perpetuated (*Figure 6.4*). An example is distemper virus infection of dogs, with an incubation period of four to five days. This disease therefore is endemic only in urban areas where there is a high density of dogs. In contrast, infectious diseases with

		Characteristic of host population		
		Low density	Mixed or changing densities	High density
Characteristic of infectious agent	Short incubation period	□	▼	▼▼▼▼▼ ▼▼
	Mixed incubation periods	▼▼▼	▼▼▼▼▼▼	▼▼▼▼▼▼
	Long incubation	▼▼▼▼▼	▼▼▼▼	▼▼▼▼▼

Fig. 6.4 The relationship between duration of incubation period of an infectious agent, density of the host, and the potential of the infectious agent to exist in a population. □: Conditions unfavourable for the existence of infectious agent. ▼: Conditions favourable for the existence of infectious agent; the number of triangles indicates the relative degree to which the conditions are favourable. (Modified from Macdonald and Bacon, 1980.)

*'Latent period' is also used for this time interval for infectious diseases in general. For non-infectious diseases, it is the interval between exposure to a cause and appearance of manifestations of disease. The latent period of canine bladder cancer, for example, is approximately four years (see Chapter 18).

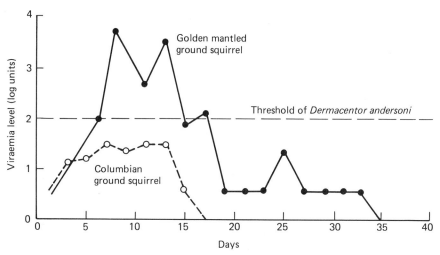

Fig. 6.5 Colorado tick fever: the relationships between viraemia levels in a maintenance host (the golden mantled ground squirrel) and an accidental host (the Columbian ground squirrel) and the threshold of infection of the arthropod maintenance host (*Dermacentor andersoni*). (From Gordon Smith, 1976, after Burgdorfer, 1960.)

long incubation periods can maintain their cycles of infection in varying animal densities (*Figure 6.4*); rabies is an example.

The time between infection and availability of an infectious agent in an arthropod vector is the agent's **extrinsic incubation period**.

For transmission to occur between a vertebrate host and an arthropod vector, an infectious agent must be present to a minimum concentration in the vertebrate host's circulation. This is the **threshold level**. Some vertebrate hosts may become infected, but are unable to transmit infection to arthropods because the threshold level is not achieved. These are therefore 'dead-end' hosts. For example (*Figure 6.5*), the Columbian ground squirrel is an incidental (dead-end) host for Colorado tick fever. However, when the virus infects and multiplies in the golden mantled ground squirrel, the threshold level is attained; therefore the vector, the tick *Dermacentor andersoni*, can ingest virus particles, and this squirrel can act as a maintenance host.

Characteristics of pathogens

Three important characteristics of pathogens that affect transmission of infectious agents are **infectivity**, **virulence** and **stability**.

Infectivity relates to the amount of an organism that is required to initiate infection. The infectivity of different organisms varies considerably. For example, the **particle:infectivity ratio** (the number of virus particles required

to instigate infection) of bacterial viruses (bacteriophages) in tissue culture is approximately 1:1, indicating a high degree of infectivity. Lower degrees of infectivity are demonstrated by animal viruses, with ratios of between 10:1 and 100:1. Plant viruses have an even lower infectivity, with a ratio of approximately 1000:1. Infectivity can vary between different strains of the same organism, and can depend upon the route of the infection, and the age and innate resistance of the host.

When an agent is capable of infecting more than one species, its infectivity for different hosts is often quite different. For instance, the infective dose of strains of *Campylobacter jejuni* isolated from chickens is only 500 bacteria for chickens, whereas the infective dose of strains of the same bacterium isolated from seagulls is above 10^7 for chickens. This example illustrates that the infectivity of an agent cannot be specified without reference to the host that it infects.

Virulence (see Chapter 5) also affects transmission and can change. Repeated passage through the same species of animal tends to increase virulence for that species but to simultaneously lower virulence for the original natural host. Thus, serial passage of Ross River virus in suckling mice increases its virulence for mice (Taylor and Marshall, 1975), but alternate passage in mice and the mosquito *Aedes aegypti* does not alter virulence. In contrast, when Edwards (1928) passaged rinderpest virus of bovine origin serially through several hundred goats, its virulence for cattle dramatically decreased, enabling production of the first veterinary modified live virus vaccine.

The length of time for which an organism can remain infective outside its host is the organism's **stability**. Some organisms survive only for short periods of time, that is they are very **labile** (e.g., *Leptospira* spp. in dry environments). Stability is frequently facilitated by protective capsules, such as those forming the outer layer of bacterial spores (e.g., *Bacillus anthracis*). The hazards presented to infectious agents by the external environment, and techniques of achieving stability, are discussed later in this chapter.

Effective contact

Effective contact describes the conditions under which infection is likely to occur. For a particular infection, it depends on the stability of the organism and the routes by which the organism leaves an infected host and enters a susceptible one.

Effective contact may be very short (e.g., seasonally transmitted, vector-borne diseases) or potentially of many years' duration (e.g., anthrax spores in soil). The duration of infectiousness determines the number of susceptibles that can be infected by an infected animal. Thus, upper respiratory tract infections (e.g., kennel cough in dogs) result in short periods of infectiousness of several days' duration, whereas cows infected with bovine tuberculosis may excrete the bacterium in their milk for several years.

Behaviour, which may be changed during infection, can also affect the likelihood of effective contact. Thus, feral animals that are naturally shy of man may enter houses when they contract rabies, therefore increasing the likelihood of human infection.

The pathogenesis of disease may increase the likelihood of transmission; for example, respiratory diseases may induce coughing and sneezing, thereby spreading respiratory pathogens to near neighbours.

Routes of infection

The site or sites by which an infectious agent gains entry to a host, and by which it leaves the host, are the agent's routes of infection. *Figure 6.6* illustrates the main sites of infection of mammalian hosts.

The oral route

Infection via the mouth is one of the more common routes of entry, especially in relation to the enteric organisms which often 'escape' from an infected animal in the faeces. Organisms such as rotaviruses, *Salmonella* spp.

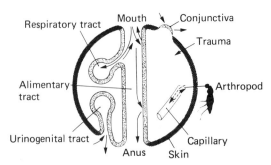

Fig. 6.6 Body surfaces as sites of horizontal infection and shedding of infectious agents. (Modified from Mims, 1987.)

and gastrointestinal parasites may contaminate water and foodstuffs, which then act as fomites. Ingested agents may be excreted in the faeces, producing the **faecal−oral** transmission cycle.

Agents that gain entry to the body orally may be disseminated from the infected animal by a variety of routes, apart from in the faeces. *Brucella abortus* often infects cows orally but is excreted later in the milk and uterine discharges. Similar circumstances occur in relation to infection of ruminants with the rickettsia *Coxiella burnetii*, the cause of Q fever. Such agents may then be retransmitted by both the oral and other routes. Although some organisms can be transmitted by the oral route, the low pH of gastric secretions is an effective barrier against this method of transmission for a wide variety of organisms.

The respiratory route

The respiratory route is also a common method of transmission for many infectious agents, including those that are not restricted to the respiratory tract (e.g., *Salmonella typhimurium*: Wathes *et al.*, 1988). Infectious agents seldom occur as individual airborne particles, but are usually associated with other organic matter in the form of droplets or dust. The nature and size of such composite particles affect their dispersal and stability. Particles of a diameter of 5 nm or greater do not reach the alveoli of the lung and therefore initially cause infection only of the upper respiratory tract.

Infections spread by the respiratory route are more likely to occur where population densities are high and ventilation is poor. Examples of such conditions are enzootic pneumonia in intensively reared pigs, and occupationally acquired brucellosis in meat workers. In environmental extremes, diseases that are rarely spread by the respiratory route become transmissible by this method. These circumstances arise in the airborne transmission of rabies from insectivorous bats to animals and man within the confines of a cave. Similarly, African swine fever virus, which is usually transmitted by *Ornithodoros* spp. ticks, spreads rapidly by the oral route in piggeries. In crowded and poor living conditions, pneumonic plague is transmitted directly between people, rather than by the bites of infected fleas, the latter method of transmission inducing the less severe bubonic plague.

Infection via skin, cornea and mucous membranes

Transmission via the skin is **percutaneous** (Latin: *per* = through, across; *cut* = skin). Certain agents infect only the skin and transmission is always by direct contact with either another infected animal or a fomes; examples are 'ringworm' and ectoparasitic infestations. The incidence of such infections and infestations is particularly influenced by the population density of the susceptible hosts. Intact skin acts as an effective barrier to the majority of infectious agents, but some, particularly the immature stages of some nematodes and trematodes, can penetrate this barrier and cause infection. Examples include blood fluke (*Schistosoma* spp.) and hookworm (*Ancylostoma* spp.) infections, the latter infection also being zoonotic and the cause of cutaneous larva migrans in man.

If the skin is cut or abraded then infection by a variety of organisms can occur, resulting in localized infections of the skin (e.g. by *Staphylococcus* spp. and the cutaneous form of human anthrax). Other agents, such as leptospires and swine vesicular disease virus) may gain entry to the body percutaneously and then develop a more generalized infection.

Another important form of percutaneous infection is from bites by both vertebrates and arthropods. Agents that are present in the saliva, such as the viruses of rabies and lymphocytic choriomeningitis, and bacteria such as *Streptobacillus moniliformis* (a common inhabitant of the oropharynx of rats), are transmitted by animal bites. Diseases transmitted by the bites of infected arthropod vectors constitute a particular class of infections that was introduced earlier in this chapter during the description of hosts and vectors.

Infection of the cornea may remain localized; for example, bovine keratoconjunctivitis caused by *Moraxella bovis*. Alternatively, the infection may spread to other parts of the body; for instance, corneal infection of birds with Newcastle disease virus.

Although few diseases can be transmitted through intact skin, several can infect undamaged mucous membranes. An important class of such agents is those that are very labile in the external environment, and require intimate sexual contact during coitus to be transmitted to the urogenital tract; for example, *Trypanosoma equiperdum* in horses.

Methods of transmission

Six main methods of transmission, which bring infectious agents into contact with the sites of infection, can be identified:

1. ingestion;
2. aerial transmission;
3. contact;
4. inoculation;
5. iatrogenic transmission;
6. coitus.

Ingestion

This may occur via a mechanical vehicle (fomes), for example contaminated water, or by ingestion of intermediate hosts, such as cestode cysts in meat. Ingested agents are usually excreted in the faeces, producing the faecal–oral transmission cycle. Some agents are excreted only faecally because they are localized to the intestine (e.g., the Johne's disease bacillus in cattle). Other agents, if they invade the bloodstream, can be excreted by additional means, such as the urine (e.g., *Salmonella* spp.). Sometimes, agents are excreted on the breath (e.g., reoviruses and rinderpest virus).

Aerial transmission

This involves airborne transmission of infectious agents via contaminated air. It is the usual method of transmission with the hardy spores of fungi and some bacteria, and also occurs with pathogens of the respiratory tract that are expired on the breath of infected animals and enter susceptible ones during inspiration.

Quasistable suspensions of liquids or solids in gases, which are capable of floating for some time, are formed only when droplet diameters do not exceed 5 nm. Expiratory droplets range in size from 15 to 100 nm and thus even the smallest sediment rapidly (within 3 s). Therefore, they cannot travel far. Direct infection from expiratory droplets is thus limited to the area directly in front of the infected individual (the 'expiratory cone'). Very localized droplet infection can occur on food bowls and by sniffing.

Aerosol transmission is a type of airborne transmission involving transmission via an aerosol, which is defined variously as (1) any solution in the form of a fine spray in

Table 6.1 Common pathogens of pigs and poultry known to be transmitted aerially. (From Wathes, 1987.)

Bacteria

Bordetella bronchiseptica	*Mycobacterium tuberculosis*
Brucella suis	*Mycoplasma gallisepticum*
Corynebacterium equi	*Mycoplasma hyorhinus*
Erysipelothrix rhusiopathiae	*Mycoplasma suipneumoniae*
Escherichia coli	*Pasteurella multicoda*
Haemophilus gallinarus	*Pasteurella pseudotuberculosis*
Haemophilus parasuis	*Salmonella pullorum*
Haemophilus pleuropneumoniae	*Salmonella typhimurium*
Listeria monocytogenes	*Staphylococcus aureus*
Leptospira pomona	*Streptococcus suis* type II
Mycobacterium avium	

Fungi

Aspergillus flavus	*Coccidioides immitis*
Aspergillus fumigatus	*Cryptococcus neoformans*
Aspergillus nidulans	*Histoplasma farcinorum*
Aspergillus niger	*Rhinosporidium seeberi*

Rickettsia

Coxiella burnetii

Protozoa

Toxoplasma gondii

Viruses

African swine fever	Infectious nephrosis of fowls
Avian encephalomyelitis	Infectious porcine encephalomyelitis
Avian leukosis	Marek's disease
Foot-and-mouth disease	Newcastle disease
Fowl plague	Ornithosis
Hog cholera	Porcine enterovirus
Inclusion body rhinitis	Swine influenza
Infectious bronchitis of fowls	Transmissible gastroenteritis of swine
Infectious laryngotracheitis of fowls	

which the droplets approximate colloidal size (1 − 100 nm), and (2) finely divided virus particles hanging or floating in air. Thus, quasistable suspensions and expiratory droplets can both be involved in aerosol transmission.

Some agents that are not primarily pathogens of the respiratory tract can contaminate the air and therefore may also be airborne. An example is foot-and-mouth disease virus shed from ruptured vesicles (Gloster *et al.*, 1981). (See also 'Long-distance transmission of infection' below.) Similarly, some *Salmonella* spp. infections are airborne and infect animals via the conjunctiva (Moore, 1957).

Table 6.1 lists some common pathogens of pigs and poultry that can be transmitted aerially.

Contact

Contact transmission is transmission without transmission factors (e.g., mechanical vectors) and without participa-

tion of an external medium. This is particularly important in relation to infectious agents that are shed from the body surfaces, such as vesicular viruses, and with agents that gain entry through the body surface. Very few agents are transmitted merely by touch; some degree of trauma is necessary, albeit microscopic. Transmission may be by bites (e.g., rabies and rat bite fever), or by scratches (e.g., cat scratch fever).

Diseases transmitted by contact may be described as 'contagious' (Latin: *contagio* = to touch closely) but this term now is used less commonly than previously.

Inoculation

Inoculation (Latin: *inoculatus* = engrafted, or implanted) is the introduction into the body, by puncture of the skin or through a wound, of infectious agents.

Although classified separately here, inoculation is frequently associated with contact transmission (e.g., bites from rabid dogs). Arthropods that act as vectors may inoculate infectious agents into the blood by biting (e.g., tsetse flies infected with *Trypanosoma* spp., in which development of the parasite occurs in the salivary gland, gut and mouth parts).

Iatrogenic transmission

Iatrogenic literally means 'created by a doctor'. Thus, an iatrogenically transmitted infection is one that is tranferred during surgical and medical practice.

There are two main types, involving:

1. introduction of pathogens by dirty instruments (e.g., during non-aseptic surgery and tattooing) or by contaminated body surfaces;
2. introduction of pathogens contaminating prophylactic or therapeutic preparations (e.g., *Pseudomonas aeruginosa* in intramammary dry-cow antibiotic preparations: Nicholls *et al.*, 1981; lumpy skin disease in anaplasmosis vaccine; scrapie in louping ill vaccine; human hepatitis B virus in serum preparations) and, more rarely, by organ transplantation (e.g., rabies virus by corneal transplants).

Coitus

Some infectious agents may be transmitted during coitus. Certain diseases are transmitted only in this way. These were called venereal diseases (Latin: *venereus* = pertaining to sexual love). In human medicine they are now referred to as sexually transmitted diseases (STDs). Sexual transmission can occur not only in vertebrates but also in arthropods. For example, African swine fever virus can be sexually transmitted from male to female ticks of the genus *Ornithodoros* (Plowright *et al.*, 1974).

The mode of transmission of agents frequently governs the epidemic picture. Thus, agents that are transmitted by the faecal–oral and airborne modes often produce sudden explosive epidemics, whereas coitally transmitted diseases spread more slowly, over a long period of time.

Long-distance transmission of infection

Infectious diseases can be transmitted by the methods described above over long distances as a result of the mobility of infected animals, microorganisms and parasites, vectors and fomites. Previously, transportation by sea provided a period of quarantine, but the increasing use

of air transport means that animals incubating infections can arrive at their destination before clinical signs of infection have appeared. The movement of horses, in connection with their sale, breeding and competition, has spread a variety of equine infections, including contagious equine metritis, equine infectious anaemia, piroplasmosis and influenza, between continents (Powell, 1985). The movement of people, for example by aeroplane, can also distribute exotic human diseases over all parts of the world (Prothro, 1977).

There is concern that the screw-worm fly, *Chrysomyia bezziana*, which is endemic in Papua New Guinea, may be imported into Australia as an inadvertent passenger on international flights, or by animal movement between the Torres Strait Islands (see the case study in Chapter 20 for further details). The importation of infested animals from Uruguay to Libya has also spread this fly.

Airborne transmission over long distances cannot occur with expiratory droplets because they sediment rapidly (see above). Transmission of respiratory and vesicular infections through the air over long distances (aerial transmission) must, therefore, be effected by other means. The evaporation of water from droplets (which can occur when droplets are airborne or on the ground) produces desiccated **droplet nuclei**, ranging in diameter from 2 nm to 10 nm. The smallest of these are quasistable and can travel over long distances, assisted by wind. The rate of formation of these nuclei depends on the temperature and relative humidity. Rain sediments the nuclei.

The distribution pattern of the nuclei can be complex. During the 1967–68 foot-and-mouth disease epidemic in England, a series of secondary outbreaks followed the primary one (*Figure 6.7a*). Initially, it was suggested that this was due to infected imported lamb, because no human or mechanical links could be established between the secondary outbreaks and the primary outreak at Bryn Farm. However, a complex meteorological hypothesis has been presented (Tinline, 1970, 1972) suggesting that the secondary outbreaks were caused by virus particles being pulled downwards in a current of air, which is forced into vertical oscillation as it flows over a hill. This phenomenon is called a **lee wave** (*Figure 6.7b*).

Another, more general model of airborne transmission of foot-and-mouth disease virus uses the meteorological **Gaussian plume** model for atmospheric diffusion (Hanna *et al.*, 1982) which is the basic model for dispersion calculations. This predicts horizontal elliptical spread, the shape of the virus-laden plume depending on wind speed, downwind distance from the source of infection, and air stability.

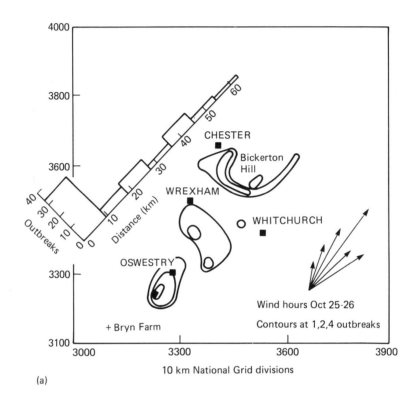

(a)

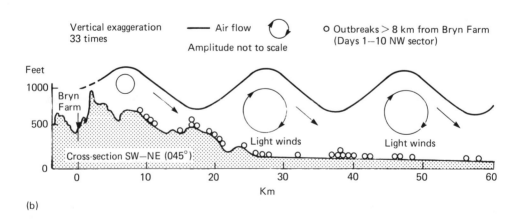

(b)

Fig. 6.7 1967–68 English foot-and-mouth disease epidemic: (a) outbreaks for days 1–10: (b) profile through Bryn Farm illustrating the lee wave hypothesis of aerial spread of virus. (Reprinted by permission from *Nature*, Vol. 227, pp. 860–862. Copyright © 1970 Macmillan Journals Limited.)

Identification of isolates of Aujeszky's disease virus using molecular epidemiological techniques has also suggested that airborne transmission of this virus over long distances can occur (Christensen *et al.*, 1990, 1993). Similarly, studies of outbreaks of vesicular stomatitis, based on nucleotide fingerprinting and trajectory analysis of winds, suggest that wind could have been responsible for carrying infection from Mexico to the US (Sellers and Maarouf, 1990). There is also evidence for airborne transmission of the virus causing porcine reproductive and respiratory syndrome (Beilage *et al.*, 1991; Mortensen and Madsen, 1992).

Wind can also carry vectors over long distances. The outbreak of bluetongue in Portugal in 1956 (point map: see *Figure 4.6*) may have been caused by windborne transfer of the African vector, *Culicoides imicola*, from North Africa, although the latter is now permanently established in Portugal (Mellor *et al.*, 1985). African horse sickness can also be transferred in a similar way.

Transmission can also involve more complex relationships. Thus, Crimean–Congo haemorrhagic fever virus infects its vector, *Hyalomma* spp. ticks, which are then carried by migrating birds from the Crimea to Africa where they are responsible for outbreaks of the disease (Hoogstraal, 1979).

Vertical transmission

Types and methods of vertical transmission

There are two types of vertical transmission: **hereditary** and **congenital**.

Hereditarily transmitted diseases are carried within the genome of either parent. Thus, retroviruses, which have integrated DNA copies of the virus in the host's genome, are transferred hereditarily.

Congenitally transmitted diseases are, literally, those present at birth. According to strict etymology, hereditarily transmitted diseases are a part of this group. However, by common usage, 'congenital' refers to diseases **acquired** either *in utero* or *in ovo*, rather than inherited.

Transmission can occur at various stages of embryonic development. It may produce either abortion, if incompatible with life, or teratoma (literally 'monsters'). Alternatively, infection which is inapparent and continuous after birth (**innate infection**) can occur.

Germinative transmission

This involves either infection of the superficial layers of the ovary, or infection of the ovum itself. Examples include the chicken leucosis viruses, spontaneous lymphoid leukaemias of mice (Gross, 1955), murine lymphocytic choriomeningitis and avian salmonellosis.

Transmission to the embryo

This is via the placenta (transplacentally) or via the foetal circulation, through the placenta, to the foetus. For example, kittens can be transplacentally infected with feline panleucopenia virus (Csiza *et al.*, 1971). Viruses, being small, cross the placenta with greater ease and earlier in pregnancy than larger microbes. The foetal circulation, however, can carry most microbes. Infection of the placenta does not always produce infection of the foetus. Q fever particles, for instance, may be found in large quantities in bovine placentae without infection of the developing calves.

Ascending infection

This is infection that is transmitted from the lower genital canal to the amnion and placenta (e.g., some *Staphylococcus* and *Streptococcus* spp. infections).

Infection at parturition

This is infection acquired from the lower genital canal at birth (e.g., human herpes simplex infection).

Immunological status and vertical transmission

The immunological status of the foetus is important when agents are transmitted vertically. Immune tolerance of microbial antigens by the foetus can be detrimental in postnatal life, because 'non-self' antigens are then recognized as 'self'. The result is a lack of a protective immune response, sometimes with the development of a carrier state with the subsequent dangers to other susceptible animals, as in the case of feline panleucopenia. However, immune tolerance by the foetus can occasionally be advantageous when infections have clinical and pathological effects mediated by the immune response. The paradigm of this is lymphocytic choriomeningitis (LCM) infection of mice. In adults the disease is mediated by a lethal infiltration of the brain by responsive T lymphocytes. Prenatal infection induces a tolerance to LCM virion antigens; therefore no lymphocytic infiltration occurs in adult infections, and thus there is no clinical disease.

Transovarial and trans-stadial transmission in arthropods

Some arthropods, notably ticks and mites, transmit bacteria, viruses and protozoa from one generation to

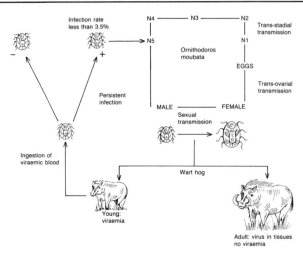

Fig. 6.8 Transmission cycle of African swine fever virus in warthogs and *Ornithodoros moubata* N = Nymphal stage. (Modified from Wilkinson, 1984.)

another via their eggs; this is **transovarial** transmission. Examples of transovarially transmitted infections include bovine anaplasmosis (a protozoan disease causing anaemia in cattle in the tropics and subtropics, transmitted by several genera of ticks) and canine babesiosis (another protozoan disease causing anaemia in dogs, transmitted by ticks of the genera *Dermacentor* and *Haemaphysalis*).

In contrast, some arthropods only transmit infections from one developmental stage to another (e.g., in ticks: larva to nymph, nymph to adult); this is **trans-stadial** transmission. An example of a trans-stadially transmitted disease is theileriosis, caused by protozoa of the genus *Theileria*, occurring in cattle, sheep and goats, and transmitted by ticks of the genus *Rhipicephalus*.

Some infections are spread both transovarially and trans-stadially; for example, Nairobi sheep disease, a virus infection transmitted by the brown tick, *Rhipicephalus appendiculatus*. Investigations of tick-transmitted diseases are revealing that many infections, once thought to be transmitted by only one of these methods, are transmitted by both.

Some infections involve transovarial, trans-stadial and sexual transmission in arthropods. Thus, in Africa, African swine fever virus is primarily maintained in the tick *Ornithodoros moubata* by these three methods of transmission (*Figure 6.8*). Warthogs are infected by the bite of the tick, but there is neither horizontal nor vertical transmission between them, and only a small proportion of nymphal ticks are persistently infected when they bite young warthogs during a brief viraemic phase.

Maintenance of infection

Hazards to infectious agents

The transmission of infection involves some stages when the infectious agent is in the host, and others when it is in the external environment or in a vector, or in both (*Figure 6.1*). Both internal and external environments present hazards to infectious agents.

The environment within the host

The host has its natural defence mechanisms: surface-active chemicals, specific reactive cells, phagocytes and humoral antibodies. The successful parasite must be able to avoid, in part, these mechanisms, and must also avoid competition with other agents that may simultaneously infect the host in a similar niche (see Chapter 7). Parasites have evolved strategies to resist the host's protective mechanisms, such as acid-resistant helminth cuticles (to resist gastric acid) and an intracellular mode of life (to avoid humoral antibodies). Some bacteria possess capsules that protect them against phagocytosis, for example *Pneumococcus* spp. (*Figure 6.9*). Many parasitic nematodes have a greater fecundity than their free-living counterparts (*Table 6.2*), thus ensuring that some offspring will survive the host's immune response and potentially lethal conditions in the external environment.

The external environment

The two main hazards presented by the external environment are desiccation and ultraviolet light. Desiccation is

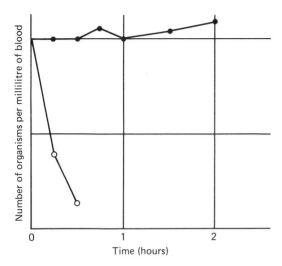

Fig. 6.9 The protective action of bacterial capsules: pneumococci, capsulated (●) and not capsulated (○), injected intravenously into mice; blood of mice then sampled every 15 minutes. (From Boycott, 1971.)

not always lethal, but frequently inhibits multiplication. Low temperatures are not usually lethal, but can inhibit multiplication. The high temperatures attained in temperate climates are probably not lethal but those reached in tropical countries may be more effective. Many agents may be partially protected from desiccation by being discharged in moist carriers such as faeces and urine. They may also persist by being shed into favourable surroundings; leptospires, for example, persist longer in paddy fields than in semi-arid regions. Some agents (e.g., the pox viruses) are resistant to desiccation and can survive for long periods in dry infected scab material. Agents may also survive in inanimate material in the environment, which may therefore act as a fomes; for example, animal foodstuffs contaminated with *Salmonella* spp.

Maintenance strategies

The ways in which infectious agents are maintained can be considered as **strategies** for maintenance. Five main strategies can be identified:

1. avoidance of a stage in the external environment;
2. the development of resistant forms;
3. a 'rapidly-in, rapidly-out' strategy;
4. persistence within the host;
5. extension of host range.

Avoidance of a stage in the external environment

Some agents avoid transfer via the environment. There are four main methods:

1. by vertical transmission;
2. by venereal transmission;
3. by vector transmission;
4. by transmission by sarcophagy (flesh eating); for example, the helminth *Trichinella spiralis* occurs in cysts in the muscle of pigs, rats and other animals, and is only transmitted when these animals are eaten by predators and scavengers, including man; 'salmon poisoning' is another example (see *Figure 7.7*).

Resistant forms

The harshness of the external environment can be buffered by surrounding the infectious agent with a shell that is resistant to heat and desiccation. Some bacteria form such shells (spores). Examples include members of the genera *Clostridium* and *Bacillus*, which can survive boiling water, even flames, for short periods of time, and may survive in the external environment for decades. Fungi may also produce spores. Generally these are less resistant than bacterial spores. Some helminths and protozoa form resistant shells (cysts). These can protect the agent from the host's defence mechanisms; the protozoan parasite, *Toxoplasma gondii*, for example, can survive for many years in its cystic form in the host, until the latter is eaten. Thick-shelled helminth eggs can resist the external environment and may overwinter on pasture.

'Rapidly-in, rapidly-out' strategy

Some agents enter the host, replicate and leave very quickly, before the host has time to mount an immune response or die. Many viruses of the upper respiratory tract can do this within 24 hours. The strategy requires a continuous supply of susceptible hosts. This may be one reason why respiratory and enteric infections, such as the common cold virus in man, are not present in primitive societies of low population density, and may not have occurred in small prehistoric societies (Brothwell and Sandison, 1967; Black, 1975).

Persistence within the host

Infectious agents may persist within the host, sometimes for life. Persistence occurs because the host's defence mechanisms fail to eliminate agents. This failure may arise because microorganisms adapt to the host's phago-

Table 6.2 The comparative fecundity of *Platyhelminthes* and *Nemathelminthes*. (From Dobson *et al.*, 1992.)

Species	Fecundity	Host
Free-living species	(young/adult/breeding season)	
Turbellaria		
Polycelis nigra	2.5	
P. tenuis	1.0	
Dugesia polychroa	0.8 – 1.7	
Planaria torva	4.9 – 15.2	
Dendrocoelom lacteum	4.9 – 10.3	
Bdellocephala punctata	16.0	
Parasitic species	(eggs/worm/day)	
Digenea		
Schistosoma mansoni	100	Hamster
Cestoda		
Echinococcus granulosus	600	Dog
Hymenolepis diminuta	200 000	Rat
Taenia saginata	720 000	Man
Acanthocephala		
Moniliformis moniliformis	5 000	Rat
Nematoda		
Ascaris lumbricoides	200 000	Pig
Enterbius vermicularis	11 000	Man
Wuchereria bancrofti	12 500	Man

cytic cells, or develop strategies for avoiding the host's immune response (Mims, 1987). The latter include **immunosuppression** and **tolerance**.

Immunosuppression results in the agents being maintained in the host for varying periods of time. It may be general or antigen-specific. General immunosuppression is demonstrated by some viruses (e.g., rinderpest) and protozoa (e.g., *T. gondii*), and facilitates survival of these and other agents in the host. Antigen-specific immunosuppression only involves the response to the infecting microorganism, the responses to other agents being unaffected. Human leprosy and tuberculosis induce this type of immunosuppression.

Tolerance is due to a primary lack of responsiveness by the host, rather than active suppression. This can occur prenatally; the example of LCM has been given earlier in this chapter. It can also occur when there are large amounts of circulating antigen or antigen–antibody complexes; for instance, in human leishmaniasis and cryptococcosis. Tolerance is sometimes found in infections with microorganisms that have antigens similar to normal host antigens (e.g., *Bacterioides* spp. infections in

mice). It has been suggested that such 'molecular mimicry' is generally associated with tolerance, but the evidence is equivocal.

Other means of avoiding the host's immune response are **antigenic variation** (see Chapter 5), **intracellular parasitism** (see Chapter 7), multiplication in **sites inaccessible** to the immune response (e.g., mammary tumour virus of mice, infecting the lumenal surface of the mammary gland), and the induction of **ineffective antibodies** (e.g., Aleutian disease virus of mink).

Other examples of persistent infections are *Mycobacterium johnei*, tapeworm infections of the gut, and *T. spiralis* in tissues. Specific types of persistent infection (latent and chronic infection, and the carrier state) have already been discussed in Chapter 5.

Persistence can be associated with a long incubation or prepatent period. A group of virus diseases, termed 'slow virus diseases' because of their long incubation period, fall into this category. Maedi-visna, for example, is a slow virus disease of sheep, producing neurological and respiratory signs, with an incubation period of 2 – 8 years. Similarly, scrapie is a virus-like disease, also of

Table 6.3 Some characteristics of host/parasite relationships between fleas, acting as vectors, and infectious agents. (Simplified from Bibikova, 1977.)

Disease and pathogen	Site of pathogen in flea	Reproduction of pathogen in flea	Duration of pathogen in flea	Pathogenic effect on flea
Myxomatosis *Fibromavirus myxomatosis*	Digestive tract	No	Up to 100 days	Yes
Tularaemia *Francisella tularensis*	Digestive tract	No	Several days	No
Murine typhus *Rickettsia mooseri*	Digestive tract	Yes	Lifetime	No
Murine trypanosomiasis *Trypanosoma lewisi*	Digestive tract	Yes	Lifetime	No
Salmonellosis *Salmonella enteritidis*	Digestive tract	Yes	Up to 40 days	Yes
Plague *Yersinia pestis*	Digestive tract	Yes	Several months to over 1 year	Yes

sheep, which produces neurological signs and has an incubation period of 1−5 years. Its persistence within its host facilitates vertical and possibly horizontal transmission in a flock.

Alternatively, an agent's prepatent period may be relatively short, but excretion of the agent may continue for a long time (i.e., the period of infectiousness is long). Excretion may be intermittent; for example, *Salmonella* spp. infection can be associated with intermittent clinical episodes or subclinical infection, both associated with occasional excretion of the bacterium. Infection may also result in continuous excretion. For instance, infection of cattle by *Leptospira*, serovar *hardjo*, results in urinary excretion of the bacterium that can last for 12−24 months. The long period of infectiousness of hosts infected with such agents ensures that a susceptible population, resulting from regular births, is always available. Some endogenous agents (see Chapter 5) may persist as the bacterial flora of hosts.

Agents may persist not only within vertebrate hosts but also in arthropod vectors. African swine fever virus, for example, persists in ticks for up to 8 months (Haresnape and Wilkinson, 1989). *Table 6.3* lists the duration of infection of fleas by various microbial agents. Note that some agents (e.g., murine typhus) can persist in fleas for the latter's lifetime, which can be very long — over 500 days in the case of unfed *Pulex irritans* (Soulsby, 1982). Additionally, agents can persist in flea excreta for long periods; murine typhus, for example, can persist for over nine years (Smith, 1973).

Extension of host range

Many infectious agents can infect more than one host. Indeed, their number exceeds that of one-host agents. In man, for example, over 80% of infectious agents to which he is susceptible are shared by other species of animal. An important role of the veterinarian is to control these zoonoses (e.g., tuberculosis and canine ascarid infections). Some infections of various hosts are inapparent, increasing the difficulty of control. For example, the bacterium *Borrellia burgdorferi*, the tick-transmitted cause of Lyme disease in man and other animals, also inapparently infects several wild and domestic mammals and birds which maintain the infection in Europe and the US (Anderson, 1988).

Extension of host range is an obvious way of maintaining infection. It is facilitated by the presence of the various hosts in the same area. However, if an agent is present in two different species in the same region, it should not be assumed that transfer between these species always occurs. In Africa, for example, foot-and-mouth disease virus infections occur in both cattle and wild buffalo, but the virus rarely spreads from one species to the other (*Figure 6.10a*). Other possible relationships between cattle and game are illustrated in *Figure 6.10*. Antelope cannot maintain the infection in their own

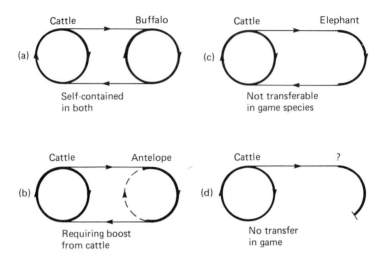

Fig. 6.10 Hypothetical interrelationship of foot-and-mouth disease in cattle and game species; see text for explanation. (From Brooksby, 1972.)

species unless it is boosted by occasional transmission to cattle (*Figure 6.10b*). Elephant can carry the virus from cattle to cattle, but cannot transmit it to members of their own species (*Figure 6.10c*). Several species of wild animals also act as dead-end hosts and are incapable of transmitting the virus to other animals (*Figure 6.10d*).

Further Reading

Appel, M.J. (Ed.) (1987) *Virus Infections of Vertebrates*, Vol. 1. *Virus Infections of Carnivores*. Elsevier, Amsterdam

Blaha, T. (Ed.) (1989) *Applied Veterinary Epidemiology*. Elsevier, Amsterdam. (*Includes details of the transmission and maintenance of the major infectious diseases of domestic animals*)

Fine, P.E.M. (1975) Vectors and vertical transmission: an epidemiologic perspective. *Annals of the New York Academy of Sciences*, **266**, 173–194

Gordon Smith, C.E. (1982) Major factors in the spread of infections. In: *Animal Disease in Relation to Animal Conservation*. Symposium of the Zoological Society of London No. 50. Eds Edwards, M.A. and McDonnell, U., pp. 207–235. Academic Press, London and New York

Matumoto, M. (1969) Mechanisms of perpetuation of animal viruses in nature. *Bacteriological Reviews*, **33**, 404–418

Mims, C.A., Playfair, J.H.L., Roitt, I.M., Wakelin, D. and Williams, R. (1993) *Medical Microbiology*. Mosby Europe, London. (*A description of host/parasite relationships, host defence mechanisms and microbial strategies for transmission*)

Mims, C.A. (1987) *The Pathogenesis of Infectious Disease*, 3rd edn. Academic Press, London and New York

Sewell, M.M.H. and Brocklesby, D.W. (Eds) (1990) *Handbook on Animal Diseases in the Tropics*, 4th edn. Ballière Tindall, London. (*A description of tropical infectious diseases of animals, including concise summaries of transmission and maintenance*)

Woldehiwet, Z. and Ristic, M. (Eds) (1993) *Rickettsial and Chlamydial Diseases of Domestic Animals*. Pergamon Press, Oxford

7 The ecology of disease

The study of disease in populations requires an understanding of the relationships between organisms (hosts and agents) and their environment. These relationships govern the spatial and temporal occurrence of disease. Climate, for example, affects the survival of hosts and infectious agents and the distribution of the latter's vectors either directly or, more subtly, by regulating the occurrence of plants that support the organisms. Similarly, the type of plant can affect the availability of minerals and trace elements and therefore the occurrence of disease associated with a deficiency, an excess, or an imbalance of these chemicals. For instance, white clover (*Trifolium repens*) absorbs relatively small amounts of selenium, whereas brown top (*Agrostis tenuis*) absorbs large amounts (Davies and Watkinson, 1966). Therefore, when pasture is top-dressed with selenium salts to prevent selenium deficiency in animals, the risk of selenium toxicity is greater if the latter plant predominates.

The study of animals and plants in relation to their habits and habitation (habitat) is **ecology** (Greek: *oikos* = house; *logo-* = discoursing). Ecology developed as a discipline relating to animals and plants, but has been extended to include microorganisms (e.g., Alexander, 1971). The scale of ecological studies therefore ranges from an investigation of leptospires in the 'environment' of the renal tubules to the distribution of sylvatic hosts of foot-and-mouth disease in the African savannahs. The study of a disease's ecology (also termed its natural history) is frequently a part of epidemiological investigations. This has two objectives:

1. an increase in the understanding of the pathogenesis, maintenance and, for infectious agents, transmission of disease;
2. the use of knowledge of a disease's ecology to predict when and where a disease may occur, to enable the development of suitable control techniques.

This chapter introduces basic ecological concepts and relates them to epidemiology.

Basic ecological concepts

Two major factors that determine the occurrence of disease are the distribution and size of animal populations. The former depends on the distribution of suitable food; the latter depends on availability of food and mates, and the species' breeding potential.

The distribution of populations

Vegetational zones

Botanists were among the first to note the division of the earth into different vegetational zones. In some parts of the world this division is clear, for example the border between forest and tundra in northern regions, and the zoning of forests as one ascends mountains. In other areas the change is more gradual, for instance the transition from deserts to prairies. Early 18th century naturalists suggested that the world was divided into discrete **formations** of vegetation, such as tundra, savannah and desert, and they drew maps that neatly but erroneously separated formations by lines.

The first serious attempt to explain these apparent neat formations was made by de Candolle (1874), who argued that climate, particularly temperature, dictated vegetation. He drew the first vegetational map based on isotherms. Rain forests were described as formations of **megatherms**, deciduous forests of **mesotherms**, and deserts of **xerophiles**. At the beginning of the 20th century, Koppen used de Candolle's classification as the basis of the modern system (*Table 7.1*) which provides a

Table 7.1 Koppen's system of classification of climate based on de Candolle's plant groups. (From Colinvaux, 1973.)

De Candolle's plant group	Postulated plant requirements	Formation	Koppen's climatic division
Megatherms (most heat)	Continuous high temperature and abundant moisture	Tropical rain forest	A (rainy with no winter)
Xerophiles (dry-loving)	Tolerate drought, need minimum hot season	Hot desert such as Sonoran	B (dry)
Mesotherms (middle heat)	Moderate temperature and moderate moisture	Temperate deciduous forest	C (rainy with mild winters)
Microtherms (little heat)	Less heat, less moisture, tolerate long cold winters	Boreal forest	D (rainy climates with severe winters)
Hekistotherms (least heat)	Tolerate polar regions 'beyond tree-line'	Tundra	E (polar climates with no warm season)

good correlation between climatic and vegetational regions. Climate may dictate boundaries, but in a much more complex way than merely by ground-level temperature changes and rainfall. Meteorological work using satellites, and long-term studies of the thermal composition of air masses, however, have suggested that the mean positions of air fronts over the earth roughly coincide with vegetational types.

Biomes

In the 19th century, zoologists noted that the broad divisions of the earth were populated by similar animals. Even if the divisions were discontinuous (e.g., Africa and South America), some animals, especially birds, showed similar features. This assisted the evolutionists in adding credence to their theory of **convergent evolution** which states that animals of different ancestral stock evolve similar features to suit similar environments.

Zoologists attempted to classify different areas of the world according to the types of animal and plant that were present, because the distribution of animals appeared to be related to vegetation. One such person was the American Merriam (1893) who defined **life zones** in North America after studying the distribution of animals and plants at various altitudes on North American mountains.

Merriam proposed four main life zones (*Figure 7.1*):

1. Boreal (northern), involving the Canadian, Hudsonian and Alpine Arctic;
2. Transition, containing animals and plants from the Boreal and Sonoran;
3. Sonoran (named after Sonora, a state in north-west Mexico), comprising the Upper and Lower;

4. Tropical.

A fifth, minor one (the Lower Californian) is also indicated in *Figure 7.1*.

It is important to note that there is a gradual transition from one zone to another; the apparent boundary on the life-zone map is set sharply by the cartographer. African ecological zones, based on climate, vegetation and potential for agricultural use, are described by Pratt *et al.* (1966).

Merriam, like de Candolle, thought that temperature governed the distribution of animals. He argued that, in the Northern Hemisphere, an animal's northern boundary was drawn by the threshold temperature below which reproduction was not possible. The animal's southern boundary was drawn by the threshold temperature above which the heat was intolerable. Although Merriam spent much time measuring mean temperatures, he was never able to match isotherms with life zones. Although reasons for the transition from one life zone to another are not available, the existence of these zones is clear. They are now commonly called **biomes**. Examples of biomes include tropical rain forest, savannah and tundra, each with its own particular range of plants and animals.

The distribution of infectious agents and their vectors, and therefore of the diseases produced by the former, may be limited by the environmental conditions of biomes. Thus, the fungus *Coccidioides immitis*, which systemically infects man, dogs, cattle and pigs, producing primary respiratory signs in man and dogs, appears to be endemically limited to the Lower Sonoran life zone (*Figure 7.2*: Schmelzer and Tabershaw, 1968). This zone is characterized by hot summers, mild winters, sparse vegetation, an annual rainfall of 6−8 inches, an alkaline

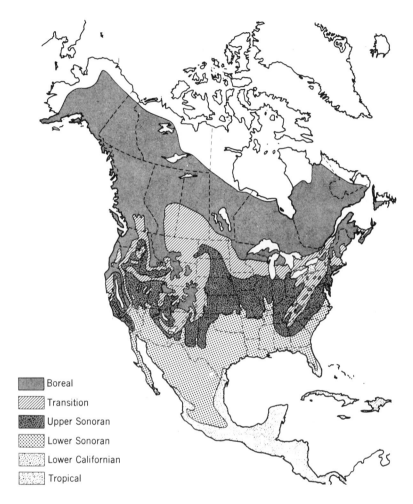

	Boreal
	Transition
	Upper Sonoran
	Lower Sonoran
	Lower Californian
	Tropical

Fig. 7.1 Map of the life zones of North America proposed by Merriam.

soil pH and wind conditions that are conducive to maintenance and dissemination of the fungus (Egeberg, 1954). The distribution of Rift Valley fever (a virus disease of sheep and cattle) is associated with the wetter African ecological zones. This may be related to the abundance of mosquito vectors in these zones (Davies, 1975).

The nature of an ecological zone also has a major influence on animal husbandry which, in turn, can affect morbidity and mortality (Carles, 1992). For example, animals reared on rangelands throughout the the world experience marked climatic and nutritional changes (e.g., in forage type and availability), and inadequate nutrition therefore occurs. Fertility is particularly sensitive to the status of the body's reserves, and so infertility is a common problem on rangelands (Carles, 1986). The practice of trekking may pose additional stress, and so diseases in which stress is a component cause (e.g., pasteurellosis; see *Figure 3.5b*) are also rangeland problems. Localized environments, such as night enclosures and watering points, become heavily contaminated with microorganisms which are responsible for septicaemias in neonatal kids and lambs in some African pastoral systems. The high prevalence of brucellosis among livestock kept on rangelands may be associated with difficulties in the adequate disposal of aborted foetuses. Pre-weaning and post-weaning mortality rates are therefore often high: in sheep and goats reared extensively on tropical rangelands in Africa, India and Australia they often exceed 30%.

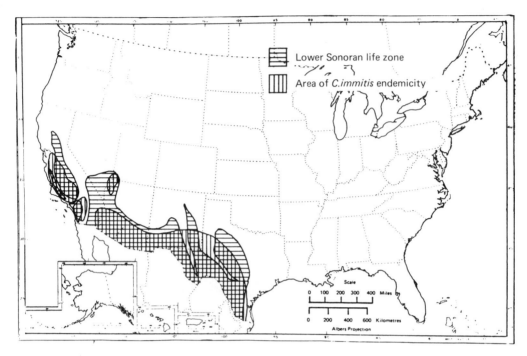

Fig. 7.2 Lower Sonoran life zone and area of endemic *Coccidioides immitis* (nosoarea) in the US. (From Schmelzer and Tabershaw, 1968.)

Regulation of population size

The 'balance of nature'

The early biologists were impressed by the stability of animal and plant populations. Populations grow, reach a certain size, and then stop growing. The population becomes stable and **balanced**, with the rate of reproduction equalling the death rate.

Control of population size by competition

Two hypotheses have been formulated to explain the balance of nature. Chapman (1928) argued that there was **environmental resistance**. Animal populations had an intrinsic rate of increase but there was some quality of the environment that resisted the increase. This theory may be good but there is no evidence to support it. The currently accepted theory is that populations are brought into balance by **competition** for the resources of the habitat, the most common of which is food. Competition therefore is **density-dependent**.

In order to test this hypothesis it is necessary to conduct an experiment with food supply controlled. Such an experiment was conducted by Gause (1934), using one

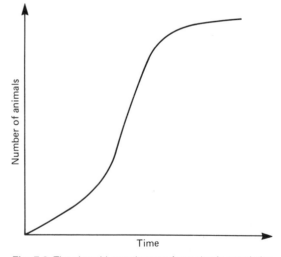

Fig. 7.3 The sigmoid growth curve for a simple population in a confined space with a limited input of energy.

species of *Paramecium* with a constant supply of food. The growth curve for this protozoon is a sigmoid (*Figure 7.3*) that approximates to a mathematical equation, called the **logistic equation** (see also Chapter 15).

The logistic equation is derived thus: if R = observed rate of increase, r = intrinsic rate of increase, N = number of animals, then, for the slope of the curve:

$$R = rN.$$

If K = saturation number, then, with increasing competition, when $N = K$, $R = 0$.

The complete history of the sigmoid curve is:

$$R = rN \left(1 - \frac{N}{K}\right).$$

Early in growth, when growth is rapid because much food is available, N is small; therefore the quotient N/K is small:

$$1 - \frac{N}{K} \text{ approaches } 1,$$

and R approaches rN.

Later, as growth decreases (because less food is available):

$$\frac{N}{K} \text{ approaches } \frac{K}{K} = 1.$$

Thus $1 - \dfrac{N}{K}$ approaches 0.

Thus:

$$R = rN \times 0$$
$$= 0.$$

Further laboratory studies, for example with the fruit fly *Drosophila*, supported the hypothesis of density-dependent competition for food. Parasite populations may also be regulated by this mechanism. Reproduction of *Ascaris* spp., for example, is density-dependent (Croll *et al.*, 1982). However, experiments with other insects, notably the flour beetle, showed that density-dependent factors other than food availability may control the size of populations, for instance the build-up of metabolic excretory products and decreased reproduction due to crowding. Thus, the competition model is a useful theoretical concept that has aided understanding of regulatory mechanisms, but in the real world other factors may also control population size.

Dispersal

In some parts of the world, there may be dramatic seasonal variations in climate. An Australian species of grasshopper overwinters in its egg. The warmth of spring causes the eggs to hatch. The adults that develop then lay eggs as long as the weather is wet. A drought kills all of the adults. This is not density-dependent; it occurs long before competition occurs. Such insects survive only by **dispersal** over large areas to different climates so that at least some are in an area that is wet. This phenomenon led Andrewartha and Birch (1954) to suggest that large animals too were controlled by climate, not competition for food. They emphasized the dangers of oversimplification using the logistic model.

Predation

Predation has an obvious plausible role in controlling the size of populations, but most of the evidence suggests that this is not true for large animals because predators take only the sick and weak and young animals. Since the latter probably would not die otherwise (a small number of deaths may occur, for example by drowning during migration), predation could have some effect on population size. There is, however, contradictory evidence. In the Serengeti of Africa there are about 200 000 wildebeests, but lions kill only 12 000 – 18 000 each year, an insignificant number, and mostly of newborn animals that become lost.

However, small predators, notably of insects, are efficient controllers of populations. Predators have been used to control insect pests; for example, the use of ladybirds to control cotton cushony-scale insects.

Infectious disease

Considerable interest is developing in the role of infectious disease in determining and regulating the size of populations (Anderson and May, 1986, 1991). There is circumstantial evidence, for instance, that the approximate decadal fluctuations in populations of forest-dwelling Lepidoptera are caused by epidemics of disease (Myers, 1988), and there may be similar effects in mammalian and avian populations.

Infectious agents can be divided into two groups according to their generation dynamics: **microparasites** and **macroparasites** (May and Anderson, 1979). This is a useful classification when considering the effects of parasites on host populations. The microparasites multiply directly when inside the hosts, increasing the level of parasitism. They include viruses, bacteria and protozoa. Macroparasites, in contrast, do not increase the level of parasitism: they grow in the host, but multiply by producing infective stages which are released from the host to infect new hosts. They include helminths and arthropods.

Microparasitic infections can obviously depress host population size when they occur as epidemics or pandemics with high case fatality rates. Such effects are usually transient, but they do indicate a potential for more general regulation of the host population akin to that of predators.

The intrinsic growth rate of a population must be influenced by parasites if they are to regulate population size. This rate is governed by host survival and reproductive capacity. Microparasites are frequently pathogenic organisms of high virulence. Their obvious regulatory potential therefore lies in their capacity to kill hosts, but they may also have less direct effects such as inducing susceptibilty to opportunistic infections and rendering infected hosts 'less competitive' than their peers.

There are certain experimentally and theoretically identified conditions under which microparasites can regulate host population size (Anderson, 1981). Disease-induced mortality must be high compared with the disease-free rate of growth. The influence of high pathogenicity and virulence, however, is often moderated by a short period of infectiousness because fewer individuals are likely to be infected. Moreover, enduring immunity in recovered individuals prevents recurrence of disease. These last two factors therefore mitigate the regulatory effects of virus and bacterial infections in vertebrates. (Invertebrates cannot develop acquired immunity, and the capacity of pathogenic bacteria and viruses to regulate invertebrate populations is generally acknowledged.) Epidemiological studies have indicated that human immunodeficiency virus (the cause of AIDS) may be able to reverse positive population growth (Anderson and May, 1988). Characteristics of the infection that contribute to this effect are the virus' high pathogenicity, the lack of an immune response in the host (and, consequently, the invariably fatal outcome of the disease), the long period of infectiousness, and vertical transmission.

Infections with macroparasites, particularly helminths, are ubiquitous in the animal kingdom (*Table 7.2*). Therefore, they could have a widespread regulatory effect on animal populations, although the effect may not be as overt as those induced by microparasites. Helminths not only significantly decrease an animal's growth rate, but can also reduce host survival and reproductive capacity. For example, sheep mortality is related to intensity of infection with *Fasciola hepatica* (Smith, 1984); and red grouse infected with *Trichostrongylus tenuis* produce smaller clutch sizes than uninfected birds (Hudson, 1986).

Table 7.2 The average parasite burdens of North American mammals.* (From Dobson *et al.*, 1992.)

	Mean burden per individual host	Mean number of species per host population
Trematodes	108	1.8
Cestodes	140	2.8
Nematodes	117	5.3
Acanthocephalans	1	0.3
Number of parasite species	3	10

* The data are from 76 populations of mammals comprising 10 species of lagomorphs, 22 species of rodents, 35 species of carnivores and 11 species of artiodactyls. Carnivores generally had the most diverse range of parasites, and lagomorphs the least. Gregarious species had the highest mean parasite burdens.

Infections may also act more subtly; for example, by increasing a host's susceptibilty to predation (Anderson, 1979). Thus, cormorants capture a disproportionately large number of roach infected with the tapeworm, *Ligula intestinalis*, compared to the prevalence of infected fish in the population as a whole (Dobben, 1952).

Microparasites and macroparasites have been identified as suitable candidates for the control of rats, dogs, cats and goats that are introduced to oceanic islands; parasitic nematodes and viruses of low to intermediate pathogenicity being the most appropriate (Dobson, 1988).

The population dynamics of microparasites and macroparasites are discussed by Nokes (1992) and Dobson *et al.* (1992), respectively.

Home range

Certain animals have a natural restriction to the area over which they roam; this is their **home range**. This may control the population and has implications for the transmission of infectious disease; infected animals may transmit infection over their home range, but no further. For example, rats are the maintenance hosts of the rickettsial disease scrub typhus. Trombiculid mites (chiggers) are the vectors; they parasitize mammals and birds. The small home range of the rats results in the mite's lifecycle being restricted to small areas, called 'mite islands' (Audy, 1961). When the mites are infected with the rickettsia, localized endemic areas of scrub typhus, associated with the mite islands, occur. Extension of the infection occurs only by dispersal of infected mites by wider-ranging incidental hosts such as birds and man, in whom the infection causes serious disease.

Territoriality

The part of an animal's home range that it defends aggressively from invaders is the animal's **territory**. This behavioural response is **territoriality**. This has an advantage, economizing movement when searching for food. Territoriality may also control the population because there is a minimum size to a territory and a finite amount of space, and therefore a finite number of animals that can exist in the territory. The sizes of territories vary for the same and different species. For example, arctic birds have a larger territory when food is scarce than when it is plentiful.

Social dominance

In the 1920s, a social hierarchy called the 'peck order' was discovered among birds. Some gregarious species, especially rodents, inhabit favourable places. When crowding occurs, the socially weaker animals are forced out. This may be a population control mechanism.

The 'Wynne-Edwards' hypothesis

The population control consequence of territoriality, social hierarchy and behaviour may be just a side-effect. The Aberdeen zoologist, Wynne-Edwards, suggested that population control was the main purpose of **group behaviour** (Wynne-Edwards, 1962), which sometimes causes physiological stress (see Chapter 5). The crowding of rats results in associated fighting, cannibalism and reduced fecundity. Such experimentally stressed animals, and those that are naturally stressed (e.g., sewer-dwelling rats), have hypertrophied adrenals, indicative of the general adaptation syndrome (see Chapter 5).

At certain times of the year animals congregate, although there are no obvious spatial restrictions (e.g., deer during the rutting season). Wynne-Edwards suggested that this 'head count' of the population evoked, by feedback, the general adaptation syndrome and controlled reproduction. There are two problems with this theory: evolution tends to select individuals, not groups, and the hypothesis suggests that birth-controllers are favoured, whereas evolution usually selects the efficient producers. This theory is not fashionable today.

For whatever reason animals congregate, the increased contact can aid transmission of infectious agents, and can produce seasonal trends in disease occurrence (see Chapter 8). Thus, when North American leopard frogs congregate to spawn during the winter, there is seasonal transmission of Lucké's frog virus (McKinnell and Ellis, 1972).

Behaviour of rabid foxes	Grouping of foxes				
	Solitary	Pair	Family	Social groups	Mixed society
Dumb	□□□□	▼	▼▼	▼▼▼	▼▼
Furious	▼	▼▼	▼▼▼	▼▼▼▼	▼▼▼
Mixed	▼	▼▼	▼▼▼▼▼	▼▼▼▼▼▼▼	▼▼▼▼▼

Fig. 7.4 Social group behaviour and behaviour of rabid foxes as determinants of rabies in foxes. □: Condition unfavourable for existence of rabies virus; number of squares indicates the relative degree to which conditions are unfavourable. ▼: Conditions favourable for the existence of rabies virus; number of triangles indicates the relative degree to which conditions are favourable. (From Macdonald and Bacon, 1980.)

It is difficult to produce a general theory of population control. Food availability is important, and energy availability limits the supportable biomass (see 'The distribution of energy between trophic levels' below). Infectious disease also may have a role. However, different mechanisms probably operate in different circumstances.

The implications for disease occurrence of the distribution and control of populations

The distribution, the home range of animals, and other behavioural activities of hosts of infectious agents affect the latter's transmission. An example is vulpine rabies. The infection is maintained in Europe in foxes (Wachendörfer and Frost, 1992). The behaviour of foxes during the year alters the association between foxes. The animals may be solitary, paired, or part of a family unit. Similarly, rabid foxes' behaviour depends on the type of rabies that they display; foxes with dumb rabies may seek a solitary existence, whereas furious rabies may cause foxes to approach other animals readily. *Figure 7.4* illustrates how these different behaviour patterns affect the survival and spread of rabies virus between animals.

Increases in home range also may increase spread of infection. Thus, during the summer months, rabies may be confined to foxes in the northern tundra and forests of Canada, but in winter, as food supplies become scarce, infected foxes may invade more southerly regions and introduce rabies to such areas.

The niche

Gause's work with *Paramecium*, mentioned earlier in this chapter, is an example of **intraspecific competition**, that is, competition between members of the same species. **Interspecific** competition also can occur when two species live together, in which circumstance either they might both thrive, or one may be exterminated by the other.

The solving, simultaneously (in the mathematical sense), of the logistic equation for each species to find the relative size of each population produces pairs of equations that were derived independently in the US by Lotka (1925) and in Italy by Volterra (Chapman, 1931). These equations are therefore called **Lotka – Volterra equations**. They can be derived for varying degrees of competition. The conclusion drawn from these equations is of fundamental importance in ecology. It is that *the coexistence of two strongly competing species is impossible*. Coexistence is possible only if competition is weak. This was tested again by Gause using two different species of *Paramecium* in a test-tube culture. He found that either one or the other species triumphed, depending on the composition of the environment. This led to the principle of **competitive exclusion**: that competition will exclude all but one species from a particular position defined by an animal's feeding habits, physiology, mechanical abilities and behaviour. This position is an animal's **niche** (Elton, 1927). The principle of competitive exclusion can therefore be summarized as 'one species, one niche'. (This implies that Charles Darwin's original concept of the survival of animals most suited to their environment, as a result of competition, should be modified to one of survival by the avoidance of competition.)

There are examples of competition leading to exclusion in the real world as a result of strong competition, although they are few. Probably the best-documented one is of the Abington turtles. Abington is an island in the South Atlantic that had an indigenous species of turtle. During the 19th century, sailors introduced goats to the island. The goats had exactly the same requirements as the turtles for food. Therefore there was strong competition, which led to the extinction of one of the species, in this case the turtles, according to the Lotka – Volterra prediction.

Competitive exclusion has been used as a means of disease control. The snail *Biomphalaria glabrata*, which is an intermediate host for schistosomiasis, has been replaced by the more competitive snail *Marisa cornuarietis*, which is not an intermediate host for the helminth (Lord, 1983). *Marisa cornuarietis* is reared and then released into streams and ponds which are the habitat of *B. glabrata*. *Marisa cornuarietis* dominates within a few months of its release, and *B. glabrata* virtually disappears.

However, the real world is very diverse and there are many opportunities for animals to avoid competition by finding their own niche. Sometimes the mechanism of avoidance is not obvious; for example, marine zooplankton are all filter feeders but actually filter particles of different sizes and therefore do not compete.

Avoidance of competition is usual in **sympatric species**, that is, species found in the same country or area. Giraffes, Thompson's gazelles and wildebeests are sympatric species in East Africa. They avoid competition for food: the giraffe, with its long neck, feeds high up; the gazelle and wildebeest, although of similar stature, eat differently: the gazelle eats ground-hugging leaves, while the wildebeest eats side shoots.

There are two sympatric species of cormorant in England: the common cormorant and the shag. Both species look alike, occupy the same stretches of shore, are submarine feeders, nest on cliffs, and are fairly abundant. They appear to occupy the same niche, but do not. The common cormorant has a mixed diet, but excluding sand eels and sprats. It fishes out to sea and nests high on cliffs on broad ledges. The shag, in contrast, eats mostly sand eels and sprats, fishes in the shallows, and nests low on cliffs or on shallow ledges.

There are many other examples of sympatric species occupying different niches, ranging from cone shells that occupy different sublittoral zones, to warblers that occupy different parts of the same tree. Short-lived animals (e.g., insects) can occupy the same niche and avoid competition by pursuing their activities during different seasons.

Gause noted a laboratory example of the development of a mechanism to avoid competition. During an experiment with two species of *Paramecium*, he noticed that both species survived in the same test-tube because one species had changed its mode of living to inhabit only the top half of the test-tube, while the other species had moved to the bottom of the tube, thus avoiding competition. This process was explained first by Darwin when he developed the concept of **divergence of character**: characters must diverge when closely related species live in the same region, be it test-tube or prairie. The synonymous term **character displacement** was first used in the 1950s.

One would expect displacement to be more common than exclusion because the world offers many ways of subtly changing niches. Displacement is also a mechanism of increasing species diversity. One example illustrates this phenomenon. Two species of nuthatch occur in Greece, Turkey and other parts of Asia: *Sitta neumeyer* and *Sitta tephronota*. The external appearance of *S. neumayer* in Greece, and *S. tephronota* in Central Asia, where the species do not overlap, is similar. However, in Iran, where the two species overlap and coexist, the external appearance of each species is different. This external divergence of characters probably reflects other changes that avoid competition.

Some examples of niches relating to disease

Louse infestations

Lice tend to be host-species-specific; pig lice do not live on man or dogs, and vice versa. By being host-specific, species of lice avoid competition: they have their own niche. The human louse also demonstrates character displacement. Two types of louse live on man: the head louse and the body louse. These each parasitize the two different parts of the body, rather like Gause's two species of *Paramecium* living in the top and the bottom of the test-tube.

Intracellular parasitism

Intracellular parasites occupy a niche in cells. They include all viruses, some bacteria (e.g., *Brucella* spp., *Mycobacterium tuberculosis* and rickettsiae) and some protozoa (e.g., *Babesia* spp.). There are several advantages to this type of existence, such as safety from humoral antibodies and the avoidance of competition with extracellular agents. The intracellular environment is harsh: the agents must protect themselves from the lytic enzymes released by lysosomes. This harshness is reflected in the relatively low generation times of intracellular parasites compared with extracellular ones. The intracellular environment shares this characteristic with larger extreme environments such as snowfields and salt lakes (Moulder, 1974: *Table 7.3*).

Epidemiological interference

Studies in India (Bang, 1975) have shown that the presence, in a human community, of one type of respiratory adenovirus prevents infection with other types, even though the latter are common in surrounding communities. This is because the first type occupies a niche (the lower respiratory tract) which therefore cannot be filled by other agents. This phenomenon is **epidemiological interference**. Similarly, there is evidence that

Table 7.3 Comparison of the intracellular environment with terrestrial extreme environments. (After Moulder, 1974.)

	Terrestrial extreme environments (e.g. deserts, salt lakes, hot springs, snowfields)	*The cell*
Diversity of inhabiting species is low	+	+
Dominant forms have evolved unique fitness traits	+	+
Dominant forms dependent on species diversity limiting factors	Factor is **abiotic**, e.g. heat, salinity, dryness	Factor is **biotic**: the cell

infection of laboratory animals and domestic livestock with one serodeme (a population demonstrating the same range of variable antigens: WHO, 1978) of *Trypanosoma congolense* delays the establishment of infection with a different serodeme in the same animals (Luckins and Gray, 1983).

Interference can affect the time of occurrence of disease. An epidemic caused by one agent may suppress epidemics caused by other similar agents. This is true of certain human respiratory infections in North America and India (Bang, 1975). Some diseases are common in the young. Interference by other agents during early life causes the diseases of the young to occur in older age cohorts, altering the age-specific incidence rates. There is evidence that this occurs with certain virus infections in man (Bang, 1975).

Interference can also affect the rate of natural immunization. If an infectious agent is present at continued high levels, and infection is followed by immunity, then there is usually a decreased incidence in older age groups. However, if other agents interfere with the agent in the young, then immunity induced by the agent is delayed, producing continued infection in older subjects. There is evidence, for example, that interference by other enteroviruses delays natural poliovirus immunization in man (Bang, 1975).

Epidemiological interference may be a general phenomenon. The delay in its discovery is probably due to the lack of long-term surveys on the incidence of infections. The phenomenon has an obvious place in the evolution of disease: it prevents massive multiple and possibly fatal infections of the young. An example of the application of epidemiological interference to the control of enteric diseases is given in Chapter 22.

The relationships between different types of animals and plants

A particular biome contains different types of animals and plants. Some are common, others are scarce. Some are large, others are small. Reasons for these variations have been suggested by ecological studies.

Animals tend to move about *en masse*, and so it is difficult to study them all simultaneously. Ecologists therefore chose to look in detail at one species of animal, in conditions that favoured easy observation. Charles Elton (1927) visited Bear Island near Spitzbergen and observed Arctic foxes, with particular reference to what they ate. Bear Island was essentially a tundra biome, thus foxes were easy to observe.

Food chains

Elton noted what the foxes ate in the summer and the winter. In the summer, the foxes ate birds (e.g., ptarmigan and sandpiper). The birds ate berries, tundra, leaves and insects. The insects also ate leaves. Thus, Elton noted that there was a **food chain**: tundra — insects — birds — fox. In addition, the foxes ate marine birds, which in turn ate smaller marine animals, which in turn ate marine plants. Thus, there was a further food chain: marine plants — marine animals — seabird — fox.

In the winter, the birds migrated to the south, leaving only polar bear dung and the remains of carcasses of seals that had been killed by polar bears. Thus, in the winter, there was a different food chain: marine animal — seal — polar bear — fox. In animal communities, therefore, a complex system has evolved, with food chains linking animals.

The size of animals and food webs

Elton observed that animals fed at different levels in the food chain. These levels he termed **trophic levels**. He also noted that animals occupying different trophic levels generally were of different sizes. The foxes were the largest, and the birds (one level down) were smaller. Similarly, those further down the pyramid (e.g., the insects) were even smaller. Also, moving down the food chain (e.g., from foxes to insects), the animals were **more abundant**. There were more birds than foxes, and more insects than birds. A histogram depicting animal size against number of individuals is shown in *Figure 7.5a*. If the vertical axis of the histogram is moved to the centre,

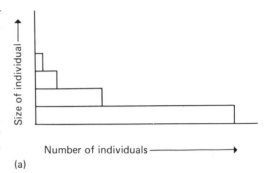

(a)

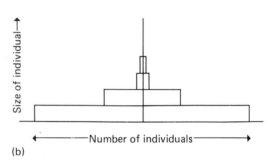

(b)

Fig. 7.5 (a) The relationship between size of animals and size of populations; (b) the Eltonian 'pyramid of numbers'.

and the bars are arranged symmetrically, a pyramid is produced (*Figure 7.5b*); this is the Eltonian **pyramid of numbers**. As animals become larger and rarer, they have larger home ranges and therefore, if shedding an infectious agent, transmit infections over larger areas than small animals. Thus, although hedgehogs (relatively small animals) can be infected with foot-and-mouth disease virus (McLaughlan and Henderson, 1947), they have relatively small home ranges, and so probably play only a minor role in the dissemination of the virus during epidemics.

The food chain is a simplistic view of the relationship between an animal and its food. In reality, an animal usually eats a variety of food, and so there are generally many linked food chains radiating outwards from the lower plant trophic levels to the herbivores, and then inwards towards the top carnivores, producing **food webs** (*Figure 7.6*). In addition, parasitic food webs can be identified in which the small parasites occupy a level in the food web higher than the organisms that they parasitize.

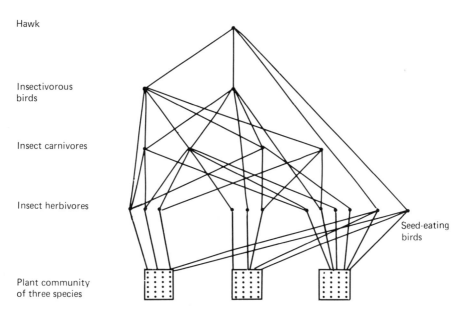

Hawk

Insectivorous
birds

Insect carnivores

Insect herbivores

Seed-eating
birds

Plant community
of three species

Fig. 7.6 Hypothetical food web involving carnivorous, insectivorous and herbivorous birds, carnivorous and herbivorous insects, and plants.

An animal's feeding habits and its place in the trophic hierarchy place restrictions on its mode of life; this led Elton to define the niche: 'an animal's place in the biotic environment; its relation to food and enemies'.

The significance of food webs to disease transmission

The food web of an animal can determine to which orally-transmitted infectious agents an animal acts as host, and from which food poisoning toxins it is at risk. Helminth diseases, for which there are definitive and intermediate hosts, are frequently transmitted via food webs. For example, the tapeworm, *Echinococcus granulosus*, includes the sheep as an intermediate host and the dog as the definitive host. The cysts in the liver and lungs of the intermediate host are transmitted to dogs when the latter eat sheep offal; hence the recommendations that raw sheep offal should not be fed to dogs.

Figure 7.7 illustrates the life-cycle of *Neorickettsia helminthoeca*. This rickettsia produces a febrile disease in dogs and foxes. The disease is called 'salmon poisoning' because it is associated with the feeding of salmon to dogs. This agent's life-cycle also illustrates a parasitic food chain, in which the smallest member, the rickettsia, parasitizes a fluke which in turn parasitizes a snail for part of its life-cycle. The snail in turn releases infected miracidia which parasitize the salmon. Feeding salmon to dogs transmits the rickettsia to the latter, where the microbe produces clinical disease.

Ingestion of intermediate stages of parasites sometimes may control, rather than transmit, infection. For example, members of the genus *Utricularia* (carnivorous bladderworts) have been shown to ingest cercariae and miracidia of *Schistosoma mansoni* (Gibson and Warren, 1970). It has been suggested (Lord, 1983) that the absence of schistosomiasis from Cuba, which has 17 species of *Utricularia*, may be related to this activity.

Parasitic food chains might also be exploited in the control of other helminth parasites (Waller, 1992). Some bacteria are effective controllers of plant nematode parasites (Tribe, 1980). The fungus *Arthrobotrys oligospora*, a predator of infective larvae of the bovine nematode *Ostertagia ostertagi*, has reduced the level of parasitism in cattle when applied to dung pats (Gronvøld et al., 1989, 1993), although oral administration has had little benefit yet (Hashmi and Connan, 1989).

The distribution of energy between trophic levels

Elton's theory explained why animals occupying different trophic levels were of different sizes, but it did not explain why there were so few animals higher up the pyramid. There could be geometric restrictions: more small

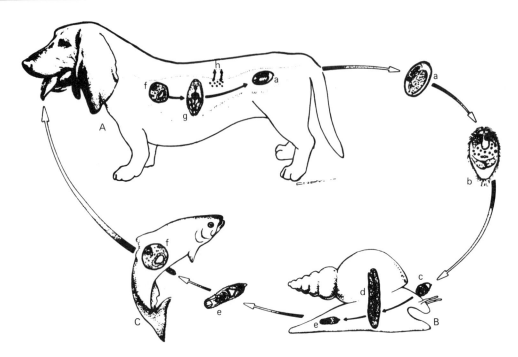

Fig. 7.7 Life-cycle of the fluke *Nanophyetus salmincola salmincola* and the microorganism *Neorickettsia helminthoeca*. A, dog (definitive host); B, *Oxytrema silicula* (first intermediate host); C, Salmonidae fish (second intermediate host); a, *Nanophyetus salmincola salmincola* egg in dog faeces; b, miracidium; c, miracidium enters snail by skin penetration; d, redia; e, cercaria; f, encysted metacercaria in salmon, ingested by the dog in raw salmon meat; g, adult fluke develops in duodenal mucosa; h, *Neorickettsia helminthoeca* leave the fluke and infect the dog systemically. (From Booth *et al.*, 1984.)

animals can be packed into a fixed space than larger ones. However, the sea contains few predators (e.g., sharks) at the top of the pyramid even though the sea is very large.

Lindemann (1942) explained population density at different levels of the pyramid by considering the food chain, not in terms of particulate food, but in terms of **calorific energy flow**. According to the second law of thermodynamics, the process of converting energy from one state to another is wasteful, that is, there is not 100% conversion of energy. Thus, moving up from one level to another in the Eltonian pyramid, conversion at each level wastes energy and so less protoplasm can be supported at progressively higher levels. Therefore, even if animals at different levels were of the same size, there would be fewer higher up. Since those higher up are larger, the packaging of a supportable amount of protoplasm produces even fewer animals.

It is because of the greater availability of energy at lower levels that ungulates are often bigger than their carnivorous predators. The biggest animals tend to be those that feed very low in the pyramid (e.g., filter feeders like blue whales) because much energy is

available to them. When civilization dawned and man ceased to be a hunter—gatherer and began cultivating crops, he 'climbed down' the pyramid, tapping more energy. This is one reason for the increase in the world's population in the cradle of civilization in early Egypt and the associated development of horticulture and livestock farming (see Chapter 1).

The analysis of predation

The association between predator and prey is a special case of interaction in a food chain. Many mathematical models have been devised to analyse predator—prey interactions. The one to be discussed here is that devised independently by Lotka and Volterra (Lotka, 1925; Chapman, 1931). They reasoned that predator—prey interactions were similar to interactions between competing species and so adapted their formulae accordingly.

The three predictions of this model are:

1. the fluctuation of two species, one of which feeds on the other, is periodic, and the periods depend only on the coefficient of growth;

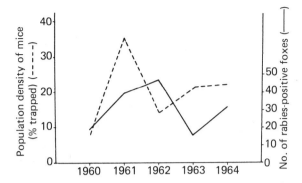

Fig. 7.8 The relationship between the population density of mice and the prevalence of fox rabies. The relationship arises from a predator/prey relationship between foxes and mice (see text). (From Sinnecker, 1976.)

2. the ultimate mean values of the numbers of individuals of the two species are, with fixed coefficients, independent of the initial numbers of individuals;
3. if individuals of the two species are eliminated in proportion to their total number, then the recovery potential of the prey is greater than that of the predator; conversely, increased protection of the prey from all risks, including the predator, allows both species to increase.

Thus, applying the first prediction, the prevalence of rabies in foxes is related to the population density of foxes (a predator) and, therefore, to the population density of mice (a prey). *Figure 7.8* illustrates this relationship, using demographic and disease prevalence data collected in Germany.

There are also similarities between predator/prey interactions and parasite/host interactions. For example, cyclic patterns of measles and other childhood diseases (Yorke and London, 1973) are equivalent to Lotka–Volterra cycles because the development of immunity by infected individuals is equivalent, in its effect on parasite populations, to the effects of removal of prey on predator populations.

Ecosystems

The relationship between animals linked by food chains defines the variety of animals in a particular area. Similarly, climate and vegetation govern the distribution of plants and therefore of the animals that live off them. These areas are characterized by the animals and plants that occupy them, and by their physical and climatic features. This unique interacting complex is called an **ecosystem** (Tansley, 1935). The components of an ecosystem can be considered separately, and ecosystems themselves can vary in size. Various terms have been devised to describe these components (Schwabe, 1984) including **biotope** and **biocenosis**.

Biotope

A biotope is the smallest spatial unit providing uniform conditions for life. An organism's biotope therefore describes its location. This contrasts with a niche, which describes the functional position of an organism in a community. A biotope can vary in size. For example, it may be the caeca of a chicken for coccidia, or an area of poorly drained land for *Fasciola hepatica* infection of cattle.

Biocenosis

A biocenosis is the collection of living organisms in a biotope. The organisms include plants, animals and the microorganisms in the biotope. Sometimes **biotic community** is used synonymously with biocenosis. On other occasions, 'biotic community' refers to a large biocenosis. Major biotic communities are biomes.

Types of ecosystem

Three types of ecosystem can be identified according to their origin: **autochthonous, anthropurgic** and **synanthropic**.

Autochthonous ecosystems

'Autochthonous' derives from the Greek adjective *autos*, meaning 'oneself' or 'itself'; the Greek noun *chthon*, meaning 'the earth' or 'the land'; and the adjectival suffix *-ous*, meaning 'deriving from'. Hence an autochthonous ecosystem is one 'coming from the land itself'. Examples are to be found in biomes such as tropical rain forests and deserts.

Anthropurgic ecosystems

'Anthropurgic' is derived from the Greek noun *anthropos*, meaning 'man': and the Greek verb root *erg*, meaning 'to work at, to create, to produce'. Thus, an anthropurgic ecosystem is one created by man (strictly, it can also mean 'creating man'). Examples are those found in cultivated pastures and towns.

Synanthropic ecosystems

'Synanthropic' originates from the Greek preposition *syn*, meaning 'along with, together with'; and the Greek noun *anthropos*, meaning 'man'. Thus, a synanthropic ecosystem is one that is in contact with man. An example is a rubbish tip, harbouring a variety of vermin. It follows that some synanthropic ecosystems, such as rubbish tips, are anthropurgic.

Synanthropic ecosystems facilitate the transmission of zoonotic infections from their lower animal hosts to man. For example, the brown rat, *Rattus norvegicus*, inhabits rubbish dumps and can be inapparently infected with *Leptospira*, serovar *ballum*. Humans in proximity to rubbish dumps that harbour infected rats may therefore be infected with the baterium.

An ecological climax

An ecological climax traditionally is said to have occurred when plants, animals, microbes, soil and macroclimate (see Chapter 5) have evolved to a stable, balanced relationship.*

Characteristically, when infections are present, they too are stable and therefore are usually endemic. Also, the balance between host and parasite usually results in inapparent infections. Such stable situations can be disrupted, frequently by man, resulting in epidemics. For example, bluetongue, a virus disease of sheep, was recognized only after the importation of European breeds of sheep into South Africa towards the end of the 19th century (Neitz, 1948). The virus, however, was present in indigenous sheep before that time, but was part of an

*In some ecosystems (e.g., tropical rain forests) an ecological climax is determined exclusively by plant/arthropod relationships (Janzen, 1971; Way, 1977).

ecological climax in which it produced only inapparent infections. The importation of exotic sheep represented a disturbance of the stable climax.

A climax involving endemic infectious agents indicates that all factors for maintenance and transmission of the agent are present. Sometimes changes in local ecology may tip the balance in favour of parasites, thus increasing disease incidence. For example, the seasonal periodicity of foot-and-mouth disease in South America may be as a result of seasonal increases in the size of the susceptible cattle population when animals are brought into an endemic area for fattening (Rosenberg *et al.*, 1980).

Ecological interfaces

An ecological interface is a junction of two ecosystems. Infectious diseases can be transmitted across these interfaces. An example is the transmission of yellow fever, an arbovirus disease of man. The virus is maintained in apes in Africa in an autochthonous forest ecosystem in the forest canopy (*Figure 7.9*). The canopy-dwelling mosquito, *Aedes africanus*, transmits the virus between apes. The mosquito, *A. simpsoni*, bridges the interface between the autochthonous forest ecosystem and the anthropurgic cultivated savannahs. This mosquito therefore maintains a plantation cycle in which man and apes may be infected. Finally, the urban mosquito, *A. aegypti*, can maintain an urban cycle in man. People who enter forests may also contract the infection from *A. africanus*.

Ecological mosaics

An ecological mosaic is a modified patch of vegetation, created by man, within a biome that has reached a climax.

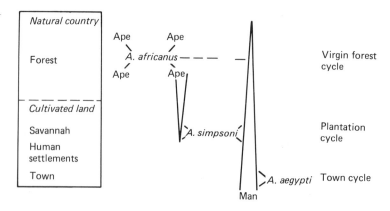

Fig. 7.9 The transmission of yellow fever between apes (primary hosts) and man (the secondary host). (From Sinnecker, 1976.)

Infection may spread from wild animals to man in such circumstances. For example (Schwabe, 1984), the helminth infection, loiasis, is transmitted by arthropods between man, living in small forest clearings, and canopy-dwelling monkeys. Similarly, clearing of the forest canopy encourages a close cover of weeds on the ground, creating conditions that are favourable for the incursion of field rats with mites infected with scrub typhus, which form mite islands and the resulting local areas of endemic scrub typhus (Audy, 1961).

However, transmission does not always occur in the mosaics because suitable vectors may not be available. Thus, in Malaya, man lives unharmed in forests in mosaics with monkeys infected with a variety of species of *Plasmodium* (a protozoon) that are pathogenic to man. Transmission to man from monkeys does not occur because vectors that bite both types of primate are not present in the ecosystem.

Landscape epidemiology

The study of diseases in relation to the ecosystems in which they are found is **landscape epidemiology**. Terms conveying the same meaning are **medical ecology, horizontal epidemiology** (Ferris, 1967) and **medical geography**. Investigations are frequently qualitative, involving the study of the ecological factors that affect the occurrence, maintenance and, in the case of infectious agents, transmission of disease. This contrasts with the study of quantitative associations between specific diseases and hypothesized factors — sometimes termed 'vertical' epidemiology — as described in Chapters 14, 15, 18 and 19. Landscape epidemiology was developed by the Russian, Pavlovsky (1964), and later expanded by Audy (1958, 1960, 1962) and Galuzo (1975); it involves application of the ecological concepts described above in the study of disease.

Nidality

The Russian steppe biome was the home of the great plagues such as rinderpest. Many arthropod-transmitted infections present in the steppes were also limited to distinct geographical areas. These foci were natural homes of these diseases and were called **nidi** (Latin: *nidus* = nest). The presence of a nidus depends on its limitation to particular ecosystems. An area that has ecological, social and environmental conditions that can support a disease is a **nosogenic territory** (Greek: *noso-* =

sickness, disease; *gen-* = to produce, to create). A **nosoarea** is a nosogenic territory in which a particular disease is present. Thus, Britain is a nosogenic territory for rabies and foot-and-mouth disease, but is not a nosoarea for these diseases, because the microbes are prevented from entering the country by quarantine of imported animals. Diseases that show strict geographical boundaries within an ecosystem or series of ecosystems are nidal because they are confined to a specific nidus. Salmonellosis is endemic in most parts of the world because virtually all vertebrates and some invertebrates (see *Table 6.3*) can act as hosts for the various species of *Salmonella*. Rabies, when maintained in foxes, is endemic in a large zone around the Northern Hemisphere because this large area supports a fox population of high density (*Figure 7.10*). The nosoarea for coccidioidomycosis was described earlier in this chapter (see *Figure 7.2*).

When diseases are vector-transmitted, they are often restricted to more precise geographical boundaries than other infectious diseases. This is because the ecosystem has to satisfy the requirements of both the vertebrate host and the arthropod vector. Thus, Rocky Mountain spotted fever, a rickettsial disease of rodents transmitted by ticks, is essentially restricted to particular areas of North America, as the name of the disease suggests.

At the opposite end of the spectrum from diseases with a wide distribution are those that may be confined to relatively small areas within a town or on a farm. An isolated clump of trees that is used as a roost by starlings may be the only reservoir of infection for histoplasmosis within a large area. The faeces from these birds provide an ideal environment in which the fungal agent can survive and replicate (Di Salvo and Johnson, 1979). Even smaller nidi can be identified. For example, a focus of infestation with the tropical dog tick, *Rhipicephalus sanguineus*, has been identified in a house in London (Fox and Sykes, 1985), the warm conditions of the house providing a suitable environment for the tick. The affected dog had not been imported from abroad, but probably contracted the infestation from a quarantine kennel where it had been boarded.

Objectives of landscape epidemiology

Landscape epidemiology is founded on the concept that if the nidality of diseases is based on ecological factors then a study of ecosystems enables predictions to be made about the occurrence of disease and facilitates the development of appropriate control strategies. Three examples will illustrate this concept.

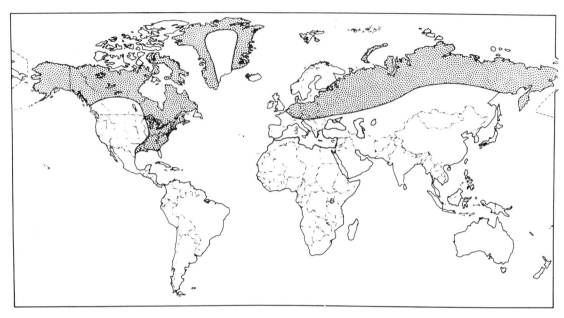

Fig. 7.10 Nosoarea (shaded) of endemic fox rabies. (From Winkler, 1975).

Leptospirosis

It is known that the prevalence of *Leptospira*, serovar *ballum*, in the brown rat is density-dependent; an estimation of the number of rats inhabiting an area enables a prediction of the prevalence of serovar *ballum* infections to be made (Blackmore and Hathaway, 1980: *Figure 7.11*). The number of rat burrows in an area is a good indicator of the number of rats, and these burrows are seldom more than 100 m from the major feeding ground, and are seldom more than 40 cm deep (Pisano and Storer, 1948). Thus, if inspection of the area reveals a large number of burrows and evidence of recent rat activity, it is likely that the area constitutes a reservoir of infection for serovar *ballum*. Conversely, if the rubbish dump is well managed and the area surrounding it shows evidence of regular bulldozing and few inhabited burrows, then the rat population is likely to be small, and any rats present are unlikely to constitute a maintenance population for this leptospiral serovar.

Tularaemia

In 1967 in Sweden, an epidemic of tularaemia occurred with more than 2000 human cases and a high mortality rate of hares (Borg and Hugoson, 1980). This epidemic was associated with the clearing of small areas of forest to create areas of grazing, which led to a sudden increase in

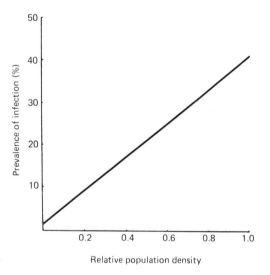

Fig. 7.11 Relationship between the relative population density and prevalence of *Leptospira*, serovar *ballum*, infection in the brown rat (*Rattus norvegicus*). (Simplified from Blackmore and Hathaway, 1980.)

the population density of hares and rodents. A consideration of local ecology in this instance would have suggested that the creation of these synanthropic ecosystems, in which man can be infected either by handling dead hares or through bites of infected mosquitoes, could result in such consequences.

Kyasanur Forest disease

Kyasanur Forest disease is caused by an arbovirus. Symptoms in man include headache, fever, back and limb pains, vomiting, diarrhoea and intestinal bleeding. Death due to dehydration can occur in untreated cases. It is apparently restricted to an area 600 miles square in the Indian state of Mysore. The virus endemically and inapparently infects some small mammals, including rats and shrews, in the local rain forest. The virus is transmitted by several species of tick (Singh *et al.*, 1964), only one of which, *Haemaphysalis spinigera*, will infest man. The usual host of the tick is the ox. Thus, when man creates ecological mosaics by cultivating areas for rice, his cattle roam into the surrounding rain forest and may become infested with virus-infected ticks. Dense populations of ticks therefore build up around villages and, when infected, these ticks can transmit the infection to man (Hoogstraal, 1966).

Further reading

Anderson, R.M. (1982) Epidemiology. In: *Modern Parasitology*. Ed. Cox, F.E.G., pp. 204–251. Blackwell Scientific Publications, Oxford. (*Includes a discussion of parasite dynamics*)

Begon, M., Harper, J.L. and Townsend, C.R. (1990) *Ecology: Individuals, Populations and Communities*. Blackwell Scientific Publications, Oxford. (*A general ecology text which also includes a discussion of parasitism and disease*)

Burnet, F.M. and White, D.O. (1962) *Natural History of Infectious Disease*. Cambridge University Press, Cambridge

Cherrett, J.M. (Ed.) (1989) *Ecological Concepts*. Blackwell Scientific Pubications, Oxford. (*A general ecology text which also includes a discussion of predator/prey and host/pathogen interactions*)

Crawley, M.J. (Ed.) (1992) *Natural Enemies: The Population Biology of Predators, Parasites and Diseases*. Blackwell Scientific Publications, Oxford

Desowitz, R.S. (1981) *New Guinea Tapeworms and Jewish Grandmothers. Tales of Parasites and People*. W. Norton and Company, New York and London. (*Essays on ecological and anthropological aspects of some parasitic diseases*)

Edwards, M.A. and McDonnell, U. (Eds) (1982) *Animal Disease in Relation to Animal Conservation*. Symposia of the Zoological Society of London No. 50. Academic Press, London

Galuzo, I.G. (1975) Landscape epidemiology (epizootiology). *Advances in Veterinary Science and Comparative Medicine*, **19**, 73–96

Lord, R.D. (1973) Ecological strategies for the prevention and control of health problems. *Bulletin of the Pan American Health Organization*, **17**, 19–34

May, R.M. (1981) Population biology of parasitic infections. In: *The Current Status and Future of Parasitology*. Eds Warren, K.S. and Purcell, E., pp. 208–235. Josiah Macy Jnr. Foundation, New York

Pavlovsky, E.N. (1964) *Prirodnaya Ochagovost Transmissivnykh Bolezney v Svyazi s Landshoftnoy Epidemiologiey Zooantroponozov*. Translated as *Natural Nidality of Transmissible Disease with Special Reference to the Landscape Epidemiology of Zooanthroponoses*. Plous, F.K. (Translator), Levine, N.D. (Ed.) (1966). University of Illinois Press, Urbana

Schneider, R. (1991) Wildlife epidemiology. In: Waltner-Toews, D. (Ed.) *Veterinary Epidemiology in the Real World: a Canadian Potpourri*, pp. 41–47. Canadian Association of Veterinary Epidemiology and Preventive Medicine, Ontario Veterinary College, Guelph. (*A concise discussion of the role of disease in regulating animal populations*)

Schwabe, C.E. (1984) *Veterinary Medicine and Human Health*, 3rd edn. Williams and Wilkins, Baltimore. (*Includes a section on medical ecology*)

Sinnecker, H. (1976) *General Epidemiology* (Translated by Walker, N.). John Wiley and Sons, London. (*An ecological approach to epidemiology*)

8 Patterns of disease

Methods of expressing the temporal and spatial distribution of disease were described in Chapter 4. The various patterns of disease that can be detected when disease distribution is recorded are discussed in this chapter. A considerable bulk of mathematical theory has been formulated to explain disease patterns (e.g., Bailey, 1975). Most of this is beyond the scope of this book, but a brief introduction will be given in this chapter. Additionally, the application of mathematics to the development of predictive models, of practical value to disease control, is described in Chapter 19.

Epidemic curves

The representation of the number of new cases of a disease by a graph, with the number of new cases on the vertical axis, and calendar time on the horizontal axis, is the most common means of expressing disease occurrence. The graphing of an epidemic in this way produces an **epidemic curve**. *Figure 8.1* depicts the various parts of an epidemic curve, stylized to a symmetric shape for the purpose of illustration. An epidemic curve is given for foot-and-mouth disease in *Figure 3.1*, with the number of new outbreaks (Appendix I) approximately indicating the number of new cases. Note that the culmination point (peak) is shifted to the left, that is, the curve is positively skewed.

Factors affecting the shape of the curve

The shape of the curve and the time-scale depend on:

1. the incubation period of the disease;
2. the infectivity of the agent;
3. the proportion of susceptible animals in the population;
4. the distance between animals (i.e., animal density).

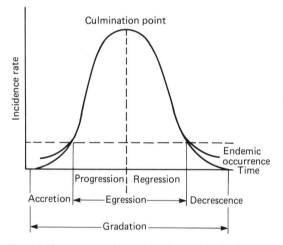

Fig. 8.1 Components of an epidemic curve (stylized to a symmetric shape). The horizontal dotted line indicates the average number of new cases. (From Sinnecker, 1976).

Thus, a highly infectious agent with a short incubation period infecting a population with a large proportion of susceptible animals at high density produces a curve with a steep initial slope on a relatively small time-scale, representing a rapid spread of infection among the population.

A minimum density of susceptible animals is required to allow a contact-transmitted epidemic to commence. This is called the **threshold level**, and is defined mathematically by **Kendall's Threshold Theorem** (in Discussion to Bartlett, 1957). *Figure 8.2* illustrates application of the theorem in relation to rabies in foxes. Above a certain density of susceptible animals, one infected fox can, on average, infect more than one susceptible fox, and an epidemic can occur; the greater the density, the steeper the slope of the progressive stage of the epidemic curve. Few threshold values relating to animal diseases are known. Wierup (1983) has estimated that a minimum density of 12 dogs/km² is required before a canine parvovirus epidemic can occur.

The threshold level is more generally defined in terms of the **basic reproduction ratio (basic reproductive rate)** R_0: the average number of secondary cases caused by one typical infectious individual during its entire infectious period (Diekmann *et al.*, 1990). If $R_0 > 1$ an infection will invade a population; whereas if $R_0 < 1$ it cannot. The basic reproduction ratio can also be applied to macroparasitic diseases (see Chapter 7), where it refers to the average number of offspring produced throughout the life span of a mature parasite (Anderson and May, 1991); a parasite population will establish within a host community only when $R_0 > 1$.

As an epidemic proceeds, the number of susceptible animals decreases, either as a result of death of infected animals, or by increasing immunity following infection (*Figure 8.3*). Eventually, the epidemic cannot continue

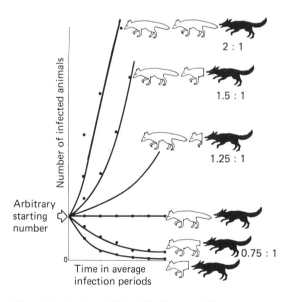

Fig. 8.2 Application of Kendall's Threshold Theorem to rabies in foxes: the theorem predicts that, if a rabid fox infects more than one other before it dies, the disease increases exponentially; if each animal infects less than one other, the disease decreases exponentially. White animals: susceptible; black animals: infected and infectious. Numbers refer to the **contact rate**: the number of susceptible animals that are infected by an infected animal per unit time (a parameter related to the basic reproduction ratio). (From Macdonald and Bacon, 1980.)

because there are insufficient susceptible animals available for infection. In the case of canine parvovirus, for instance, an epidemic stops when the density of susceptible dogs falls below 6 dogs/km² (Wierup, 1983). A period of time is then necessary to allow replacement of susceptible animals before another epidemic can commence. This explains the cyclicity of some epidemics.

Common source and propagating epidemics

A **common source epidemic** is one in which all cases are infected from a source that is common to all individuals. If the period of exposure is brief, then a common source epidemic is a **point-source** (or, more briefly, just a **point**) epidemic. A food-poisoning outbreak, in which a single batch of food is contaminated, is a typical point-source epidemic. *Figure 8.4* illustrates a point-source epidemic of human leptospirosis in the USSR in 1955 associated with the contamination of the water supply with the urine of infected dogs. An epidemic of leptospirosis was occurring in dogs, and contaminated urine was discharged onto fields. A cloudburst occurred on 28 June during a brief period of heavy rainfall. This washed off the topsoil. Some of the soil entered a water pumping station inspection shaft which was open for repair. Thus, the water supply was contaminated, resulting in the human epidemic.

A **propagating epidemic** is an epidemic caused by an infectious agent in which initial (i.e., **primary**) cases excrete the agent, and thus infect susceptible individuals which constitute **secondary** cases. Epidemics of foot-and-mouth disease are examples (*Figure 3.1*). One of the primary cases is frequently the **index case**, that is, the first case to come to the attention of investigators.

The time intervals between peaks of successive temporal clusters of cases, separating the primary from subsequent secondary cases, reflect the incubation period of the infection. Typically, all cases of a point-source epidemic occur within one incubation period of the causal agent. Thus, if the period between subsequent peaks is less than the most common incubation period then it is difficult to differentiate between a propagating epidemic and a series of point-source epidemics. Sartwell (1950, 1966) describes a suitable technique of differentiation, based on the statistical distribution of incubation periods.

The Reed–Frost model

The shape of the epidemic curve in a propagating epidemic in a defined population can be mathematically modelled (Bailey, 1975). One of the basic models is the **Reed–Frost model** (Abbey, 1952; Frost, 1976). In this

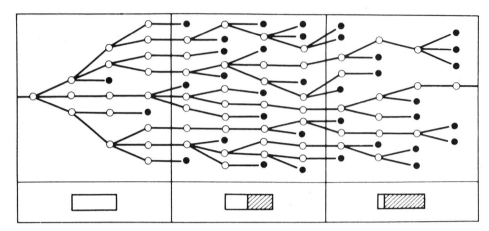

Fig. 8.3 The course of a typical epidemic caused by an infectious agent infecting a totally susceptible population. Each circle represents an infection, and the connecting lines indicate transfer from one case to the next. Black circles represent infected individuals who fail to infect others. Three periods are shown, the first when practically the whole population is susceptible, the second at the height of the epidemic, and the third at the close, when most individuals are immune. The proportions of susceptible (white) and immune (hatched) individuals are indicated in rectangles beneath the main diagram. (From Burnet and White, 1972.)

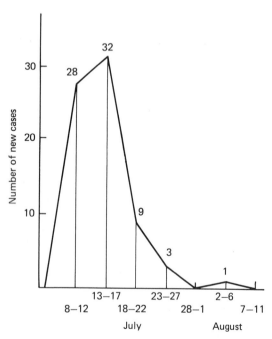

Fig. 8.4 A point-source epidemic: human leptospirosis associated with contaminated water supply, Rostov-on-Don, USSR, 1955. (From Ianovich *et al.*, 1957.)

model's classical simple form, the population is divided into three groups, comprising:

1. infected animals (cases);
2. susceptible animals;
3. immune animals.

The number of individuals in each group determines the shape of the epidemic curve and the pattern of immunity in the population.

Assuming that the period of infectiousness of infected animals is short, and the incubation period or latent period is constant, then, starting with a single case (or several simultaneously infected cases), new cases will occur in a series of stages. Cases occurring at each stage can be expected to have a binomial distribution (see Chapter 12), depending on the number of susceptible and infectious animals at the previous stage. A **chain** of **binomial** distributions thus can be expected; this model is therefore termed a 'chain-binomial model'. The model also assumes that all infected animals develop disease, become infectious in the next stage, and then become immune.

The model is constructed using the formula:

$$C_{t+1} = S_t (1 - q^{C_t}),$$

where:

t = the time period: usually defined as the incubation period or latent period of the infectious agent;

Table 8.1 Simulation of an epidemic using the classical Reed—Frost model.

Time (t)	Number of Cases (C_t)	Number of susceptible animals (S_t)	Number of immune animals (I_t)	Totals	Probability of effective contact (p)	pS_t
0	1	100	0	101	0.06	6.00
1	6	94	1	101	0.06	5.64
2	29	65	7	101	0.06	3.90
3	54	11	36	101	0.06	0.66
4	11	0	90	101	0.06	0.00
5	0	0	101	101	0.06	0.00

C_{t+1} = the number of infectious cases in time period, $t+1$;

S_t = the number of susceptible animals in the time period, t;

q = the probability (see Chapter 12) of an individual not making effective contact.

The value, q, is given by $(1-p)$, where p = the probability of a specific individual making effective contact (see Chapter 6) with another individual which would result in infection if one were susceptible and the other were infectious. The term $(1-q^{C_t})$ arises because it represents the probability that at least one of the C_t infectious cases makes effective contact. The magnitude of p is a matter of chance, and depends on a variety of factors, including those already described in Chapter 6. It is usually estimated empirically from real epidemics (Bailey, 1975).

If at time t (the beginning of an epidemic), there are 100 susceptible animals, no immune animals, and one case, then $S_t = 100$ and $C_t = 1$.

If $p = 0.06$, then $q = (1-0.06) = 0.94$.

At time $t+1$:

$$C_{t+1} = 100 \ (1-0.94^1)$$
$$= 6,$$

and

$$S_{t+1} = 100-6$$
$$= 94.$$

At time $t+2$:

$$C_{t+2} = 94 \ (1-0.94^6)$$
$$= 29,$$

and

$$S_{t+2} = 94-29$$
$$= 65.$$

At time $t+3$:

$$C_{t+3} = 65 \ (1-0.94^{29})$$
$$= 54,$$

and

$$S_{t+3} = 65-54$$
$$= 11,$$

and so on.

The number of immune animals at any time period is the cumulative total of infected animals during the preceding time periods. Thus, at time $t+1$, the number of immune animals $I_{t+1} = 1$ (the 1 case from time $t = 0$); at time $t+2$, $I_{t+2} = 6+1 = 7$; at time $t+3$, $I_{t+3} = 7+29 = 36$, and so on.

Table 8.1 presents the results of the Reed—Frost model, using the above parameters, for the complete course of the modelled epidemic. The results are also plotted in *Figure 8.5*. Note that an epidemic can only occur when $p \times S_t > 1$, and declines (or cannot initially occur) when $p \times S_t < 1$. The likelihood of an epidemic occurring, and the shape of the epidemic curve, are therefore functions of the probability of effective contact and the number of susceptible animals.

The **proportion** of the population that is susceptible is often used as a general guide to the likelihood of an infection spreading — commonly, at least 20—30% of the population; with the corollary that, if 70—80% of the population is immune, infection will not spread. Although the latter level of protection will prevent a major epidemic, infection can spread with a relatively low

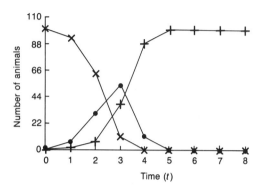

Fig. 8.5 An epidemic curve, number of susceptible animals and number of immune animals simulated by the classical Reed−Frost model. —•— Cases; —+— immune animals; —x— susceptible animals. (Data from *Table 8.1*.)

proportion of susceptible animals if there are sufficient susceptible animals to render $p \times S_t$ greater than 1.

Figure 8.6 depicts epidemic curves that are simulated using various values for the number of susceptible and immune animals, and the parameter, p. A number of immune animals at the beginning of an epidemic can decrease the amplitude of the epidemic and delay its peak; a change in effective contact can also alter the amplitude.

The basic Reed−Frost model can be modified to include control components, such as vaccination with a

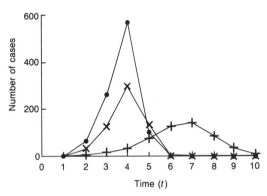

	Initial number of susceptible animals	Initial number of immune animals	Probability of effective contact
—•—	1000	0	0.007
—+—	600	400	0.007
—x—	600	400	0.015

Fig. 8.6 Some epidemic curves simulated by the classical Reed−Frost model. Population size = 1000; a single case is introduced into the population.

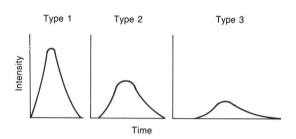

Fig. 8.7 Kendall's concept of changing wave shape over time. (From Cliff and Haggett, 1988.)

varying duration of immunity (Carpenter, 1988), and varying periods of infectiousness (Bailey, 1975).*

Kendall's waves

Some epidemics — notably those caused by viruses — occur as a series of outbreaks which can be considered as a series of epidemic **waves**: a **wave-train**. Three types of wave, representing particular stages of a continuum, were identified by Kendall (1957); these are called **Kendall's waves** (*Figure 8.7*). There are three main differences between these waves (Cliff and Haggett, 1988):

1. **amplitude** — decreasing intensity from type 1 to type 3;
2. **peakedness** (concentration of cases) — also decreasing from type 1 to type 3;
3. **skewness** — noticeable in type 1, but decreasing in succeeding types.

The shape of each wave in the wave-train at a given time or place in a population at risk of size, S, depends on the rate of infection, β, and the rate of removal, μ. Removal occurs when infected animals die, are isolated, or recover and become immune. These two parameters are related in a third, S_c: the **relative removal rate**.

$$S_c = \mu/\beta.$$

The relative removal rate defines a critical susceptible threshold population size, whose magnitude compared with S determines the wave's shape. When S is much greater than S_c, a type 1 wave occurs. Type 3 waves occur

*Some models of the age distribution of cancer also show remarkable similarities to the Reed−Frost model (Burch, 1966), reflecting underlying biological similarities. Contact between an infectious and a susceptible individual is similar to an environmental carcinogen effectively 'hitting' a cell; and the conversion of a susceptible individual to a case is similar to a mutation that converts a normal cell to a malignant one (see Chapter 5).

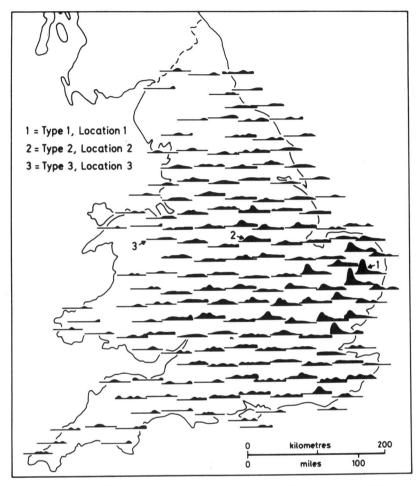

Fig. 8.8 Newcastle disease epidemic of 1970−71 in England and Wales. (From Cliff and Haggett, 1988.)

when the number of animals at risk is low, and consequently S is only slightly greater than S_c. These waves are characterized by relatively lengthy outbreaks of low amplitude. Type 2 waves are intermediate to types 1 and 3.

The shape of the waves changes as an epidemic spreads over time and space. This is exemplified by the epidemic of the virus disease, Newcastle disease, which occurred in England and Wales in 1970−71, and which is charted in *Figures 8.8* and *8.9*. The infection is spread by movement of live birds and other animals, fomites, poultry products and airborne transmission (Calnek, 1991). Although the disease is preventable by vaccination, the previous epidemic had occurred six years earlier, and the subsequent casual attitude to vaccination resulted in a level of population immunity well below the 75%

required to prevent a major epidemic. The epidemic began in the east of England and spread westwards. Initially, the amplitude was great, but succeeding waves showed a transition over time and space from type 1 to type 3; locations 1, 2 and 3 in *Figure 8.8* corresponding to the wave types predicted by Kendall. The contours in *Figure 8.9* are time contours of 15-day periods (15 days is a rough multiple of the average incubation period, calculated from a range of 3−10 days). Thus, the contour with the value 9 marks the 135th day of the epidemic. These contours suggest that the 'velocity' of the epidemic temporarily decreased as the epidemic moved westwards.

The changes in the shape of these waves must result from a decrease in the value of S/S_c over time and space. This could occur either because S decreases and/or S_c increases. An increase in the latter could occur because of

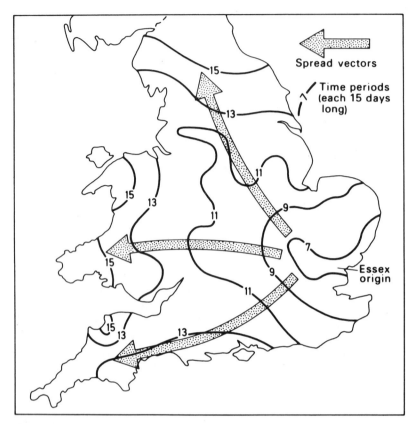

Fig. 8.9 Progress of the Newcastle disease epidemic of 1970–71 in England and Wales from its origins to the rest of the country. (From Cliff and Haggett, 1988.)

a change in the value of the removal rate, μ, but this is unlikely for a specific disease. Alternatively, the rate of infection, β, could alter, but this is equally unlikely, necessitating a change in virulence or infectiouness of the agent during the course of the epidemic. Thus, the most probable reason for the change in the wave shape is a reduction in S, which could plausibly be brought about by isolation of animals and vaccination. This is consistent with the pattern of the Newcastle disease epidemic, in which increased vaccinations and mandatory restrictions on poultry movement during the epidemic would have decreased the value of S.

Trends in the temporal distribution of disease

The temporal changes and fluctuations in disease occurrence can be classified into three major trends (*Figure 8.10*):

1. short-term;
2. cyclical (including seasonal);
3. long-term (secular).

Short-term trends

Short-term trends (*Figure 8.10b*) are typical epidemics, which have already been discussed.

Cyclical trends

Cyclical trends (*Figure 8.10c*) are associated with regular, periodic fluctuations in the level of disease occurrence. They are associated with periodic changes in the size of the susceptible host population and/or effective contact, and may produce **recurrent epidemics** or **endemic pulsations** (regular, **predictable** cyclical fluctuations). Thus, the 3–4 year cycle of foot-and-mouth disease in Paraguay (see *Figure 8.16*), and the predicted 4-year periodicity of fox rabies in Britain, with

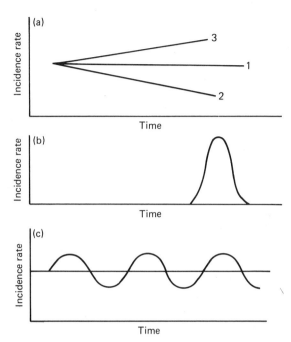

Fig. 8.10 Temporal trends in disease occurrence. (a) Long-term trend: (1) with equilibrium between infectious agent and host; (2) host/agent interaction biased to the host; (3) host/agent interaction biased to the agent. (b) Short-term trend. (c) Cyclical trend. (From Sinnecker, 1976.)

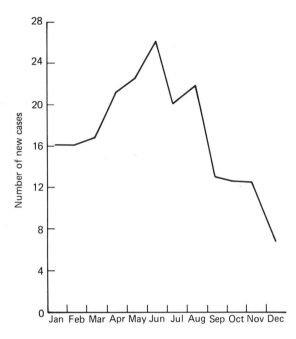

Fig. 8.11 Time trend graph depicting the seasonal occurrence of human brucellosis in the US: average annual occurrence, 1965–70. (Simplified from Steele *et al.*, 1972.)

a contact rate of 1.9 (see *Figure 19.4a*), are probably related to the time taken for the susceptible population to reach the threshold level.

Seasonal trends

A seasonal trend is a special case of a cyclical trend, where the periodic fluctuations in disease incidence are related to particular seasons. Fluctuations may be caused by changes in host density, management practices, survival of infectious agents, vector dynamics and other ecological factors. Thus, rinderpest occurs in Africa more commonly in the dry than the wet season because animals congregate at water holes, increasing the local animal density.

The prevalence of Lassa virus infection of the multimammate mouse (see Chapter 6) is related to density-dependent variations in mortality, competition with other rodents, and seasonal factors. The mouse may seek shelter in homes during the wet season, and this may partly explain the increased incidence of human Lassa fever during the wet season.

Human brucellosis in the US is more common during summer than winter (*Figure 8.11*), being associated with

the spring peak in calving of dairy cows and the concomitant increased risk of contracting infection from infected uterine discharges.

Rat plague demonstrates a seasonal incidence, being associated with climatically determined fluctuations in the population size of certain fleas that are vectors of the disease. Additionally, the rat population increases during the interepidemic season, thereby exacerbating the seasonal trend (Pollitzer and Meyer, 1961).

Leptospirosis is more common in the summer and early autumn than in the winter in temperate climates (*Figure 8.12*) because the warm, moist conditions during the summer predispose to survival of the pathogen (Diesch and Ellinghausen, 1975).

In contrast, transmissible gastroenteritis of pigs is more common in winter than summer (*Figure 8.13*). This may be because the survival time of the virus is very short in summer because of the stronger ultraviolet light and higher temperatures then (Haelterman, 1963).

In the US, feline panleucopenia shows a seasonal peak in August and September (Reif, 1976). This is associated with a peak in the number of births in the cat population in June, which increases the number of susceptible cats in the population at risk. The kittens are protected passively

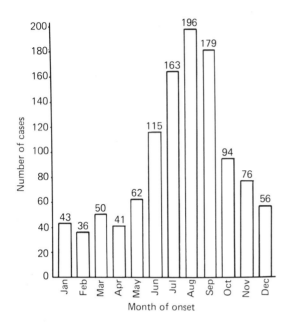

Fig. 8.12 Bar chart depicting the seasonal occurrence of human leptospirosis in the US. (From Diesch and Ellinghausen, 1975.)

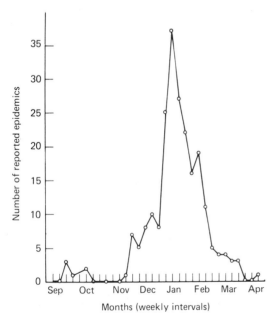

Fig. 8.13 Seasonal trend of transmissible gastroenteritis of pigs: reported epidemics in Illinois, 1968–69. (From Ferris, 1971.)

by maternal antibody for approximately the first two months of life, therefore the peak 'herd' susceptibility occurs two months after the birth peak. Such seasonal fluctuations are less likely in canine than in feline populations because births of puppies are distributed more evenly throughout the year than those of kittens (Tedor and Reif, 1978).

Some non-infectious diseases may also show seasonal trends. Thus, bovine hypomagnesaemia is common in spring and is associated, among other factors, with low levels of magnesium in rapidly-growing pastures (see *Figure 3.6*).

Sometimes seasonal determinants may be unidentified. For example, canine diabetes mellitus, like human insulin-dependent diabetes, is more common in winter than in summer (Marmor *et al.*, 1982).

Long-term (secular) trends

Secular trends (*Figure 8.10a*) occur over a long period of time and represent a long-term interaction between host and parasite. If a balance occurs, then a stable, endemic level of disease is maintained (1 in *Figure 8.10a*); if the interaction is biased to the host, then there is a gradual decrease in disease occurrence (2); and if the interaction is biased to the parasite, there is a gradual increase in disease occurrence (3).

Figure 8.14 illustrates a **reported** increasing long-term trend in the annual prevalence of rabies in wildlife in the US, whereas the prevalence in dogs is decreasing due to adequate control. 'Reported' is emphasized to stress that accurate estimation of trends is open to errors, some of which are described below.

Upward trends may also result from the intervention of man and changing human habits. Such trends occur with

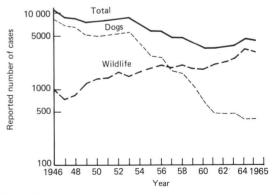

Fig. 8.14 An example of a secular trend: reported cases of rabies in the US, 1946–65. (From West, 1972.)

Table 8.2 Reasons for true and false temporal changes in incidence and prevalence according to changes in the numerator (cases) and denominator (animal-years at risk etc./population at risk).

True changes

Incidence:	change in incidence
Prevalence:	(a) change in incidence
	(b) change in duration of disease

False changes

Prevalence and incidence:

1. Errors in the numerator:
   (a) changes in the recognition of disease
   (b) changes in the procedures for classifying disease

2. Errors in the denominator:
   (a) errors in enumeration of the animal-years at risk etc./population at risk

---

the so-called 'diseases of civilization' and 'urbanization' in man (e.g., coronary heart disease) and the diseases of intensive production in animals. Secular decreases in morbidity may be the product of prophylaxis (e.g., vaccination). Mortality may show a secular decrease due to improved therapeutic techniques.

True and false changes in morbidity and mortality

The temporal changes that occur in recorded morbidity and mortality rates may be either true or false. The recording of mortality rates is rarer in veterinary than in human medicine because recording death in animals is not compulsory. Thus, details of trends in mortality in animals are usually unavailable.

The common measures of morbidity — prevalence, cumulative incidence and incidence rate — comprise a numerator (number of cases) and a denominator ('population at risk' for the first two measures, and 'animal-years at risk' etc. or a suitable approximation, for the third: Chapter 4). Changes in either numerator or denominator induce changes in these measures that may be either true or false (*Table 8.2*). True changes in incidence can affect these recorded measures and prevalence; additionally, changes in disease duration affect prevalence (see Chapter 4).

A major cause of false changes is variation in the recognition and reporting of disease. Thus, the increasing secular trend in wildlife rabies in the US between 1946

and 1965 (*Figure 8.14*) may have resulted from increased recognition and reporting of affected animals, rather than a genuine increase in incidence. Similarly, in the US reports of feline heartworm disease have increased over the years (Guerrero *et al.*, 1992), but it is difficult to say if this is due to increased awareness, improved methods of diagnosis, or a true rise in the disease's incidence.

The sampling of an animal population to record morbidity is also subject to inherent **variation** in the samples (see Chapter 12), and so appropriate statistical analysis should be undertaken (see Chapter 13).

Apparently changing patterns therefore should be interpreted with due regard to the possibility that they are artificial.

Detecting temporal trends: time series analysis

Short-term, seasonal and secular changes are temporal trends that can occur simultaneously, and may be mixed with random variation. In such circumstances, the various changes can be identified by statistical investigation. One method, originally applied in commerce, that is used in epidemiology to detect temporal trends, is **time series analysis**.

A time series is a record of events that occur over a period of time; cases of disease are typical events. The events are plotted as points on a graph, with 'time' along the horizontal axis. *Table 8.3*, for instance, records the percentage of sheep lungs condemned monthly because of pneumonia or pleurisy at a Scottish slaughterhouse. *Figure 8.15a* plots these monthly values. There is considerable variation in the location of the points, but, by eye, an annual cycle is suggested, and there appears to be a slight secular trend of increased prevalence from 1979 to 1983. Trends in these data may be detected by three methods:

1. free-hand drawing;
2. calculation of rolling (moving) averages;
3. regression analysis;

the object being to identify, and, if required, to remove, random variation, and seasonal and secular trends.

Free-hand drawing

The joining of points by eye is an obvious, easy method of indicating a trend. However, it is susceptible to subjective interpretation and cannot counteract random variation readily.

Calculation of rolling (moving) averages

A rolling average is the arithmetic average of consecutive

Table 8.3 Percentage of sheep lungs condemned monthly because of pneumonia and/or pleurisy, and average monthly and yearly percentage condemnation rates (1979–83) at a Scottish abattoir. (From Simmonds and Cuthbertson, 1985.)

	Jan %	Feb %	Mar %	Apr %	May %	Jun %	Jul %	Aug %	Sep %	Oct %	Nov %	Dec %	Yearly % condemnation rate
1979	0.33	0.24	0.46	0.57	0.65	0.23	0.27	0.37	0.14	0.30	0.24	0.14	0.33
1980	0.40	0.38	0.39	0.65	0.58	0.49	0.49	0.19	0.27	0.34	0.30	0.44	0.41
1981	0.48	0.58	0.62	0.75	0.51	0.44	0.21	0.17	0.18	0.21	0.35	0.27	0.40
1982	0.72	0.71*	0.75*	0.85	0.45	0.34	0.26	0.43	0.95	0.60	1.41	0.63	0.68
1983	0.71	0.64	0.48	0.84	0.38	0.48	0.69	0.80	1.09	0.76	1.25	0.97	0.76
Average monthly % condemnation rate	0.53	0.51	0.54	0.73	0.51	0.40	0.38	0.39	0.53	0.44	0.71	0.49	

*Estimated

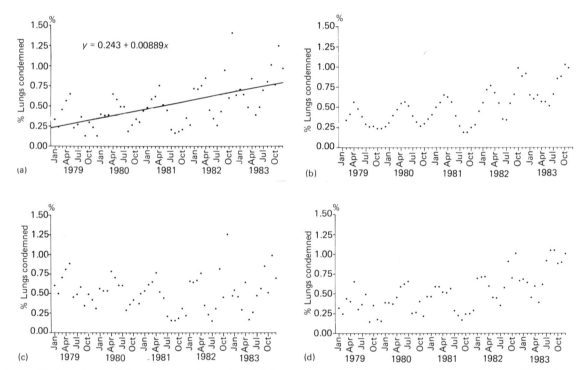

Fig. 8.15 Percentages of sheep lungs condemned monthly because of pneumonia and/or pleurisy and average monthly and yearly percentage condemnation rates (1979–83) at a Scottish abattoir. (a) Percentages of lungs condemned monthly because of pneumonia and/or pleurisy (data from *Table 8.3*) with regression line. (b) Three-monthly rolling average percentage lung condemnation rate because of pneumonia and/or pleurisy (data from *Table 8.4*). (c) Percentages of lungs condemned monthly (corrected to remove secular trend) because of pneumonia and/or pleurisy. (d) Percentages of lungs condemned monthly (corrected to remove seasonal trend) because of pneumonia and/or pleurisy. (From Simmons and Cuthbertson, 1985.)

groups of measurements. Thus, to construct a rolling three-month average of the monthly data in *Table 8.3*, sequential sets of three adjacent values are averaged. For example, the rolling average for February 1979 is calculated by summing the monthly averages for January, February and March and dividing by 3:

Table 8.4 Three-month rolling average percentage condemnation rates because of pneumonia and/or pleurisy (1979–83) at a Scottish abattoir. (Calculated from the data in *Table 8.3*.)

	Jan %	Feb %	Mar %	Apr %	May %	Jun %	Jul %	Aug %	Sep %	Oct %	Nov %	Dec %
1979		0.34	0.42	0.56	0.48	0.38	0.29	0.26	0.27	0.23	0.23	0.26
1980	0.31	0.39	0.47	0.54	0.57	0.52	0.39	0.32	0.27	0.30	0.36	0.41
1981	0.50	0.56	0.65	0.63	0.57	0.39	0.27	0.19	0.19	0.25	0.28	0.45
1982	0.56	0.72	0.77	0.68	0.55	0.35	0.34	0.55	0.66	0.99	0.88	0.92
1983	0.66	0.61	0.65	0.57	0.57	0.52	0.66	0.86	0.88	1.03	0.99	

$$\text{three-month rolling average (February 1979)} = \frac{0.33 + 0.24 + 0.46}{3}$$
$$= 0.34$$

The three-month rolling average for March 1979 likewise is calculated by summing the values for February, March and April 1979 and dividing by 3. *Table 8.4* presents three-month rolling averages using the data in *Table 8.3*, and *Figure 8.15b* presents these averages graphically. This technique reduces random variation, and therefore may reveal underlying trends; an annual cyclic trend is clearly visible in *Figure 8.15b*.

The seasonal trend in this example cannot be explained readily. However, it is known that the prevalence of atypical pneumonia increases as the stocking density increases and as the altitude at which sheep are reared decreases (Jones and Gilmour, 1983). Thus, lowland, intensively reared sheep are more likely to develop pneumonia than hill sheep. Lambs slaughtered in the spring are most frequently from the lowlands, and lambs slaughtered in the late summer and autumn are most frequently from the hills; this policy could therefore explain the seasonal trend.

Two disadvantages of rolling averages are that the first and last elements of a data set cannot be averaged (January 1979 and December 1983 in *Table 8.4*), and the averages can be affected unduly by extreme values.

Regression analysis

Regression analysis is a statistical technique for investigating relationships between two or more variables. It requires a knowledge of statistics and so the reader who is unfamiliar with basic statistics should read Chapters 12 and 14 before proceeding further.

Regression and correlation (the latter described in Chapter 14) are related. However, there is one major difference: a correlation coefficient may be evaluated if both or all variables exhibit random variation. Regression, however, involves the **selection** of individuals on the basis of one or more measurements (the explanatory variables) and then records the others (the response variables); therefore the explanatory variables should have no random variation. Discussion here will consider only one explanatory variable and one response variable.

When observations are made at defined intervals, these **selected** intervals of time represent the explanatory variable, x, which is why regression, not correlation, is applied to detecting an association between events and time. The technique can be applied to the data in *Table 8.3*.

A graph showing the variation of the mean of y in relation to x would show the relationship between y and x that is observed, in practice, with random variation. If it is assumed that the true values of y, for each value of x, lie in a straight line, then this line is known as the **regression line** of the linear regression of y on x. The slope of the line is termed the **regression coefficient** of y on x. This may be positive, negative, or, if x and y are unassociated, zero. The estimation of the regression coefficient and the intercept with the vertical axis, and the interpretation of the values of these estimates, is called **regression analysis**. If the relationship is not a linear one then a suitable transformation of x or y or both, such as their squares or logarithms, may transform the relationship to linearity.

Assume that the equation of the true regression line is:

$$y = \alpha + \beta x,$$

where β is the regression coefficient, and α is the intercept defining the point of interception of the y axis by the regression line. A set of n points (x, y) of observations is available to estimate this line. The regression coefficient, β, is estimated by:

$$b = \frac{\Sigma(x-\bar{x})(y-\bar{y})}{\Sigma(x-\bar{x})^2}$$

$$= \frac{\Sigma(xy)-(\Sigma x)(\Sigma y)/n}{\Sigma x^2-(\Sigma x)^2/n}$$

The intercept, α, is estimated by:

$$a = \bar{y} - b\bar{x}.$$

Using the data in *Table 8.3*, the values of x being integers from 1 to 60 (i.e., monthly intervals for 5 years) and of y being the respective monthly condemnation rates:

Σx	= 1830.0	Σy	= 30.820
$(\Sigma x)^2$	= 3 348 900	Σx^2	= 73 810
$\Sigma(xy)$	= 1 100.0	n	= 60
$\bar{x}$	= 30.500	$\bar{y}$	= 0.51367.

Thus:

$$b = \frac{1100.0 - (1830.0 \times 30.820)/60}{73\ 810 - 3\ 348\ 900/60},$$

$$= 0.008\ 89,$$

and:

$$a = 0.573\ 67 - (0.008\ 89 \times 30.500)$$
$$= 0.2425.$$

The regression line can now be plotted, substituting the values of x, from 1 to 60, in the formula for the regression line, to determine the respective values of y (*Figure 8.15a*).

Thus, when $x = 1$ (January 1979):

$$y = 0.2425 + (0.008\ 89 \times 1)$$
$$= 0.2514;$$

when $x = 2$ (February 1979):

$$y = 0.2425 + (0.008\ 89 \times 2)$$
$$= 0.2603;$$

and so on.

Note that, in this example, the relationship between x and y is linear.

The effect of the secular trend can be removed by subtracting $b(x-\bar{x})$ from each value of y. Thus, for July 1979, $x = 7$ and:

$$b(x-\bar{x}) = 0.008\ 89(7-30.500)$$
$$= 0.008\ 89 \times -23.500$$
$$= -0.2089;$$

and the value of y with the secular trend removed is:

$$0.27 - (-0.2089) = 0.4789.$$

The results for the 60-month period, with the secular trend removed, are depicted in *Figure 8.15c*.

The effect of seasonal variation can be removed by calculating a 'seasonal index', in this example for each month. The value of y for each month of a year is taken as a proportion of the total of y for that year; these proportions are averaged for a particular month over the period of study (five years in this instance) to give a seasonal index for each month of the year. The results are 'de-seasonalized' by dividing each value of y by the relevant monthly index multiplied by 12. Thus, for July 1979, the proportion of the total of y contributed by July is:

$$0.27/(0.33+0.24+0.46+0.57+0.65+0.23+$$
$$0.27+0.37+0.14+0.30+0.24+0.14)$$

$$= \frac{0.27}{3.95} = 0.0684.$$

The proportions for July 1980, 1981, 1982 and 1983 are 0.0995, 0.0440, 0.0320 and 0.0759, respectively. The July seasonal index therefore is:

$$(0.0684 + 0.0995 + 0.0440 + 0.0320 + 0.0759)/5$$
$$= 0.3199/5 = 0.0640,$$

and the 'de-seasonalized' value for July 1979 is:

$$0.27/(0.0640 \times 12) = 0.352.$$

The 'de-seasonalized' results for the period of study are shown in *Figure 8.10d*.

Note that a considerable amount of random variation remains when the secular and seasonal trends are removed (*Figures 8.15c* and *d*, respectively); this variation tends to obscure the seasonal trend in *Figure 8.15c*, and the secular trend in *Figure 8.15d*. In such circumstances, calculation of rolling averages provides a rapid means of reducing random variation. An increase in sample size also should reduce the effects of this variation. A formal significance test may be required when the effects of random variation are considerable. A description of a suitable test, and the estimation of the standard error and confidence limits of β, is given by Bailey (1981).

Figure 8.16 shows the results of a time series analysis of foot-and-mouth disease in Paraguay (Peralta *et al.*, 1982). The disease shows a cycle with a periodicity of 3−4 years (peaks in 1972, 1975−76 and 1979), due to type O virus. The small peak in 1974, which was not consistent with the cycle, was caused by a sporadic outbreak due to type C virus. The reason for the cyclicity may be the changes in the proportion of the susceptible

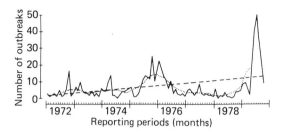

Fig. 8.16 Foot-and-mouth disease outbreaks reported by month, 12-month rolling average and trend; Paraguay, 1972–79. ———— Raw data: ···· 12-month moving average; – – – trend. (From Peralta *et al.*, 1982.)

cattle population, 3–4 years being necessary to increase the number again to the threshold level. Identification of this temporal pattern can indicate times when particular attention should be paid to control.

A similar time series analysis of rabies in Chile, comparing the disease's temporal pattern before and after implementation of a control campaign (Ernst and Fabrega, 1989), is depicted in *Figure 8.17*. There was a slight, but statistically significant, secular increase in rabies between 1950 and 1960, attributable to cases in dogs, when no control was undertaken (*Figure 8.17a*). A national control programme, involving vaccination of humans and dogs, was instituted in 1961, and rabies declined between 1961 and 1970 (*Figure 8.17b*). The steady decline continued between 1971 and 1986 (*Figure 8.17c*). No cases were reported in 1982, but a previously undescribed sylvatic cycle was reported in insectivorous bats in 1985, and resulted in cases in dogs and cats (*Figure 8.17c*). This study also revealed a seasonal trend, and five-year cyclical trend, possibly associated with fluctuations in the size of the susceptible dog population.

Regression is discussed in standard introductory statistics texts such as that by Bailey (1981) and, in the context of time series analysis, in those by Sard (1979) and Wheelwright and Makridakis (1973).

Trends in the spatial and temporal distribution of disease

Spatial trends in disease occurrence

An epidemic represents not only the clustering of cases over a period of time, but also a clustering of cases in a defined area. An infectious disease that propagates through a population results in a **contagious** spatial pattern, in contrast to sporadic outbreaks, which are

distributed **randomly**. These two patterns can be compared with **regular** spatial occurrence (*Figure 8.18*). 'Contagious' can also be applied, in a general sense, to the spatial clustering of disease, whether or not it is infectious (ecologists sometimes use 'over-dispersion' to refer to this type of spatial clustering in animal populations, with 'under-dispersion' referring to more regular spacing).

A variety of statistical distributions (see Chapter 12) serve as models for the spatial distribution of events (Southwood, 1978). The Poisson distribution has commonly been applied. The goodness of fit of a set of

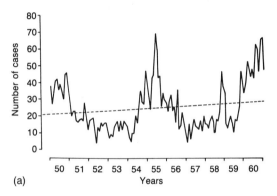

(a)

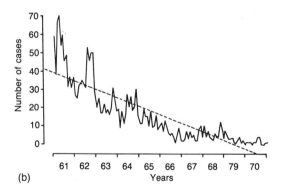

(b)

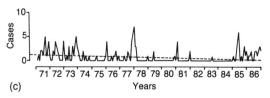

(c)

Fig. 8.17 Total number of laboratory-confirmed cases of rabies reported by month, and trend, Chile, 1950–86: (a) 1950–60, (b) 1961–70, (c) 1971–86. ———— Raw data: – – – trend. (From Ernst and Fabrega, 1989.)

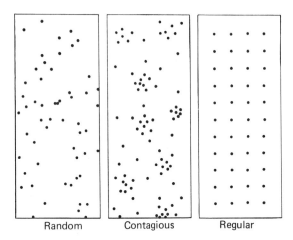

Random   Contagious   Regular

Fig. 8.18 Patterns of the spatial distribution of disease. (From Southwood, 1978.)

data to the Poisson distribution can be tested by performing a χ^2-test on the observed and expected values; standard statistical texts, such as Bailey (1981), give details. If the variance is less than the mean, it implies the occurrence of a more regular distribution than is described by a Poisson series. If the variance is greater than the mean, it implies that a 'contagious' distribution is present.

Identification of spatial clustering can assist in the identification of the cause of disease (Rothman, 1987). Thus, the clustering of feline leukaemia among genetically unrelated cats provided early evidence of

horizontal transmission and therefore of the disease's infectious nature (Brodey *et al.*, 1970).

The statistical methods for identifying different spatial patterns are described in detail by Cliff and Ord (1981).

Space−time clustering

Space−time clustering is an interaction between the places of onset and the times of onset of a disease; cases that are close in space tending to be close in time. The Poisson distribution can sometimes, but not always, be applied to this type of interaction — particularly for large samples (David and Barton, 1966). Techniques for detecting time−space clustering are beyond the scope of this book. They are described by Knox (1964), David and Barton (1966), Mantel (1967), and Pike and Smith (1968). They are reviewed by Williams (1984) and Schukken *et al.* (1990) who also give an example relating to winter dysentery in dairy cattle.

Further reading

Bailey, N.T.J. (1975) *The Mathematical Theory of Infectious Diseases*, 2nd edn. Charles Griffin and Company, London and High Wycombe

Cliff, A.D. and Haggett, P. (1988) *Atlas of Disease Distributions: Analytic Approaches to Epidemiological Data*. Basil Blackwell, Oxford

Halpin, B. (1975) *Patterns of Animal Disease*. Baillière Tindall, London

Sinnecker, H. (1976) *General Epidemiology* (translated by Walker, N). John Wiley and Sons, London

9 The nature of data

The epidemiologist investigates the frequency and distribution of disease (and sometimes other characteristics, such as performance) in groups of animals. This involves the collection and analysis of **data** (singular: datum): 'facts, especially numerical facts, collected together for reference or information' (*Oxford English Dictionary*, 1972). These data may relate to clinical signs, therapy, and post-mortem and laboratory examinations. If an investigation is undertaken prospectively, the epidemiologist has to decide what data should be collected. If an investigation is undertaken retrospectively, the epidemiologist may use data that have been collected by veterinary practices, abattoirs, laboratories, clinics, and other organizations (see Chapter 10). Therefore, it is necessary to know whether the types of data that are collected are suitable for a particular investigation.

Inferences about the cause of disease involve categorizing individuals into a group that has a disease and a group that does not have the disease, the object being to decide whether these two groups differ with respect to possible determinants. This is the basis of observational studies (outlined in Chapter 2 and detailed in Chapter 15). Animals are put into the diseased category because they possess certain attributes, such as clinical signs and lesions, that are used to define, and sometimes to name, the disease. A knowledge of the various features that are pertinent to the classification of disease is therefore necessary.

Some data are observations; for example, the recording of diarrhoea. Other data are interpretations of observations; for instance, a diagnosis, which represents an interpretation of a set of clinical signs, lesions and laboratory results. The interpretation, and therefore the diagnosis, may be incorrect; this could result in an animal being erroneously categorized as having a particular disease. Any inferences on association between possible causal factors and disease, drawn from a study of this animal, may therefore be erroneous.

Additionally, some data that epidemiologists use nowadays are stored in computers as codes.

Classification of data

Data can be broadly classified into **qualitative** and **quantitative** (*Figure 9.1*).

Qualitative data describe a property of an animal, that is, its membership of a group or class. Such data therefore are termed **categorical**. Examples are the breed and sex of an animal.

Quantitative data relate to **amounts**, rather than just indicating classes. Examples are prevalence, incidence, body weight, milk yield, temperature and antibody titre. These data may be further divided into **discrete** and **continuous**.

Discrete data can have only one of a specified set of values, such as whole numbers (1, 2, 7, 9, etc.), for example, the number of teats on a sow. Discrete data generate **counts**. Thus, aggregates of qualitative (categorical) data are counted (e.g., the total number of male dogs or Friesian cows).

Continuous data may have any value within a defined range (though the range can be infinite). Examples are the girth of a cow and its body weight. Continuous data are quantified by comparison with a fixed unit, that is, they are measured. Continuous data therefore generate **measurements**.

Scales (levels) of measurement

Although measurement can be applied strictly only to quantitative, continuous data, 'scale of measurement' is also conventionally used to describe the 'strength' of values that can be attached to both qualitative and quantitative data. There are four main scales (levels) of measurement: **nominal, ordinal, interval** and **ratio** (*Figure 9.1*), and a **visual analogue scale** is also sometimes used.

The nominal (classificatory) scale

The nominal scale involves the use of numbers (or other symbols) to classify objects. Thus, male and female can be **coded** 1 and 2, respectively. A non-veterinary example is the use of numbers or letters on aircraft to indicate their origin. The property of a nominal scale is **equivalence**: members in a class must possess the same property.

The only legitimate operation that can be performed on a nominal scale is transformation of the symbols. For example, if the disease, diabetes, was numerically coded as 671 then this value could be transformed or changed to 932 for **all** diabetics. This scale is a 'weak' form of 'measurement'.

The ordinal (ranking) scale

The ordinal scale allows groups to be related to other groups. Most commonly, the relation can be expressed in terms of equal to, greater than ($>$) or less than ($<$). Examples are the use of body condition scores for sheep, and clinical grading of severity of disease.

The difference between the nominal and the ordinal scale therefore is that the ordinal includes not only equivalence but also the 'greater than' and 'less than' property.

In the ordinal scale, any transformation must preserve the order. It does not matter what number is attached to a class, as long as the relationship with other classes is consistent. Thus, a carcass condition score scale can include 5 = 'good' and 1 = 'poor', and equally 1 = 'good' and 5 = 'poor', as long as the numbers between 1 and 5 maintain the same order of ranking. Although 'stronger' than the nominal scale, the ordinal scale is still a relatively 'weak' form of 'measurement'.

The interval scale

In an interval scale, the distance between the ranked values is known with some accuracy. A good example is body temperature. Two thermal interval scales are commonly used — Celsius and Fahrenheit — each containing the same amount of information. The ratios of the intervals (temperature differences in this example) are independent of the zero point ($0°C = 32°F$) and are equal to the ratios of the differences on the other interval scales. For example:

$37°C = 99°F$ (approximately)
$22°C = 72°F$ (approximately)
$6°C = 43°F$ (approximately).

Thus $(°C)$ $\dfrac{37-22}{22-6} = \dfrac{15}{16} = 0.9375$

and $(°F)$ $\dfrac{99-72}{72-43} = \dfrac{27}{29} = 0.931\ 034\ 4\ldots$

that is, the ratios are approximately the same (0.9).

The interval scale therefore includes equivalence, 'greater than' relationships, and ratios of intervals. Because the ratios are independent of the zero point, arithmetic calculations can be performed only on differences between numbers. The interval scale is a relatively 'strong' form of (actual) measurement.

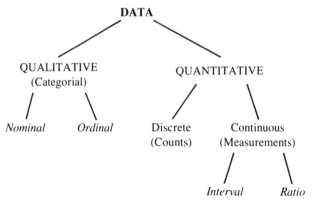

Fig. 9.1 A broad classification of data. Scales (levels) of measurement are italicized.

The ratio scale

The ratio scale is an interval scale with a true zero point. Weight is a ratio scale. The various weight ratio scales may have units of kilograms, grams, pounds or ounces, but they all start from the same zero point. This means that arithmetic operations can be performed not only on the ratios of differences but also on the numbers themselves. Note that a ratio scale is not necessarily associated with ratios, many of which are ratios of counts (e.g., prevalence; see Chapter 4). Weight, for instance, is a ratio scale that is not a ratio.

The visual analogue scale

The visual analogue scale (VAS) uses a straight line, usually 100 mm long, the extreme limits of which are marked with perpendicular lines. Each end has a verbal description of one extreme of the variable that is being measured; *Figure 9.2* is an example of a VAS for recording severity of lameness in sheep. The observer marks the line in a position corresponding to the 'severity' of the variable that is being evaluated. The line is subsequently divided into 100 equal divisions for the purpose of analysis. The VAS is commonly used in human medicine to assess pain, and has been similarly applied in veterinary medicine (Reid and Nolan, 1991).

Ordinal and visual analogue scales are relatively simple, non-invasive ways of recording severity of lesions and clinical signs, and so are attractive options for recording changes in patients' status in clinical trials (see Chapter 16). However, both scales are subjective, and their accuracy and repeatability (see below) are complex; for example, the latter can vary along the length of a VAS (Dixon and Bird, 1981). Welsh *et al*. (1993) demonstrated good correlation* between the two scales, and between repeated measurements on the same animals, when assessing lameness in sheep.

These scales of measurement have been considered in detail because of their importance in determining appropriate statistical methods. Most statistical tests can be used with interval, ratio and visual analogue scales. However, not all tests can be applied to nominal and ordinal scales. This point will be expanded in Chapter 14.

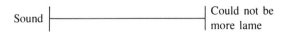

Sound ├─────────────────────┤ Could not be
                                  more lame

Fig. 9.2 An example of a visual analogue scale: severity of lameness in sheep (reduced). (From Welsh *et al*., 1993.)

*Note, however, that *correlation* is not the same as *agreement* (see Chapter17).

Data elements

Nomenclature and classification of disease

Nominal data relating to disease frequently include the names of diseases. The name given to a disease is closely associated with the way in which a disease is classified. Diseases are defined at three levels (*Figure 9.3a*) in relation to:

1. specific causes;
2. lesions or deranged functions;
3. presenting problems.

Diseases are generally named according to their allocation to one of these three levels; for example, parvovirus infection (specific cause), hepatitis (lesion) and ataxia (presenting problem). A fourth method of naming involves the use of eponyms, for example, Rubarth's disease and Newcastle disease.

The situation is frequently more complicated: a presenting problem may have more than one set of lesions and specific causes (*Figures 9.3b* and *9.3c*). Similarly, one specific cause may produce more than one lesion and therefore more than one presenting sign (*Figure 9.3d*).

Veterinarians usually define (and therefore record) disease as a diagnosis in terms of a combination of specific cause, lesion and presenting problem. Sometimes one or more levels may be missing; thus, the dilated pupil syndrome in cats (feline dysautonomia) is defined in terms of lesions and presenting problem, although the specific cause is unknown (Gaskell, 1983). Initially this disease was eponymously named the 'Key-Gaskell syndrome'.

The significance of the nomenclature and classification of disease in epidemiological investigations

Different sectors of the veterinary profession require different types of information for their work. Pathologists have a major interest in lesions. When notifiable diseases occur, administrators act according to sets of rules that are defined by legislation; the classification of these diseases is of little consequence to the action that is taken. Similarly, epidemiologists who undertake surveys of morbidity that do not involve the testing of a causal hypothesis are concerned only with identification of a disease, irrespective of the way in which it is classified or named. However, the method of classifying disease is important in causal investigations.

The classification shown in *Figure 9.3* can be simplified to two methods:

1. by **manifestations**, namely signs and lesions;

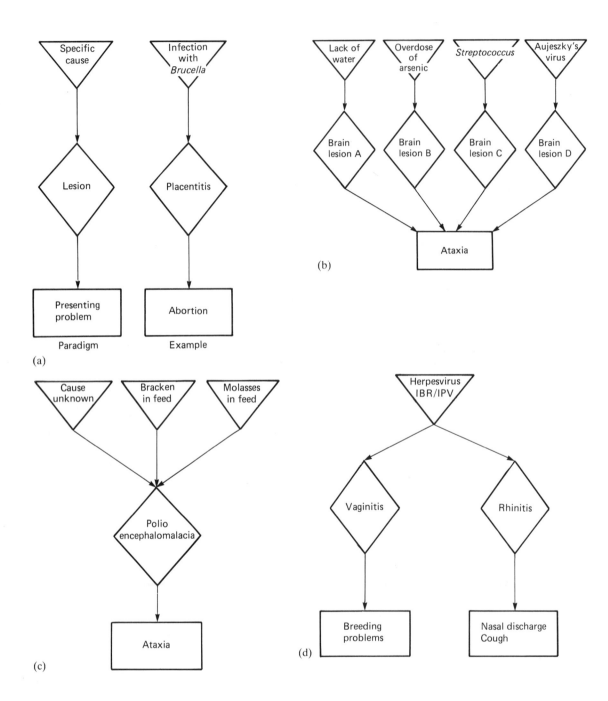

Fig. 9.3 (a) The three levels of disease classification. (b) A presenting problem common to multiple sets of lesions and specific causes. (c) A presenting problem and a lesion common to multiple specific causes. (d) A specific cause with divergent sets of lesions and presenting problems. In terms of causal model 1 (Chapter 3), a specific cause represents a major component of a sufficient cause. ((a) Modified from Hall, 1978; (b) (c) and (d) from Hall, 1978.)

2. by **cause**.

An epidemiological causal investigation attempts to detect associations between causal factors and disease. The investigation therefore is conducted because one or more specific causes are not known. In such a case, the disease that is being studied is frequently named according to manifestations. For example, considering *Figure 9.3b*, if the disease being studied were defined as ataxia (a presenting sign which is a manifestation), then ataxic animals would be heterogeneous with respect to cause; four separate specific causes could be involved. This would make causal inference more difficult than if there were only a single specific cause that was common to all animals classified as diseased. Similarly, in *Figure 9.3c*, if disease were defined as polioencephalomalacia (a lesion, which is a manifestation), then the animals with the lesion could also be heterogeneous with respect to cause. Classification by cause in *Figure 9.3a* assists causal inference, because a common specific cause and associated component causes may be demonstrated in all cases of animals that are classified as diseased.

Frequently, only suboptimal data relating just to manifestations (often just signs) are available, and they must be used with due regard to their defects, or as the basis of more detailed investigations. Russell *et al.* (1982), for example, were aware that lameness (a datum defining disease in terms of presenting signs, and frequently involving several lesions and causes) was a problem in British dairy herds, and used this as the starting point for an investigation in which they attempted to elucidate the underlying lesions and causes, by means of a questionnaire, before trying to develop suitable control strategies.

Diagnostic criteria

Disease can be diagnosed using one or more of four criteria:

1. clinical signs and symptoms;*
2. detection of specific agents;
3. reactions to diagnostic tests;
4. identification of lesions.

Observational and interpretative data

Records relating to the four diagnostic criteria may be of either **observations** or **interpretations** (Leech, 1980).

---

*A sign is an abnormal feature of the patient that is observed; a symptom is a subjective abnormal feature that is described by the patient himself in human medicine.

The terms overlap in that observations usually imply a comparison with the normal which itself is often a matter of judgement. For example, to observe and record that a cow is diarrhoeic implies that its faeces are less firm than its peers, and must also take into account that cows at peak yield, receiving much concentrate, usually have loose faeces.

A clinical sign may represent an observation, for example nasal discharge. A diagnosis represents an interpretation of one or several observations. Distemper, for example, is a diagnosis that implicitly involves the interpretation of several signs, including perhaps nasal discharge, diarrhoea and coughing.

Specific agents may be observed, for instance species of *Babesia* may be identified in a blood smear. Alternatively, the presence of agents may be recorded interpretatively, for example the presence of *Escherichia coli* in the faeces of an animal with diarrhoea may be recorded as being 'not clinically significant'.

Test reactions may be observed, for example the recording of antibody titres in serological tests. Results may also be interpreted, for example the result of an intradermal tuberculin test may be recorded as 'inconclusive'.

Pathological lesions may be observed, for example a histological description of a skin tumour may be given. This description may then be interpreted as a diagnosis, for example defining a skin tumour as equine sarcoid.

Interpretation involves the use of currently acceptable diagnostic criteria. The recording of 'distemper', mentioned above, assumes a causal association between a particular virus and several signs. This assumption, based upon previous experimental work and many field observations, has been acceptable for many years. Similarly, the recording of *E. coli* as being 'not clinically significant' in some diarrhoea cases uses a criterion based upon current knowledge of commensalism.

Sometimes, however, diagnostic criteria may be difficult to define; for example, when the histological appearance of a tumour can vary considerably (e.g., equine sarcoid: Ragland *et al.*, 1970). Additionally, criteria may be complex and subject to change. Thus, navicular disease has historically had several criteria for its diagnosis, including heel pain, soundness following palmar digital nerve block, and radiological evidence of enlarged vacular foramina, cystic formations, thinning of the flexor cortex, marginal osteophytosis and remodelling of the normal shape of the bone (McClure, 1988). However, many conditions causing heel pain can be blocked by palmar digital nerve block, and recent studies suggest that there is no difference between the frequency of radiographically identified lesions of navicular disease in clinically affected animals and animals with no history of lameness (Turner *et al.*, 1987).

An observational datum is easily recorded in full. However, it is difficult to record an interpretative datum fully; this would require not only the interpretation (e.g., a diagnosis) but also a record of the criteria used in the interpretation. In many cases the criteria are implicit, as in the case of distemper, and so are not recorded explicitly. In others, where diagnostic criteria are complex (e.g., navicular disease), the criteria should be listed, otherwise comparison between cases (past, present and future) is impossible.

Observational and interpretative data are applied in different ways. Veterinary administrators, organizing national disease control campaigns, frequently use interpretative data to make decisions. For example, an animal's future may depend upon whether it reacts 'negatively', 'inconclusively' or 'positively' to screening tests.

Epidemiological investigations, particularly of diseases of unknown aetiology, require data such as details of diet, exposure to possible causal agents, and the various stages of a disease's pathogenesis, that are unambiguous. In this context, interpretative data may be misleading. Thus, when investigating obesity, it is better to have even an approximate estimate of an animal's body weight and food intake, than to have a subjective (interpretative) impression of its weight as 'heavy' or 'light', and its food intake as 'a little' or 'a lot', because these terms may represent different weights and amounts of food to different people. Observational studies also require an unambiguous, consistent definition of cases, and so the diagnostic criteria used to classify animals as diseased and healthy should be specified.

Sensitivity and specificity

Events may be recorded as being true when, actually, they are not. Thus, a dog may be diagnosed as having diabetes mellitus when it does not. This constitutes a **false positive** record, and renders the diagnosis inaccurate. The error in this case may have resulted from an improper inference based upon only a few clinical signs such as polyphagia and polydipsia, with no supporting biochemical evidence. Alternatively, diabetes may not be diagnosed when it is actually present. This constitutes a **false negative** record. Such errors inevitably lead to misclassification of 'diseased' and 'non-diseased' animals. These errors can occur when using clinical signs,

Table 9.1 Possible results of a diagnostic test exemplified by application of a centrifugation/flotation technique to horses of known tapeworm status. (From Proudman and Edwards, 1992.)

Test status	True status		Totals
	Positive	Negative	
Flotation positive	22(*a*)	1(*b*)	23
Flotation negative	14(*c*)	43(*d*)	57
Total	36	44	

Sensitivity = $a/(a+c)$ = 22/36 = 0.61 (61%)
Specificity = $d/(b+d)$ = 43/44 = 0.98 (98%)

detection of specific agents and reactions to diagnostic tests as diagnostic criteria.

These errors can be quantified by comparing results obtained by the diagnostic method with those obtained from an independent valid criterion. For example (*Table 9.1*), the validity of a faecal centrifugation/flotation technique in diagnosing equine cestodiasis can be determined by comparing the results of the test with those obtained from post-mortem examination of the intestinal tract to identify tapeworms (the independent valid criterion).

The **sensitivity** of a diagnostic method is the proportion of true positives that are detected by the method. The **specificity** of the method is the proportion of true negatives that are detected. Sensitivity and specificity can be quoted either as a probability between zero and one, or as a percentage. Thus, the sensitivity and specificity of the centrifugation/flotation technique are 0.61 and 0.98, respectively (*Table 9.1*).

The sensitivity and specificity of a diagnostic test are important in deciding the value of the test in disease control campaigns (see Chapter 17) and in categorizing animals in observational studies (see Chapter 15).

Accuracy, refinement, precision, reliability and validity

These terms can be used in relation to qualitative data (e.g., the description of a disease) and to quantitative measures (e.g., of prevalence and weight).

Accuracy

Accuracy is an indication of the extent to which an investigation or measurement conforms to the truth.

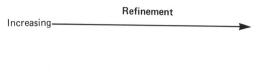

Otitis externa

Otitis externa caused by bacteria

Otitis externa caused by *Pseudomonas* spp.

Fig. 9.4 Example of increasing refinement of a diagnosis.

Thus, if a set of scales records an animal's weight at 15 kg and this is the actual weight of the animal, then the measurement is accurate.

Refinement

The degree of detail in a datum is its **refinement**. Thus, 13 kg and 13.781 kg may both represent the accurate weight of an animal, but the second record is more refined than the first. Similarly, 'orthopaedic surgery' is a less refined description of a surgical technique than is 'bone plating'. In *Figure 9.4*, 'otitis externa' is a less refined diagnosis than either 'otitis externa caused by bacteria' or 'otitis externa caused by *Pseudomonas* spp.' The less refined definition may be described as 'coarse grained' and the more refined definitions as 'fine grained' by analogy with photographic film. Specificity is sometimes used synonymously with refinement.

Increasing the refinement of descriptive diagnostic data may improve their epidemiological value because it usually moves towards a definition of disease in terms of particular specific causes, whereas a less refined definition in terms of manifestations can include several specific causes (*Figure 9.3c*).

Auxiliary tests are frequently required to increase the refinement of a diagnosis. Thus, physical examination may facilitate the diagnosis of otitis externa, but a more refined diagnosis of otitis externa involving *Pseudomonas* spp. infection would require the use of microbiological techniques. The refinement of auxiliary techniques may also vary. For example, the complement fixation test will detect types of influenza A virus, but will not detect subtypes. Identification of the latter requires more refined tests, for example haemagglutination and neuraminidase inhibition (see Chapter 17).

Precision

Precision can be used in two senses. First, it can be used as a synonym for refinement. Secondly, it can be used statistically to indicate the consistency of a series of measurements. Thus, repeated sampling of a population may allow estimation of a prevalence value of, say, 40% ± 2%. Alternatively, the value may be estimated as 40% ± 5%. The first estimation is more precise than the second. Precision, in the second sense, is discussed in more detail in Chapter 12.

Reliability

A diagnostic technique is **reliable** if it produces similar results when it is repeated. Thus **repeatability** is a characteristic of a reliable technique. This is defined in terms of the degree of agreement between sets of observations made on the same animals by the same observer (see Chapter 17). (This contrasts with **reproducibility**, which can be defined in terms of agreement between sets of observations made on the same animals by **different** observers: BSI, 1979.)*

Validity

If a diagnostic technique measures what it purports to measure, it is **valid**. Validity is a long-term characteristic of a technique, of which sensitivity and specificity are indicators. The validity of a technique depends upon the disease that is being investigated and the method of diagnosis. A midshaft femoral fracture, for example, may be diagnosed very accurately when using only physical examination (*Figure 9.5*): the lesion is rarely misdiagnosed; thus physical examination, as a diagnostic technique, is highly valid in this instance. However, physical examination alone may not be considered sufficiently error-free when used to diagnose diabetes mellitus. Biochemical examination, in this case urine analysis, may be used to decrease error, and fasting blood

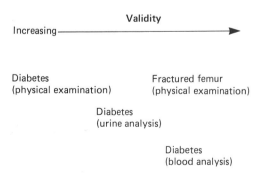

Fig. 9.5 Validity of diagnostic techniques in relation to the disease being studied.

*Some authorities (e.g., Last, 1988) do not distinguish between repeatability and reproducibility.

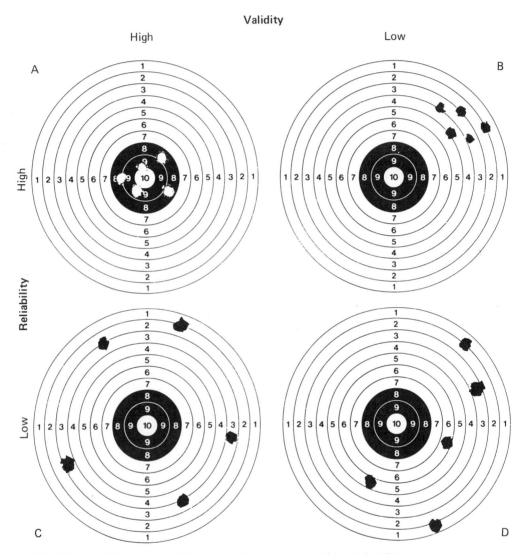

Fig. 9.6 Reliability and validity of diagnostic tests presented as analogues of target shooting.

sugar estimation to decrease it further. The use of auxiliary diagnostic aids, such as biochemical, radiological and microbiological investigation, is simply a means of increasing the accuracy of a diagnosis by selecting diagnostic techniques of higher validity.

The value of a diagnostic technique is judged in terms of its **reliability** and **validity**. This can be exemplified using target shooting as an analogy (*Figure 9.6*). In target A, each shot is accurate (i.e., close to the bull's-eye, which represents the true value), therefore validity and repeatability are high. In target B, none of the shots is

accurate, but the result is repeatable. In target D, none of the shots is accurate, and reliability is low because the shots are inconsistent with one another. Target C illustrates that, **on average**, it is possible to obtain high validity when the accuracy of individual shots is low. Thus, high validity corresponds to shots, on average, hitting the bull's-eye, whereas high reliability corresponds to shots being tightly packed.

Although there has been ambiguity in the use of these five terms (Last, 1988), accuracy is best considered as the property of a single diagnosis (i.e., of one shot at the bull's-eye) whereas validity should be considered as a long-term characteristic of a diagnostic technique (i.e., the average result of several shots).

Sensitivity, specificity and repeatability are discussed further in Chapter 17.

Bias

The shots fired at target B in *Figure 9.6* are not accurate, but they are repeatable. Thus, the results are reliable, but of low validity. In this example, the results may have occurred because the sights on the gun were **biased** to the right of the centre of the target. A similar bias can occur in diagnostic tests and epidemiological studies. Bias is any systematic (as opposed to random) error in the design, conduct or analysis of a study that renders results invalid.

Several types of bias can be identified (Last, 1988). Major ones are:

1. **bias due to confounding** (see Chapter 3);
2. **interviewer bias**, where an interviewer's opinions may affect accurate reporting of data;
3. **measurement bias**, involving inaccurate measurements or the misclassification of animals as diseased and non-diseased (e.g., when sensitivity and specificity are less than 100%);
4. **selection bias**, where animals selected for study have systematically different characteristics from those that are not selected for study; for example, animals selected from an abattoir are unlikely to have clinical disease, whereas the general population will include some clinically diseased individuals.

Bias is a **long-run** effect. Any individual shot in target B could have been one of those in targets C or D. Only when all of the shots have been fired can the bias be detected, because it requires demonstration of reliability. Thus, an individual observation from a population cannot be biased. Similarly, if many samples produce repeatable inaccurate results then bias is present in the **population** from which the sample was drawn.

Bias can be corrected if its extent is known. Thus, the sights on the gun can be adjusted to compensate for the bias; shots will then be accurate. Similarly, biased estimates of prevalence, resulting from a test's specificity and sensitivity being less than 100%, can be corrected if the sensitivity and specificity are known (see Chapter 17).

Representation of data: coding

Data are usually represented by both words and numbers. An alternative type of notation involves **coding**. This is a means of representing text and numerals in a **standardized**, usually abbreviated, form. Such standardization enables veterinary and medical data to be recorded in a consistent, unambiguous and uniform way. Codes are easier and more economic to handle by a computer than plain text and so are commonly used in modern computerized recording systems, from which the standardized data can be distributed (see Chapter 11). Representation may be by letters (**alpha codes**), numbers (**numeric codes**), a combination of each (**alphanumeric codes**) and, less frequently, by **symbols**.

Codes are a form of shorthand; they are briefer than their textual equivalents. Thus, it is easier and quicker to record the code number 274 than to write its possible textual equivalent, 'contagious bovine pleuropneumonia'.

Code structure

Data about animals divide into two groups; any system of coding must cope with both groups. The first includes categories that relate to **permanent** data such as details of species, breed, date of birth and sex. These data have been termed 'tombstone data' because they remain unchanged during the whole of an animal's life. The second group comprises data relating to events that **vary** during life, such as date of occurrence, lesions, test results, signs and diagnoses. The various categories sometimes are called **descriptors** or **specifier types**. Other data can be derived from these categories, for example, the animal's age at the onset of disease.

Components

The data that define disease can comprise a single component, called an **axis**, for example 'bronchiolitis'. Alternatively, the definition can be broken down into constituent parts. In the case of a lesion, two convenient axes are the underlying pathological process and its site (topography). Using this **biaxial** system (two axes), bronchiolitis can be recorded as 'inflammation' and 'bronchiole'. Similarly, surgical procedures can be coded biaxially, in terms of procedure and site; for example, 'intramedullary pinning' and 'femur'. It is therefore possible to build up disease definitions from basic components in various axes.

Numeric codes

Numeric codes represent text by numbers, for example: seborrhoea = 6327.

Most of the early veterinary and medical coding systems were numeric. A veterinary system, developed in

North America, is the *Standard Nomenclature of Veterinary Diseases and Operations* (*SNVDO*: Priester, 1964, 1971), which is based on the medical *Standard Nomenclature of Diseases and Operations* (*SNDO*: Thompson and Hayden, 1961). This codes diseases and operations (treatments) biaxially: diseases by topography and either aetiology or lesion, and operations by topography and procedure. Examples are:

diagnosis: 3530   3900.0 = bronchiolitis due to allergy,

treatment: 723   52 = ureteric anastomosis.

In these examples, the diagnosis includes a topographical part (3530 = bronchiole) and an aetiological part (3900.0 = allergy). Similarly, treatment is defined in terms of topography (723) and procedure (52).

Multiaxial systems have also been developed that allow the summarizing of recorded data under several axes; for example, the *Systematized Nomenclature of Veterinary Medicine* (*SNOVET*), which was originally based on six axes: topography, morphology, aetiology, function, disease and procedure (Pilchard, 1985). This has now been modified and combined with *SNOMED* (Systematized Nomenclature of Medicine) to form *SNOMED III* (Cote *et al.*, 1993). Despite shortcomings, *SNOMED III* is considered a sound base for coding veterinary findings, phrases, terms and concepts (Case, 1994; Klimczak, 1994).

Consecutive and hierarchic codes

A **consecutive** code is one in which consecutive numbers are drawn up to represent data, for example: 001 = distemper, 002 = infectious hepatitis, 003 = acute cystitis.

It is also possible to draw up a list of codes with a **hierarchic** structure, that is, with initial digits representing broad categories, and succeeding digits indicating more refined categories; the more digits used, the more refined the definition. An example is given in *Table 9.2*, and its hierarchic structure, resembling the roots of a tree, is illustrated in *Figure 9.7*. The use of initial digits alone produces 'coarse grain' definitions; use of additional succeeding digits produces 'fine grain' (i.e., more detailed) definitions.

There are three advantages to hierarchic codes. First, if accurate auxiliary diagnostic techniques are not available and therefore refined diagnoses are not definable, then a coarse grain code may be used without succumbing to the temptation of offering a more refined diagnosis than can be substantiated. Secondly, the individual interests of data collectors can be accommodated. For example, someone

Table 9.2 An example of hierarchic numeric codes.

	Code	Meaning
Treatment	100	General medical therapy
	110	Antibiotic
	112	Oxytetracycline
	120	Parasiticide
	122	Thiabendazole
Species and breed	100	Horse
	110	Pony
	111	Welsh mountain pony
	120	Warm blooded
	121	English thoroughbred
	200	Dog
	300	Cat
	400	Cow
	410	Friesian

with a specialist interest in chemotherapy may be able to record the use of a particular antibiotic, whereas those who are content with recording just that an antibiotic has been used may record in the coarser grain. Thirdly, most computerized recording systems allow flexible querying at various levels of a hierarchy using a 'wild card' facility. This uses a character which, when positioned on the right of specified codes, indicates that the codes specified on the left of it, and **all** codes on its right, are to be selected. For instance, if '%' is the wild card character, and a query is conducted on the treatment codes in *Table 9.2*, thus:

'select 1%'

then all records of medical therapy at all levels of the hierarchy would be selected (all antibiotics, all parasiticides, etc.). In contrast, if '12%' were specified, only all parasiticides would be selected.

In addition to recording qualitative data, it is possible to use code to record quantitative data such as test results. There is some loss of refinement compared with the use of the results themselves because coding often involves the grouping of individual values into ranges of values (blocks). *Table 9.3*, for example, illustrates the numeric codes for ranges of numbers of helminth eggs isolated from faeces. Some test results are already blocked, although the blocking is often concealed by the mode of expression. Thus, a serological test quoted as positive at a dilution of 1:1024 implies that it was negative at 1:1025, whereas the next dilution tested that yielded a negative result was probably 1:2048. Blocking converts interval and ratio data to ordinal data, and this must be considered when selecting statistical methods for analysing the coded data (see Chapter 14).

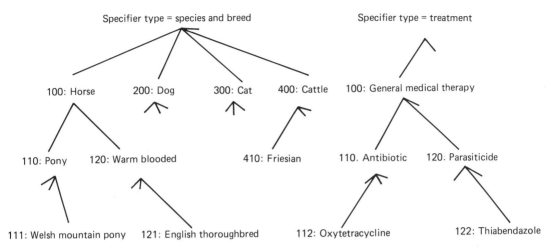

Fig. 9.7 Diagrammatic representation of a hierarchic code (code listed in *Table 9.2*).

Table 9.3 An example of numeric coding of quantitative data: frequency codes for numbers of eggs per gram of faeces (epg) for use on a parasitology data report form. (From Slocombe, 1975.)

Code	epg	Code	epg
004	1– 500	014	5001– 5500
005	501–1000	015	5501– 6000
006	1001–1500	016	6001– 6500
007	1501–2000	017	6501– 7000
008	2001–2500	018	7001– 7500
009	2501–3000	019	7501– 8000
010	3001–3500	020	8001– 8500
011	3501–4000	021	8501– 9000
012	4001–4500	022	9001– 9500
013	4501–5000	023	9501–10000

Alpha codes

Alpha codes represent plain text by alphabetical abbreviations or acronyms, for example: FN = Female neuter, M = Male.

Table 9.4 lists some components of a hierarchic alpha coding system for diagnoses. It has two axes: location and abnormality. Thus, displaced abomasum is coded DA PD, retained placenta is coded GL PR, and hepatitis is coded DH B.

Alphanumeric codes

Alphanumeric codes have evolved more recently than numeric codes. An example is given in *Table 9.5*, where the disease is located in three axes: the disease's name, its topography and its aetiology. The first axis classifies the disease according to its name. In the first example in the

table, the first (alpha) part of the first axis relates to the broad disease category (abomasitis) and the second (numeric) component produces a 'finer grain' description (mycotic abomasitis); this is therefore a simple hierarchy. The second axis classifies the disease according to the anatomical system that it affects (UDIG = upper digestive system). The third axis classifies the disease according to cause (MYCO = mycosis).

Signs may also be coded alphanumerically. *Table 9.6* illustrates a hierarchic alphanumeric code of signs.

Symbols

Symbols can be used as codes. Thus ↑ and ↓ are frequently used to represent elevated and lowered body temperature respectively. Symbols may be combined with letters such as D+ and D− to indicate the presence and absence, respectively, of diarrhoea. *Table 9.7* lists some examples of symbolic codes used in the international veterinary disease reporting system of the Office International des Epizooties (see Chapter 11). These may appear to represent very vague descriptions. However, they reflect the level of knowledge of morbidity in many countries, where reliable, accurate, quantitative data are unavailable. The value of such general terms was noted in the last century by a notable medical epidemiologist William Farr: 'The refusal to recognize terms that express imperfect knowledge has an obvious tendency to encourage reckless conjecture'.

Choosing a code

The choice of a code is partly subjective. Some people find numbers easier to handle; others are more content

Table 9.4 An example of hierarchic alpha diagnostic codes (two axes). (From Williams and Ward, 1989a).

Axis 1 Location		Axis 2 Abnormality	
Code	Meaning	Code	Meaning
D	Digestive system	B	Inflammation
DA	Abomasum	E	Exudate
DE	Oesophagus	EBH	Haemorrhage
DH	Liver		
		P	Position
G	Reproductive system	PD	Displaced
GO	Ovary	PL	Dislocation
GU	Uterus	PR	Retention
GL	Placenta	PP	Prolapse
GS	Scrotum		

Table 9.5 An example of alphanumeric diagnostic codes (three axes). (From Stephen, 1980.)

Code	Axis 1 Name of disease	Axis 2 Anatomical system involved	Axis 3 Aetiological agent or other indicated cause
ABO 10	Abomasitis, mycotic	UDIG (upper digestive)	MYCO (mycotic)
BRA 10	Brachygnathia	BOJOS (bones, joints, etc.)	CONGEN (congenital)
ENC 45	Encephalomyelitis, equine, Western	NERVO (nervous)	VIRO (virus)
EPI 10	Epidermitis, porcine, exudative	SKAP (skin and appendages)	BACTE (bacterial)
TOX 64	Seneciosis (including pyrrolizidine poisoning)	LIVBIP (liver and biliary)	TOXO (toxicosis)

with letters. There are, however, several definable advantages and disadvantages to numeric and alpha codes.

If acronyms or abbreviations are used (e.g., ABO for abomasum) they may be easier to relate to the plain text data and easier to remember than numeric codes (Williams and Ward, 1989a).

In some cases, alpha codes, in order to be acronymic, may require more characters than their numeric counterparts, even though 26 alternatives are available for each alpha character, and 36 for alphanumeric, compared with only 10 for numeric systems. This may be an important space consideration in computerized systems which, in any case, can pack numeric data more tightly than either alpha or alphanumeric strings.

Numeric codes can be entered into computers more quickly than alpha codes. Most computer keyboards have a nine-digit numeric keypad which can be depressed more quickly than the alphabetic typewriter-style keyboard, especially if the user cannot type.

If a consecutive numeric code is used, care should be taken to ensure that it is long enough to accommodate all definitions of a specifier type. A four-digit code (e.g., 0000 − 9999) can accommodate 10 000 definitions (1000, if the last digit is a 'check digit' — see below), and then would be 'full'. If more than 10 000 definitions were required, a five-digit code would have to be used.

If there is a requirement for a variable 'grain' in the definition, then a hierarchic code is the most suitable. Alpha codes can be used, although numeric codes are more common. Numeric codes can have ten categories (0 − 9) at each level of the hierarchy. Alpha codes, based on the Roman alphabet, can have 26 categories (A − Z) at each level of the hierarchy.

Numeric codes are not subject to language differences. Alpha codes, however, if acronymic, may need to vary according to the language of the user.

When all of these merits are considered, subjective assessment is still a major factor. This is a reason for the

Table 9.6 An example of hierarchic alphanumeric codes for signs. (From White and Vellake, 1980.)

Acoustic sense signs
A00 Deafness

| | A01 Complete deafness |
| | A02 Partial deafness |

A10 Discharge from ear

| | A11 Bloody discharge from ear |
| | A12 Purulent discharge from ear |

A20 Excess wax/cerumen in ear

A30 Abnormal ear size

A40 Other signs referrable to the ear

	A41 Mite infestation of ear, parasite, dirt
	A42 Odour bad ear
	A43 Cold ears

Digestive system signs

D00 Abnormal appetite

	D01 Decreased appetite
	D02 Polyphagia—excessive appetite
	D03 Anorexia—loss of appetite
	D04 Pica—Depraved appetite

D10 Difficulty in prehension, cannot get food in mouth

D20 Chewing difficulty

D30 Signs of the jaw

	D31 Weakness of jaw
	D32 Inability to close jaw
	D33 Inability to open jaw
	D34 Malformation of jaw

D40 Odour from mouth

D50 Signs referrable to the oral mucosa

	D51 Bleeding oral mucosa
	D52 Ecchymosis oral mucosa
	D53 Petechia oral mucosa
	D54 Dryness oral mucosa
	D55 Cold oral mucosa

Table 9.7 An example of symbolic codes. (From FAO-WHO-OIE, 1992.)

Code	Disease occurrence
-	Not reported
?	Suspected but not confirmed
(+)	Exceptional occurrence
+	Low sporadic occurrence
+ +	Endemic
+ + +	High occurrence
+?	Serological evidence and/or isolation of causative agent, no clinical disease
+..	Disease exists, distribution and cocurrence unknown
()	Confined to certain regions
)(	Ubiquitous
!	Recognized in country for the first time
< =	Only in imported animals (quarantine)
...	No information available

have satisfied the criteria. This is important when combining data from different sources and when combining data that have satisfied different, perhaps incompatible, sets of criteria.

Consistency

Initially, checks should be made that the codes are recognizable, and then that they are internally consistent. Thus, it is illogical to record an elevated body temperature and a lowered body temperature at the same time. Placing the event in the context of what else is known about the animal's life history may reveal other inappropriate data. For instance, the recording of 'dystocia' becomes unacceptable when the animal's existing record shows it to be either male, or juvenile, or to have undergone an ovariohysterectomy some time ago. All of these inconsistencies would suggest that the animal may have been misidentified.

The initial check that the code is recognizable is simple if consecutive codes are employed: the check is that the code which is offered is neither less than the lowest nor greater than the highest code that is in use. Alphanumeric codes may need to be checked against a list held within the computer containing all permissible codes. Some codes (e.g., *Table 9.5*) use combinations of code elements taken from different lists; for example, representing organs, pathological processes and causes. Each element must be identified and checked against the appropriate list; further

considerable range of codes that are available and for the lack of a universally acceptable one.

Error detection

Provision must be made for verifying data during the process of combining them with an existing collection of data. In general, as many checks as possible should be made on each datum, and the criteria used for checking should remain a permanent characteristic of the data that

checks are required to ensure that any particular combination of organ, pathological process and cause is feasible and, for quantitative data, that extreme values are plausible.

'Finger trouble'

Data that are entered via keyboards (a common form of data entry in computerized systems — see Chapter 11) are subject to four types of error, collectively and colloquially termed 'finger trouble'. These errors are:

1. **insertion**, where extra characters are erroneously added;
2. **deletion**, where characters are omitted;
3. **substitution**, where the wrong character is typed;
4. **transposition**, where the correct characters are typed in the wrong order.

The danger is that the incorrect version may be an allowable code that means something totally different from the intended code. If the codes have the same number of characters then insertion and deletion are easily detected because the incorrectly entered code is the wrong length. The likelihood of entry of an incorrect code can be reduced by increasing the 'redundancy' of the code, that is, by adding more characters to the code. Unfortunately, highly redundant codes with many characters require many keystrokes which itself increases the chance of error. A balance must be found between these conficting requirements.

Data that are transmitted electronically, for example from one computer to another via telephone links or computer networks (see Chapter 11), can be corrupted during transit by the 'noise' of the transmission medium. There are several ways of protecting data from this degradation, including the use of 'parity bits' and 'check bytes' (bits and bytes are defined in Chapter 11) to signal corruption of each character. Alternatively or additionally a 'check digit' may be incorporated in numeric codes to perform the same function while also increasing the codes' length and redundancy.

Check digits

Check digits are mathematical functions of the preceding digits of the code. For example:

5029 = anaemia.

The first three digits (502) are a consecutively ordered code which relates to anaemia, and the fourth digit (9) is a check digit which is a function of the code numbers. The check digit, in this case, may have been generated using the formula:

$$(\text{first digit} \times 2) + \text{second digit} - \frac{\text{third digit}}{2}$$
$$= \text{check digit}.$$

The computer will not accept 5028 or 5020 since it recognizes that the last digit is not the correct function of 502. Similarly it will not accept 5019 or 5039 which represent two totally different diagnoses. This is therefore a useful validation check against corruption to incorrect codes. (Of course, in this example, 4229 and 4109 would be consistent with the formula used to produce the check digit, but these are so unlike 5028 and 5020 that it is very improbable that they would be entered.)

Further reading

Cimino, J.J. (1993) Saying what you mean and meaning what you say: coupling biomedical terminology and knowledge. *Academic Medicine*, **68**, 257–260. (*A critique of medical terminology, nomenclature and coding*)

Hall, S.A. (1978) Farm animal disease data banks. *Advances in Veterinary Science and Comparative Medicine*, **22**, 265–286. (*Includes a discussion of disease nomenclature*)

Leech, F.B. (1980). Relations between objectives and observations in epidemiological studies. In: *Veterinary Epidemiology and Economics*. Proceedings of the Second International Symposium, Canberra, 7–11 May 1979, Eds Geering, W.A., Roe, R.T. and Chapman, L.A., pp. 254–257. Australian Government Publishing Services, Canberra

10 Sources of data

Epidemiological investigations utilize data relating to disease and its determinants, performance and population size. These data can be collected from many sources, including veterinary practices, farms, diagnostic laboratories, abattoirs and university clinics. These organizations can supply data that they already have recorded, for use in retrospective studies. They can also co-operate in the collection of data in prospective studies.

The collection of data always incurs a cost. This includes postal charges when the data are collected by postal questionnaire (see Chapter 13) and laboratory examination charges. The value of data therefore has to be judged in the context of the cost of collecting them.

Some general considerations

Nature of data

Data from some sources may be unsuitable because they are **inaccurate**. Also, they may be of the **wrong type**. For example, a record that just notes 'lameness' would be useful in a general estimation of the prevalence of bovine foot problems, but would be of little value to a detailed study of the various lesions and their causes that produce lameness (see Chapter 9).

Co-operation

The lack of co-operation can pose a problem to epidemiological investigations. There are several reasons why people may not be willing to supply data.

The **reasons** for undertaking a study or survey may not be clear to potential suppliers of data, and so they may be discouraged. This emphasizes that the **objectives** of an investigation should be explained to all who are involved

with it. Co-operation is more likely if the investigation is part of a planned animal health programme than if it is undertaken in isolation. For example, Sudanese farmers co-operated in a survey of mortality due to schistosomiasis, conducted by interview, because this survey was part of an investigation of the financial viability of a new vaccine against *Schistosoma bovis* (McCauley *et al.*, 1983a,b). However, surveys in Haiti, conducted without a concomitant animal health programme, eventually met with resistance from local animal owners (Perry and McCauley, 1984). Some studies, particularly prospective ones (e.g., cohort studies: see Chapter 15), may also take several years to complete, during which time **motivation** may be difficult to maintain.

The collection of information may risk a breach of **confidentiality**; for example, if practitioners' records that contain details of financial transactions of practices are examined. This, too, may prevent co-operation.

Co-operation is unlikely if data collection is laborious or time-consuming, for instance, completing a complex or cumbersome questionnaire. The method of data collection therefore should be as simple as possible, within the constraints of the requirements of the investigation.

Trace-back

Data on the geographical distribution of disease may be difficult to gather because of an inability to trace animals back to their origin. This can be a major problem at abattoirs where carcasses may not be clearly identified. Trace-back can be very valuable. An obvious example is tracing contacts with rabid dogs. Similarly, the control of chlamydiosis in Californian parakeets has been facilitated by a state law requiring all parakeets to be banded with details of their year of birth and breeding establishment (Schachter *et al.*, 1978).

Bias

Sources of veterinary data may be biased (see Chapter 9); a common type being selection bias. The bias in the sources of data listed below is indicated when each source is described.

The cost of data collection

In most countries the collection of information on diseases of national importance is supported by government funds. Similarly, in many countries funds are available for research on diseases of economically important livestock. However, investigation of companion animals' diseases, especially if they are not demonstrably of public health significance, relies on the limited financial support available from welfare societies and charities. Lack of funds, therefore, can restrict companion animal data collection.

Problems unique to developing countries

Data collection in developing countries may face additional difficulties (Broadbent, 1979). There may be poor laboratory diagnostic support and insufficient manpower. The terrain may be difficult. In these cases, it is often advisable to collect as much information and as many specimens (e.g., faeces for the counting of helminth eggs, and serum for antibody titration) as possible during a survey to investigate several diseases at once, thus avoiding the need for repeated journeys to difficult areas. The prevalence of some diseases can be measured directly while conducting surveys, such as tuberculosis using the intradermal test, and trichomoniasis by examining preputial washings.

The general and unique problems in developing countries highlight the need for methods of data collection and analysis that are powerful, quick, careful and cheap. A range of **rapid rural appraisal** techniques, using multidisciplinary teams, has evolved to fulfil these requirements in the agricultural sector in developing countries (McCracken *et al.*, 1988), and these techniques can be applied to animal health issues (Ghirotti, 1992).

Sources of epidemiological data

The organizations and groups described below represent a comprehensive list of possible sources of data. The membership of the list will vary between countries. Some countries, particularly the developed ones, have veterinary infrastructures that facilitate potential or actual data collection from the majority of these sources. The developing countries may be able to utilize only a few of them.

Some organizations record and store data routinely and therefore provide structured collections of data (databases) to which reference can be made when mounting epidemiological studies. Some of these established pools of data are discussed in greater detail in Chapter 11. The *International Directory of Animal Health and Disease Data Banks* (USDA, 1982) lists and briefly describes epidemiological, laboratory, clinical and bibliographic databases and databases of research in progress. These databases have also been reviewed by Pilchard (1979).

Government veterinary organizations

Most countries have organized government veterinary services. These services investigate diseases of national importance, particularly those infectious ones for which legislation enforces reporting (the notifiable diseases). Many governments also operate diagnostic laboratories. Reports are sometimes prepared and published routinely; for example, records of diagnoses made at diagnostic laboratories in the UK (Hall *et al.*, 1980). Submissions to diagnostic laboratories from practitioners are often voluntary and may therefore reflect personal interest and motivation, causing selection bias. Reports of notifiable diseases, similarly, depend upon the conscientiousness of observers.

Publications that collate information from a variety of government sources, including 'field' and laboratory investigations, are also available routinely. In some cases routine reports are prepared but are confidential and therefore not readily available. An international bulletin of animal diseases, covering most countries of the world, is published by the Paris-based Office International des Epizooties (OIE: Blajan and Chillaud, 1991). The bulletin provides a statement of disease prevalence, based on regular reports of member countries of OIE (see Chapter 11).

Sometimes surveys have been undertaken that use data collated from several sources. A good example is the survey of livestock diseases in Northern Ireland that was undertaken in 1954 and 1955 (Gracey, 1960). This included demographic and disease data relating to a wide range of infectious and non-infectious diseases in cattle, sheep and pigs. It included data collected from 70% of farms in the country by field officers, and abbatoir data.

Veterinary practices

In countries with private veterinary practices (notably the developed countries) practitioners have contact with farm and companion animals, although the extent of contact varies. Farm animal veterinarians have the greatest contact with dairy cattle, less contact with pigs and beef cattle, and the least contact with sheep. Problems in ruminants tend to be seasonal and related to parturition.

Owners of companion animals usually attend private clinics. Thus the practitioner is a major potential source of small animal and equine data that relate to a reasonably representative cross-section of animals. In companion animal practice the cost of therapy may prevent animals being presented for treatment, and so diseases of animals owned by the poor may be under-represented, therefore inducing selection bias.

In large animal practices mild diseases and hopeless cases are not usually brought to the practitioner's attention by the farmer and so may be under-represented. Similarly, the farmer may treat some animals himself and so some diseased animals may not be recorded.

The data may not be accurate because of incorrect diagnoses. If the purpose of an investigation is unclear to a practitioner and its results are not presented to him with obvious benefit, he is unlikely to participate in data recording, especially over a long period of time, which may be necessary in prospective studies.

Even when information is freely available, it usually exists as separate accumulations of records in the individual practices and therefore may be difficult to collect and collate. Questionnaires can be used (see Chapter 13), but are time consuming. Veterinary practitioners have conducted surveys relating to either total clinic populations, for example, nematode infections in dogs (Turner and Pegg, 1977), or in defined cohorts of populations, for example, *Toxocara canis* infection in puppies (Holt, 1976). These surveys inevitably are limited geographically to the vicinity of the practices concerned.

Continuous monitoring programmes have also been instigated using veterinary practice data (see also *Table 11.3*).

Table 10.1 lists the categories of data routinely recorded by some practices in the Bay of Plenty region of New Zealand. Most of the data are categorical. They relate to diagnoses (e.g., ketosis), treatments or procedures (e.g., induced calving) and, occasionally, simply to the reason for presentation of the animal (e.g., road accident). The listed diagnoses may be named according to cause (e.g., salmonellosis), lesion (e.g., metritis) or

presenting sign (e.g., unthrift). They may be highly refined (e.g., vasectomy) or less refined (e.g., parasitic). They may relate to observations (e.g., prolapsed uterus) or interpretations (e.g., photosensitivity). Also, in all cases referring to diagnoses, accuracy is not indicated, because the criteria on which the diagnoses were based are not cited. In all cases, the numerator in morbidity and mortality calculations (i.e., number affected) is recorded, but in only one instance (lepto-redwater) is the denominator specified.

Computerized practice records

Modern developments in computer technology are increasing accessibility of data (see Chapter 11), and present the possibility of using routinely collected veterinary practice data for epidemiological research. There are several computerized livestock health and productivity recording schemes operated by veterinary practices, bureaux and universities (see Chapters 11 and 21). Computerized data, pooled from many farms, have been used in epidemiological studies and surveys of, for example, bovine lameness (Russell *et al.*, 1982; Whitaker et al., 1983a) and fertility (Esslemont, 1993). However, there have been few attempts to pool small animal data from computerized practice records (Thrusfield, 1991).

The use of pre-existing data is attractive because these data can be extensive, covering a representative cross-section of the population, and are less expensive than data that are collected for a particular purpose (*ad hoc*). However, there are problems associated with routinely collected computerized data. First, some of the data may be of insufficient refinement for a proposed study (e.g., some presenting signs listed in *Table 10.1*). Secondly, data from various recording systems may be difficult to unify and compare because the systems contain varying categories of data of varying degree of refinement. For example, one computerized system records lesions of the bovine foot in considerable detail (Russell *et al.*, 1982) whereas another simply records that lameness is present (Smith *et al.*, 1983). Thirdly, the researcher has little control of the collection, and therefore the quality, of the data (Willeberg, 1986); this may result in inaccurate records (e.g., caused by 'finger trouble': see Chapter 9), incomplete data, selection bias, misclassification and confounding.* Fourthly, conversion of the records into a form that is suitable for analysis can be complex (Mulder *et al.*, 1994).

---

*For accounts of assessment of the quality of data, see also Canner *et al.* (1983), Neaton *et al.* (1990), Roos *et al.* (1989) and Willeberg (1986).

Table 10.1 An example of routine disease reporting in general veterinary practice: categories recorded by practitioners in the Bay of Plenty region of New Zealand. (From MAFF, 1976.)

Cattle	*Mastitis:*
Metabolic:	Individual
Milk fever	Herd advice
Ketosis	*Abortion investigations*
Grass staggers	(Total number of accessions)
General:	*Lepto-redwater:*
Actinomycosis	Cases
Arthritis	Farms
Bloat	Animals at risk
Blood testing	*Male:*
Castration	Bull soundness
Dehorning	Semen examinations
Hernia	Vasectomies
Indigestion	Other faults
Miscellaneous	
Postmortem examination	**Calf losses**
Starvation	**Sheep**
Unthrift	Dystocias
Respiratory:	Facial eczema
Upper respiratory tract	Foot-rot
Pneumonias etc.	*Neonatal losses:*
Gastroenteritis:	('Brucellosis')
Colic	('Toxoplasmosis')
Colibacillosis	Pneumonia
Parasitic	Post mortems
Salmonellosis	Prolapsed uterus
Other or unspecified	Salmonellosis
Skin:	Other
Facial eczema	*Rams:*
Photosensitivity	Palpation
(excluding facial eczema)	
Other dermatoses	**Horses**
Vaccinations:	Branding
Brucellosis	Castration
Leptospirosis	Colic
Other (including IPV/BVD)	Foaling
Lameness:	Foals
Feet—foot-rot	Tubing
Abscess	Wounds
Other .	Other
Female:	
Anoestrus	**Pigs**
Calving	Castration
Herd advice	Abscesses
Induced calving	Reproductive
Metritis/uterine irrigation	Respiratory
Paresis	Salmonellosis
Pregnancy diagnosis	Other
Prolapsed uterus	
Retained fetal membranes	**Small animals**
Teat surgery	Road accidents

Abattoirs

Red meat abattoirs process large numbers of animals for human consumption and identify some diseases during meat inspection. Only clinically healthy animals usually are presented for slaughter, therefore the majority of diseases that are diagnosed at meat inspection are subclinical. Most reports relate to helminth diseases and internal lesions such as hepatic abscesses.

The objective of meat inspection is to safeguard the health of the human population. Traditionally this is practised by preventing the sale of meat and offal that are **obviously** unfit for human consumption. Therefore, most conditions are diagnosed only by macroscopic post-mortem examination; experience has shown that this approach is adequate.

A secondary objective is to record details of abnormalities that are found, because these findings may be of epidemiological value, for example, in associating outbreaks of disease in man with infections in animals (Watson, 1982). Thus an increase in the prevalence of tuberculosis lesions in cattle at slaughter was the first indication of a human tuberculosis epidemic in Barbados (Wilson and Howes, 1980).

Abattoirs therefore can be primary sources of data for disease surveillance for conditions for which other diagnostic methods are not appropriate. In Europe, for example, clinical signs are not reliable indicators of contagious bovine pleuropneumonia, and the probably low prevalence of antibodies makes serological screening inefficient. Thus, in Switzerland, examination of lungs at slaughter has been proposed as the basis of a surveillance system for this disease (Stärk *et al.*, 1994).

Epidemiological investigations are essentially a subordinate goal of meat inspection at abattoirs, although it is possible to conduct auxiliary investigations of blood, sputum, lymph nodes and other tissues for specific surveys and studies. Thus, in Ireland, bovine kidneys condemned at meat inspection by the usual macroscopic techniques have been subjected to electron-microscopic examination to determine the nature of the lesions (Monaghan and Hannan, 1983). This is an example of using auxiliary aids to increase refinement of a diagnosis. Similarly, a survey of *Cysticercus tenuicollis* infection of sheep in Britain has been undertaken (Stallbaumer, 1983). This was necessary because the condition was not routinely recorded separately but was included in the 'coarse grained' category: 'other conditions'.

Animals examined at meat inspection do not originate from the abattoir; they have travelled there. Trace-back is therefore desirable if the diseases that are identified are to be associated with their farm or area of origin. This is relatively easy in countries that have a simple marketing system. In Denmark, for example, pigs are shipped directly from producers to co-operative slaughterhouses from which data are collectively pooled, thereby allowing rapid trace-back and surveillance of disease (Willeberg, 1980a; Willeberg *et al.*, 1984). In contrast, in Britain, marketing involves many sellers and purchasers; this makes trace-back difficult when it is epidemiologically

desirable (e.g., Sunguya, 1981).

Even when trace-back from the abattoir is possible, improper identification of viscera can be a further problem. Carcasses may be identified by ear tag or tattoo, but viscera containing lesions may not be labelled adequately and it may therefore be impossible to associate them with the carcasses from which they were removed.

Some countries publish routine meat inspection findings. These include Australia, Cyprus, Denmark, India, Luxembourg, New Zealand, Nigeria, Norway, the UK and the US. The published data may originate from the majority of abattoirs (e.g., in Denmark); from a sample of abattoirs (e.g., in Britain: Blamire *et al.*, 1970, 1980); or from only a single abattoir (e.g., in India: Prabhakaran *et al.*, 1980). These sources have been used for epidemiological surveys; for instance, surveys of reasons for condemnation of sheep at Scottish abattoirs (Cuthbertson, 1983) and of numerous diseases identified in animals in English abattoirs (Blamire *et al.*, 1970, 1980).

Abattoir investigations can also be used to indicate faults in husbandry. A survey of hoof and pedal horn lesions in sows at a Budapest abattoir has assisted in the identification of defects in floor construction in pig houses (Kovacs and Beer, 1979).

Poultry packing plants

In several countries, poultry are slaughtered separately from the larger food animals on poultry packing plants. Post-mortem examination results from these premises constitute another source of information. Again, the population is biased, comprising only young healthy birds, although some culled hens might also be included. Most clinically diseased and dead birds are excluded before slaughter.

Knacker yards

In some countries, animals that are ill or have died, and are therefore unfit for human consumption, are sent for slaughter to premises other than abattoirs. These premises are called 'knacker yards'. The carcasses may be fed to animals. In Europe, dogs kennelled for hunting (e.g., fox hunting in Britain) are often supplied with flesh from these sources. Knacker yards also handle horses in countries in which horse flesh is not routinely eaten by man.

Data from knacker yards are biased, but in quite a different way from those obtained from abattoirs and poultry packing plants: animals sent to knacker yards are usually either ill or dead — not alive and healthy. Data from this source are difficult to acquire; they are distributed over many premises and would require professional veterinary inspection of lesions to ensure accuracy.

Serum banks

Stored collections of serum samples are called serum banks. Such samples are collected routinely during mandatory control and eradication campaigns in which serological tests are used to diagnose infection (e.g., brucellosis eradication). They may also be collected during specific surveys. For example, in a serological survey of warble fly infestation of cattle in England and Wales (Sinclair *et al.*, 1989), over 74 000 specimens, from over 3000 farms, were collected. Much of the serum is not used, particularly now that diagnostic techniques using very small volumes of serum are available, and so the unused serum is usually discarded. Serum samples can provide useful epidemiological information on vaccination priorities, the periodicity of epidemics, the spatial distribution of infections and the origin of newly discovered infectious diseases. Serum banks are described in detail in Chapter 17.

Registries

A registry is a reference list (more commonly, the word describes the building in which the list is kept). In human medicine, registries of diseases (notably of tumours) are maintained using hospital and death certificate data as numerators and census data as denominators in morbidity and mortality rates. There are some veterinary tumour registries but these usually lack census data and so the denominators tend to be biased by non-response. For instance, when using estimates of population size based on the enumeration of licensed or vaccinated dogs (e.g., Cohen *et al.*, 1959), the denominator will tend to be underestimated because of a low public response to licensing and vaccination.

Some registries reduce the non-response bias by utilizing demographic surveys in specified areas. A Californian tumour registry (Dorn, 1966) defines a 'veterinarian using' reference population, counted by household survey, as the denominator. The Tulsa (US) *Registry of Canine and Feline Neoplasms* (MacVean *et al.*, 1978) defines a 'veterinarian using' reference population, enumerated by a census of all veterinary practices in the Tulsa area, which includes not only sick animals but also healthy animals presented for routine

examination, vaccination and elective surgery; the numerator comprises diagnoses made by registry pathologists from specimens submitted by practitioners. Although these registries reduce the selection bias inherent in specialized populations (e.g., of clinical cases), the true population at risk may not be estimated. In the previous example, animals may not attend veterinary practices and therefore would be undetected, and some animals may attend more than one practice, one animal therefore counting twice in the denominator. The extent of these inaccuracies is difficult to assess, but is probably small.

Pharmaceutical and agricultural sales

The sales records of pharmaceutical companies provide an indirect means of assessing the amount of disease. The sale of antibiotics, for example, is a rough guide to the prevalence of bacterial diseases, although estimates made from this information may be inaccurate. Antibiotics may be used without isolating specific bacteria — indeed, without even positively incriminating a bacterium — and so may be used when a bacterial infection is not present. They may also be used prophylactically; for example, following routine surgery. Similarly, they may be used for a purpose other than that for which they were intended: some small animal practitioners, for instance, sometimes use bovine intramammary antibiotics to treat otitis externa. The extent of unjustifiable and unusual use of some drugs is difficult to estimate.

Zoological gardens

Most zoos maintain detailed records of animals and their diseases (e.g., Griner, 1980; Pugsley, 1981). Several zoos send their data to a central registry in Geneva as part of an international database — the *International Veterinary Record of Zoo Animals* (Roth *et al.*, 1973).

Agricultural organizations

There are many agricultural bodies associated with the livestock industry that record information on animal production, such as liveweight gain, food conversion and milk yield. Although these data are not related directly to disease, they can provide information on the composition and distribution of populations that can be of value in defining populations that can be studied. For example, the British National Milk Records File has been used to locate Friesian herds for a survey of reasons for culling and wastage in dairy cows (Young *et al.*, 1983).

Commercial livestock enterprises

The intensification of animal industries mentioned in Chapter 1 has resulted in the establishment of commercial enterprises, particularly in the pig and poultry sector, where large units are common (see *Table 1.9*). Many of these enterprises have their own recording systems, although again some data may be confidential. These sources have been utilized in some surveys; for example, mortality in broiler chickens in Australia (Reece and Beddome, 1983), losses in commercially reared rabbits (Hugh-Jones *et al.*, 1975), unthriftiness in weaned pigs (Jackson and Baker, 1981) and lesions associated with the movement of weaners (Walters, 1978).

Non-veterinary government departments

There are non-veterinary government departments that collect data relating to animals. These include economic and statistical units. The latter record the numbers and distribution of animals in Britain, enabling the drawing of choroplethic density maps of cattle, sheep and pigs in England and Wales (MAFF/ADAS, 1976a,b,c).

Farm records

Many farmers, particularly those keeping dairy cattle and pigs, routinely record production data. Some record information on disease. The recorded data may be computerized, and computerized schemes operated by bureaux, universities and veterinary practices have already been discussed above (see 'Veterinary Practices').

Veterinary schools

Veterinary schools have clinics that record the results of consultations. Many have established databases, often using computerized techniques that allow rapid access to records; for instance, the Florida (Burridge and McCarthy, 1979), Edinburgh (Stone and Thrusfield, 1989) and Liverpool (Williams and Ward, 1989b) schools. The study population is frequently biased, especially when clinicians have specialist interests resulting in a high proportion of referred cases.

Feral animal organizations

Wildlife and animal conservation organizations and pest control centres record data on feral animals, particularly relating to the size of populations. Wildlife can be important sources of infection to domestic animals and man (e.g., rabies-infected skunks and foxes in the US and Europe, respectively), and may be potential sources of infection (e.g., if hares were infected with *Brucella suis* in the UK). Routine monitoring of disease in these animals would be expensive. However, *ad hoc* surveys can be undertaken. Demographic data are also valuable when investigating the actual and potential spread of infection (see, for example, the discussion of potential fox rabies in Britain in Chapter 19).

Research laboratories

Research laboratories record data on primates, lagomorphs, rodents and cavies that are used in experiments. These sources are very specialized, closed communities, and therefore are obviously biased.

Pet-food manufacturers

Manufacturers of pet food sometimes collect animal demographic data as part of their market research (e.g., Anderson, 1983), although commercial interests may prevent release of all of these data.

Certification schemes

Schemes certifying freedom from disease involve compulsory and often regular examination of animals belonging to participating owners, and can therefore provide morbidity figures for a range of diseases. For example, under the British Veterinary Association/Kennel Club eye examination scheme, certificates attesting to freedom from canine hereditary eye disease are issued for one year and are subject to renewal throughout a dog's life. This scheme therefore guarantees routine examination of dogs, and has facilitated estimation of the incidence of cataracts (Curtis and Barnett, 1989).

Pet shops

Pet shops are potential sources of information on conditions of young animals, such as congenital lesions (Ruble and Hird, 1993), but trace-back (e.g., for genetic studies) is difficult or impossible.

Breed societies

Companion animal breed societies have information on breed numbers and distribution. The extent of co-operation can vary. If a survey could highlight a certain problem in a particular breed then that breed's society may be unwilling to help. This fear is real, although it is based on the false notion that epidemiological investigations just produce incriminating morbidity figures. The main goal of these investigations, however, is to detect causes, with a view to developing beneficial preventive strategies.

Further reading

Curtis, C.R. and Farrar, J.A. (Eds) (1990) The National Animal Health Monitoring System in the United States. *Preventive Veterinary Medicine*, **8**, 87−225

Hinman, A.R. (1977) Analysis, interpretation, use and dissemination of surveillance information. *Bulletin of the Pan American Health Organization*, **11** (4), 338−343

Hutton, N.E. and Halvorson, L.C. (1974) *A Nationwide System for Animal Health Surveillance*. National Academy of Sciences, Washington, DC

International Directory of Animal Health and Disease Data Banks (1982) National Agriculture Library. United States Department of Agriculture, Miscellaneous Publication No. 1423

Konigshofer, H.O. (1972) *The Organisation of Surveillance of Animal Diseases*. World Health Organization inter-regional seminar on methods of epidemiological surveillance of communicable diseases including zoonoses and food-borne diseases, Nairobi, 9−20 October 1972. Working Paper No. 8

Poppensiek, G.C., Budd, D.E. and Scholtens, R.G. (1966) *A Historical Survey of Animal-Disease Morbidity and Mortality Reporting*. National Academy of Sciences, Washington, DC. Publication No. 1346

Report of a Ministry of Agriculture, Fisheries and Food Working Party (1976) *Animal Disease Surveillance in Great Britain*. MAFF, UK

Schilf, B.A. (1975) Meat inspection service as an element of epidemiologic surveillance and a component of animal disease control programmes. Seventh Inter-American Meeting on Disease and Zoonosis Control, April 1974, pp. 149−153. Pan American Health Organization—World Health Organization Scientific Publication No. 295

11 Data management

Earlier chapters have described some of the sources of veterinary data and the methods of collecting them. Data may need to be stored for a long time if they are to be available for future use, for example in retrospective surveys. This chapter is concerned with the techniques that are used to store and retrieve veterinary data, and with the principles underlying the distribution of data as useful information. Emphasis will be placed on the suitability of the techniques to epidemiological studies, although some of the standard methods of clinical case recording will be outlined. Methods of physically storing and ordering records have been described in detail elsewhere (Duppong and Ettinger, 1983; Thrusfield, 1985b; Nelson and White, 1990). Finally, some examples of veterinary recording systems will be given.

Database models

A **database** is a structured collection of data, and is the basis of an organized data storage and retrieval system. A database containing animal records includes different types of data that comprise different components of the records. The data consist of several categories (**specifier types**), for example, breed, sex, age and clinical signs, that are attributes (**features**) of the animal (**item**). Some of these are permanent attributes (i.e. 'tombstone data': see Chapter 9) and therefore are **case-specific**; for example, breed and date of birth. Others, such as diagnoses and signs, change from one consultation (and therefore record of consultation) to another, thus being **record-specific**.

The association between the various components of a record can be viewed in several ways, depending on the way in which the data are stored, producing four models of a database.

The 'record' model

The **record** model is the traditional way of structuring

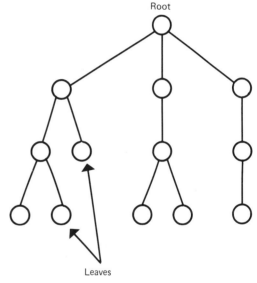

Fig. 11.1 The 'tree' structure of a hierarchic database.

data. The central component is the individual record which contains case- and record-specific data. This is a useful approach for the clinician concerned mainly with individual patient care. However, it is difficult to correlate specifier types between records. Correlation is very useful in epidemiological studies: for example, correlation of breed, age and sex with disease.

The 'hierarchic' model

The **hierarchic** model and the two models that follow are used to explain how data are stored and handled in computerized systems. In this model, data components are stored in **nodes** which are arranged in a tree-like structure (*Figure 11.1*). The uppermost level of the hierarchy has only one node; it is called a **root**. With the

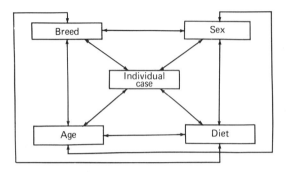

Fig. 11.2 An example of some possible relations in a simple 'network' database. (From Thrusfield, 1983a.)

Table 11.1 The structure of data components in a simple 'relational' database.

Animal's name	Age	Sex
Patch	7	M
Sally	5	F
Thor	13	M
.		
.		
.		
.		
Arthur	4	M
Liz	15	F
Brenda	9	F
.		
.		
.		

exception of the root, every node has one node related to it at a higher level; the latter is called the former's **parent**. No component can have more than one parent. Each component can have one or more components related to it at a lower level; these are called **children**. Components at the end of the branches (i.e., with no children) are called **leaves**. *Figure 11.1* shows a hierarchy with four levels. An example of a hierarchy with only two levels would be one with 'veterinary practice' (the root) and 'veterinary surgeons in the practice' (the children).

The 'network' model*

Using the terminology of tree structures, if a child in a data relationship has more than one parent, then the relationship cannot be a strict hierarchic one. In these circumstances, the structure is described as a **network**. The network model therefore includes and extends the hierarchic model. An example is illustrated in *Figure 11.2*. This model allows relationships to occur between many data components and is therefore of considerable epidemiological value because it allows correlation of determinants (e.g., age and sex) with disease if the determinants and diseases are stored as components of the network.

The 'relational' model

In the relational model, all data are represented by two-dimensional tables which have the following properties:

1. entries in the table are single-valued; neither repeating groups nor arrays are allowable;
2. the entries in any one column must all be of the same kind (e.g., one column might contain animals' sexes, and another contain animals' ages);
3. each column has a unique name and the order of columns is immaterial;
4. each row of the table is unique and the order of the rows is immaterial.

An example is given in *Table 11.1*.

The relational approach is different from that of the hierarchic and network models. The principal difference is that in the hierarchic and network models, relationships are expressed explicitly and are predefined. In the relational model, the basic data structure is predefined but record relationships are not defined until they are used. This ability to dynamically reflect relationships, combined with the simplicity of the relational model, makes it potentially more flexible than the other models, which it can also represent. The main disadvantage of the relational model is its inefficiency relative to the other two, because, although the model is simple, it is complex to implement on computers. However, with increasing sophistication of computer technology, the model has become widely used in computerized data recording systems.

Non-computerized recording techniques

Longhand recording techniques

The recording of data in longhand is a common technique

---

* The term 'network' model, in this context, should not be confused with mathematical network models of infectious disease, described in Chapter 19, or with communications networks, described later in this chapter.

in general veterinary practice where computerized storage methods may not be available.

Day books

The day book is a long-established type of longhand record. It is an 'open' record of cases examined during the day, that is, it allows any data to be recorded in any form, usually as a narrative description. This type of record is now used infrequently for epidemiological purposes. It is bulky and does not allow either an animal's previous consultations to be located rapidly or correlation of components of different records.

Record cards

Cards, stored in drawers or boxes, are a common means of storing clinical records. They use a 'record' model of a database, each card often referring to one animal. They are usually stored alphabetically according to owners' names. The record-specific data are ordered chronologically on each card, providing a complete history of the patient. Cards may be blank, in which case they can be used to provide an 'open' record. Alternatively, they can be printed as a 'closed' record, that is, with a fixed number of options (see 'Collecting information: questionnaires' in Chapter 13). These options commonly include details of specifier types such as breed, sex and date of birth. They are usually partially closed, consisting of a closed section, but with a blank area for the 'open' recording of additional details.

Pro formas

A pro forma is an extension of the partially closed record. It is a mainly closed record, comprising a checklist of many features (*Figure 11.3*). This can produce a very detailed record of observational and interpretative data. However, the merits of producing a comprehensive record must be weighed against the unwillingness of busy clinicians to complete them, and against the value of the data. Completion of all components of the record, especially if a 'mandatory' part of the running of a clinic or laboratory, can rapidly lead to rejection of the system (Darke, 1982). Pro formas should always have an open section to accommodate any salient details that are not included in the closed part. The closed section can be coded and therefore readily entered into a computer.

Punched card recording techniques

Record cards can have their items (patients) and features coded by associating these with circular or rectangular holes punched in the cards. This facilitates correlation of features and items. There are two main types of punched card: **item** and **feature** (Jolley, 1968).

Item cards

Each item card represents an animal. The features (attributes) of the patient are associated with circular holes around the edge of the card. A hole is converted to a notch when the item concerned has the relevant feature. For example, if a dog is male then the hole corresponding to male on the dog's item card will be changed to a notch. To search for all items with a particular feature, the cards are held in register and a needle is passed through the appropriate hole. The cards representing items possessing the feature will have been notched in this position so that when the needle is lifted the notched cards fall from the pack. Eighty-column cards, with rectangular holes, corresponding to relevant features, punched over the face of the card, were common in the 1960s and 1970s because they were 'readable' by early computers.

Feature cards

In a feature card system, one card is allocated to a single feature. All patients with this feature are each allocated unique reference numbers that are part of a matrix of numbers printed on the card. The corresponding numbers are centre-punched out of the card when animals possess that feature. The search is usually made by laying the cards on an illuminated screen. Eighty-column cards were also adapted for use as feature cards.

Punched card recording has been applied to veterinary data storage and retrieval in veterinary schools, government diagnostic laboratories (Hugh-Jones *et al.*, 1969) and zoos (Griner, 1980), but is now of mainly historical interest because it has been superseded by computerized recording techniques.

Computerized recording techniques

Computers are an efficient means of storing, analysing and retrieving data, in addition to acting as complex calculators. The components of early computers included many valves and transistors and so the machines were necessarily expensive. They were therefore found only in sizeable organizations. The invention and subsequent development of silicon microchips has decreased the size and cost of computers and has made them readily available to a wide range of users including general veterinary practitioners. Although the initial reason for a

ROYAL (DICK) SCHOOL OF VETERINARY STUDIES
UNIVERSITY OF EDINBURGH

100,006

OWNER	Mr. Mrs. Miss	Surname **CAMPBELL, Mrs.**	Initials **H.**	Address **42, Glenayre Place**		
	Phone home business		clinician **A.B.Jones**	student	animals name **Petra**	

ANIMAL	species **Dog**	breed **Shetland Collie**	sex **F.**	age **4yrs.**	colour **Champagne/White**	weight **9kg**

ATTENDANCE: date **1/6/77**   hour   ADMITTANCE ☐   DISCHARGE ☐   date   hour

PRIMARY COMPLAINT: **Pruritus**

REFERRED BY	Name	reply sent	admitting clinician
	Address	phone No.	attending clinician

MEDICAL HISTORY

IMMUNISATION : state age, none or ?   Initial : C.D.   C.V.H.

Repeats : C.D.   C.V.H.

Initial : Lep. can/ict.   Other

Repeats : Lep. can/ict.

PREVIOUS ILLNESS, injury or surgery (specify +age, or none)

DURATION OF ILLNESS   **1 Month**   Length of time owned   **4 Years** | duration

APPETITE : anorexia   variable   fair   good ✓ excessive   depraved

THIRST : normal ✓ decreased   increased   excessive

RESPIRATION : normal ✓ shallow   dyspnoeic   abdominal   painful

SNEEZING : Nasal discharge   (nature)   Salivation (nature)

COUGH : none   dry   soft   persistent   paroxysmal

VOMITION : none   occasional   frequent   persistent   haematemesis   retching only

Vomitus : character and when occurs

FAECES : none   normal ✓ soft (not formed)   fluid   blood   mucus   other

Defaecation :   normal ✓ difficult   painful   frequency   colour

URINATION : none   normal ✓ frequent   difficult   painful   incontinent   haematuria

Volume :   normal ✓ decreased   increased   colour :

TEMPERAMENT : normal   listless   depressed   cantankerous   restless   excitable ✓ neurotic

NERVOUS : normal ✓ excitement   hysteria   convulsions   chorea   nystagmus   ataxia   paraplegia

Paralysis (define)

SKIN : normal   inflamed   pruritus ✓ loss of hair   alopoecia   pigmentation   hyperkeratosis   Licking   rubbing

Biting (site)   Ectoparasites :

Wounds (site)

Tumour (site)   Other lesions :

MUSCULO-SKELETAL : normal ✓ Lameness (limb)   Injuries (site):

Swellings (site) :   Deformities (site)

SEXUAL : Fertility : proven   apparently infertile   unknown

Libido : normal   none   excessive   unknown

OESTRUS : age of onset   last oestrus   normal   abnormal (define)

intervals   false preg.   Last litter   No. of litters

Any discharge (define)

EYES : normal ✓ discharge (specify)   Blindness   Other lesions

EARS : normal ✓ rubbing ear   head shaking   smell   discharge   other

DIET : Daily amount   Meat (specify)   Fish

Carbohydrate :   Vegetables :   Other

OTHER RELEVANT INFORMATION : **Synthetic fibre bedding**

MEDICAL HISTORY

Fig. 11.3 An example of a clinical case record pro forma. (From Thrusfield, 1983a.)

practitioner's acquiring a computer may be as an aid to practice management (e.g., Pinney, 1981), the machine can also manipulate clinical data very efficiently.

There are two types of computer: **digital** and **analogue**. They allow alternatives to be asked, such as this **and** that, **either/or**, or **neither/nor**. The digital computer stores data in a discrete fashion, usually in the binary scale (i.e., 0 or 1: 'on' or 'off'). The analogue computer allows quantities to be represented as infinitely variable physical measurements, rather like a slide rule. Most computers with which veterinarians are concerned are digital.

Hardware

The physical parts of a computer are termed **hardware**. This comprises **peripheral units** and the **central processing unit** (CPU). The peripheral units include the **input units** and the **output units**.

Data enter through the input unit. If they are textual or numerical data, they are entered using a **keyboard** or a **keypad**. Additionally, **optical character readers** may be used; these interpret ordinary printed paper in much the same way as a photocopier. A **mark sense document reader** is used to interpret marks on completed questionnaires. Pictorial information (e.g., maps) can be transferred to a computer using **digitizers** and **graphics tablets** which convert the images to a binary form. A **joystick** or, more commonly, a **mouse**, can also be used to input pictorial information.

Data leave the computer through the output unit. This may be a **video display unit**, **graph plotter**, or **printer**.

The CPU includes:

1. a **storage (memory) unit**, which records the instructions (program) and data;
2. the **arithmetic unit**, which performs operations (additions, multiplications, comparisons) on data that the program selects from the storage unit;
3. the **control unit**, which examines the storage unit's instructions sequentially and interprets them.

The capacity of a computer's database depends on the size of the memory unit, which gives immediate access to data, and the size of any **auxiliary storage units**, which store data that can be fed into the main memory bank.

Handling capacity

A computer's storage and handling capacity is measured in **bits** and **bytes**. A bit holds the basic binary doublet: 0 and 1. Bits are formed into bytes. Contiguous bytes are grouped together to form **words** (normally 2 or 4 bytes, depending on the particular computer). A word can be used to store a simple integer or a real number (two words for the latter in the case of a 2-byte word). Complex numbers thus will require either four 2-byte words or two 4-byte words. For the purposes of storing data in auxiliary stores and transferring data between auxiliary storage and the CPU's memory unit, words are formed into **blocks**. The size of a block varies from one computer system to another. In a small computer, typically, there are in the order of 500 bytes (i.e., 250 2-byte words) in one block. Two such blocks therefore constitute 1 kilobyte, abbreviated to 1 Kb. There are 1000 Kb in 1 Megabyte (Mb), and 1000 Mb in 1 Gigabyte (Gb).

Auxiliary storage

There are several types of auxiliary storage. Some common ones are magnetic tape, hard magnetic disks (usually stacked vertically), 'floppy' magnetic disks, mini-floppy disks, magnetic tape cassettes and laser disks. The main form of storage is usually a hard disk. (Early methods involved punched paper tape and cards, and magnetic drums, but these are now largely obsolescent.) Floppy disks are 5¼ ″ or 3½ ″ in diameter, most holding up to 2 Mb.

The format also dictates the speed of access. If one wishes to access data at the beginning and end of a tape or cassette, then it is necessary to wind the tape from beginning to end; this can take several minutes, whereas any part of a disk can be accessed relatively quickly. Tapes are therefore now usually used for 'archiving' and producing secure back-up copies of data, rather than as a routine working medium.

Types of computer

There are currently three main types of computer. Their classification originally was based on their physical size, although, with increasing miniaturization, this is no longer a valid criterion; the distinction now relates to the number of users who can access the computer simultaneously.

1. The **mainframe** computer has one or more large capacity CPUs and an auxiliary store. It can be used simultaneously by many people, often over 100, and can usually run many programs simultaneously. The CPU is usually distant from the many input and output units to which it is connected by electrical or fibre-optic cables. Mainframes use drums, hard disks and magnetic tapes as auxiliary stores.
2. The **minicomputer** is similar to the mainframe, but usually supports fewer users simultaneously. Auxiliary storage is similar to that of the mainframe.

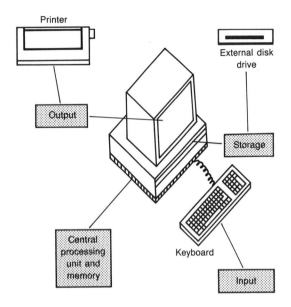

Printer

External disk drive

Output

Storage

Central processing unit and memory

Keyboard

Input

Fig. 11.4 The components of a modern microcomputer.

3. The **microcomputer** is a self-contained unit, with CPU and input and output units (usually a keyboard and video display unit, respectively) located together (*Figure 11.4*). The microcomputer is now widely used in veterinary medicine, including general practice, because of its relatively low cost and increasing power. Its capacity is sometimes described in terms of **RAM** (random access memory), which corresponds to the immediate access memory of the mainframe, into which data can be put, and from which they can be extracted. Additionally, it has **ROM** (read-only memory) which contains fixed information (e.g., the sequence of instructions which have to be carried out when the microcomputer is switched on). Floppy disks, magnetic tape cassettes and hard disks are used for auxiliary storage, the latter currently with a capacity of up to 3 Gb, and either built into the computer housing (internal hard disks) or designed to stack on top of it (external hard disks).

Software

A computer cannot learn; it lacks intelligence. Therefore it must be supplied with a complete set of unambiguous instructions that cause it to perform more or less intelligently. The set of instructions is called a **program**. Programs constitute a computer's **software** (cf. hardware). Problems must be broken down into a form with

which the computer will be able to deal, usually by producing a step-by-step sequence of unambiguous rules for the computer to follow. The complete set of rules for solving a problem is called an **algorithm**. This is the basis of a computer program.

Languages

Programs have to be written in a recognizable **language**. The most fundamental language, similar to the binary coding, is called **machine code**. In order to avoid the awkwardness of humans reading and writing binary coding, most computers use a fundamental language system similar to the machine codes, but representing the binary notation by mnemonics or acronyms, and numerals in decimal notation, so that the instructions are understood more readily. This type of language is **low level**; a common example is Assembler.

However, to allow programs to be written more quickly, languages with a more familiar structure have been devised. These are called **high level** languages. Some of them accept ordinary sentences. These languages must be translated into the machine code, and so a translation program, called either an **interpreter** or a **compiler**, must be used. Interpreters translate the program line by line as it is executed and are therefore slow to run; translation is performed each time that the program is run. Compilers translate the whole program once, and the machine code is kept to run rapidly whenever required.

There are several types of high level language. These include FORTRAN, which is commonly used by scientists and mathematicians; BASIC, which is used on many home computers; and Pascal and C, which are multipurpose languages. *Table 11.2* indicates the criteria for suitability of some languages for implementation on microcomputers.

Operating systems

It is necessary to communicate with the computer via a resident program, called an **operating system**, that does 'house-keeping' jobs such as remembering the location of data and arranging for programs to be loaded and run, with access to appropriate input and output units. The operating system comprises:

1. a **user interface** which allows the user to 'converse' with the computer either by typing simple **commands** or using a mouse;
2. a file system for recording bodies of information (files) on storage devices, and naming them;

Table 11.2 Summary of general criteria for choosing a language for microcomputers.

Criteria	Languages					
	Assembler	BASIC	FORTRAN	COBOL	C	Pascal
1. Embedded in a support environment	−	++	−	−	−	+++++
2. Portable	+	++	+++	+++	+++	++++
3. Good data structure	−	+	++	+++	+++	++++
4. Support for structured code design	−	−	++	++	++++	++++
5. Flexible input/output	−	+	++++	++++	*	+++
6. Standardization	+	+	++++	**	++++	++++
7. Stable	−	−	++++	++++	++++	+++
8. Easy to teach***	−	+++	+++	++	+	+++++
9. Simple, easy to use and learn***	−	++++	+++	+++	++	+++++
10. Flexible storage structures	−	−	−	−	−	+++
11. Suitability for packages	+	+	++++	+	+++	+
12. Suitable for business data processing (record handling) etc.	−	+	++	++++	+++	+++
13. Flexible file handling	−	−	+++	++++	+	++
14. Suitability for systems programming	++	−	−	−	++++	+
15. Compiler availability	−	+++	++++	++	+++	++++
16. Implemented on mini, micro and mainframe computers	−	+++	++++	+++	+++	+++

*Depends on the system on which the language is implemented.
**Variable, depending on the compiler.
***The grading is subjective and also reflects the aims and capacity of the pupil.
− Language unsuited to criterion.
+ to +++++ Degree of suitability of language to criterion.

3. **language systems** using some of the languages described above.

Currently common operating systems for microcomputers are MS DOS ('Microsoft' Disk Operating System), and MS Windows. Others, including UNIX and VMS, are used on mainframe computers and some microcomputers.

Applications software

Applications software carries out tasks for the user (in contrast to the programs which comprise the operating system and which direct the working of the computer), and many ready-written programs, designed for specific tasks, are now available. These are software packages, which are aimed at the ordinary user with little or no knowledge of computer languages. Geographical information systems (see Chapter 4), word-processing packages, network and relational database management systems (DBMSs), graphics packages, expert systems (see Chapter 2) and statistical packages are examples. Some modern packages combine different tasks (e.g., statistical, word-processing and graphics packages), providing the user with comprehensive data-analysis and presentation facilities. Some packages are also designed

so that data can be easily 'exported' from them and 'imported' to other packages.

Appendix III lists some useful packages for data storage and analysis in epidemiological studies.

Changing approaches to computing

Since the 1950s, when computers were initially developed, the way in which data are stored and handled inside a computer, and the ways by which data can be accessed, have changed.

Storing and manipulating data

Initially, programs were written to perform one particular purpose (e.g., 'extract all data about Hereford cows from the database'); the programs (applications) were considered central to the system, with the data merely passing through the application in a convenient form (*Figure 11.5a*). This 'systems analysis' approach has several disadvantages. The main one is the rigidity of the program. If a new application (e.g., 'extract all data about Charolais cows from the database') is required, then a new program may have to be written. This means that different correlations often require new programs.

A more recent approach — the 'database' approach — is more flexible. The data are considered central, and the

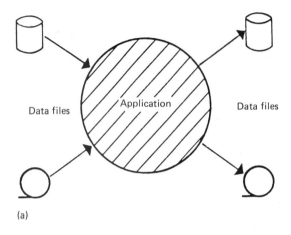

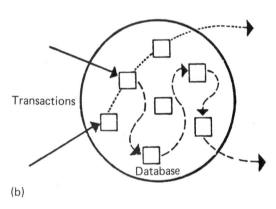

Fig. 11.5 Approaches to data storage and manipulation: **(a)** the 'systems analysis' approach; **(b)** the 'database' approach. (From Thrusfield, 1983a.)

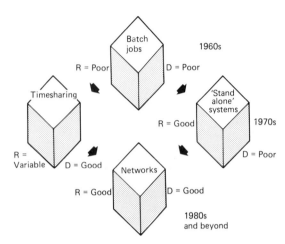

Fig. 11.6 Changing approaches to computerized data access. D = resource and data sharing; R = responsiveness. (From Thrusfield, 1983b.)

applications can constantly change (*Figure 11.5b*). The database approach enables flexible querying and correlation of data. This approach is used in constructing network and relational computerized databases, and many of these database management systems (DBMSs), usually with their own special languages for querying data (e.g., SQL), are now available on mainframes and microcomputers. Most DBMSs facilitate the design of applications as well as controlling the storage and access of data. Additionally, standardization of database languages and software for linking computers allows data stored on a mainframe or minicomputer to be easily accessed locally by microcomputers.

Accessing computerized data

Figure 11.6 illustrates how the approach to computing has developed, and how it affects access to data. In the 1960s,

work was run on mainframe computers, usually by inputting work on paper tapes or cards to be run overnight as batch jobs. Response was poor (i.e., the process was slow) and it was very difficult for users to share their data and resources.

In the 1970s, a division took place. Mainframe users began to share time on computers and it was possible to share data and resources, although response varied according to the number of users and the tasks being performed at any one time. Separate 'stand-alone' microcomputer systems developed with good response, but data and resources could not be shared because the systems were not linked.

In the 1980s, developments in communications technology allowed data to be accessed rapidly from several places. Initially, computers could be linked using acoustic signals sent via conventional telephone handsets. However, the rate of data transfer was slow. Now, using communications 'networks', direct cable, fibre-optic and satellite links between computers (mainframes and microcomputers) are available, operating at up to 10 million characters per second. For example, in Japan, emergency reports of outbreaks of infectious diseases, and routine reports, are sent electronically from local animal health centres to a central, national database (Tanaka, 1992).

Future trends aim at expanding links between many users and speeding up response. The concept is one of a network of individual microcomputers linked to one another and to mainframes by fast communication systems, the mainframes being reserved mainly for complex calculations ('number crunching') and the processing of very large volumes of data.

The development of database management systems and improved communications technology increases the potential for epidemiological investigation considerably. Data from a wide cross-section of veterinary sources, ranging from veterinary practices to government services, are likely to be more representative because of reduced selection bias, and should therefore produce more accurate morbidity and mortality rates for use in epidemiological surveys. However, collection and analysis of this range of data face several difficulties, including the absence of a standardized recording and coding scheme (Thrusfield, 1981), differences in data format between the files in which data are initially stored and subsequently analysed (Mulder *et al.*, 1994), and assessment of the quality of the recorded data (see Chapter 10).

Veterinary recording schemes

Scales of recording

The types of veterinary recording scheme were classified by Hugh-Jones (1975):

1. microscale schemes (*Figure 11.7a*) concerned with internal disease problems in separated populations such as those on farms and research institutes;
2. mesoscale schemes (*Figure 11.7b*) involved with more widely distributed disease problems; for example, data collection at abattoirs, diagnostic laboratories and clinics;
3. macroscale schemes (*Figure 11.7c*) designed to collect data with the purpose of gaining an international or national view of disease.

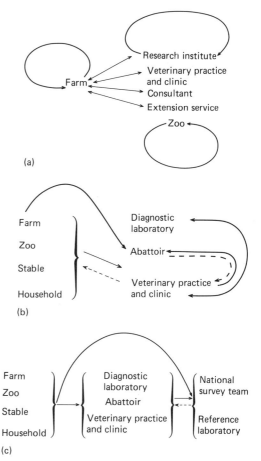

Fig. 11.7 Veterinary data recording schemes defined according to flow of data: **(a)** microscale schemes; **(b)** mesoscale schemes; **(c)** macroscale schemes. Solid arrows indicate main paths of data flow. Broken arrows indicate paths of limited or no data flow. (From Thrusfield, 1983b, after Hugh-Jones, 1975.)

Microscale schemes

In the microscale scheme, information is transferred from the farm to the practice or consulting organization where it is analysed and the results are necessarily fed back to the farm to effect health improvement. With an 'on-farm' system, data may be manipulated and analysed without leaving the farm's confines. Herd health and productivity schemes are typically microscale. Essentially, they record individual and herd performance and productivity and sometimes disease occurrence, and relate productivity to disease in an attempt to improve the former. These will be considered in greater detail in Chapter 21.

Mesoscale schemes

In the mesoscale scheme, data are transmitted from their source to the organizations responsible for analysis. The data are usually of more direct value to the analysing institution than to their source. Therefore, feedback of data is a less important component of the system (although still desirable). Small animal practice records are an example of this type of recording system.

Macroscale schemes

Macroscale schemes are designed to gain a global, globally regional, national, or nationally regional picture, and therefore are not designed primarily to help specific animal units. There is thus little flow of data back to their origin. National and international monitoring and surveillance programmes are typically macroscale.

Several contemporary recording projects now have various combinations of macroscale, mesoscale and microscale elements. For example, the Canadian Animal Productivity and Health Information Network, APHIN (see *Table 11.3*, and further details below), includes on-farm microcomputers that record herd health and productivity (microscale), but these are also linked to a central database which can provide a regional view of animal health (macroscale). This triple classification, however, still provides a useful focus on the broad objectives, flow of data and general geographical scope of a recording scheme.

Veterinary information systems

Databases themselves only have limited value. Maximum benefit from the data is obtained only when they are converted to **information**. Data and information are not synonymous, and, when they are treated as such, confusingly similar terms like 'information processing' and 'data processing' arise. **Information** comprises data that have been processed and organized for some purpose so that someone can extract **meaning** from them. A **system** is generally defined as an entity comprising at least two related components (Ackoff, 1971). A precise definition of an **information system** is difficult to achieve (Avgerou and Cornford, 1993) but, in a practical veterinary context, may be considered as collections of disease-related data that are integrated to satisfy the informational requirements of its users (e.g., farmers, veterinary practitioners, epidemiologists and administrators). The borderline between a simple database and an information system is also indistinct because stored data, even before they are processed, can have value as information. However, an important characteristic of an information system is its ability to deal with large, complex issues (e.g., the national control of epidemics).

An extension of the information system is the **decision support system** (Sprague and Carlson, 1982). Its two key components are:

1. a focus on decision makers — at both policy and implementation levels — rather than on the system itself;
2. 'seamless integration' of all components of the system so that all features can be accessed via a single user interface without regard to which component of the system is providing the answers; this represents a logical development from the simple database where data analysis may be handled quite separately from data entry and storage — often not even on the same computer.

Decision support systems have the following characteristics (Morris *et al.*, 1993):

1. they tend to be directed at relatively unstructured, poorly specified problems;
2. they combine models and analytical techniques with traditional data storage and retrieval functions;
3. they focus on features that make them easy to use by people whose computer 'literacy' is low;
4. they emphasize flexibility and adaptability to accommodate changing circumstances (e.g., changes in approaches to decision making) and therefore can be valuable parts of a national animal health information system.

Data collection

Data may be collected either **passively** or **actively**. Passive collection utilizes existing data sources, such as diagnostic laboratory submissions or abattoir records. Data collected in this way are prone to selection bias (see Chapters 9 and 10). However, the use of passively collected data involves little extra cost. Actively collected data, in contrast, are gathered specifically to fulfill the requirements of the information system, are not available from pre-existing sets of data, and therefore have a cost attached to them. Therefore, the technical and economic feasibility of active collection needs to be considered.

Many epidemiological studies require details of the population at risk, as well as diseased animals (e.g., for calculation of morbidity and mortality values). Thus, census data may also be an important part of an information system. These data are collected routinely in many countries and therefore are passively available for use in information systems. However, the accuracy of these data needs to be assessed before they are used.

The value of collected data

The value of collected data needs to be judged in terms of the objectives of the information system. Some pitfalls associated with inappropriate data collection are summarized by **Finagle's 'Laws'** (Opit, 1987):

1. the information one **has** is not what one **wants**;
2. the information one **wants** is not what one **needs**;
3. the information one **needs** is not what one **can get**;

4. the information one **can get** costs more than one **wants** to pay.

Thus, the objectives of an information system should be clearly defined **before** the system is designed, and **before** active data collection begins.

Objectives

There are several objectives of a comprehensive information system:

1. surveillance of endemic diseases;
2. fulfilling international reporting needs;
3. monitoring productivity;
4. identifying new syndromes;
5. supporting and monitoring the technical efficacy of control programmes;
6. managing laboratory data;
7. providing information for the economic assessment of disease and its control.

These objectives can be fulfilled at three levels: **farm**, **national** and **international**, and the information required at each level therefore needs to be identified. The **flow** of information in the information system can then be defined.

Farm level: This includes individual producers, producer groups (e.g., farm co-operatives), and product processors. Individual producers generally need records of diseases on their farms, and details of productivity (e.g., milk production and reproductive efficiency). Producer groups require similar information on productivity, although it may be prudent to keep details of an individual farm's disease problems confidential. Product processors need details of hazards such as zoonotic diseases and residues (e.g., for milk processors, details of milk-borne infections and antibiotic contamination).

National level: At this level, several organizations have different information requirements. Departments of agriculture utilize aggregated data on farm productivity. Veterinary services need a national view of animal disease, including the monitoring of zoonoses, and a log of veterinary activity. The agricultural industry needs details of product sales. National banks may require information on productivity potential before awarding loans; similar information may also be needed by insurance companies.

International level: Various regional and global agencies utilize information on animal health and productivity. Examples of the former are the European Union, the Pan-American Health Organization (PAHO), the South Asian

Association for Regional Co-operation (SAARC) and the Animal Production and Health Commission for Asia (APHCA). The latter include the World Health Organization (WHO) and the Food and Agriculture Organization of the United Nations (FAO).

The United Nations also has several regional and global agencies which are particularly concerned with funding agricultural projects in **developing countries**, and for which information on animal health and productivity is therefore valuable. These include the World Bank, the International Fund for Agricultural Development (IFAD), the Economic Commission for Latin America and the Caribbean (ECLAC), the United Nations Development Programme (UNDP), and the Inter-American Development Bank (IDB).

Information system implementation

Implementation of an information system is undertaken in several stages:

1. definition of the data requirements and flow of information;
2. identification of areas where passive and active data collection are appropriate;
3. identification of areas where computerization is desirable;
4. construction of a work plan, including any incremental steps in computerization (e.g., national centres first, followed by local centres) and in fulfilling information requirements (e.g., international needs may need to be supplied before national or local needs);
5. training;
6. assessment of progress;
7. modification of the system, if necessary.

Each stage must be considered in the context of the availability of data generated by existing data-collection procedures, and the circumstances of the country or region in which the system is to be implemented. For example, a developing country may have greater restrictions on manpower and financial and technical resources than a developed one.

Modern information systems are usually partly or totally computerized. Attention therefore needs to be given to the selection of appropriate hardware and software. Servicing and maintenance of the former should be available locally, and it should have sufficient RAM and auxiliary storage to run the software and store the amount of data that is anticipated. Additionally, in developing countries, an uninterruptible power supply unit (UPS) is desirable to prevent damage to hardware and loss of data during power fluctuations and interruptions.

Various types of software may be required, and should be well supported by suppliers. A DBMS is suitable for storing, handling and extracting data, and for generating reports. Statistical packages may also be required for the analysis of data (Appendix III); and a word-processing package is invaluable for producing reports and other communications. A geographical information system (see Chapter 4) may also be useful. The portability of files between packages is an important consideration, and so packages should not be selected in isolation, but in relation to one another. Ideally, all components should be 'seamlessly integrated'.

Some examples of veterinary databases and information systems

Table 11.3 lists some examples of veterinary databases and information systems. A brief outline of some of them will indicate their scope and the techniques employed in updating and using them.

The Office International des Epizooties international disease reporting system

The Paris-based Office International des Epizooties (OIE) is an international organization concerned with the global control of animal disease. It was founded in 1924 following an outbreak of rinderpest in Belgium in 1920, and has a macroscale reporting system that records data on the major infectious epidemic diseases of animals throughout the world.

Its objectives are:

1. to alert countries threatened by an epidemic;
2. to strengthen international co-operation on animal disease control;
3. to facilitate international trade.

It is therefore necessary to know the natural history of diseases relevant to trade, the risk of transmission, and the biological and economic consequences of introduction of a pathogen. Two categories of disease are defined (OIE, 1987):

1. 'List A': communicable diseases which have the potential for very serious and rapid spread, irrespective of national borders, which are of serious socio-economic or public health consequence, and which are of major importance in the international trade of animals and animal products (e.g., African horse

sickness, foot-and-mouth disease, fowl plague, Newcastle disease, rinderpest and swine fever);
2. 'List B': communicable diseases which are considered to be of socio-economic and/or public health importance within countries and which are significant in the international trade of animals and animal products (e.g., anthrax, contagious equine metritis, foul brood, glanders, Johne's disease, leptospirosis and rabies).

Collaborating countries are required to submit alert messages for outbreaks of List A diseases and exceptionally important List B and unlisted diseases. These messages comprise:

1. an initial report of the event (on form SR1);
2. additional information on the event and control measures (on form SR2).

Additionally, a standard monthly report (form SR3) and an annual report are requested. The Office issues an International Animal Health Code in an attempt to standardize reporting procedures (OIE, 1992). It also defines minimum health guarantees required of trading partners to avoid the risk of spreading animal disease.

NAHMS

NAHMS (National Animal Health Monitoring System) is a macroscale system, designed to measure the incidence, prevalence and cost of health-related events in livestock in the US, and to identify determinants of disease in modern production systems. It has evolved in response to calls in the US for a national surveillance system for endemic conditions of livestock, which began in the 1920s and continued during the 1960s and 1970s (Poppensiek *et al.*, 1966; Hutton and Halvorson, 1974). An important requirement is that farm enterprises are randomly selected so that representative, unbiased results are obtained (see Chapter 13). Following early random selection schemes (e.g., the Minnesota disease recording system: *Table 11.3*), a pilot project involving pig producers, and called NADS (National Animal Disease Surveillance System), began in the states of Ohio and Tennessee in 1983, and NAHMS is now being extended over the country to cover the full range of livestock species. Data relating to disease occurrence, demography and costs (e.g., of preventive measures) are collected from the selected farms. Samples of blood, faeces, feed and water are collected from some participating farms to validate clinical diagnoses and producers' observations. Following local data collection and analysis, records are forwarded to a national co-ordinating centre for aggregation and regional and

Table 11.3 Some veterinary databases and information systems.

Macroscale	Mesoscale	Microscale *†
ANADIS (Roe, 1980; Andrews, 1988; Cannon, 1993)	Australian slaughter check scheme (Pointon and Hueston, 1990)	APHIN [Cattle, pigs] (Dohoo, 1988, 1992)
APHIN (Dohoo, 1988, 1992)	Danish pig health and production surveillance system (Christensen et al., 1994)	Australian slaughter check scheme [Pigs] (Pointon and Hueston, 1990)
Australian State animal disease information systems (Andrews, 1988)	Danish swine slaughter inspection bank (Willeberg, 1979)	Bristol sheep health and productivity scheme [Sheep] (Morgan and Tuppen, 1988)
BENCHMARK (Martin et al., 1990)	Edinburgh SAPTU clinical record summary system (Stone and Thrusfield, 1989)	Checkmate [Dairy cattle] (Booth and Warren, 1984)
Californian turkey flock monitoring system (Hird and Christiansen, 1991)	FAHRMX (Bartlett et al., 1982, 1985, 1986; FAHRMX, 1984)	CHESS [Pigs] (Huirne and Dijkhuizen, 1994)
Danish pig health and production surveillance system (Christensen et al., 1994)	Florida teaching hospital data retrieval system (Burridge and McCarthy, 1979)	COSREEL [Cattle, sheep, pigs] (Russell and Rowlands, 1983)
Danish pig health scheme (Willeberg et al., 1984; Mousing, 1988; Willeberg, 1992)	Liverpool clinical recording and herd health system (Williams and Ward, 1989b)	DairyCHAMP [Dairy cattle] (Udomprasert and Williamson, 1990)
Danish swine slaughter inspection data bank (Willeberg, 1979; Willeberg et al., 1984)	Minnesota disease recording system (Diesch, 1979)	Danish pig efficiency control system [Pigs] (Herløv and Vedel, 1992)
Japanese disease reporting system (Tanaka, 1992)	Parasitology diagnostic data program (Slocombe, 1975)	Danish pig health and production surveillance system [Pigs] (Christensen et al., 1994)
Management and disease information retrieval system for broiler chickens in Northern Ireland (McIlroy et al., 1988)	Queensland veterinary diagnostic data recording system (Elder, 1976)	Danish pig health scheme [Pigs] (Willeberg et al., 1984; Mousing, 1988; Willeberg, 1992)
Management and disease information retrieval system for farmed Atlantic salmon in Northern Ireland (Menzies et al., 1992)	Slovakian Veterinary Service management system (Haladej and Hurcik, 1988)	DAISY [Dairy cattle] (Pharo, 1983; Esslemont et al., 1991)
NAHIS (Morley, 1988)	Veterinary Recording of Zoo Animals (Roth et al., 1973)	Edinburgh DHHPS [Dairy cattle] (Smith et al., 1983)
NAHMS (King, 1985; Glosser, 1988; Curtis and Farrar, 1990)	VIDA II (Hall et al., 1980)	FAHRMX [Dairy cattle] (Bartlett et al., 1982, 1985, 1986; FAHRMX, 1984)
New South Wales animal disease information system (Rolfe, 1986)	VMDB (Priester, 1975; Warble, 1994)	Liverpool clinical recording and herd health system [Dairy cattle] (Williams and Ward, 1989b)
New Zealand laboratory management and disease surveillance information system (Christiansen, 1980)		Ontario dairy monitoring and analysis program [Dairy cattle] (Kelton et al., 1992)
OIE international disease reporting system (Blajan and Chillaud, 1991)		PigCHAMP [Pigs] (Stein, 1988)
Ontario dairy monitoring and analysis program (Kelton et al., 1992)		SIRO [Dairy cattle] (Goodall et al., 1984)
Slovakian Veterinary Service management system (Haladej and Hurcik, 1988)		VAMP [Dairy cattle] (Noordhuizen and Buurman, 1984)
Swiss national animal health information system (Riggenbach, 1988)		VIRUS [Dairy cattle] (Martin et al., 1982a)
Taiwanese disease reporting system (Sung, 1992)		

*These systems are health and productivity schemes. They may also function to varying degrees as mesoscale and macroscale systems.
†The type of livestock recorded in each system is in square brackets.

national analysis. Individual-producer and state summary reports are also produced.

APHIN

APHIN (Animal Productivity and Health Information Network) was established in the late 1980s at the Atlantic

Veterinary College, Prince Edward Island, Canada, to provide pig, beef and dairy farmers on Prince Edward Island with information to increase production efficiency. It comprises microcomputers situated on farms and in veterinary practices, the processing industry, government agricultural laboratories and the veterinary college.

Microscale health and productivity packages (e.g., Pig-CHAMP: *Table 11.3*) record data on individual farms. Other data sources, at varying stages of incorporation into APHIN, include abattoir records, diagnostic and nutritional laboratory records, and milk quality data.

The separate microcomputers usually operate independently, providing local users with the information that they require. Additionally, relevant data are transferred on floppy disks (proposed developments include electronic transmission) to a central mainframe relational database on which the data are collated, analyses conducted, and summaries produced for participating farmers.

Danish swine slaughter inspection data bank

This database comprises post-mortem information on pigs collected at slaughter. Most Danish fattening pigs are recorded in the database and so not only does the database act as a mesoscale scheme but also it performs the function of a national macroscale monitoring scheme.

VMDB

The VMDB (Veterinary Medical Data Base) — formerly the VMDP (Veterinary Medical Data Program) — is a collaborative mesoscale database involving several veterinary schools in North America. Data are coded using SNVDO codes (described in Chapter 9). The data sources, like many of the others that have been described (see Chapter 10), demonstrate selection bias but the database has provided a considerable amount of material for epidemiological investigations, including observational studies (see Chapter 15).

VIDA II

VIDA II (Veterinary Investigation Diagnosis Analyses) is a mesoscale database comprising records of specimen submissions to veterinary investigation laboratories in Great Britain. These submissions are voluntary and constitute only a proportion of all post-mortem and laboratory specimens. The system stores data on a central mainframe computer. The individual laboratories code diagnostic data on pro formas using a modification of SNVDO codes, and the pro formas are then posted to a centre where the data are put into the computer.

Edinburgh SAPTU clinical recording system

This system records clinical case summaries from the veterinary school's Small Animal Practice Teaching Unit (SAPTU) on a mainframe computer. It is therefore a mesoscale scheme. Data are entered as consecutive numeric codes. It uses a relational DBMS, facilitating correlation of case record components.

DairyCHAMP

DairyCHAMP is a microcomputerized dairy herd health and productivity scheme to assist daily animal management, herd performance monitoring, and problem analysis. It is therefore a microscale scheme. Events related to individual cows are recorded in relation to reproductive and lactation cycles and health records (e.g., records of service, pregnancy diagnosis, and mastitis). There is also a bull record, and a record of farm-related data, such as type of housing, and feed and drug inventories and use. Three categories of report are generated: management aids, performance monitors (e.g., conception rate and heifer growth charts), and problem analysis reports which are used in conjunction with the performance monitors to detect problems such as excessive calving to conception intervals.

DairyCHAMP can be fully integrated with a decision support system, DairyORACLE (Marsh *et al.*, 1987). A similar degree of 'seamless integration' is also possible between other dairy herd health and productivity schemes and decision support systems (e.g., Williams and Esslemont, 1993), and the pig herd health and productivity scheme, PigCHAMP; a decision support system for pig breeding enterprises, PigORACLE; an economic expert system for assessing breeding herd performance, CHESS (Computerised Herd Evaluation System for Sows: Huirne *et al.*, 1992); and an expert system for evaluating herd culling and replacement policy, PorkCHOP (Dijkhuizen *et al.*, 1986; Huirne *et al.*, 1991).

EpiMAN

EpiMAN (Morris *et al.*, 1992, 1993) is a decision support system for the control of diseases that require national control or eradication procedures. It was developed in New Zealand, initially for the control of exotic diseases. The system is mounted on microcomputers that can be linked by communications networks, and is portable so that it can be moved easily to required locations.

The main components of EpiMAN, applied to foot-and-mouth disease control, are illustrated in *Figure 11.8*. Spatial and textual data relating to infected areas are stored in a relational DBMS. The spatial data are handled by a geographical information system. There is provision to store information on all farms in a country in which the system is used (the 'Agribase'). A Monte Carlo model

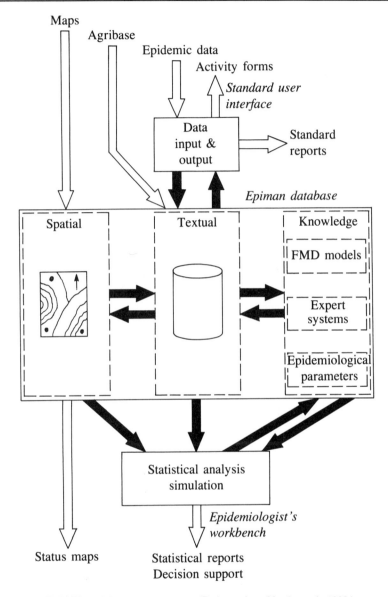

Fig. 11.8 The structure of the EpiMAN decision support system. (Redrawn from Morris *et al.*, 1993.)

(see Chapter 19) simulates spread of infection on individual farms; airborne transmission is modelled using the Gaussian plume dispersion model (see Chapter 6); and a third model predicts spread between farms, using parameters such as the size of infected areas, contact slaughter and 'ring' vaccination (vaccinating animals in a ring around an infected area). Finally, expert systems assign priorities to tracing animals and people who moved on to or off infected premises prior to diagnosis of the disease, and rate the risk of infection on unaffected farms so that daily patrol schedules can be planned.

Further reading

Blissmer, R.H. (Ed.) (1991) *Introducing Computers: Concepts, Systems and Applications*. John Wiley, New York. (*A general introduction to computers*)

Blood, D.C. and Brightling, P. (1988) *Veterinary Information Management*. Baillière Tindall, London

Date, C.J. (1990) *An Introduction to Database Systems*, 5th edn. Addison Wesley Publishing, Reading, Massachusetts

Davis, W.S. (1991) *Computing Fundamentals: Concepts*, 3rd edn. Addison-Wesley Publishing, Reading, Massachusetts. (*A general introduction to computer hardware, operating systems, applications software and communications*)

Frerichs, R.R. and Selwyn, B.J. (1991) Microcomputer applications in epidemiology. In: *Oxford Textbook of Public Health*, 2nd edn, Vol. 2. Eds Holland, W.W., Detels, R. and Knox, G., pp. 271–284. Oxford University Press, Oxford

Geering, W.A. (1992) Some epidemiological principles in disease surveillance and reporting. *Office International des Epizooties Quarterly Report (Asian and Pacific Region)*, **1**, 31–35. (*A brief discussion of information requirements for disease surveillance systems*)

Martinez, T.A., Kaneene, J.B., Lloyd, J.W. and Brown, M.I. (1992) Potential users and user requirements of an animal-health monitoring system in a developing country: case study of Honduras. *Preventive Veterinary Medicine*, **13**, 1–11

Menzies, P.I., Meek, A.H., Stahlbaum, B.W. and Etherington, W.G. (1988) An assessment of the utility of microcomputers and dairy herd management software for dairy farms and veterinary practices. *Canadian Veterinary Journal*, **29**, 287–293

Morris, R.S. (Ed.) (1991) Epidemiological information systems. *Revue Scientifique et Technique, Office International des Epizooties*, **10**, 1–231

Morris, R.S., Nimis, G. and Stein, T.E. (1986) The computer as a tool in epidemiological studies — an appraisal of trends. In Proceedings of the 4th International Symposium on Veterinary Epidemiology and Economics, Singapore, 18–22 November 1985, pp. 34–39. (*A discussion of data collection, storage and analysis with microcomputers*)

Smith, R.D. (Ed.) *American Veterinary Computer Society Newsletter*. (College of Veterinary Medicine, University of Illinois, 2001 South Lincoln, Urbana, IL 61801, USA)

12 Presenting numerical data

The epidemiologist makes inferences from data collected from groups of animals. The data are frequently quantitative, comprising numerical values. A fundamental characteristic of numerical biological data is their inherent **variability**. The weights of 100 Friesian cows, for example, will not be identical; there will be a range of values. If the 100 cows were a sample of a much larger group — say the national herd — then a different sample of 100, drawn from the same national herd, is almost certain to have a different set of weight values.

Variability is of importance to the epidemiologist in two circumstances: when a **sample** is taken and when different groups of animals are being **compared**. In the first circumstance, it is necessary to assess to what extent the sample's values are representative of those in the larger population from which the sample was drawn. This is relevant to surveys, which are discussed in the next chapter. In the second circumstance, it is often necessary to decide whether or not a difference between two groups is due to a particular factor. In epidemiology this frequently involves detecting an association between disease and hypothesized causal factors, and is discussed in Chapters 14 and 15. For example, if the effect of ketosis on milk yield were being investigated, then two groups of cows — one comprising cows with ketosis and one consisting of cows without ketosis — could be compared with respect to milk yield. A detected difference in yield could be due to:

1. the effect of ketosis;
2. inherent natural variation in milk yield between the two groups;
3. confounding variables (see Chapter 3) such as breed: cows of different breeds may be present in different proportions in each group, when the different breeds produce different milk yields.

In this example, the second and third reasons for the difference can confuse the investigation by contributing to differences in the milk yields of the two groups.

Statistical methods exist to separate the effects of the factors that are being investigated from random variation and confounding. Essentially, these involve estimating the **probability** of an event taking place. Probability is a numerical measure taking values between zero and 1. An event that is impossible has a probability of zero, whereas an event that is certain has a probability of 1. Probability also may be thought of as the frequency of certain events relative to the total number of events that can occur. Thus, the probability of throwing a 'head' with an unbiased coin is 1/2 (0.5). The probability of throwing either a 'head' or a 'tail' (i.e., the total probability) is 1. Similarly, prevalence is a measure of probability (see Chapter 4). A specific prevalence value is an estimation of **conditional probability**; a male sex-specific prevalence of 30% means that there is a probability of 0.3 of any one animal having a disease at a given point in time, conditional on its being male.

This chapter deals with the probability distributions of numerical data that are the basis of many statistical tests (some of which are described in Chapter 14) and with the methods of displaying numerical values. The statistical content of this book is not comprehensive; it is designed to give the reader a basic knowledge of some relevant concepts and techniques. The reader who is unfamiliar with elementary mathematical notation should first consult Appendix II.

Some basic definitions

Variable: any observable event that can vary. Variables may be either continuous or discrete (see Chapter 9). An example of a continuous variable is the weight of an animal. An example of a discrete variable is the number of cases of disease. In some circumstances, the numerical values of the variable are called **variates**.

Study variable: any variable that is being considered in an investigation.

Response and explanatory variables: a response variable is one that is affected by another (explanatory) variable; for instance, an animal's weight may be a response variable and food intake an explanatory variable, because weight is assumed to depend on the amount of food consumed. In epidemiological investigations, disease is often considered as the response variable, for example when studying the effects of dry cat food (the explanatory variable) on the incidence of feline urolithiasis. There may also be circumstances in which disease is considered as the explanatory variable, for instance when studying the effect of disease on weight. Response variables are sometimes called **dependent variables** and explanatory variables called **independent variables**.

Parameter: a quantity that can differ in different circumstances, but is constant in the case that is being considered. It may be a **constant** in a mathematical formula or model. For example, a survey may be designed to detect a minimum disease prevalence, such as 20%. Although prevalence can vary, the minimum detectable prevalence is defined for the objectives of the survey as a single unvarying value, and is therefore a parameter of the survey which is incorporated in the appropriate formula to detect the specified minimum disease prevalence (see Chapter 13). A parameter may also be a **measurable characteristic** of a population such as the average milk yield of a herd of dairy cows.

Data set: a collection of data.

Raw data: the initial measurements that form the basis of analyses.

Some descriptive statistics

Table 12.1 lists sample weights of two groups (A and B) of piglets, when weaned at three weeks of age. These can be considered as random samples of a much larger group of piglets, namely all piglets at three weeks of age. The inherent variability is obvious. The number of piglets with weights within defined intervals (i.e., the group **frequency distribution** of the weights) for group B is recorded in *Table 12.2* and depicted in *Figure 12.1*. This figure, which summarizes the data, is called a **histogram**. The intervals on the horizontal axis are 0.5 kg wide. The

Table 12.1 Specimen three-week weaning weights (kg) of two groups (A and B) of piglets.

Group A				
4.2	5.3	5.6	6.0	6.4
4.6	5.3	5.7	6.0	6.4
4.7	5.4**	5.7	6.1	6.4
4.8	5.4	5.7	6.1	6.5
4.9	5.4	5.9*	6.1	6.5
5.1	5.4	5.9	6.1	6.5
5.2	5.4	5.9	6.1**	6.8
5.2	5.5	5.9	6.2	6.8
5.2	5.5	6.0	6.3	6.8
5.3	5.5	6.0	6.4	

$n=49$; $\bar{x}=5.76$ kg; $s=0.60$ kg; $Q_2 = 5.9$ kg; $SIR = 0.35$ kg.

Group B				
2.6	4.3	4.6	4.8	5.3
3.4	4.3	4.6	5.0	5.5
3.6	4.3**	4.6	5.0	5.5
3.8	4.4	4.6	5.0	5.6
3.9	4.4	4.7*	5.0	5.6
4.0	4.4	4.7	5.1	5.6
4.0	4.4	4.7	5.1**	5.6
4.1	4.5	4.8	5.2	5.7
4.1	4.5	4.8	5.2	6.3
4.2	4.5	4.8	5.2	

$n=49$; $\bar{x}=4.69$ kg; $s=0.67$ kg; $Q_2 = 4.7$ kg; $SIR = 0.40$ kg.

*Median
**Quartiles

number of piglets within each interval is proportional to the area of the vertical bars. If the intervals on the horizontal axis are equal, as in this example, then the number of piglets within each interval is also proportional to the height of the bars. Alternatively, the vertical plots and the mid-points of the horizontal intervals can be joined, rather than constructing bars, in which case a

Table 12.2 Grouped frequency distribution for the three-week weaning weights of piglets in group B of *Table 12.1*.

Weight (kg)	Number of piglets
2.6–3.0	1
3.1–3.5	1
3.6–4.0	5
4.1–4.5	13
4.6–5.0	15
5.1–5.5	8
5.6–6.0	5
6.1–6.5	1

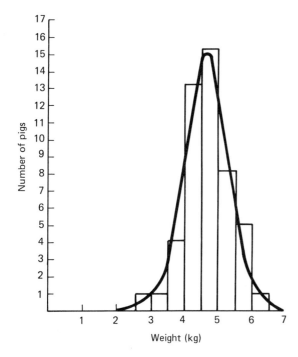

Fig. 12.1 Observed distribution of the weights of the 49 piglets in group B depicted as a histogram (rectangles) and fitted 'Normal' curve (smooth curve). (Data from *Table 12.1*.)

frequency polygon is constructed. These data can be summarized further by the use of descriptive statistics that are measures of **position** and **spread** of the histogram.

Measures of position

A commonly adopted measure of position is the **mean** of the sample, denoted by $\bar{x}$ (pronounced *x*-bar). It is calculated using:

$$\bar{x} = \frac{\Sigma x}{n}$$

where n is the number of values in the random sample. In *Table 12.1*, $n = 49$ in each group, and $\bar{x} = 5.76$ kg in Group A and 4.69 kg in Group B.

Each sample has been assumed, implicitly, to be drawn from a much larger population; thus the mean of the sample is only an **estimate** of the true population mean, μ. Only if all the population is investigated can the parameter μ be known. As the sample size increases, $\bar{x}$ will be a better estimator of μ, that is, the precision of $\bar{x}$ as an estimator of μ will increase.

The **median** of the sample, sometimes denoted by Q_2, is another measure of position. It is the value below which half, and therefore above which half, of the observations lie. It divides the distribution into equal, ordered subgroups and is termed a **quantile**. Quantiles that divide the distribution into hundredths are centiles (percentiles). The median therefore is the 50th centile (percentile).

The median values in *Table 12.1* for Groups A and B respectively are marked with an asterisk, '*'. If the data set contains an even number of values then the median is defined as the average of the two middle values. Again, the sample median is an estimator of the true population median.

The lower and upper quartiles, Q_1 and Q_3 respectively, are defined as the two values that are midway between the lower and upper extreme values and the median. For Groups A and B they are marked with two asterisks, '**'. Thus, 25% of values fall below Q_1, and 75% of values lie above it; Q_1 is therefore the 25th centile. Similarly, 75% of values fall below Q_3 and 25% of values lie above it; Q_3 is therefore the 75th centile.

Measures of spread

Measures of spread are a little more difficult to calculate than those of position. Two examples of simple measures of spread are the range and the mean of the absolute deviations of the individual values from the mean. However, these measures often do not distinguish different sets of data.

A commonly adopted measure is the **sample variance**, s^2, which is calculated by:

$$s^2 = \frac{\Sigma(x - \bar{x})^2}{n - 1}$$

This formula may be rewritten in a form that is more easily calculated with small calculators, namely:

$$s^2 = \frac{\Sigma x^2 - \{(\Sigma x)^2/n\}}{n - 1}$$

The square root of the sample variance is called the sample **standard deviation**. Using the values from *Table 12.1*, Group B, and the formula for s^2 above, the sample standard deviation, s, is given by:

$$s = \sqrt{\left[\frac{\Sigma x^2 - \{(\Sigma x)^2/n\}}{n - 1}\right]}$$

$$= \sqrt{\left[\frac{1099.16 - (229.8^2/49)}{48}\right]}$$

$$= \sqrt{\frac{21.45}{48}}$$

$$= 0.67 \text{ kg.}$$

Just as the sample mean is an estimate of the population mean, so the sample variance and sample standard deviation are estimates of the **population variance**, σ^2 and the population **standard deviation**, σ (sigma).

When summary statistics are presented, the sample standard deviation should be presented as well as the sample mean in order to indicate the variability within the population.

A measure of spread that often accompanies the median is the **semi-interquartile range** (*SIR*). This is half of the range between the quartiles, Q_1 and Q_3:

$$SIR = \frac{Q_3 - Q_1}{2}.$$

This is an estimator for the population semi-interquartile range.

Alternatively, and increasingly, a sample may be summarized by a **five-point summary** consisting of the minimum, lower quartile, median, upper quartile and maximum.

Interval estimation

The mean

The sample mean gives a single estimate for the population parameter μ and is therefore called a **point estimate**. Repeated sampling of the population will produce different sample means as estimates of the population mean. The sample mean has a distribution; the mean of this distribution is equal to the population mean, but its variance is σ^2/n, the population variance divided by the sample size. The square root of the variance of the sample means is termed the **standard error of the mean** (s.e.m.) to avoid confusion with the standard deviation of the individual values. It is given by:

$$\text{s.e.m.} = \sigma/\sqrt{n}.$$

This may be estimated by what is termed the **estimated standard error of the mean** (e.s.e.m.), obtained by replacing σ by s:

$$\text{e.s.e.m.} = s/\sqrt{n}.$$

The e.s.e.m. is an indication of the **precision** (see Chapter 9) of the sample's estimate of the population mean: the smaller the e.s.e.m., the greater the precision.

It is sometimes more useful to quote a range within which one is reasonably confident that the true mean will lie. This range is known as a **confidence interval**. It combines a measure of location (the mean) with a measure of spread (the s.e.m.). For example, on 95% of occasions that samples are taken from a population of Normally* distributed values, the confidence interval given by the sample mean, $\bar{x} \pm 1.96$ s.e.m will contain the true population mean. For a single sample, the interval $\bar{x} \pm 1.96$ s.e.m. is known as the **95% confidence interval**. The upper and lower points of a confidence interval are **confidence limits**.

When the s.e.m. is estimated by the e.s.e.m. (which is nearly always the case), the multiplier 1.96 must be replaced by an appropriate value to take account of sampling variability. The value is obtained from tables (Student's *t*-distribution: Appendix IV). It depends on the required level of confidence, the sample size and a related figure known as the **degrees of freedom**. If a sample consists of n **independent** observations (the value of one observation does not influence the value of another) then there are, in a sense, n independent 'pieces of information'. Calculating the mean uses one piece of information, leaving $(n - 1)$ for the variance. This is because knowledge of $(n - 1)$ observations and the mean fixes the value of the remaining observation. The number $(n - 1)$ is the number of degrees of freedom.

Using the values from Group B (*Table 12.1*):

$$\text{e.s.e.m.} = s/\sqrt{n}$$

$$= \frac{0.67}{\sqrt{49}}$$

$$= 0.096.$$

To select the value of the appropriate multiplier for a 95% confidence interval from Appendix IV, the column headed '0.05' $(1 - 95/100)$ is chosen. There are 48 degrees of freedom $(49 - 1)$. This number is not represented in the table, and so the highest value, not greater than 48, which is represented in the table, is picked: 40. The appropriate multiplier is therefore 2.021, and the 95% confidence interval is

$$\bar{x} \pm 2.02 \text{ e.s.e.m.} = 4.69 \pm 0.194 \text{ kg}$$

*The 'Normal' distribution is one of several families of statistical distributions, some of which are described later in this chapter.

= 4.496, 4.884 kg,

assuming that the three-week weaning weights are Normally distributed. (A comma conventionally separates the lower and upper limits of a confidence interval.)

Other confidence intervals can be estimated. To select the value of the appropriate multiplier for a 90% confidence interval from Appendix IV, the column headed '0.10' (1 − 90/100) is chosen, and the appropriate multiplier is 1.684. The 90% confidence interval therefore is:

$$\bar{x} \pm 1.68 \text{ e.s.e.m.} = 4.69 \pm 0.161 \text{ kg}$$
$$= 4.529, 4.851 \text{ kg.}$$

The appropriate multiplier for a 99% confidence interval is 2.704 (selected from the column headed '0.01': 1 − 99/100).

Note that, with a given data set, greater confidence is associated with a wider confidence interval.

Other parameters

Confidence intervals can be calculated for many parameters, including medians and other quantiles (Gardner and Altman, 1989) and parameters whose point estimates have already been described in Chapter 4: incidence rate (Kahn and Sempos, 1989) and adjusted (standardized) measures (Gardner and Altman, 1989). Calculation of confidence intervals for prevalence is discussed in detail in Chapter 13, and the same methods can be applied to cumulative incidence and cumulative mortality. Calculation of confidence intervals for other parameters is discussed in the succeeding chapters in which the parameters are encountered.

Statistical distributions

The Normal distribution

If many piglets were weighed, rather than just the 49 in the data set shown in *Table 12.1*, and if the intervals used in the histogram in *Figure 12.1* were reduced, then the bars would become narrower. Eventually, the corresponding frequency polygon would trace a smooth curve. One such curve has been fitted over the bars in *Figure 12.1*, using a computer program which identifies the curve, using the weights in *Table 12.1*. The curve has one peak in the middle and is symmetrical. This bell shape is typical of a family of frequency distributions known as the **Normal** family of distributions. It is better spelled with an upper case N to avoid confusion with other meanings of the word. Another name for this distribution is the

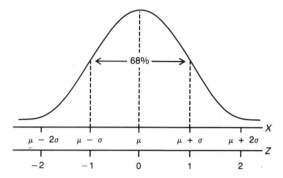

Fig. 12.2 A Normal density curve showing the relationship between μ, σ, z and the proportion of observations for Normally distributed data.

Gaussian distribution. This distribution is described by two parameters: its mean, μ, and its standard deviation, σ.

The Normal curve can be used as a smooth approximation to a histogram based on a sample of values, as in *Figure 12.1*, or as the paradigm of the population distribution of a variable. The latter can be described mathematically as a **density function** (Samuels, 1989), and plotted graphically as a **density curve** which can be interpreted quantitatively in terms of areas under the curve (*Figure 12.2*). All Normal curves can be made equivalent with respect to areas under them by rescaling the horizontal axis. The rescaled variable is denoted by z, the **standardized Normal deviate**:

$$z = \frac{x - \mu}{\sigma}.$$

The values $z = 0$, 1, 2, 3 correspond to $x = \mu$, $\mu + \sigma$, $\mu + 2\sigma$ and $\mu + 3\sigma$, respectively.

The z scale can be used to ascertain the proportion of observations that fall within a specified range of values. Approximately 68% of all Normally distributed values lie within one standard deviation of the mean of the population from which they were sampled ($\mu - \sigma$ to $\mu + \sigma$; $z = -1$ to $z = 1$), and 95% within approximately two standard deviations of the mean (precisely: $\mu - 1.96\sigma$ to $\mu + 1.96\sigma$; $z = -1.96$ to $z = 1.96$) (*Figure. 12.2*).

In many cases, the Normal distribution provides a workable approximation to the distribution of biological variables; for this reason it is a very important distribution. However, this distribution cannot be applied to all variables. Measurements to which Normality does not apply (although it can do as an approximation for large samples) are counts of nominal data and ordinal data that only have a small number of intervals on the scale (*Figure*

Table 12.3 Possible series of calves born to a cow during three successive uniparous gestations (M = male; F = female).

First gestation	Second gestation	Third gestation	Total male	Total female
M	M	M	3	0
M	M	F	2	1
M	F	M	2	1
M	F	F	1	2
F	M	M	2	1
F	M	F	1	2
F	F	M	1	2
F	F	F	0	3

9.1). Visual analogue measurements also may not be Normally distributed.

The binomial distribution

The binomial distribution relates to discrete data when there are only two possible outcomes on each occasion; for instance, the sex of a calf at birth can only be either male or female. An example is given in *Table 12.3*. The two outcomes may be of any kind but, for convenience, here are termed 'success' and 'failure'. On n occasions, the probability $Pr(r)$ of r successes out of n trials is found to be:

$$Pr(r) = \frac{n!}{r!(n-r)!} \; p^r(1-p)^{n-r} \quad [r = 0, 1, 2, \ldots$$
$$n, 0 < p < 1]$$

where p = probability of success on a single occasion assuming **no association** between the outcomes occurring on different occasions. In this example, two males (outcomes, $r = 2$) may be born during three pregnancies (occasions, $n = 3$). If it is assumed that the sex of the first calf does not affect the sex of future calves, and $p = 0.52$, then the probability, $Pr(2)$, will be:

$$Pr(2) = \frac{3!}{2!1!} (0.52)^2(0.48) \quad [\text{Note: } n - r = 1]$$

$$= 0.39.$$

The value of p can vary considerably between 0 and 1; for example, in some genetically determined diseases.

The Poisson distribution

The Poisson distribution is concerned with counts. It is applicable when events occur randomly in space or time. Some commonly quoted examples are the distribution of

blood cells in a haemocytometer and the distribution of virus particles infecting cells in tissue culture. This distribution is important in epidemiology because it relates to the spatial and temporal distribution of disease. The random occurrence of cases of disease in unit time or in unit area can follow a Poisson distribution. A significant departure from this distribution therefore indicates temporal and geographical departures from randomness (see Chapter 8).

The distribution is characterized by one parameter, λ (lambda): the average count per unit area or per unit time.

The probability of counts of $r = 0, 1, 2, 3, 4,$ and so on, is given by the formula:

$$Pr(r) = \frac{e^{-\lambda}\lambda^r}{r!} \quad [\lambda > 0, r = 0, 1, 2, \ldots]$$

where e is a constant: the base of natural (Napierian) logarithms = 2.718 28. The value of $e^{-\lambda}$ can be found in published tables and is determined on many pocket calculators.

For example, suppose that a tissue culture monolayer is being infected with virus particles. If there are 1×10^6 cells to which are added 3×10^6 virus particles, then the average count/cell (λ) is 3. The proportion of cells expected to be infected with, for example, two particles can be calculated using the formula above, with $\lambda = 3$ and $r = 2$. Substituting in the formula:

$$Pr(2) = e^{-3}3^2/2!$$

From tables, $e^{-3} = 0.0498$.

Thus: $Pr(2) = 0.0498 \times 3^2/2!$
$$= 0.2241.$$

This means that the expected proportion of cells infected with two virus particles is 22.41%.

Other distributions

There are many other statistical distributions. Some deviate from Normality; some of these deviations are illustrated in *Figure 12.3*. The mean and median are equal when a variable is symetrically distributed; and the mean and standard deviation provide good measures of position and spread. However, when frequency distributions deviate from Normality, this may not be true. Thus, with a positive skew the mean is located to the right of the peak of the frequency distribution. In such cases, the median and semi-interquartile range are better measures of position and location. Some distributions are neither Normal nor binomial nor Poisson. Two other distributions are compared with the Normal in *Figure 12.4*. If

Asymmetry   Kurtosis

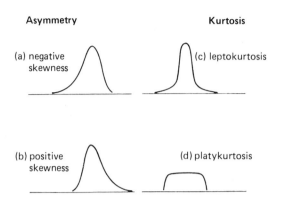

Fig. 12.3 Some deviations from the Normal distribution. (From Sard, 1979.)

unusual distributions are suspected, then expert statistical advice should always be obtained.

Transformations

Natural scales of measurement are not always the simplest to analyse and interpret because they may produce non-

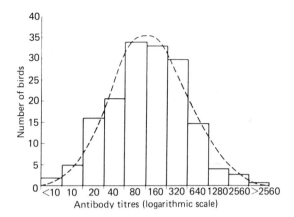

Fig. 12.5 An example of a transformed lognormal distribution. Distribution of the haemagglutination-inhibiting antibody titres of a group of 165 domestic fowls, six weeks after having been inoculated with a single dose of an inactivated Newcastle disease virus vaccine. The broken line shows a Normal curve fitted to these results. (From Herbert, 1970.)

Normal distributions. However, it is sometimes possible to transform these distributions to approximate Normality by changing the way in which the variables are expressed — usually by raising the variables to a simple power or by converting them to logarithms. The distribution for which the logarithms of the data are Normally distributed is called the **lognormal distribution**. This distribution occurs in biology. It is characterized by a positive skew to the untransformed data. An example is given in *Figure 12.5*, which shows the frequency distribution of antibody titres to Newcastle disease virus in vaccinated birds, plotted on a logarithmic scale. In this case, a transformation was performed by diluting serum samples logarithmically before the titration was performed, initially to base 10 (1/10) and thereafter to base 2 (1/20, 1/40, 1/80, etc.). The application of logarithmic scales to serological investigations is discussed in Chapter 17. Epidemic curves (see Chapter 8) and incubation periods are often lognormal (Sartwell, 1950, 1966; Armenian and Lilienfeld, 1974). In the case of epidemic curves, the data (numbers of new cases) are discrete, but are treated as continuous measurements, because the numbers are frequently large.

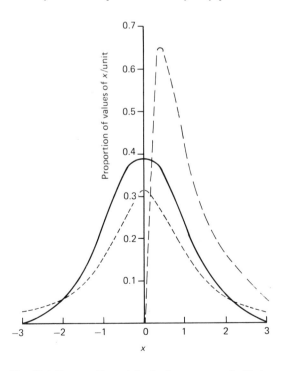

Fig. 12.4 Two non-Normal distributions compared with the Normal distribution. ——— Normal distribution; - - - - - *t*-distribution; — — — lognormal distribution.

Normal approximations to the binomial and Poisson distributions

When samples are large, and *p* is not too close to 0 or 1, the binomial distribution can be approximated to the

Normal. The approximation is better when a 'continuity correction' is applied to binomial data, to allow for the discrete nature of the data, while the Normal distribution relates to continuous data. Similarly, when samples are large, the Normal distribution provides a good approximation to the Poisson distribution. Therefore, techniques that are used to analyse Normally distributed data can sometimes be applied to the binomial and Poisson distributions. Such techniques, which become more accurate as sample size increases, are termed **asymptotic** (**large-sample**) methods.

Using the Normal approximations to the binomial and Poisson distributions, confidence limits can be defined for the parameters of these two distributions, that is, p and λ (Bailey, 1981), and asymptotic methods also can be applied to confidence interval estimation for other parameters. The multipliers used in calculating asymptotic confidence intervals correspond to those for the Normal distribution (e.g., 1.960 for 95%, 2.576 for 99%, as in Appendix V). These correspond to the values given for Student's t-distribution when the number of degrees of freedom is infinite (the last row in Appendix IV).

Displaying numerical data

Data should be represented in a form that is easy to interpret and to analyse in detail. This presentation may reveal interesting facts about the data and their distributions. Some of the methods of displaying data have, of necessity, been described (see Chapter 4). These include tables, bar charts, graphs and frequency polygons. A further method is the histogram, already depicted in *Figure 12.1*. The histogram is used for continuous variables, whereas the bar chart is used for discrete data.

'Pie' charts

A 'pie chart' is a circle (the 'pie') in which individual characteristics are represented as 'slices', the angle of a segment being proportional to the relative frequency of the corresponding characteristic. An example is given in *Figure 12.6*.

'Box and whisker' plots

Frequency distributions can be compared visually using a 'box and whisker' plot (Tukey, 1977; Erickson and Nosanchuk, 1979), which is based on a five-point summary, described earlier. An example is shown in *Figure 12.7* using the data in *Table 12.1*. The central horizontal line indicates the median; the upper and lower extremities of the vertical lines (the 'whiskers') mark the

maximum and minimum values of the data set; the horizontal sides of the large rectangles (the 'boxes') represent the quartiles.

Monitoring performance: control charts

It is sometimes desirable to monitor aspects of livestock production, such as mean litter size in a herd of pigs, so that any significant negative or undesirable deviations in the values from a **predefined standard** or **acceptable range** can be detected. It is then possible to undertake appropriate remedial action. When data are recorded in tables, it is often difficult to appreciate the full significance of values or of their differences from one another. A suitable technique for monitoring data when they accrue sequentially is the use of **control charts**, which are graphs on which successive results are plotted in sequence while production is proceeding. These charts are important in modern Statistical Process Control methods (Owen, 1989). The significance of changes can then be evaluated, and corrective action taken at the earliest possible moment, thereby ensuring a smooth level of production.

Shewhart charts

The change in a variable's value can be monitored easily over a period of time by plotting values on squared graph paper (or, more likely nowadays, displaying the data

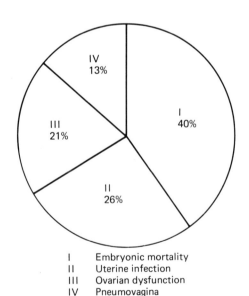

I	Embryonic mortality
II	Uterine infection
III	Ovarian dysfunction
IV	Pneumovagina

Fig. 12.6 An example of a 'pie' chart: proportions of principal mare infertilities detected in over 100 clinical cases reported and presented. (From Fraser, 1976.)

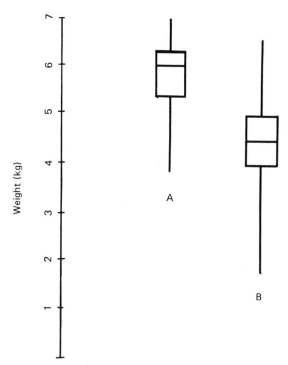

Fig. 12.7 'Box and whisker' plots of three-week weaning weights (kg) of two groups (A and B) of piglets. The central horizontal line indicates the median. The upper and lower extremities of the vertical lines (the 'whiskers') mark the maximum and minimum values of the data set. The horizontal sides of the large rectangles (the 'boxes') represent the quartiles. (Data from *Table 12.1*.)

graphically, using a computer program), with 'time' as the horizontal axis. This technique was developed by Shewhart (1931) to control the quality of manufactured articles, and an example is given in *Figure 12.8* which charts the mean of the number of piglets born alive per litter in a herd of pigs over a two-year period (Wrathall and Hebert, 1982).

Before the results are plotted, a **standard** or **reference value** is ruled as a horizontal line on the chart. This value is derived from the average of (ideally, at least 100) previous observations of the plotted variable in the herd. Alternatively, a composite value from other herds of a similar type in the national population may be used.

Decision boundaries (also termed **action levels** or **interference levels**: see Chapter 21) are also ruled on the chart, and remedial action is taken if a value of the variable crosses these boundaries. A mathematically derived decision boundary is based on the e.s.e.m. of a typical sample. It requires knowledge not only of the

standard deviation of the reference figure but also of the average batch size. In some applications, two decision boundaries above and two below the target level may be used. The inner pair give 'warning' and the outer pair indicate 'action'. Selection of boundaries is discussed by Goulden (1952).

In *Figure 12.8* (with only one pair of decision boundaries) the decision boundary is set at 2 e.s.e.m (2 here used as an approximation to 1.96; visually the difference should be of little consequence). A problem was detected in September 1977, and another, more severe problem was detected six months later. Such a problem may have been caused by reproductive disease in the sow, and subsequent microbiological investigations identified parvovirus in mummified foetuses.

If two standard errors are selected, it is expected that 2.5% of observations from the population will lie outside each boundary by chance alone. Therefore, remedial action will be taken on 2.5% of occasions when it is not justified. Similarly, if 2.33 standard errors are chosen as the boundary, then action will be unjustifiably taken on approximately 2% of occasions; if three standard errors are chosen, then unjustifiable action will be taken on approximately 0.28% of occasions. While an interval of three standard errors may seem attractive, this is accompanied by a greater probability of failing to take action, when desirable, than if a smaller number of standard errors had been chosen.

Although a decision boundary based on the e.s.e.m. is valuable, rigid adherence to such boundaries is not always valid because batch sizes tend to vary over time and so the e.s.e.m. will vary. However, average batch sizes can be used in calculating the e.s.e.m.; and this approach is more valuable than the arbitrary selection of a boundary level where individual values may cross the boundary level purely at random.

Cusum charts

The Shewhart chart is effective for detecting large, abrupt changes in the value of a monitored variable. However, it is less effective when the change is small and results from a slight shift or 'drift' away from the reference or standard value over a period of time. The 'cumulative sum' technique is a more sensitive method for detecting such trends, and control charts incorporating this technique are known as **cusum charts** (Woodward and Goldsmith, 1964). The technique is useful for detecting changes in average levels, determining the point of onset of these changes, obtaining reliable estimates of current average values, and making short-term predictions of future average levels.

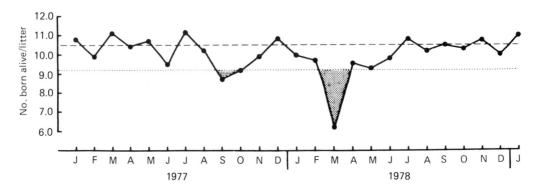

Fig. 12.8 Shewhart chart: number of piglets born alive/litter in a herd of pigs, 1977 and 1978. ---- Reference value; ..... decision boundary. (From Wrathall and Hebert, 1982; data from *Table 12.4*.)

Table 12.4 Mean monthly values for piglets born alive per litter in a 125-sow herd, January 1977 – December 1978. (From Wrathall and Hebert, 1982; raw data supplied by the authors.) The reference value, $k = 10.5$; the cumulative sum, $C_j = C_{j-1} + (x_j - k)$. (See text for explanation.)

j	Month	Mean number of piglets born alive/litter (x_j)	$x_j - k$	C_j
1	1977 Jan	10.9	0.4	0.4
2	Feb	9.9	−0.6	−0.2
3	Mar	11.1	0.6	0.4
4	Apr	10.5	0.0	0.4
5	May	10.7	0.2	0.6
6	June	9.4	−1.1	−0.5
7	July	11.0	0.5	0.0
8	Aug	10.3	−0.2	−0.2
9	Sept	8.7	−1.8	−2.0
10	Oct	9.2	−1.3	−3.3
11	Nov	9.9	−0.6	−3.9
12	Dec	10.7	0.2	−3.7
13	1978 Jan	9.8	−0.7	−4.4
14	Feb	9.6	−0.9	−5.3
15	Mar	6.5	−4.0	−9.3
16	Apr	9.4	−1.1	−10.4
17	May	9.3	−1.2	−11.6
18	June	9.6	−0.9	−12.5
19	July	10.7	0.2	−12.3
20	Aug	10.1	−0.4	−12.7
21	Sept	10.5	0.0	−12.7
22	Oct	10.3	−0.2	−12.9
23	Nov	10.7	0.2	−12.7
24	Dec	10.1	−0.4	−13.1

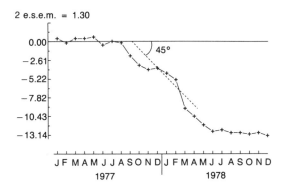

2 e.s.e.m. = 1.30

Fig. 12.9 Plot of the cumulative sum values (cusum) for the mean monthly number of piglets born alive per litter in a herd of pigs in a 125-sow herd, January 1977–December 1978. (Data from *Table 12.4*.)

A cusum chart consists of a continuous plot (usually against time) of deviations of the cumulative value of the monitored variable from its reference value, k. *Table 12.4* lists the mean monthly number of piglets born alive in a pig herd over a two-year period. The selected reference value (obtained, for example, from previous production data on the farm) is 10.5.

In each successive time period, as values $x_1, x_2, \ldots$ for the batches become known, the cumulative sums, $C_1, C_2, \ldots$ are calculated thus:

Period 1: $C_1 = x_1 - k$
$= 10.9 - 10.5$
$= 0.4;$

Period 2: $C_2 = (x_1 - k) + (x_2 - k)$
$= C_1 + (x_2 - k)$
$= 0.4 - 0.6$
$= -0.2;$

Period 3: $C_3 = C_2 + (x_3 - k)$
$= -0.2 + 0.6$
$= 0.4;$

and so on (see the last column in *Table 12.4*).

The cusum is plotted in *Figure 12.9*. So long as the mean for a series of batch values remains close to the reference value, k, some of the individual cusum values will be positive, and some negative, and so they will tend to cancel each other out. The cusum plot will then be essentially horizontal, indicating that the monitored variable is in a state of control.

Important indicators of abnormality on the cusum chart are changes in direction and slope of the plotted line. The scales of the horizontal and vertical axes must therefore be chosen carefully. If one time period equals one unit on the horizontal axis, and 2 e.s.e.m. of cusum are equal to one unit on the vertical axis (the e.s.e.m. being obtained from previous production data), then a plot's slope of 45° or more will indicate a change which is significant at the 2.5% level (see Chapter 14). Often, the slope is examined over a period of 10 time points (Owen, 1989). Thus (*Figure 12.9*), it can be seen that in the 10 months preceding May 1978, the slope is approximately 45°. Consequently, this cusum analysis suggests a drift from the reference value. If smaller changes are of interest — and this is quite likely — then techniques such as the use of a 'V-mask' (Barnard, 1959) and a decision interval scheme (Wetherill, 1969) are available. Page (1961), Davies and Goldsmith (1972) and Wrathall and Hebert (1982) discuss this topic in detail.

Cusum charts do not detect steady trends and regular cyclical variations. These can be detected by other techniques such as time-series analysis (see Chapter 8).

Further reading

Brown, R.A. and Swanson Beck, J. (1990) *Medical Statistics on Microcomputers*. British Medical Journal, London
Erickson, B.H. and Nosanchuk, T.A. (1979) *Understanding Data*. Open University Press, Milton Keynes
Fowler, J. and Cohen, L. (1992) *Practical Statistics for Field Biology*. John Wiley, Chichester
Gardner, M.J. and Altman, D.G. (1989) *Statistics with Confidence*. British Medical Journal, London. (*Estimation of confidence intervals and statistical guidelines*)
Mead, R., Curnow, R.N. and Hasted, A.M. (1993) *Statistical Methods in Agriculture and Experimental Biology*, 2nd edn. Chapman and Hall, London
Sard, D.M. (1979) *Dealing with Data. The Practical Use of Numerical Information*. BVA Publications, London

13 Surveys

Information on disease and associated events, such as productivity, can be obtained from **surveys** (introduced in Chapter 2). These involve **counting** members of an aggregate of units and measuring their characteristics. They may be conducted to estimate either a continuous variable such as weight and milk yield, or discrete events such as diseased animals. An important application of surveys in epidemiology is estimation of the **prevalence** of clinical disease, infection, or seropositive animals from samples of an animal population.

A survey of prevalence can involve:

1. a single sample, either to determine prevalence or to determine whether or not disease is present in a group of animals;
2. two samples, to compare prevalence;
3. three or more samples.

The first situation is commonly encountered in epidemiological investigations and is the main subject of this chapter; the statistical methods are those used in estimating proportions.* Comparisons between two samples are described in the next chapter.

Censuses and sample surveys

If all animals in a population are investigated then the survey is a **census**. Demographic censuses of human and animal populations are conducted regularly in many countries to determine the size and structure of the populations. A census is the only means of measuring **exactly** the distribution of a variable in a population. Some prevalence surveys that are 'almost' censuses have been conducted. For example, Jasper *et al.* (1979) surveyed 2,400 out of 2,800 farms in California to

---

*Surveys of continuous variables are not discussed here. Appropriate methods are described in the general texts on survey methods, listed at the end of this chapter.

---

determine the prevalence of mycoplasmal mastitis in dairy cows. Censuses can be expensive and may be difficult or impossible to conduct. However, if a survey is designed well then a reasonably accurate and acceptable **estimate** of a variable can be made by examining some of the animals in the relevant population, that is, a **sample**.

Sampling: some basic concepts

The validity of sampling theory is based on the assumption that an aggregate of units can be divided into representative subunits, and that characteristics of the aggregate can be estimated from the subunits.

Some definitions

The **target population** is the total population about which information is required. Ideally, this should be the population at risk. The **study population** is the population from which a sample is drawn. These two populations should be the same. However, for reasons of practicality, this may not be possible. For instance, if an investigation of periodontitis in Maltese terriers were to be undertaken, then, ideally, all Maltese terriers (the target population) should be sampled, although it may only be possible to investigate animals at dog shows or attending veterinary practices (the study population). If the study population is not 'representative' of the target population, then results should not be generalized beyond the study population.

The study population consists of **elementary units** which cannot be divided further. In veterinary surveys, these are usually individual animals.

A collection of elementary units, grouped according to a common characteristic, is a **stratum**. Thus, a dairy farm is a stratum comprising cows.

Before a sample is taken, members of the study population must be identified by constructing a list; this is the **sampling frame**. Each member of the sampling frame is a **sampling unit**. Thus, a list of hunting licence receipts was used as the sampling frame to identify hunters in an investigation of the recreational importance of feral pigs in relation to the possible control of African swine fever in the US (Degner *et al.*, 1983). A register of veterinarians can provide a sampling frame for sampling veterinary practices.

In areas in which telephone ownership is widespread, a sampling frame can be constructed from the list of names and numbers in telephone directories. Alternatively, all possible numbers can be used as the basis of sample selection. This second approach uses **random-digit dialling** (Waksberg, 1978) and is preferred to the first because it can include unlisted numbers and therefore reduces the likelihood of selection bias (Roslow and Roslow, 1972). It is a useful sampling method for surveys of pet populations (e.g., Lengerich *et al.*, 1992; Teclaw *et al.*, 1992).

The **sampling fraction** is the ratio of sample size to study population size. Thus, if 10 animals were chosen from 1,000 the sampling fraction would be 1%.

Veterinary sampling frames include lists of abattoirs, farms and veterinary practices, and can be constructed from some of the other sources of data described in Chapter 10. The objective of sampling is to provide an **unbiased** estimate of the variable that is being measured in the population. Many veterinary sampling frames (e.g., abattoirs) themselves relate to biased sectors of the total animal population and so caution must be exercised when extrapolating results to other sectors (e.g., farms). However, biased estimates also can be produced **within** a sampling frame when:

1. lists of members of the frame are incomplete;
2. information is obsolescent;
3. segments of the frame are untraceable;
4. there is lack of co-operation by some members of the frame;
5. sampling procedures are not random (see 'Types of sampling' below).

These sources of bias are **non-compensating errors** because they cannot be reduced by increasing the size of the sample.

The nature of sampling units

Sampling units may be individual animals (i.e., elementary units) or they may be aggregates such as herds, farms, or administrative regions, and prevalence may be calculated in relation to these different units. Thus, individual animal prevalence (the proportion of affected animals) may be quoted, or herd prevalence (the proportion of affected herds) may be cited.

It is important to distinguish between the 'epidemiological unit' and the 'sampling unit' when dealing with infectious diseases such as rinderpest (Tyler, 1991). The former unit is the group of animals which is of epidemiological significance in terms of the transmission and maintenance of infection, and therefore of disease control. It is convenient if the two units are identical. Thus, large herds that are managed independently constitute different epidemiological units that may be considered as separate sampling units. In contrast, in developing countries, several small village herds that are put together and are herded on common grazing constitute a single epidemiological unit, and the village could be considered as the sampling unit.

Types of sampling

There are two main types of sampling:

1. **non-probability sampling** in which the choice of the sample is left to the investigator;
2. **probability sampling** in which the selection of the sample is made using a **deliberate**, **unbiased** process, so that **each sampling unit in a group has an equal probability of being selected**; this is the basis of **random sampling**.

Selecting a random sample

There are several ways of selecting a random sample. For instance, each animal in the study population could be represented by a numbered piece of paper in a hat. The desired number of pieces of paper, corresponding to the sample size, could then be drawn from the hat to identify the sample's members. This method assumes that selection is random, and could be laborious for large study populations. A more convenient and less haphazard way of random selection uses **random numbers**. These are listed in published tables, one of which is given in Appendix VI, which also includes an example of random number selection.

Random numbers can also be generated by pocket calculators and computers. The former generate random numbers between 0 and 1. These values can be multiplied by the study population size to produce the required numbers. For example, if a random sample of 50 animals were required from a population of 2,000 amimals, then the calculator's random number generator might produce the values:

0.969, 0.519, 0.670 and 0.164, . . .,

which, when multiplied by 2,000, produce the sample numbers:

1,938, 1,038, 1,340 and 328, . . .,

respectively; and so on, until 50 animals are selected.

Non-probability sampling methods

Convenience sampling

Convenience sampling is the collection of easily accessible sampling units. When convenience is the main criterion for selecting a sample, it is very unlikely that the sample will be truly representative of the study population, resulting in biased estimates. For instance, if a survey were undertaken to estimate the prevalence of lameness in cattle, and if a sample were selected by choosing the first 10 out of 100 animals that entered a milking parlour, the sample probably would underestimate the prevalence because the leading animals would be less likely to be lame than those who entered the parlour last. In other cases, the selection procedure may not induce bias as obviously as in this example, but bias may nevertheless occur.

Despite its disadvantages, convenience sampling may be the only means of providing information quickly and cheaply, and may be necessary when financial resources are limited. However, care must be taken in extrapolating the results of surveys based on this method of sampling to the target population.

Purposive selection

Purposive (judgemental) selection is the choice of a sample, the averages of whose quantitative characteristics (e.g., weight) or distribution of whose qualitative characteristics (e.g., sex and breed) are similar to those of the target population. The object is to select a sample where characteristics are **balanced** with those of the target population. For example, a veterinarian who is undertaking a tuberculosis test on several herds may be asked to take blood samples from a 'representative' (i.e., balanced) sample for titration of antibodies against various bacteria and viruses. Purposive selection of so-called 'average' samples can produce a sample, none of whose members is far from the population mean. This sample, therefore, will only be representative of those collections of sampling units for which none of the members is far from the population mean. The sample will not be representative of all the possible samples that

may be taken from the population, some of which will have means far from the population mean. Therefore, the variability of the population that is being sampled may be underestimated. Additionally, experience and experimental evidence have demonstrated that consciously selected 'representative' samples are always biased. Yates (1981) discusses the disadvantages of purposive selection in detail.

Probability sampling methods

Simple random sampling

A simple random sample is selected by drawing up a list of all animals or other relevant sampling units (e.g., herds) in the study population, and then selecting the sampling units randomly, as described above.

Systematic sampling

Systematic sampling involves selection of sampling units at equal intervals, the first animal being selected randomly. For example, if one animal in every 100 were required, then the first animal would be selected randomly from the first 100. If this were animal 63, then the sample would comprise animals, 63, 163, 263, 363 and so on. Systematic sampling is used frequently in industrial quality control, such as selecting samples of goods on a conveyor belt.

Simple random versus systematic sampling

A systematic sample does not require knowledge of the total size of the study population. A simple random sample, however, can only be selected when all of the animals in the study population are identified. If lists are available with which to compile the sampling frame (e.g., lists of farms), then the random sample can be selected relatively easily. However, if lists are not available it may be difficult — even impossible — to draw up the sampling frame and therefore to select the random sample.

Systematic samples tend to be more evenly spread in the population than random samples, but in practice give results similar to simple random samples (Armitage and Berry, 1987). However, the technique can be dangerous if there is periodicity in the sampling frame. For example, if a farmer only sends his animals to slaughter on Tuesdays, and abattoir samples are only selected on Wednesdays, then that farmer's animals will not be represented in the samples.

Stratified sampling

A stratified random sample is obtained by dividing the

Table 13.1 An example of stratification: selection of a stratified random sample of cows from different regions of Great Britain based on a 5% sample of all cows (147 000). (Data extracted from Wilson *et al.*, 1983.)

Region	Number of cows	Number sampled
Devon and Cornwall	302 647	$302\ 647 \times 0.05 = 15\ 132$
SW England other than Devon and Cornwall	469 486	$469\ 486 \times 0.05 = 23\ 474$
S England	271 225	$271\ 225 \times 0.05 = 13\ 561$
E England	119 835	$119\ 835 \times 0.05 = 5\ 992$
East Midlands	189 817	$189\ 817 \times 0.05 = 9\ 491$
West Midlands	462 826	$462\ 826 \times 0.05 = 23\ 141$
Wales	342 346	$342\ 346 \times 0.05 = 17\ 117$
Yorkshire/Lancashire	255 626	$255\ 626 \times 0.05 = 12\ 781$
N England	273 838	$273\ 838 \times 0.05 = 13\ 692$
Scotland	260 366	$260\ 366 \times 0.05 = 13\ 018$
Totals	2 948 012	147 399

study population into exclusive groups (**strata**), then randomly sampling units from all of the individual strata. For example, the strata may be different ranges of herd or flock size. Stratification can improve the accuracy of a sample because it overcomes the tendency of a simple random sample to either over- or under-represent some sections of the sampling frame. Thus, if a simple random sample of animals in all herds in a country were selected, it is possible that no animals in very small herds would be chosen. Stratification, which ensures that each group in the population is represented, overcomes this problem.

The number of sampling units selected from each stratum can be determined by several methods. A common method is **proportional allocation**, where the number of sampling units selected is proportional to the number in each stratum. For instance, if a sample of cows were required from the British dairy herd by region, the number of cows selected from each region would be proportional to the number of cows in each region to ensure that cows in regions with large numbers of dairy cattle are not under-represented. *Table 13.1* illustrates this method of selection based on a 5% sampling fraction. Proportional allocation is the most efficient method of selection if there is equal cost in sampling each stratum. If this assumption is not true, then other, more complex, allocation methods should be used (Levy and Lemeshow, 1991).

Cluster sampling

Sometimes, strata are defined by geographical locations,

such as different countries, shires, parishes and villages, or by other categories such as veterinary practices or periods of time during which samples are selected. The strata are then termed **clusters**. Sampling from all of these clusters can be time-consuming and costly. This disadvantage can be overcome by selecting a few clusters, and sampling the animals only in these clusters; for example, animals in a few villages or herds could be sampled. This is **cluster sampling**. Commonly, **all** animals in each selected cluster are sampled; this is **one-stage cluster sampling**.

A sample may also be selected in more than one stage. Thus, a sample of clusters can be selected, followed by sub-sampling of **some** animals in the clusters (in contrast to **all** animals in one-stage cluster sampling). This procedure is therefore called **two-stage cluster sampling**; the clusters are the **primary units**, and the selected members of the sub-samples are the **secondary units**.

If the secondary units are the individual members of the study population, (i.e. elementary units), there is no point in going further. However, if they consist of **groups** of population members, either all of their constituent members could be sampled or further stages of sampling could be undertaken, corresponding to progressively higher levels of sub-sampling; for example, sampling regions, then dairy farms in each selected region, then cows on each selected farm. This is **multistage cluster sampling**. The sampling technique at each stage is usually simple random sampling.

Cluster sampling is sometimes used when there is an incomplete list of all members of a population: a list of primary units is required, but secondary units need only be listed within the selected primary units. The technique is therefore convenient and relatively cheap because resources can be concentrated on limited parts of the full sampling frame. However, information is less precise than if either a systematic or random sample comprising the same number of animals were selected, because disease prevalence tends to be more variable **between** groups than **within** them — particularly with contagious diseases where herds are likely to have either high or low levels of infection.

Sometimes it is impossible to construct a sampling frame because reliable demographic data are not available. In such circumstances, clusters can be defined using coordinates of a map grid. Grids may need to be constructed on maps that lack them, and grid lines identified by letters should be relabelled with numbers. *Figure 13.1* is an example. The coordinates 37 ('latitude') and 34 ('longitude') are chosen randomly (e.g., using random number tables). If herds are being selected, all

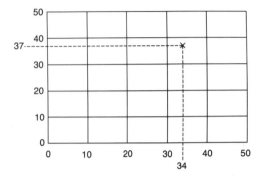

Fig. 13.1 An example of sampling using map grids.

herds within a defined radius of the selected coordinates should be sampled, the radius depending on the density of herds. If no herds are present within the radius, then no animals are sampled. The nearest herd to selected coordinates should **not** be the only herd sampled because this would bias the result by including too many herds from sparsely populated areas, and too few from densely populated ones.

What sample size should be selected?

The question that should be answered in all sample surveys is 'how many animals should be chosen for the survey?' An answer cannot be given without considering the objectives and circumstances of the investigation.

The choosing of sample size depends on non-statistical and statistical considerations. The former include the availability of manpower and sampling frames. The latter are the desired **precision** of the estimate of prevalence and the **expected frequency** of the disease.

Precision of the estimate of prevalence

The ability of an estimator to determine the true population value of a variable (i.e., the estimator's precision) can be expressed in terms of the bound on the error of estimation that can be tolerated. The error can be defined either absolutely or relatively. For example, an acceptable absolute error of ±2% of a prevalence of 40% represents an acceptable range of 38−42%. A relative error of ±2% of the same prevalence corresponds to 2% of 40%, that is 40% ± 0.8%, representing an acceptable range of 39.2−40.8%.

Expected frequency of the disease

It may appear paradoxical to suggest that some idea of disease frequency (i.e., prevalence) is necessary before a survey is undertaken, because the object of the survey is to determine the prevalence. However, a general notion is required; if the prevalence is thought to be close to either 0% or 100%, then the confidence interval for a given sample size will be narrower than if the prevalence were close to 50% (*Table 13.2*), that is, fewer animals will be required in the sample to achieve a stipulated width of confidence interval in the former case. Information on prevalence might be obtained from other related surveys. However, frequently this information is not available and so estimates have to be made that may be little more than informed guesses ('guestimates').

Table 13.2 The approximate sample size required to estimate prevalence in a large population with the desired fixed width confidence limits. (Modified from Cannon and Roe, 1982.)

Expected prevalence	Level of confidence								
	90%			95%			99%		
	Desired absolute precision			Desired absolute precision			Desired absolute precision		
	10%	5%	1%	10%	5%	1%	10%	5%	1%
10%	24	97	2435	35	138	3457	60	239	5971
20%	43	173	4329	61	246	6147	106	425	10616
30%	57	227	5682	81	323	8067	139	557	13933
40%	65	260	6494	92	369	9220	159	637	15923
50%	68	271	6764	96	384	9604	166	663	16587
60%	65	260	6494	92	369	9220	159	637	15923
70%	57	227	5682	81	323	8067	139	557	13933
80%	43	173	4329	61	246	6147	106	425	10616
90%	24	97	2435	35	138	3457	60	239	5971

Estimation of disease prevalence

Simple random sampling

The approximate sample size required to estimate prevalence in a large (theoretically 'infinite') population can be
determined for a defined precision and level of confidence. The limits of the associated interval indicate the
specified bounds within which the estimate will lie with
the defined level of confidence. The relevant formula for
a 95% confidence interval is:

$$n = \frac{1.96^2\, P_{exp}(1 - P_{exp})}{d^2},$$

where:

n = required sample size,
P_{exp} = expected prevalence,
d = desired absolute precision.

For example, if an expected prevalence of 30% is to be
estimated with a desired absolute precision of 5% (i.e.,
the limits of the associated 95% interval are 25% and
35%), then:

$$P_{exp} = 0.30,$$

and

$$d = 0.05.$$

Substituting these values in the formula:

$$n = \frac{1.96^2\, 0.30(1 - 0.30)}{0.05^2},$$

$$= \frac{3.84 \times 0.21}{0.0025},$$

$$= 323.$$

If other confidence intervals are required, then 1.96 is
replaced by the appropriate multiplier (Appendix V).
Table 13.2 can also be used. This table lists expected
prevalence values and the desired absolute precision
within 10%, 5% and 1% for three levels of confidence
(90%, 95% and 99%). Thus, if the expected prevalence is
again thought to be about 30%, and it is desired to
estimate this with an absolute precision of 5% for a 95%
confidence interval, then 323 animals are required — the
same value as that given by the formula.

In this example, the use of 30% might be based on prior
evidence. In other circumstances the approximate prevalence might not be known. A suitable procedure would be
either to choose the 50% figure to give the maximum

sample size, or to select the 20% figure and take more
samples, if necessary.

Appendix VII can also be used. The figures in this
Appendix give the sample sizes required to attain either a
95% or a 99% confidence interval for various prevalence
values at various values of absolute precision. Using the
same example of a 30% expected prevalence and absolute
precision of 5%, the sample would be selected using
Figure 4 of the appendix, giving a sample size of
approximately 400 (judged by eye from the curve) at the
95% level of confidence.

The formula and *Table 13.2* are based on the Normal
approximation to the binomial distribution. This is
acceptable if the size of the study population is large in
relation to the sample. However, as the size of the sample
relative to the study population increases, the variance of
the estimator of the mean of the study population is
decreased and the width of the confidence interval is
reduced accordingly. Therefore, in relatively small
populations, it is possible to select a smaller sample than
one from a theoretically infinite population to achieve the
same degree of precision.

The required sample size, n_{adj}, is given by the following
formula:

$$n_{adj} = (N \times n)/(N + n),$$

where n is the sample size, based on an infinite population
(obtained from the formula above or *Table 15.2*) and N is
the size of the study population.

For example, if prevalence were to be estimated using
values similar to those in the example above, but in a
small study population, say 900 animals, then

$$n = 323,$$

$$N = 900.$$

Therefore:

$$n_{adj} = (900 \times 323)/(900 + 323),$$

$$= \frac{290\,700}{1223},$$

$$= 238.$$

Thus, the number of animals required to estimate the
prevalence to the same absolute precision as the example
above (which was based on an infinite population) is 238.

It is difficult to give a strict rule regarding application
of this formula. It will always give the correct sample
size, but n_{adj} will be very close to n if adjustment is
unnecessary. A rough guideline is to calculate n_{adj} if n is
5% or more of N.

These approximate methods are usually sufficient, but, if the more complex exact methods are required, Levy and Lemeshow (1991) should be consulted.

Systematic sampling

If it is reasonable to assume that a systematic sample is as representative as a simple random sample, then sample size can be calculated using the same formulae as those used above for calculating sizes of simple random samples. However, if periodicity is likely to be present in the sampling frame, more sophisticated formulae should be applied (Levy and Lemeshow, 1991).

Stratified sampling

Sample sizes for proportionally allocated stratified samples can again be calculated using the methods appropriate to simple random samples. However, if more complex methods of allocation are adopted, then other formulae should be used (Levy and Lemeshow, 1991).

Cluster sampling

The formulae for sample size determination for simple random samples cannot be applied to cluster samples because they do not take account of the potentially large variation that can occur **between** clusters, and different methods therefore need to be applied.

An indication of the **between-cluster variance component**, V_c, is first needed. This is the variation expected between clusters if all animals in the clusters were sampled (i.e., there is no sampling variation within the clusters). If previous cluster sample data are available, then the between-cluster variance can be approximately calculated:

$$V_c = c \left(\frac{K_1 cV}{T^2(c-1)} - \frac{K_2 \hat{P}(1-\hat{P})}{T} \right)$$

where:

c = number of clusters in the sample;
T = total number of animals sampled;

$K_1 = (C - c)/C$,

where:

C = number of clusters in the population;

$K_2 = (N - T)/N$,

where:

N = total number of animals in the population; and

$V = \hat{P}^2 (\Sigma n^2) - 2\hat{P} (\Sigma nm) + (\Sigma m^2)$,

Table 13.3 An example of cluster sampling: a survey of 14 farms selected randomly from 865 farms; all animals in the selected farms investigated.

Farm	Total number of animals	Number of diseased animals	Farm prevalence
1	272	17	0.063
2	87	15	0.172
3	322	71	0.221
4	176	17	0.097
5	94	9	0.096
6	387	23	0.059
7	279	78	0.280
8	194	59	0.304
9	65	37	0.569
10	110	34	0.309
11	266	23	0.087
12	397	57	0.144
13	152	19	0.125
14	231	17	0.074
Total	3032	476	

where

$\hat{P}$ = sample estimate of overall prevalence,
n = number of animals sampled in each cluster,
m = number of diseased animals sampled in each cluster.

Table 13.3 presents information from 14 farms selected as clusters from a total of 865 farms, **all** animals in each cluster being sampled (i.e., one-stage cluster sampling). If such data are available, they can be used to determine between-cluster variance for determination of sample size for a subsequent cluster sample.

The sample estimate, $\hat{P}$, of overall prevalence
= 476/3032
0.157.

(It would be misleading to calculate the overall prevalence by taking the mean of the individual cluster prevalences. In this example, such a calculation would give a value of 0.186 i.e., [0.063 + 0.172 + ... 0.074]/14 — somewhat higher than the actual overall prevalence.)

In this example, $C = 865$ and $c = 14$. Thus, K_1 is approximately equal to 1 and so K_1 can be omitted from subsequent calculations. Similarly, N is assumed to be large, compared to T, and so K_2 is approximately equal to 1 and so can also be omitted from the calculations.

Calculate V thus:

$\Sigma n^2 = 272^2 + 87^2 + \ldots 231^2,$
$\qquad = 811\ 450.$
$\Sigma nm = (272 \times 17) + (87 \times 15) + \ldots (231 \times 17)$
$\qquad = 116\ 445.$
$\Sigma m^2 = 17^2 + 15^2 + \ldots 17^2$
$\qquad = 22\ 972.$

Thus:

$V = (0.157^2 \times 811\ 450) - \{(2 \times 0.157) \times 116\ 445\}$
$\qquad + 22\ 972$
$\quad = 20\ 001 - 36\ 564 + 22\ 972,$
$\quad = 6409.$

Now substitute the values $c = 14$, $T = 3032$ and $V = 6409$ into the formula:

$$V_c = 14\left(\frac{14 \times 6409}{3032^2 \times 13} - \frac{0.157 \times (1 - 0.157)}{3032}\right),$$

$\qquad = 14 \times 0.000\ 707,$
$\qquad = 0.009\ 90.$

This value of V_c can be used to determine sample size for a subsequent cluster sample if the expected prevalence, P_{exp}, in the latter is assumed to be the same as that in the previous sample, $\hat{P}$ (15.7%). However, if the expected prevalence is different, then an adjustment must be made:

$$V_{c,adj} = \frac{V_c P_{exp}(1 - P_{exp})}{\hat{P}(1 - \hat{P})}.$$

For example, if the expected prevalence in the new survey is 30%, then, $P_{exp} = 0.30$, $\hat{P} = 0.157$, and

$$V_{c,adj} = \frac{0.009\ 90 \times 0.3(1 - 0.3)}{0.157(1 - 0.157)}.$$

$\qquad = 0.0157.$

(Note that this value is only **coincidentally** one-tenth the value of the prevalence in the previous cluster sample.)
This value is then used for V_c.

One-stage cluster sampling: The first step in determining sample size in one-stage cluster sampling is prediction of the average number of animals per cluster. The appropriate formula for a 95% confidence interval is then:

$$g = \frac{1.96^2\{nV_c + P_{exp}(1 - P_{exp})\}}{nd^2}$$

where:

g = number of clusters to be sampled,

n = predicted average number of animals per cluster,
P_{exp} = expected prevalence,
d = desired absolute precision,
V_c = between-cluster variance.

For example, if an expected prevalence of 25% is to be estimated with a desired absolute precision of 5%, and the predicted average number of animals per cluster is 20:

n = 20,
P_{exp} = 0.25,
d = 0.05,
V_c = 0.0157.

Thus:

$$g = \frac{1.96^2\{20 \times 0.0157 + 0.25(1 - 0.25)\}}{20 \times 0.05^2},$$

$\qquad = 38.5.$

Therefore, rounding up, 39 clusters should be sampled.
If the population of clusters from which the sample is to be drawn is small, the estimated number of clusters should be adjusted by:

$$g_{adj} = Gg/(G+g)$$

where G is the total number of clusters in the population.
For instance, if the sample was to be selected from a population containing only 150 clusters:

g = 38.5,
G = 150,

and:

g_{adj} = 150 × 38.5/(150 + 38.5),
$\qquad$ = 30.6;

thus, 31 clusters are required.
If the subsequent sampling results in a value for the average number of animals in each cluster that is less than the predicted value, n, then more clusters should be sampled until the value gn is attained.
If other confidence intervals are required, the appropriate multipliers should be used in place of 1.96 (Appendix V).

Two-stage cluster sampling: Determination of sample size for two-stage cluster sampling depends on whether:

1. the total sample size is fixed, and the number of clusters to be sampled is required; or
2. the number of clusters is fixed, and the number of animals to be sampled is required.

(If neither the number of clusters nor the total sample size is fixed, then the optimum sample size can only be determined in terms of the cost of sampling from different clusters relative to the cost of sampling animals in the clusters. The relevant method is described by Levy and Lemeshow, 1991.)

(1) Number of clusters to be sampled when the total sample size is fixed: If the population of clusters is large compared to the number to be sampled, and the total number of animals is also large (which is the usual circumstance), the relevant formula for a 95% confidence interval is:

$$g = \frac{1.96^2 T_s V_c}{d^2 T_s - 1.96^2 P_{exp}(1 - P_{exp})}$$

where:

g = number of clusters to be sampled,
P_{exp} = expected prevalence,
d = desired absolute precision,
T_s = total number of animals to be sampled,
V_c = between-cluster variance.

For example, if an expected prevalence of 30% is to be estimated with a desired absolute precision of 5%, 1,000 animals are to be sampled, and the between-cluster variance is assumed to be 0.0157 (estimated from the previous cluster sample data in *Table 13.3* with an adjustment for the difference between the prevalence in the previous cluster sample and the expected prevalence in the proposed sample):

P_{exp} = 0.30,
d = 0.05,
T_s = 1000,
V_c = 0.0157.

Thus:

$$g = \frac{1.96^2 \times 1000 \times 0.0157}{(0.05^2 \times 1000) - 1.96^2\, 0.30(1 - 0.30)},$$

= 35.6.

Thus, 36 clusters need to be sampled, each sample ideally containing 28 animals ($36 \times 28 \simeq 1000 = T_s$). The selection of unequal numbers of animals from each cluster should not affect the result materially, unless there are major disparities. However, if fewer than 28 animals, on average, are sampled (i.e., $T_s < 1000$), then the desired level of precision may not be attained.

If the number of clusters to be sampled is negative, then it is not possible to obtain the desired absolute precision,

even with a very large number of clusters. It would therefore be necessary to increase the total sample size, T_s, or decrease precision (i.e., increase the value of d). If g is unrealistically high, it can be reduced by increasing d and/or increasing T_s, and then recalculating g.

If the population of clusters from which the sample is to be drawn is small, the adjustment formula, $g_{adj} = Gg/(G+g)$, should again be applied.

Thus, if the cluster sample designed above involved selection from a population of only 100 clusters, then G = 100, g = 35.6 and

$$g_{adj} = (100 \times 35.6)/(100 + 35.6)$$
$$= 26.3.$$

Therefore, rounding up, 27 clusters are required, each sample containing approximately 37 animals.

If the total number of animals in the population, N, is not large compared to T_s, then, for a 95% confidence interval, the number of clusters is approximately:

$$g = \frac{1.96^2 NT_s V_c}{d^2 NT_s - 1.96^2(N - T_s)P_{exp}(1 - P_{exp})}$$

where N = total number of animals in the population, and P_{exp}, g, d, T_s and V_c follow the same notation as before.

For example, if 1000 animals are to be sampled from a total population of 10 000 animals to estimate a prevalence of 30% with an absolute precision of 5%, then N = 10 000, T_s = 1000, d = 0.05 and, for a 95% confidence interval:

$$g = \frac{1.96^2 \times 10\,000 \times 1000 \times 0.0157}{0.05^2 \times 10\,000 \times 1000 - 1.96^2(10\,000 - 1000)}$$
$$\times 0.30(1 - 0.30)$$

$$= \frac{603\,131}{25\,000 - 7261}$$

= 34.0.

Therefore, 34 clusters are required, each containing, on average, 30 animals.

If the total number of animals and clusters in the population are both small, then the value of g obtained should be adjusted using the formula for g_{adj}, given above. Thus, if the total population of 10 000 animals is contained in 100 herds:

G = 100
g = 34

and

$$g_{adj} = (100 \times 34.0)/(100 + 34.0)$$

= 25.4.

Therefore, 26 clusters are required, each sample containing approximately 39 animals.

Again, the appropriate multipliers (Appendix V) should be used if other confidence intervals are required.

(2) Number of animals to be sampled when the number of clusters is fixed: To determine the number of **animals** to be sampled when the number of clusters is fixed, the appropriate formula for a 95% confidence interval is:

$$T_s = \frac{1.96^2 \, gP_{exp}(1 - P_{exp})}{gd^2 - 1.96^2 V_c}$$

using the same notation as before.

If the total number of clusters in the population, G, is not large compared to g, then:

$$T_s = \frac{1.96^2 \, GgP_{exp}(1 - P_{exp})}{Ggd^2 - 1.96^2 V_c(G - g)}$$

and if the total number of animals in the population, N, is not large compared to T_s, then adjust T_s thus:

$$T_{s,adj} = \frac{NT_s}{N + T_s}.$$

For example, if $V_c = 0.0157$, $P_{exp} = 0.30$, $g = 30$, $d = 0.05$, and the total population of clusters is large compared to g, then:

$T_s = (1.96^2 \times 30 \times 0.30 \times 0.70)/$
$\quad (30 \times 0.05^2 - 1.96^2 \times 0.0157) = 1648;$
$\quad$ i.e., 55 animals per cluster.

If there are only 50 clusters in the total population, then:

$T_s = (1.96^2 \times 50 \times 30 \times 0.30 \times 0.70)/$
$\quad \{50 \times 30 \times 0.05^2 - 1.96^2 \times 0.0157(50 - 30)\}$
$\quad = 476;$ i.e., 16 animals per cluster.

If there are only 2000 animals in the total population, but a large number of clusters, then:

$T_{s,adj} = (2000 \times 1648)/(2000 + 1648)$
$\quad = 904;$ i.e., 30 animals per cluster.

If there are only 2000 animals and 50 clusters in the total population, then:

$T_{s,adj} = (2000 \times 476)/(2000 + 476)$
$\quad = 385;$ i.e., 13 animals per cluster.

If the number of animals to be sampled is negative, it will be necessary to decrease precision (i.e., increase the value of d) or to sample from more clusters. If T_s is

unrealistically high, it can be reduced by increasing d and/or g, and then recalculating T_s.

Information derived from previous cluster samples is often not available. In such circumstances, a small random sample of clusters can be selected to provide a rough idea of the between-cluster variance before a full study is undertaken. Alternatively, the between-cluster variance component can be guessed. This is most easily done by guessing the standard deviation (i.e., the average difference expected between an individual cluster prevalence and the overall mean cluster prevalence), and then squaring it to give the between-cluster variance component. Thus, if an overall mean cluster prevalence of 0.30 (30%) is anticipated, and the average difference between this and the individual-cluster prevalence is guessed to be 0.09 (9%), then the between-cluster variance component would be $0.09^2 = 0.0081$. There is potential for error in determining the most appropriate sample size when there is greater variability between clusters than is guessed. It may therefore be prudent to assume a larger standard deviation than is guessed; for example 20%, giving a between-cluster variance component of 0.04 (0.2^2).

There are no simple formulae for sample size estimation involving three or more stages. If the simple random sample formula is applied, it is likely to produce conservative estimates. (Some authorities recommend applying the simple random sample formula and then, for all types of cluster sampling, multiplying the estimated sample size by between 2 and 4. This approach is empirical and can be inaccurate.)

Detecting the presence of disease

If an investigator only wishes to know whether or not a disease is present in a group of animals (rather than determining the prevalence), a suitable sample size can be selected using the formula:

$$n = \{1 - (1 - p_1)^{1/d}\} \{N - d/2\} + 1,$$

where:

N = population size,
d = number of affected animals in the population,
n = required sample size,
p_1 = probability of finding at least one case in the sample.

For example, in the Pan-African Rinderpest Campaign, at the stage of serological surveillance, it was necessary to sample herds to ascertain if unvaccinated animals had seroconverted (i.e., had been exposed to natural infection). It is unlikely that only a small number of animals would have seroconverted in infected herds, and it was considered reasonable to assume that at least 5% of animals in such herds would be seropositive. Therefore, the sampling protocol was designed to detect a seroprevalence of 5%. Thus, if p_1 is set at 0.95, and if a herd containing 200 animals is to be sampled, then, substituting these values into the formula,

$N = 200$,
$d = 10$ (5% of 200),
$p_1 = 0.95$.

Therefore:

$$n = \{1 - (1-0.95)^{1/10}\} \ \{200 - 10/2\} + 1,$$
$$= \{1 - 0.05^{1/10}\} \times 195 + 1,$$
$$= \{1 - 0.74113\} \times 195 + 1,$$
$$= 0.2589 \times 195 + 1,$$
$$= 50 + 1,$$
$$= 51.$$

Thus, if the seroprevalence is 5%, 51 animals need to be sampled to detect at least one seropositive animal with probability 0.95. *Table 13.4* can also be used. This lists the sample sizes, with p_1 set at 0.95, for detecting at least one case of disease for various prevalence values and sizes of sampling frame, offering a rapid means of determining sample size, rather than working the formula given above. For example, if the anticipated prevalence is 25%, and the population size is 120, then 10 animals need to be sampled to detect at least one case with probability 0.95.

If a sample of size n has been selected from a population of size N and **no** cases have been detected, then the upper $100\xi\%$ confidence limit, u, to the number of cases that may be present can be estimated from:

$$u = \{1 - (1-\xi)^{1/n}\} \ \{N - n/2\} + 1.$$

(ξ is the Greek letter 'xi'.)
For example, if $N = 400$, $n = 50$ and $\xi = 0.95$, then the upper 95% confidence limit, $u = 23$.

Again, *Table 13.4* can be used for this estimation. For instance, if 25% of 1400 animals are sampled and found to be disease-free, the upper 95% confidence limit of diseased animals is 11. Similar tables, constructed for 90% and 99% confidence limits, are listed in Cannon and Roe (1982).

The probability of detecting at least one positive animal, with various sampling fractions, is given in Appendix VIII. The probability of **failing** to detect

positive animals for various sample sizes and prevalence values is given in Appendix IX.

The cost of surveys

Sampling the study population incurs a cost. For example, sampling of cows to determine the prevalence of mastitis by bacteriological examination of milk specimens involves a laboratory cost. The most economic sample size can be determined with defined precision. Alternatively, if a fixed amount of money is available, then the sample size can be determined to maximize precision. Scheaffer *et al.* (1979) and Levy and Lemeshow (1991) describe techniques of estimating sample size for simple random, stratified, systematic and cluster sampling that include **cost functions** in the estimations. An example of estimation of optimum sample size for a fixed cost, relating to a national British bovine mastitis survey, is given by Wilson *et al.* (1983).

Calculation of confidence intervals

There may be occasions when sample size is predetermined (e.g., by the availability of animals). Moreover, even when an appropriate sample size has been selected before a survey is undertaken, it is unlikely that the prevalence will be exactly what is anticipated, and that the specified number of animals will be sampled. Thus, in all circumstances, a confidence interval should be calculated from the sample that is available.

Simple random sampling

A 95% confidence interval can be calculated from a simple random sample for a given sample size, n, and estimated prevalence, $\hat{P}$, using a formula based on the Normal approximation to the binomial distribution (Gardner and Altman, 1989):*

$$\hat{P} - 1.96 \sqrt{\left(\frac{\hat{P}(1-\hat{P})}{n}\right)}, \ P + 1.96 \sqrt{\left(\frac{\hat{P}(1-\hat{P})}{n}\right)}.$$

For example, if 200 animals were sampled, and 80 were found to be diseased, then the estimated prevalence would be 40%, and:

---

*This formula assumes that the population from which the sample is drawn is large, and therefore that the sampling fraction, f, is small, which is usually the case. If the sampling fraction is large (greater than 10%), then the numerator, $\hat{P}(1-\hat{P})$, needs to be multiplied by $(1 - f)$; for example, by $(1-0.2)$ if the sampling fraction is 20%.

Table 13.4 (i) Sample size required for detecting disease where the probability of finding at least one case in the sample is 0.95; (ii) upper 95% confidence limits for number of cases. (From Cannon and Roe, 1982.)

Population size (N)	(i) Percentage of diseased animals in population (d/N) OR (ii) Percentage sampled and found clean (n/N)											
	50%	40%	30%	25%	20%	15%	10%	5%	2%	1%	0.5%	0.1%
10	4	5	6	7	8	10	10	10	10	10	10	10
20	4	6	7	9	10	12	16	19	20	20	20	20
30	4	6	8	9	11	14	19	26	30	30	30	30
40	5	6	8	10	12	15	21	31	40	40	40	40
50	5	6	8	10	12	16	22	35	48	50	50	50
60	5	6	8	10	12	16	23	38	55	60	60	60
70	5	6	8	10	13	17	24	40	62	70	70	70
80	5	6	8	10	13	17	24	42	68	79	80	80
90	5	6	8	10	13	17	25	43	73	87	90	90
100	5	6	9	10	13	17	25	45	78	96	100	100
120	5	6	9	10	13	18	26	47	86	111	120	120
140	5	6	9	11	13	18	26	48	92	124	139	140
160	5	6	9	11	13	18	27	49	97	136	157	160
180	5	6	9	11	13	18	27	50	101	146	174	180
200	5	6	9	11	13	18	27	51	105	155	190	200
250	5	6	9	11	14	18	27	53	112	175	228	250
300	5	6	9	11	14	18	28	54	117	189	260	300
350	5	6	9	11	14	18	28	54	121	201	287	350
400	5	6	9	11	14	19	28	55	124	211	311	400
450	5	6	9	11	14	19	28	55	127	218	331	450
500	5	6	9	11	14	19	28	56	129	225	349	500
600	5	6	9	11	14	19	28	56	132	235	379	597
700	5	6	9	11	14	19	28	57	134	243	402	691
800	5	6	9	11	14	19	28	57	136	249	421	782
900	5	6	9	11	14	19	28	57	137	254	437	868
1000	5	6	9	11	14	19	29	57	138	258	450	950
1200	5	6	9	11	14	19	29	57	140	264	471	1102
1400	5	6	9	11	14	19	29	58	141	269	487	1236
1600	5	6	9	11	14	19	29	58	142	272	499	1354
1800	5	6	9	11	14	19	29	58	143	275	509	1459
2000	5	6	9	11	14	19	29	58	143	277	517	1553
3000	5	6	9	11	14	19	29	58	145	284	542	1895
4000	5	6	9	11	14	19	29	58	146	268	556	2108
5000	5	6	9	11	14	19	29	59	147	290	564	2253
6000	5	6	9	11	14	19	29	59	147	291	569	2358
7000	5	6	9	11	14	19	29	59	147	292	573	2437
8000	5	6	9	11	14	19	29	59	147	293	576	2498
9000	5	6	9	11	14	19	29	59	148	294	579	2548
10000	5	6	9	11	14	19	29	59	148	294	581	2588
∞	5	6	9	11	14	19	29	59	149	299	598	2995

The table gives:
(i) the sample size (n) such that the probability (p_1) of including at least one positive if the disease is present at the specified level is 0.95;
(ii) the upper 95% confidence limit (u) to the number of diseased animals in a population, given that the specified proportion were tested and found to be negative.

Examples:
(i) expected proportion of positives is 2%; the population size is 480 — use 500; from the table, a sample of 129 is required to detect at least one positive with probability 0.95;
(ii) for a population of 1000, a sample of 10% were all found to be negative; from the table, the upper 95% confidence limit for the number of positives is 29.

$\hat{P} = 0.4,$
$n = 200.$

Thus, the 95% confidence interval is

$$0.4 - 1.96 \sqrt{\left(\frac{0.4(1-0.4)}{200}\right)}, \ 0.4 + 1.96 \sqrt{\left(\frac{0.4(1-0.4)}{200}\right)},$$

$= 0.4 - 0.068, \ 0.4 + 0.068,$
$= 0.332, 0.468,$

that is, 33.2%, 46.8%.

If other confidence intervals are required, then 1.96 is replaced by the appropriate multipliers (Appendix V).

The formula assumes that:

1. $P \geq 0.05,$
2. nP and $n(1 - P) \geq 5;$

where n = sample size, and P = prevalence in the study population.

In the example just given, P is replaced by its estimate from the sample, $\hat{P}$:

$\hat{P}$ $= 0.40,$
$n\hat{P}$ $= 200 \times 0.4,$
      $= 80,$
$n(1 - \hat{P}) = 200(1 - 0.4),$
      $= 120,$

and so the formula may be applied.

Simple random sampling: small sample size

If only a small-sized sample is available, then nP or $n(1-P)$ may be less than 5. It is then necessary to calculate exact confidence intervals, based on the binomial distribution (Armitage and Berry, 1987). This also can be done conveniently by consulting Appendix X.

Simple random sampling: diseases of low prevalence

Some diseases (e.g., tumours) may be rare. If the Normal approximation to the binomial distribution is applied, then a very large sample would be required to estimate a confidence interval accurately. Moreover, Appendix X can only be used for prevalence values greater than 0.2%. Therefore, if the estimated prevalence is lower than this, an alternative method, utilizing the Poisson distribution relating to rare events (see Chapter 12), should be used;

Appendix XI gives the appropriate table for constructing a 95% confidence interval.

Systematic sampling

Confidence intervals for prevalence can be calculated for systematic samples using the formulae applied to simple random samples, assuming that there is no periodicity in the samples. More complex formulae should be applied if the latter may be present (Levy and Lemeshow, 1991).

Stratified sampling

The simple random sample formulae are also satisfactory for proportionally allocated stratified samples. However, if other methods of allocation are undertaken, more complex formulae are required (Levy and Lemeshow, 1991).

Cluster sampling

Confidence intervals for cluster samples need to be calculated differently from those for simple random samples, to take account of the variability that is likely to exist between the groups that constitute the clusters.

The data in *Table 13.3* will again be used to illustrate how confidence intervals are calculated. The sample estimate, $\hat{P}$, has already been calculated in the preceding section on sample size determination for cluster samples, and was found to be 0.157.

An **approximate** 95% confidence interval may be calculated using the formula:*

$$\hat{P} - 1.96 \left(\frac{c}{T} \sqrt{\frac{V}{c(c-1)}}\right), \ \hat{P} + 1.96 \left(\frac{c}{T} \sqrt{\frac{V}{c(c-1)}}\right),$$

where:

c = number of clusters in the sample,
T = total number of animals in the sample;

and

$$V = \hat{P}^2(\Sigma n^2) - 2\hat{P}(\Sigma nm) + (\Sigma m^2)$$

where:

n = number of animals sampled in each cluster,
m = number of diseased animals sampled in each cluster.

---

*Again, this formula assumes that the fraction of clusters sampled (f) is small (less than 10%). If the fraction is not small, the value $V/\{c(c-1)\}$ needs to be multiplied by $(1 - f)$. In this example, $f = 14/865, = 0.016$; thus $(1 - f) \approx 1$, and so $(1 - f)$ can be omitted from the formula without affecting the result materially.

Now, substitute the values $c = 14$, $T = 3032$ and $V = 6409$ (derived in the preceding section on sample size determination for cluster samples) into the formula:

$$0.157 - 1.96 \left(\frac{14}{3032} \sqrt{\frac{6409}{14(14-1)}} \right) \text{ to}$$

$$0.157 + 1.96 \left(\frac{14}{3032} \sqrt{\frac{6409}{14(14-1)}} \right)$$

$$= 0.157 - (1.96 \times 0.0046 \times \sqrt{35.214}) \text{ to}$$
$$0.157 + (1.96 \times 0.0046 \times \sqrt{35.214}),$$
$$= (0.157 - 0.0535), (0.157 + 0.0535),$$
$$= 0.1035, 0.2105,$$

i.e., 10.35%, 21.05%.

Again, if other confidence intervals are required, the appropriate multipliers should be used (Appendix V).

Note that the value for the confidence interval is much wider than that which would have been obtained if the formula for simple random sampling had been inappropriately used (14.4%, 17.0% for a 95% confidence interval), illustrating that, for a given sample size, cluster samples usually produce less precise estimates than simple random samples.

This formula can be used for both one-stage and two-stage cluster samples. In the former, $n =$ all animals in each cluster, whereas in the latter, n is a sample of animals in each cluster.

A simple rule stating when this Normal-approximation method for calculating confidence intervals may be applied does not exist. This is because the distribution of a cluster sample proportion is complex due to the presence of the two variance components (between clusters and between animals within clusters).* An indication of the validity of the method can be obtained by plotting the frequency distribution of the individual cluster prevalence values. If this has a smooth, symmetric distribution, the Normal-approximation method is likely to be valid. Otherwise, the calculated confidence intervals may only be approximate, particularly if a small number of clusters

---

*This means that it is unclear when the *central limit theorem* holds. This theorem states that, as more observations are included, eventually the mean of any distribution will tend towards a Normal distribution, providing its variance is finite. (See 'Normal approximations to the binomial and Poisson distributions' in Chapter 12.) The central limit theorem should hold before Normal-approximation methods are used with complete trust. In cluster sampling, the larger the number of clusters and the number of animals, the more likely that the theorem will hold.

has been sampled. Thus, a plot of the individual cluster prevalence values in *Table 13.3* does not show a smooth distribution, and so the confidence intervals should be regarded as approximate. In such circumstances, an alternative approach to presenting precision would be to simply state the standard error of the cluster sample's overall prevalence (i.e., the value derived in the worked example above before being multiplied by the multiplier 1.96: 0.0273). More complex methods of calculating exact confidence intervals are also available (Thomas, 1989), but would require the use of a computer program.

Samples with three or more stages require more complicated methods (Levy and Lemeshow, 1991).

Collecting information: questionnaires

Information that is required for studies and surveys may be available in existing records; for example, those kept at abattoirs, diagnostic laboratories and veterinary clinics. However, there are occasions when the appropriate unbiased information is not readily available, in which case it must be collected. A common means of collecting information is the **questionnaire**: a set of written questions. Technical information acquired from specialists, such as veterinary practitioners and laboratory staff, is recorded in a standardized fashion on a specialized questionnaire called a **pro forma**. An example has already been given (*Figure 11.3*). The person who answers the questionnaire is termed the **respondent**.

Structure of a questionnaire

The questionnaire is designed to record information:

1. in a standard format;
2. with a means of checking and editing recorded data;
3. by a standardized method of questioning;
4. with a means of coding.

Questions may be either **open-ended** or **closed**.

Open-ended questions

Open-ended questions allow the respondent freedom to answer in his or her own words; for example, 'What is your opinion of intramammary preparation X?'. The chief advantage of the open question is the freedom of expression that it allows: the respondent is allowed to comment, pass opinions and discuss other events that are related to the question's topic. The disadvantages are, first, that the open questions can increase the length of time taken to complete a questionnaire and, secondly, that the answers cannot be coded when the questionnaire is designed, because the full range of answers is not known. A range of answers may be difficult to categorize and code. Continuous variables can be grouped into intervals (e.g., 0.0−1.9 kg, 2.0−2.9 kg) for coding.

Closed questions

Closed questions have a fixed number of options of answers. The questions may be **dichotomous**, that is, with two possible answers, such as 'Do you use intramammary tube X for dry cow therapy (answer yes or no)?' Alternatively, the questions may be **multiple choice**; for example, 'When did your dog last have a litter? Within the last 3 months, 4−6 months, 7−11 months, 1−5 years?'

Closed questions are useful for ascertaining categorical, discrete data, such as breed and sex. The advantages of the closed question are ease of analysis and coding because of the limited, fixed response that is allowed. Codes can be allocated when the questionnaire is designed. The closed question is also quick to answer. A major disadvantage is that, because the options of answers are fixed, the answers may not reveal related events that may be significant.

Coding

It is advisable to store the results of a questionnaire in a computerized database (see Chapter 11). Therefore, questionnaires are frequently coded to facilitate transcription to such databases. Coding has already been discussed in detail in Chapter 9. Each question and each possible answer is coded. For example, in the question:

26. What is the sex of your animal?
    Enter 1 if male and 2 if female.

the question is coded as number 26, and the options to the answers to the dichotomous question are coded as either 1 or 2. The name of the respondent may be coded if confidentiality is required. It is also desirable to justify numeric answers to the right for transcription to computerized systems. For example, the date 8th March 1985 is coded as:

| 0 | 8 | 0 | 3 | 8 | 5 |

not

| 8 | 3 | 8 | 5 | | |

to allow for 31 days in the month and 12 months in the year.

Designing a questionnaire

The success of a questionnaire depends on careful design. Ideally, everyone who is issued with a questionnaire should complete it. The proportion of those who respond is the **response rate** (usually expressed as a percentage). The **non-response rate** is therefore 100 minus the response rate (%); for example, a response rate of 70% represents a non-response rate of 30%. Non-response from a respondent may be either total, in which the questionnaire is not returned, or partial, in which some questions are not answered but the partially answered questionnaire is returned. Good questionnaire design decreases both types of non-response.

Initial presentation

The title of the questionnaire should be brief and accurate. A polite letter, explaining the reason for producing the questionnaire, and the value of the results deriving from its completion, should be enclosed. The inclusion of a reply-paid envelope should increase the response rate.

Wording

Wording should be unambiguous, brief, polite, unemotional and (unless a pro forma is used) non-technical. If technical terms are used then they should be defined simply. Common ambiguous terms include 'often', 'occasionally', 'severe', 'mild', 'heavy' and 'light'. Double negatives should be avoided. Each question should contain only *one* idea. Sensitive, emotive and emotional questions should be avoided.

Question sequence

Related questions may need to be separated because the answer given to one question may influence that given to the succeeding question producing the phenomenon termed 'carry over'. General questions should be presented first, and specific ones later. The questionnaire can be made more interesting by 'branching out' from one question to another; for example, 'if you answer yes to question 2, then move to question 8'. However, the number of questions should be as small as possible, while achieving the objectives of the survey.

Question structure

Closed questions must be **mutually exclusive** and **exhaustive**. For example, the age of animals may be expressed as:

Age (please tick):   under 6 months   ☐
                      6−12 months   ☐
                      over 12 months   ☐

In this case, there is no overlap of ages between categories (they are mutually exclusive) and all possible ages are included (the options are exhaustive). To ensure exhaustiveness, it may be necessary to include **dumping categories** that accommodate all possibilities remaining after the specified options are considered. For example, 'other' is a dumping category in:

Against what infections has your dog been vaccinated (please tick):

distemper ☐   parvovirus ☐   hepatitis ☐
leptospirosis ☐   other ☐

Lack of confidentiality may increase the non-response rate. Total anonymity ensures confidentiality but prevents the tracing back of information (e.g., of diseased animals to a farm). A limited degree of confidentiality can be ensured by preventing identification of respondents by the majority of the data-processing staff. Three ways of doing this are

1. by having a separate sheet of paper for the respondent's name and address, with a code identifying the respondent on the questionnaire;
2. by using a coded strip down one side of the questionnaire, which can be detached;
3. by using carbon impregnated paper (NCR paper), allowing duplicates to be produced, but with the respondent's name masked off most of the copies.

Figures 13.2 and *13.3* are two examples of questionnaires. In the first example (a survey of Johne's disease in vaccinated herds) the following concepts can be demonstrated:

1. closed questions (e.g., No. 2);
2. open-ended questions (e.g., No. 19);
3. mutual exclusiveness and exhaustiveness (e.g., No. 17);
4. a clear title, with a statement of confidentiality;
5. a polite presentation (e.g., the last portion of the questionnaire that thanks the respondent for his or her co-operation).

In the second example (a lameness survey in cattle), these additional concepts are illustrated:

1. a dumping category (the inclusion of '6. other' in description of breeds);
2. confidential coding of the veterinary practice and veterinarian (two digits) and farm (three digits);
3. a clear description and definition of terms that are used (sites and nature of lesions in this example).

Questionnaires can either be completed by respondents after having been delivered to them (frequently by mail), or completed by an interviewer who presents the questions, verbally (either in person or by telephone), to the respondents.

Mailed and self-completed questionnaires

Requirements

The main requirements for a mailed or self-completed questionnaire are:

1. a list of respondents to act as the sampling frame (e.g., a register of veterinarians);
2. great clarity: no one will be present to cope with any difficulties that may arise;
3. a covering letter politely explaining the reason for sending the questionnaire.

Advantages

The main advantages of this type of questionnaire are that:

1. it is relatively cheap with potential for wide coverage;
2. it is quick and easy to organize;
3. it avoids interviewer bias (see below);
4. it allows a highly motivated respondent to 'check the facts' over a period of time;
5. respondents have the opportunity to reply anonymously, which may produce a high response rate.

Disadvantages

The disadvantages of this type of questionnaire are that:

1. clarity of question may be difficult to achieve;
2. the questionnaire cannot prevent reviewing of questions, which may lead to undesirable modification of previously answered questions;

Response rate

In mailed and self-completed questionnaires, response rates tend to be low — 50% is not uncommon, and the value can be as low as 10% (Edwards, 1990). The response rate cannot usually be increased by issuing more questionnaires.

Factors influencing the response rate are:

1. the sponsor — a respected sponsor should enhance the likelihood of obtaining a high response rate;

INVESTIGATION OF JOHNE'S VACCINATED HERDS

Conducted by: The Epidemiology Unit, Central Veterinary Laboratory, Weybridge, Surrey.

PLEASE NOTE ALL INFORMATION WILL BE TREATED AS STRICTLY CONFIDENTIAL

Herd Owner _____   1. Herd Code _____

Address _____

_____

2. Present herd type: Dairy ☐   Beef ☐   Mixed ☐

3. Replacement policy. Entirely home reared. Please write YES or NO _____

4. % breed composition of present adult herd _____

5. Present adult herd size _____

6. Present system of winter housing: Cowshed ☐   Cubicles ☐   Loose ☐   Outwintered ☐

7. Method of pasture utilization: Intensive ☐   Extensive ☐

8. Date of approval for use_____/_____/19_____

9. Year in which vaccination started 19_____

10. If vaccination has been intermittent please give the years in which either vaccine was not used or in which only some of the animals

    retained for breeding were vaccinated _____

    _____

11. Year in which vaccination ceased. 19_____   Write NA if not applicable _____

12. Average number of clinical cases of Johne's disease per year prior to vaccination _____ cases

13. Adult herd size at start of vaccination _____ _____

14. Number of clinical cases occurring in each year since vaccination started:

Years since start of vaccination	Number of clinical cases	Years since start of vaccination	Number of clinical cases
1		5	
2		6	
3		7	
4		8	

    If clinical cases occurred 9 years or more after start of vaccination please specify which year(s)

    _____

    _____

15. Have there been any major changes in breed since vaccination started? Please write YES or NO _____

    If 'YES', please specify change with approximate date from _____ to _____ in 19____

16. Have there been any changes in herd type since vaccination started? Please write YES or NO _____

    If 'YES', please specify change with approximate date from _____ to _____ in 19____

17. Have any attempts been made to identify latently infected animals? Please write YES or NO _____

    If 'YES', please specify diagnostic methods used: CFT ☐   Johnin ☐   Microsc. Exam ☐   Faeces Culture ☐

    and whether positive animals were called: Always ☐   Sometimes ☐   Never ☐

18. Please indicate which of the following control measures are practised on the farm:

    Please write YES or NO

    (a) prompt removal of confirmed clinical cases   _____

    (b) only 'bucket' rearing of calves (in dairy herds)   _____

    (c) adequate separation of calves from adults (in dairy herds)   _____

    (d) removal from herd of calves born of infected dams   _____

(e) adequate hygiene of food and water supplies to housed animals _____

(f) piped water supplies to all cattle at pasture _____

(g) prevention of access to ponds and ditches etc. _____

(h) calves grazed on pastures not used by adult cattle _____

19. Have any other changes in management been instituted to control the disease?

_____

_____

_____

20. Do you think the vaccine has had a valuable part to play in the control of Johne's disease in this herd. Please write YES or NO

_____

GENERAL COMMENTS

THANK YOU FOR YOUR CO-OPERATION IN THIS INVESTIGATION.

The completed questionnaire should be sent to:

J. W. Wilesmith, B.V.Sc., M.R.C.V.S.
Epidemiology Unit,
Central Veterinary Laboratory,
New Haw,
Weybridge,
Surrey KT14 3NB.

Fig. 13.2 A questionnaire: survey of Johne's disease in vaccinated cattle in Great Britain. (A questionnaire produced by John Wilesmith of the Central Veterinary Laboratory, UK, 1977.)

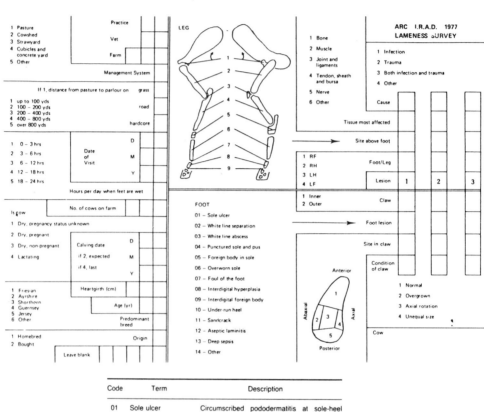

Code	Term	Description
01	Sole ulcer	Circumscribed pododermatitis at sole-heel junction, with or without protrusion of granulation tissue through horn defect
02	White line separation	Breakdown of integument of white line, usually abaxially, and impaction of foreign material into crack
03	White line abscess	Breakdown of integument of white line, usually abaxially, and occurrence of septic laminitis of wall
04	Punctured sole and pus	Traumatic penetration of solar horn with infection of laminae and pus production
05	Foreign body in sole	Self-explanatory
06	Overworn sole	Sole which is obviously flexible, horn usually not more than 3mm thick, often discoloured laminae due to haemorrhagic bruising
07	Foul of the foot	Interdigital necrosis affecting skin and, or, subcutaneous tissues
08	Interdigital hyperplasia	Thick interdigital skin fold, often with localised areas of pressure necrosis or ulceration as secondary feature
09	Interdigital foreign body	Self-explanatory
10	Underrun heel	Separation of heel horn axially towards sole-heel junction, usually with some exposure and infection of sensitive laminae; erosion of heel horn
11	Sandcrack	Vertical split in wall horn at coronet or lower down, involving sensitive tissues
12	Aseptic laminitis	Generalised digital pain and heat, often involving more than one foot, and without break in integument
13	Deep sepsis	Self-explanatory
14	Other	

Fig. 13.3 A questionnaire: survey of lameness in cattle in Great Britain. Respondents were requested to indicate which categories were appropriate to their farm and cattle. (From Russell *et al.*, 1982.)

2. the nature of the respondent population — a well-educated group should produce a higher response rate than a poorly educated group;
3. the subject and aim of the study — if the study is of obvious direct relevance and value to the respondent, then he is likely to reply;
4. appearance and length of the questionnaire — if it is attractive and concise, then response should be good;
5. confidentiality.

The results of questionnaires should be treated with caution when response rates are lower than about 70%, because there may be systematic differences between those who do, and those who do not, respond (response bias). For example, in a questionnaire survey of scrapie in the UK, the average sheep flock size was larger on farms whose owners responded than on those whose owners did not respond (Wooldridge *et al.*, 1992).

Interviews

A personal interview can overcome some of the disadvantages of mailed and self-completed questionnaires, and is particularly useful where illiteracy of the respondent is a problem. The tone of the interviewer's voice may, however, bias the respondent's answer, by implying a desirable answer (interviewer bias). Questionnaires can be longer than self-completed ones, and reponse rates of 90% can sometimes be achieved (Edwards, 1990). However, personal interviews can be costly to organize, involving training, payment and travelling expenses of interviewers.

Telephone interviews (Groves *et al.*, 1988) also generally have high response rates, and can produce results more quickly and cheaply than personal interviews and mailed questionnaires. However, questions need to be short to reduce conversation time to a minimum. Telephone interviews can be used to follow up non-responders in surveys that are initially based on mailed and self-completed questionnaires, in an attempt to reduce response bias.

The use of veterinary interviews is discussed by Ruppanner (1972) and, in developing countries, by Perry and McCauley (1984). Examples of their use include surveys of schistosomiasis in the Sudan (McCauley *et al.*, 1983b), swine fever in Honduras (McCauley, 1985), bovine health and productivity in Zambia (Perry *et al.*, 1984a) and sheep diseases in New Zealand (Simpson and Wright, 1980).

Testing questionnaires

Several drafts of a questionnaire are usually required following testing. There are normally two stages to testing: **informal** and **formal**.

Informal testing

Informal testing is carried out on colleagues, who can detect trivia, ambiguities and defects in questionnaire design.

Formal testing

Formal testing is undertaken on a small random sample of the population on which the full survey will be conducted. This testing is called a **pilot survey**. The pilot survey exposes further defects in questionnaire design. This survey should never be used as part of the full survey, and respondents used in the pilot survey should never be used again in the full one.

Criteria for success of questionnaires

The two main criteria for the success of a questionnaire are **reliability** and **validity** (Chapter 9).

Reliability

A questionnaire, like a diagnostic test, is reliable if it produces consistent results (see *Figure 9.6*). Reliability can be assessed by issuing the same questions to the same respondents more than once (e.g., Slater *et al.*, 1992; French *et al.*, 1992) and applying paired statistical tests (see Chapters 14 and 17) to the answers to each question. The type of test depends on the level of measurement and frequency distribution of the variables that are being studied (see *Tables 14.1* and *14.2*).

Validity

Validity is a measure of the degree to which answers, on average, reflect the truth (see *Figure 9.6*). Validity is therefore achieved by comparing the results of the questionnaire with an independent reliable criterion. For example, Selby *et al.* (1973, 1976) compared the results of a mailed questionnaire with information derived from farm records and diaries, when investigating congenital abnormalities in pigs; Perry *et al.* (1983), in a survey of several animal diseases in Zambia, compared the results obtained from an owner interview survey with those obtained from an investigation of sentinel herds; and the results of a telephone interview on diet and exercise in dogs were compared with subsequent written dietary records (Slater *et al.*, 1991). Sensitivity and specificity (see Chapters 9 and 17) can be calculated for questions with either a positive or negative ('yes'/'no') outcome; continuous and ordinal data require other techniques (Maclure and Willett, 1987).

Unreliability often means invalidity. However, reliable questions may not always be valid (see *Figure 9.6b*).

Further details of veterinary questionnaires can be found in Waltner-Toews (1983), Edwards (1990) and Vaillancourt *et al.* (1991).

Further reading

Atkinson, J. (1971) *Handbook for Interviewers*. Great Britain Office of Population Census and Surveys, Social Survey Division. Her Majesty's Stationery Office, London

Barnett, V. (1991) *Sample Survey Principles and Methods*. Edward Arnold, London

Bennett, A.E. and Ritchie, K. (1975) *Questionnaires in Medicine*. Published for the Nuffield Provincial Hospital Trust by the Oxford University Press, London

Casley, J.D. and Lury, D.A. (1981) *Data Collection in Developing Countries*. Clarendon Press, Oxford

Cochran, W.R. (1977) *Sampling Techniques*, 3rd edn. John Wiley, New York

Dillman, D.A. (1978) *Mail and Telephone Surveys: the Total Design Method*. John Wiley, New York

Farver, T.B. (1987) Disease prevalence estimation in animal populations using two-stage sampling designs. *Preventive Veterinary Medicine*, **5**, 1−20

Leech, F.B. and Sellers, K.C. (1979) *Statistical Epidemiology in Veterinary Science*. Charles Griffin, London and High Wycombe

Levy, P.S. and Lemeshow, S. (1991) *Sampling of Populations: Methods and Applications*. John Wiley, New York

Lwanga, S.K. and Lemeshow, S. (1991) *Sample Size Determination in Health Studies: A Practical Manual*. World Health Organization, Geneva

Moser, C.A. and Kalton, G. (1971) *Survey Methods in Social Investigation*, 2nd edn. Heinemann Educational Books, London

Yates, F. (1981) *Sampling Methods for Censuses and Surveys*, 4th edn. Charles Griffin, London and High Wycombe

Woods, A.J. (1985) Sampling in animal health surveys. In: Proceedings of a meeting held at the University of Reading, 27−29 March 1985. Ed. Thrusfield, M.V., pp. 36−54. Society for Veterinary Epidemiology and Preventive Medicine

14 Demonstrating association

A valuable step in the identification of the cause of a disease is the detection of a **statistically significant** association between the disease and hypothesized causal factors; this is the basis of the first three of Evans' postulates (see Chapter 3).

Some basic principles

Demonstration of association can be approached in three ways.

1. The difference, under two different circumstances, between the mean of the probability distribution of a set of values of a variable can be measured. If there is a significant difference between the means in the two circumstances, the different circumstances may lead to an explanation that reflects a causal association. For example, the weights of two groups of piglets, one group of which has developed neonatal diarrhoea and one group of which has not, can be measured. The effect of diarrhoea on weight can then be assessed by analysing the difference between the mean weights of the two groups. A similar approach can be adopted when comparing medians.
2. Variables can be categorized, and a significant association sought between various categories. For example, bitches can be categorized according to whether or not they have physiological urinary incontinence and whether or not they are neutered. Evidence of an association between the syndrome and neutering can then be sought.
3. A correlation between variables can be sought. For example, the incidence of lameness in cattle and the amount of rainfall can be recorded to investigate whether increased rainfall is significantly associated with an increased incidence of lameness.

Although approaches 1 and 2 are introduced in this chapter in the context of causal studies, they can be applied in any circumstance in which two groups are being **compared**.

Many of the statistical techniques that adopt these three approaches were developed for use in agricultural science. Their use is confined to epidemiological investigations in this book, but they also have a wide application to experimental and observational biological and social sciences, and therefore are described in most general statistics textbooks.

The principle of a significance test

The bell shape of the Normal distribution (see *Figure 12.1*) reveals that there is a probability, albeit a small one, of an observation occurring at the extreme tails of the distribution. This distribution may not only be used to describe the frequency distribution of the values of a continuous variable that has a Normal distribution but also of the means of repeated samples taken from that population (here termed the 'reference population'). This also includes means of parameters of other distributions, such as the binomial, when Normal approximations are applied. There is, therefore, a high probability of the mean of a sample being under the peak, and a much lower probability of this mean being close to either of the two tails. If the mean is close to a tail, this indicates either that the sample is one of those improbable samples taken from the reference population, or, more likely, that it has been drawn from a population with a different population mean.

It is necessary to decide when it is improbable that a sample mean has come from the reference population. This decision is taken when the probability, P, of obtaining a value for the sample mean at least as extreme as the one observed, **assuming that the sample is drawn from the reference population**, is less than a value corresponding to the **level of significance**. This level is represented by a probability called α (alpha). Conventionally, in biological sciences, α is taken to be 0.05, representing the 5% significance level. In the event of $P < 0.05$, the result is reported as 'significant $P < 0.05$' and supports the claim that the sample was not drawn from the reference population. The 5% significance level is purely conventional. If more caution in inferring a difference were necessary, the 1% level ($P < 0.01$) or 0.1% level ($P < 0.001$) could be chosen. Some reporting procedures use *, ** and *** to record significance at these 'critical' levels of 5%, 1% and 0.1%, respectively. This decision-making procedure is the principle of a significance test.

Significance tests were originally conducted in conjunction with tables that presented only a limited number of significance levels, including the critical ones, and this practice is still common. However, some contemporary applications software (see Chapter 11) calculates exact P values, and these should always be quoted, if available, in preference to the relevant critical levels.

The null hypothesis

In the previous discussion, a statistical test was undertaken on the basis that the sample came from a population with a mean no different to that of the reference population. This constitutes the **null hypothesis**; the null hypothesis is thus one of *no difference*. A significant result indicates that the null hypothesis is rejected in favour of an alternative one which states that the sample has been drawn from a population with characteristics that are different from the reference population. Demonstration of a significant difference implies rejection of the null hypothesis.

Notice that confidence intervals (see Chapter 12) and the outcomes of significance tests are closely related. For example, suppose that the null hypothesis states a particular value for the mean of a Normal distribution. A sample is taken and the significance test rejects the null hypothesis at the 5% level. The corresponding 95% confidence interval (sample mean $\pm$ 2 e.s.e.m.) then will **not** contain the value of the mean specified by the null hypothesis. Conversely, if the significance test does not reject the null hypothesis at the 5% level, the corresponding 95% confidence interval will contain the value of the mean specified by the null hypothesis.

Errors of inference

Five per cent of samples from the reference population lie within the region that would lead to rejection of the null hypothesis at the 5% level. If this happens it constitutes a rejection of the null hypothesis when the hypothesis is true. This error is an example of a **Type I error**: false rejection of a true null hypothesis. The probability of a Type I error is just the level of significance discussed above.

A **Type II error** is a failure to reject the null hypothesis when it is untrue. The probability of committing this error is called β (beta). Ideally, both α and β should be known by the investigator before the study begins.

Depending on the alternative hypothesis, β may or may not be determinable. In the previous discussion, if the alternative hypothesis specified the mean of the population from which the sample was drawn, then β could be determined for a stated value of α and sample size. However, if the alternative hypothesis only hypothesized that the mean of the population from which the sample was drawn took one of several values, then β cannot be calculated. It is known that β can be kept small by increasing either α or the sample size. The probabilities of Type I and II errors decrease as sample size increases. For a fixed sample size, the larger the probability of a Type I error is chosen to be, the smaller the probability of a Type II error will be, and vice versa.

Two remaining alternative decisions are possible. These represent correct inferences, rather than errors. The first inference is not rejecting the null hypothesis when it is true. The second is rejecting the null hypothesis when it is false (i.e., demonstrating a significant difference). The probability of the latter is called the **power** of a test; it is denoted by $1 - \beta$.

One- and two-tailed tests

The previous discussion has been concerned with demonstrating any differences between a sample and a reference population, irrespective of the 'direction' of the difference; that is, whether the sample differs because it comes from a distribution with a mean to the left or right of the mean of the reference population. In this case, the investigator is concerned with significant departures towards either of the two tails of the distribution. A test that considers these departures is therefore called a **two-tailed** test.

Sometimes, an investigator may be reasonably certain that significant departures only occur in one direction. An example would be investigating whether diarrhoea depressed weight gain in piglets, rather than either depressed or increased it (the latter is very unlikely). This investigation requires a **one-tailed** test. The 5% significance level in a two-tailed test represents approximately 2 standard errors to either side of the mean. If the same criterion of approximately 2 standard errors were used in a one-tailed test, then the actual significance level would only be 2.5% (corresponding to the tail with which the investigator is concerned). Therefore, rejection of the null hypothesis at the 5% level in a one-tailed test requires a deviation corresponding to that required for rejection at the 10% level in a two-tailed test.

Significance tests involving other distributions, and conducted on large samples for which Normal approximations to these distributions are valid, often compute values of the standardized Normal deviate, z (see Chapter 12). These are then compared with tabulated values using values of mean and variance specified by the null hypothesis (Appendix XII). Some examples are given later.

Independent and related samples

Groups (samples) that are compared may be **independent** or **related**, and different statistical techniques are required for these two circumstances. Independent samples require **unpaired** tests; related samples require **paired** tests.

Samples are related when:

1. comparisons are made between repeated measurements on the same individuals;
2. they are matched for other variables.

An example of the first situation is the measuring of the weights of individual calves one week, and then a week later. Similarly, the completion of a questionnaire twice by the same respondents constitutes related samples.

Matching is a feature of some observational studies (see Chapter 15) and clinical trials (see Chapter 16).

Pairing can have the benefit of removing a source of variation, therefore providing a more sensitive test than its unpaired counterpart.

Parametric and non-parametric techniques

Parametric tests

Some tests are **parametric** because they are concerned with the mean, which is one of the parameters of the Normal distribution. Parametric techniques make the following assumptions of the data that are to be analysed:

1. the distribution is Normal;
2. the variables are measured on the interval or ratio scale, that is, they are continuous (see Chapter 9);*

additionally:

3. some tests require that the two populations being compared have equal variances; if this is not the case then these tests must be modified.

Table 14.1 lists some commonly used parametric techniques that test hypotheses relating to the mean. This chapter focuses on comparing two populations (i.e., two-sample methods) and correlation.

Non-parametric tests

If the assumptions of a parametric test cannot be met then **non-parametric** techniques should be used. These can be applied to nominal and ordinal data, as well as interval and ratio data. Most of these tests are distribution-free, that is, they do not require assumptions such as the underlying distribution being Normal, but they do assume symmetry.

Table 14.2 lists some commonly used non-parametric techniques. These are described fully by Siegel and Castellan (1988).

Parametric tests are more powerful than non-parametric tests if the distributional assumptions hold; that is, the former require a smaller sample size than the latter to detect a significant difference of a given size. Moreover, parametric tests are more robust to deviations from Normality than are non-parametric tests to deviations from symmetry.

Hypothesis testing versus estimation

Comparisons have traditionally been made by **testing** the null hypothesis using an appropriate significance test. However, such tests do not indicate the *magnitude* of the difference between groups that are being compared, with defined *precision*, and it is the magnitude that may be of interest (e.g., when assessing the prophylactic or therapeutic impact of a compound in a clinical trial). An alternative approach, which **estimates** the difference with defined precision, therefore conveys more information, and is frequently preferred (Gardner and Altman, 1989). This involves calculating confidence intervals for the

---

*Although visual analogue measurements are subjective, they can be treated as continuous data for the purpose of analysis.

Table 14.1 Summary of some parametric statistical techniques for testing hypotheses relating to means of Normally distributed data.

Level of measurement	Variance	One-sample case	Parametric statistical test				Parametric measure of association
			Two-sample case		Case with three or more samples		
			Related samples	Independent samples	Related samples	Independent samples	
Interval and ratio	Known	Normal test	Normal test	Normal test			Correlation coefficient, $\rho*$
Interval and ratio	Unknown	t-test	t-test	t-test* (equal variance)	F-test (equal variance)	F-test (equal variance)	Correlation coefficient, $\rho*$
				Welch t-test* (unequal variances)	Welch F-test (unequal variances)	Welch F-test (unequal variances)	

*Indicates a technique that is exemplified in this book.

parameters that are being considered. Both approaches are outlined in this chapter.

Sample size determination

The importance of determining appropriate sample sizes before undertaking an investigation was introduced in relation to surveys (Chapter 13). It is also desirable to determine sample sizes before two groups are compared. This ensures that results will be obtained according to specified parameters. These are:

1. the acceptable level of Type I error, α (the probability of inferring a difference between the groups when one does not exist);
2. test power, $1 - \beta$ (the probability of correctly inferring a difference);
3. the magnitude of the difference to be detected (i.e., the difference between means, medians or proportions);
4. the choice of alternative hypothesis: one-tailed or two-tailed;

and, additionally, for ordinal, interval and ratio response variables:

5. the variability of the response variable between the two groups.

Conventionally, α is set at 0.05 and β at 0.20 (power = 0.80), but these values may be different, depending on inferential requirements (see, for example, Chapter 16).

Unless there is strong evidence that a one-tailed test is justifiable, it is prudent to estimate sample sizes for two-tailed conditions because the latter require a larger sample size than the former for a specified value of α, power and magnitude of the difference to be detected.

Statistical versus clinical (biological) significance

Statistical significance tests give an indication of the probability that observed differences between groups are due to chance. **Clinical (biological)** significance, however, concerns the relevance of findings to clinical veterinary practice. Because statistical significance is partly dependent on sample size, it is possible that small and clinically unimportant differences may become statistically significant. It is also possible that clinically important results may be overlooked because a study's sample size is too small to allow sound conclusions to be drawn. For example, in a clinical study to compare the effect of diet on bilirubin levels in two groups of dogs, the sample sizes may be large enough to indicate statistical significance when the difference in means between the two groups is 2 μmol/l. However, an investigator may judge a 2 μmol/l change in means to be of no clinical relevance. In contrast, if the investigator considers a 1 μmol/l change in means to be important to health, the sample sizes may not be large enough to conclude that the difference is significant. In this case, there is a serious

Table 14.2 Summary of some non-parametric statistical techniques.

Level of measurement	One-sample case	Non-parametric statistical test — Two-sample case: Related/matched samples	Non-parametric statistical test — Two-sample case: Independent samples	Case with three or more samples: Related samples	Case with three or more samples: Independent samples	Non-parametric measure of correlation
Nominal	Binomial test χ^2 goodness-of-fit test	McNemar change test	Fisher exact test for 2×2 contingency tables* χ^2 test for: 2×2 contingency tables* $r \times 2$ contingency tables	Cochran Q test*	χ^2 test for $r \times k$ tables	Cramer coefficient, C Phi coefficient, r_ϕ The kappa coefficient of agreement, K* Asymmetrical association, the lambda statistic, L_B
Ordinal	Kolmogorov–Smirnov one-sample test, $D_{m,n}$ One-sample runs test Change-point test	Sign test Wilcoxon signed ranks test, T^+*	Median test Wilcoxon–Mann–Whitney test, W_x^* Robust rank-order test, U Kolmogorov–Smirnov two-sample test, $D_{m,n}$ Siegel–Tukey test for scale differences	Friedman two-way analysis of variance by ranks, F_r Page test for ordered alternatives, L	Extension of the median test Kruskal–Wallis one-way analysis of variance, KW Jonckheere test for ordered alternatives, J	Spearman rank-order correlation coefficient, r_s Kendall rank-order correlation coefficient, T Kendall partial rank-order correlation coefficient, $T_{xy.z}$ Kendall coefficient of concordance, W Kendall coefficient of agreement, U Correlation between k judges and a criterion, T_c
Interval and ratio	Test for distributional symmetry	Permutation test for paired replicates	Permutation test for two independent samples Moses rank-like test for scale differences			Gamma statistic, G Somers' index of asymmetric association, d_{BA}

Each column lists, cumulatively downwards, the tests applicable for the given level of measurement. For example, in the case of three or more related samples, when the variables are measured on the ordinal scale, both the Friedman two-way analysis of variance and the Cochran Q test are applicable.

*Indicates a technique that is exemplified in this book.

(Reprinted, with modifications, from Siegel, S. and Castellan, N.J., *Nonparametric Statistics for the Behavioral Sciences*, 2nd edn. Copyright © 1988 McGraw-Hill Inc., New York)

risk of failing to recognize a genuine dietary effect. This is why the sample sizes for prospective studies should be justified (Lipsey, 1990).

Interval and ratio data: comparing means

Hypothesis testing

Independent samples: Student's t-test

Student's *t*-test is a parametric significance test, commonly used for small samples. This involves calculation of a test statistic called t, which measures departures from the mean that is specified by the null hypothesis. The distribution of this test statistic follows a t-distribution (illustrated in *Figure 12.4*) — hence the name of the test.

Student's t-test can be applied to samples from different populations and an hypothesis that the data come from Normal distributions with a known difference $\mu_1 - \mu_2 = \delta$ (delta) between the two population means, μ_1 and μ_2, and common unknown variance, s^2. If n_1, $\bar{x}_1$, s_1^2 are the sample size, sample mean and sample variance from the first population, and n_2, $\bar{x}_2$, s_2^2 are similar statistics from the second population, then the estimate of the common unknown variance, σ^2, is:

$$s^2 = \{(n_1 - 1)s_1^2 + (n_2 - 1)s_2^2\}/(n_1 + n_2 - 2).$$

The test statistic, t, is:

$$t = (\bar{x}_1 - \bar{x}_2 - \delta)/\sqrt{\{s^2(1/n_1 + 1/n_2)\}}$$

and there are $n_1 + n_2 - 2$ degrees of freedom (see Chapter 12). (In this two-sample case, with sample sizes of n_1 and n_2, two means are evaluated. There are thus $n_1 + n_2 - 2$ 'pieces' of information for calculation of the variance.)

This test is exemplified using the data in *Table 12.1*:

$n_1 = 49$; $\bar{x}_1 = 5.76$ kg; $s_1 = 0.60$ kg;
$n_2 = 49$; $\bar{x}_2 = 4.69$ kg; $s_2 = 0.67$ kg.

The hypothesis to be tested is that there is no difference in three-week weaning weights between the two groups of piglets; that is, $\delta = 0$.

$$\begin{aligned} s^2 &= \{(48 \times 0.60^2) + (48 \times 0.67^2)\}/96 \\ &= (17.280 + 21.547)/96 \\ &= 0.404. \end{aligned}$$

$$\begin{aligned} t &= (5.76 - 4.69 - 0)/\sqrt{\{0.404(1/49 + 1/49)\}} \\ &= 1.07/\sqrt{0.0165} \\ &= 8.33. \end{aligned}$$

There are 96 degrees of freedom $(49 + 49 - 2)$. Appendix IV is consulted. It does not have a row corresponding to 96 degrees of freedom, and so the row with the greatest number of degrees of freedom less than 96 is chosen (60 in this instance). This is a conservative procedure. The 0.1% value for 60 degrees of freedom is 3.460. This is considerably less than 8.33. Therefore, in this example, the two groups (A and B) of piglets have mean values that differ significantly at the 0.1% level. This is a two-tailed test, for which Appendix IV is directly applicable. If a one-tailed test is being conducted, the probability should be halved (the probability of a figure falling outside a certain value of t at one end only of a distribution is only half as great as the probability of it falling at either end).

Often, when sample sizes are large, the e.s.e.m. is regarded as the true s.e.m. and the t-test is conducted with degrees of freedom corresponding to infinity (∞). The test then becomes a **two-sample z-test**.

If the variances of the two samples are not equal, the test is modified as the **Welch *t*-test**, an example of which is presented in Chapter 17.

Related samples: Student's t-test

Student's t-test can also be applied to comparisons in which the observations between the two samples are related. The test assumes the difference between the members of each pair is Normally distributed with mean δ (usually zero) and an unknown variance, σ^2. If $\bar{d}$ and s^2 are the sample mean and variance of the **differences**, respectively, then the test statistic is:

$$t = (\bar{d} - \delta)/\sqrt{s^2/n}$$

where n is the sample size. There are $(n - 1)$ degrees of freedom.

Calculation of confidence intervals

Independent samples

Confidence intervals can be calculated for the difference $\mu_1 - \mu_2$ between the true population means for independent samples. The t-distribution is again used if the data have an approximately Normal distribution.

First, an estimate of the common standard deviation, s, is calculated:

$$s = \sqrt{\frac{(n_1 - 1)s_1^2 + (n_2 - 1)s_2^2}{n_1 + n_2 - 2}}$$

using the notation of Student's t-test.

The standard error of the difference between the two sample means, SE_{diff}, is then:

$$SE_{diff} = s\sqrt{1/n_1 + 1/n_2}.$$

Using the data in *Table 12* ':

$$s = \sqrt{\frac{(49 - 1)0.60^2 + (49 - 1)0.67^2}{49 + 49 - 2}}$$

$$= \sqrt{0.404},$$

$$= 0.636.$$

Therefore:

$$SE_{diff} = 0.636\sqrt{1/49 + 1/49},$$

$$= 0.128.$$

A 95% confidence interval is calculated thus:

$$\bar{x}_1 - \bar{x}_2 \pm (t_{\nu(0.95)} \times SE_{diff}),$$

where $t_{\nu(0.95)}$ is the 95% point of the t-distribution with ν (nu) degrees of freedom. This may be alternatively expressed as $t_{\nu(1-\alpha)}$, where α is the level of significance.

Consulting Appendix IV, there are 96 degrees of freedom, and 60 is again chosen conservatively; $t_{\nu(0.95)}$ is located in the column headed '0.05' ($\alpha = 0.05$); this is 2.000 for 60 degrees of freedom.

$$\bar{x}_1 = 5.76$$
$$\bar{x}_2 = 4.69.$$

The 95% confidence interval is therefore:

$$(5.76 - 4.69) \pm (2.000 \times 0.128)$$

$$= 1.07 \pm 0.256$$
$$= 0.81, 1.33.$$

If the 95% confidence interval includes zero, the two means are not significantly different at the 5% level. In this example, the confidence interval **excludes** zero, and so a significant difference can be inferred at the 5% level. This result is consistent with the results of Student's t-test which indicated a significant difference at the 1% (and therefore 5%) level.

Ninety per cent, 99% and 99.9% confidence intervals (corresponding to respective values of α of 0.10, 0.01 and 0.001) can be calculated utilizing values of t_ν of 1.671, 2.660 and 3.460, respectively.

Note that the confidence interval conveys more information than the result of the t-test. It gives an indication of the **precision** of the **magnitude** of the difference between the two means of the populations from which the samples were selected.

This method is not appropriate when the standard deviations of the two samples differ considerably; more complex methods must then be used (Armitage and Berry, 1987).

Related samples

Confidence intervals for related samples are calculated in the same way as those for a single sample (see Chapter 12), but $\bar{x}$ and s are now the mean and standard deviation of the individual **differences** between the first and second samples (Gardner and Altman, 1989).

What sample size should be selected?

The approximate sample size required to detect the difference between the true means of two populations, using a two-tailed test at significance level α, can be determined thus:

$$n = 2\left\{\frac{\sigma(M_{\alpha/2} + M_\beta)}{\mu_1 - \mu_2}\right\}^2$$

where:

n = sample size for each population;
μ_1 = true mean in population 1;
μ_2 = true mean in population 2;
σ = common standard deviation of the two populations;
$M_{\alpha/2}$ = multiplier associated with the required significance level, α;
M_β = multiplier associated with β, the probability of a Type II error.

For example, suppose that an investigator wishes to identify a difference in the mean day at which bacon pigs reach slaughter weight under two different systems of management, and that this difference is specified as a change of five days (i.e., the alternative hypothesis is two-tailed). An estimate of the mean day under the first system of management is required: say, day 160. Next, an estimate of the standard deviation is required. Previous production data indicates that this is approximately seven days, and so this value is used as an estimate of the common standard deviation, σ. These estimates are then applied to the formula.

The two multipliers, $M_{\alpha/2}$ and M_β, are obtained from Appendix XII. If the level of significance is set at 5%, α

= 0.05. The value of z corresponding to $P = 0.025$ is 1.96; this is therefore chosen as the multiplier, $M_{\alpha/2}$. If the investigator wishes to be 80% confident of detecting this difference, test power $(1 - \beta) = 0.80$, and $\beta = 0.20$.* Consulting the appendix again, the value of z corresponding to a probability of 0.20 is 0.84, and this is used as the multiplier M_{β}.

Therefore:

$$n = 2\{7(1.96 + 0.84)/(160 - 165)\}^2$$
$$= 2(7 \times 2.80/-5)^2$$
$$= 2 \times 15.37$$
$$= 30.7.$$

Under the given error criteria, 62 pigs are therefore required: 31 under each system of management.

If one specific group were expected to have an *increase* over the other of five days in the mean day to slaughter, the alternative hypothesis would be one-tailed. The multiplier $M_{\alpha/2}$ should then be replaced by M_{α} in the appropriate formula. Thus, from the same appendix, $z = 1.64$ and $M_{\alpha} = 1.64$. This would require 50 pigs: 25 under each system of management. This exemplifies that two-tailed tests require a **larger** sample size than their one-tailed counterparts.

Note that, in addition to the nature of the alternative hypothesis, the sample size is determined by the *difference* between the two means, not their absolute values: the smaller the difference to be detected, the larger the required sample size. Additionally, a large common standard deviation (indicating considerable variability within the two groups) results in a large sample size.

This formula will slightly underestimate sample sizes for independent samples, and overestimate sample sizes for related samples.

Ordinal data: comparing medians

Hypothesis testing

Independent samples: the Wilcoxon – Mann – Whitney test

The **Wilcoxon – Mann – Whitney test** is used to compare two independent groups when at least ordinal

measurement has been achieved for the study variables. It is also an appropriate test for interval and ratio data that are not Normally distributed.

Table 14.3a lists the summer body condition scores from samples of two groups of ponies on Assateague Island off the coast of Maryland, US. One group lives on the north of the island, and the other group lives on the south. The medians of the two samples are 2.5 and 3.5, respectively. The question posed is: 'Do the body condition scores of north-end and south-end ponies differ significantly?' (i.e., the test is two-tailed). Body condition score is an ordinal measurement, and the two groups of ponies are independent; therefore the Wilcoxon – Mann – Whitney test is appropriate.

The test is based on **ranking** of the scores, and tests the null hypothesis that the median values of each group are the same, the alternative hypothesis being that either (1) the median of one group is greater than the other, or vice versa (a two-tailed test), or (2) the median of **one** specified group is greater than the other (a one-tailed test).

First, the smaller group, X, of size m, is selected. If both groups are of equal size, as in this example, then either can be chosen (say, the north-end ponies). The value of the statistic used in the test, W_x, is the sum of the ranks in this group.

The scores in group X and the other group, Y, of size n (south-end ponies), are then ranked in order of increasing size, retaining their identity. Scores are relatively crude measures, usually with a limited range, and so samples may include two or more individuals with the same scores. Identical scores constitute **ties**. The rank given to such ties is the average of the tied ranks which would have been assigned if the scores had differed slightly. For example, if three individuals are given the lowest score, then they are each assigned the rank of 2, that is, $(1+2+3)/3$. The next score would then be ranked 4. If the lowest score was shared by two individuals they would each be ranked 1.5 $([1+2]/2)$ and the next score would be ranked 3.

The scores and ranks of the ponies are therefore:

Score:	1	2	2.5	2.5	3	3	3.5	3.5	4	4
Group:	X	Y	X	X	X	Y	Y	Y	X	Y
Rank:	1	2	3.5	3.5	5.5	5.5	7.5	7.5	9.5	9.5

The sum of the ranks is then calculated for the first group:

$$W_x = 1 + 3.5 + 3.5 + 5.5 + 9.5 = 23;$$

and similarly for the second group:

$$W_y = 2 + 5.5 + 7.5 + 7.5 + 9.5 = 32.$$

---

*Recall that β is conventionally set at four times the value of α.

The total sample size, $N = m + n = 10$.

If there were no difference between the two groups, then the average ranks of each group would be about the same. However, if there were a difference then the

Table 14.3 Summer body condition scores of feral ponies on the northern and southern parts of Assateague Island, 1988: (a) scores for six ponies; (b) scores and ranks for 44 ponies. (From Rudman and Keiper, 1991; raw data supplied by the authors.)

(a)

North-end ponies	South-end ponies
Score	Score
1	2
2.5	3.5
3	4
2.5	3.5
4	3

(b)

North-end ponies		South-end ponies	
Score	Rank	Score	Rank
3	35	4	44
3	35	3	35
2.5	22	3	35
2.5	22	3.5	43
1	2.5	1	2.5
2.5	22	3	35
2	11	1	2.5
2	11	3	35
2	11	3	35
2.5	22	3	35
2.5	22	2.5	22
2	11	2	11
2	11	3	35
2	11	2	11
2.5	22	3	35
2	11	3	35
1.5	5	1	2.5
3	35	3	35
2	11	3	35
3	35	2.5	22
		2.5	22
		2	11
		2.5	22
		2.5	22
Total $W_x = 367.5$		$W_y = 622.5$	

average ranks would not be the same. In this example, the average rank of group X is $23/5 = 4.6$, and the average rank of group Y is $32/5 = 6.4$, and so there is reason to suspect a difference.

The sampling distribution of W_x under the null hypothesis is given in Appendix XIII. This is used to determine the significance of the result, using the values W_x, m and n. The lower limit is used for observations at the lower end of the distribution. The table appropriate to the values $m = 5$ and $n = 5$ is selected, and the probability of observing a value of $W_x < 23$ when the null hypothesis is true is located by finding the entry to the right of the lower critical limit, c_L with a value equal to W_x (i.e., 23). This (one-tailed) probability is 0.2103. Thus, in a two-tailed test (as in this example) the probability is doubled (0.420); this is considerably greater than 0.05 and so the result is not significant at the 5% level.

If W_y is chosen to determine the significance of the results, the upper limit is used for observations at the upper end of the distribution. Thus, the probability of observing a value of $W_y > 32$ is similarly 0.2103, and the same conclusion is reached.

Large samples: Appendix XIII can only be used when m and n are less than 11 ($n < 13$ if $m = 3$ or 4). For larger values of m and n, however, the sampling distribution of W_x is approximately Normal. It is therefore possible to use Appendix XII to assess the significance of any observed differences between large samples.

A value of the standardized Normal deviate, z, can be calculated using the formula:

$$z = \frac{W_x + 0.5 - m(N + 1)/2}{\sqrt{mn(N + 1)/12}}$$

using the same notation as above.

The value 0.5 is added when looking at the lower end of the distribution, and subtracted when considering the upper end.

Table 14.3b lists a larger number of records of scores of ponies on Assateague Island than *Table 14.3a*. The median score values for north-end and south-end ponies are 2.5 and 3.0, respectively, and the significance of this sample difference can again be assessed. The total number is too great to be accommodated by Appendix XIII and so Appendix XII should be used. There are also ties which are accommodated by the ranking given in the table.

The average of the ranks for the north-end ponies is $367.5/20 = 18.4$, whereas the average for the south-end ponies is 25.9, also suggesting that the latter are in better condition in the summer than the former.

$W_x = 367.5,$
m (north-end ponies) $= 20,$
n (south-end ponies) $= 24,$
$N = m + n = 44.$

These values are substituted into the formula, adding the value 0.5 (because W_x is associated with the average rank of the smaller group, hence the lower end of the distribution is being considered), and the alternative hypothesis is again two-tailed:

$$z = \frac{367.5 + 0.5 - 20(44 + 1)/2}{\sqrt{20 \times 24(44 + 1)/12}},$$

$$= \frac{367.5 + 0.5 - 450}{\sqrt{1800}},$$

$$= -1.93.$$

The calculated value of z is negative, corresponding to the lower tail of the Normal distribution. Appendix XII tabulates only the upper tail, and so the sign is ignored. The value 1.93 corresponds to a one-tailed P value of 0.0268 (a two-tailed P value of 0.0536), and indicates that the observed condition scores between the two groups are not significantly different at the 5% level ($P > 0.05$). Note, however, the prudence of quoting the P value in view of it being so close to the 5% significance level.

Related samples: the Wilcoxon signed ranks test

Related samples can be compared using the **Wilcoxon signed ranks test**. This tests a similar hypothesis to its unpaired analogue, described above.

Table 14.4a lists the body condition scores of a group of seven sheep recorded in the summer and then again in the winter. These therefore constitute related samples. The median summer and winter scores are 4.0 and 3.5, respectively. It is reasonable to assume that scores are likely to be higher in the summer than the winter — not vice versa — and so the alternative hypothesis is one-tailed. To perform a Wilcoxon signed ranks test to assess the significance of these sample differences, the *differences* between the paired observations are determined; then the differences are ranked, without reference to sign. If there is no difference between a pair, that is, there is a tie with the value zero (e.g., sheep number 5 in *Table 14.4a*), the pair is excluded from further analysis. Ties not taking the value zero are ranked in the same way as in the Wilcoxon−Mann−Whitney test. The sign (+ or −) which the difference represents is then attached to each

rank. Next, the sum of the positive ranks, T^+, is calculated. The ranking of the differences in the sheep body condition scores is listed in *Table 14.4a*, and:

$$T^+ = 5.5 + 2 + 4 + 2 + 5.5$$
$$= 19.$$

Appendix XIV is then consulted. This gives the corresponding one-tailed significance levels for T^+ and the sample size, N, for pairs with non-zero differences. In this example, $N = 6$ and $T^+ = 19$. The table entry for this combination is 0.0469. This is less than 0.05, indicating that there is a significant difference between median summer and winter condition scores. (If the alternative hypothesis were two-tailed, the significance level would be 0.094, and the difference would not be significant at the 5% level.)

Large samples: Appendix XIV cannot be used when N is larger than 15, but the sampling distribution of T^+ is then approximately Normally distributed, and:

$$z = \frac{T^+ - N(N + 1)/4}{\sqrt{N(N + 1)(2N + 1)/24}}.$$

Table 14.4b lists the winter and summer condition scores for 25 sheep, with medians of 3.0 and 4.0, respectively. Sheep 5, 14 and 18 have no difference in winter and summer scores and so are not considered further; thus, $N = 22$ and $T^+ = 212.0$. Thus:

$$z = \frac{212.0 - 22(22 + 1)/4}{\sqrt{22(22 + 1)(2 \times 22 + 1)/24}}$$

$$= \frac{85.5}{\sqrt{948.75}}$$

$$= 2.78.$$

Appendix XII is consulted, and the alternative hypothesis is again one-tailed. The probability of obtaining a value of 2.78 if the null hypothesis were true is 0.0027. Thus, a significant difference between the summer and winter median condition scores can be inferred.

Calculation of confidence intervals

Confidence intervals for the difference between two medians can be calculated on the assumption that the two samples have frequency distributions that are identical in shape, but differ in location.

Table 14.4 Winter and summer body condition scores of sheep: (a) scores and ranks for seven sheep; (b) scores and ranks for 25 sheep. (Hypothetical data.)

(a)

Sheep no.	Winter score	Summer score	Difference in scores (summer − winter)	Rank of difference
1	3.5	5	1.5	5.5
2	3.5	4	0.5	2
3	3	4	1	4
4	3.5	4	0.5	2
5	3.5	3.5	0	—
6	3.5	3	−0.5	−2
7	3.5	5	1.5	5.5

(b)

Sheep no.	Winter score	Summer score	Difference in scores (summer − winter)	Rank of difference
1	4.5	3	−1.5	−19
2	4	3.5	−0.5	−6.5
3	2.5	3.5	1	15
4	3	3.5	0.5	6.5
5	3	3	0	—
6	3	3.5	−0.5	−6.5
7	5	4	−1	−15
8	4.5	5	0.5	6.5
9	2	2.5	0.5	6.5
10	4.5	5	0.5	6.5
11	2	3.5	1.5	19
12	2.5	3	0.5	6.5
13	4	4.5	0.5	6.5
14	4	4	0	—
15	2.5	3.5	1	15
16	3	3.5	0.5	6.5
17	2	4.5	2.5	22
18	2.5	2.5	0	—
19	3.5	4.5	2	21
20	4	4.5	0.5	6.5
21	3.5	4.5	1	15
22	2.5	4.5	2	21
23	4	4.5	0.5	6.5
24	3	4.5	1.5	19
25	3.5	4	0.5	6.5
			$T^+ = 212.0$	

Table 14.5 Differences in condition scores of two groups of ponies. (Data from *Table 14.3a*.)

South-end ponies	North-end ponies				
	1	2.5	2.5	3	4
2	−1	0.5	0.5	1	2
3	−2	−0.5	−0.5	0	1
3.5	−2.5	−1	−1	−0.5	0.5
4	−3	−1.5	−1.5	−1	0

Independent samples

If there are n_1 and n_2 observations in the two respective samples, the difference between the two medians is first estimated as the median of all possible $n_1 \times n_2$ differences. The differences for the data in *Table 14.3a* are given in *Table 14.5*. The differences are then sorted:

$$-3 \quad -2.5 \quad -2.5 \quad -2 \quad -1.5 \quad -1.5 \quad -1 \quad -1 \quad -1$$
$$-1 \quad -1 \quad -1 \quad -0.5 \quad -0.5 \quad -0.5 \quad -0.5 \quad 0 \quad 0$$
$$0.5 \quad 0.5 \quad 0.5 \quad 0.5 \quad 1 \quad 1 \quad 2.$$

The point estimate of the difference between two medians is thus -0.5.

A parameter, K, based on the Wilcoxon−Mann−Whitney test statistic, is then calculated (Gardner and Altman, 1989). This is tabulated for 95% confidence limits in Appendix XV for sample sizes between 5 and 25. The value of K for appropriate values of $n_1 = 5$ (north-end ponies) and $n_2 = 5$ (south-end ponies) is identified; this is 3. The approximate 95% limits are then the **3rd** smallest and **3rd** largest difference: -2.5 and 1, respectively. The 95% confidence interval therefore contains the value zero, and so a significant difference between condition scores cannot be inferred at the 5% level. This is in accord with the result of the Wilcoxon−Mann−Whitney test.

Gardner and Altman (1989) give appropriate values of K for determining 90% and 99% confidence intervals.

Large samples: When each sample size is greater than 25, an approximate value of K for a 95% confidence interval, based on the Normal-approximation multiplier, is:

$$K = \frac{n_1 n_2}{2} - \left\{ 1.96 \times \sqrt{\frac{n_1 n_2 (n_1 + n_2 + 1)}{12}} \right\}$$

rounding K up to the nearest integer.

Related samples

Confidence intervals for related samples are calculated in a similar way to those for unrelated samples. If there are n differences for all matched pairs, the averages of all possible differences are calculated, including each difference with itself. For example, in *Table 14.4b*, the average of the difference of sheep number 1 with itself is $(-1.5 - 1.5)/2 = -1.5$; the average of the difference of sheep number 1 with sheep number 2 is $(-1.5 - 0.5)/2 = -1$; and so on:

	Change			
Change	−1.5	−0.5	1	0.5
−1.5	−1.5	−1	−0.25	−0.5
−0.5		−0.5	0.25	0
1			1	0.75
0.5				0.5

These differences are again sorted, and the point estimate of the median identified. A parameter, K^*, based on the Wilcoxon signed ranks test statistic, is then calculated (Gardner and Altman, 1989). This is tabulated in Appendix XVI for 95% confidence limits for sample sizes, n, between 6 and 50. The value of K^* is applied to the sorted differences in the same way as K, previously. Gardner and Altman (1989) give appropriate values of K^* for determining 90% and 99% confidence intervals.

Large samples: When each sample size is greater than 50, an approximate value of K^* for a 95% confidence interval is:

$$K^* = \frac{n(n+1)}{4} - \left\{ 1.96 \sqrt{\frac{n(n+1)(2n+1)}{24}} \right\}$$

rounding K^* up to the nearest integer.

This method can also be used to determine a confidence interval for the median of a single sample, if the population distribution around the median is symmetric; otherwise, alternative methods should be used (Gardner and Altman, 1989).

What sample size should be selected?

Determination of sample sizes to detect a specified difference between two medians is complex (Khmaladze, 1975). An appropriate formula for a two-tailed test can be derived for independent samples:

$$\sqrt{T} = \sigma(M_{\alpha/2} + M_\beta)/u,$$

where:

T = total sample size ($T = 2t$, where t is the common sample size for each population);

u = prespecified difference between the two medians;

$M_{\alpha/2}$ = multiplier associated with the required significance level, α;

M_{β} = muliplier associated with β, the probability of a Type II error;

σ^2 = large-sample ($m > 10$ or $n > 10$) variance of the Wilcoxon−Mann−Whitney test statistic,

$$= \frac{mn(N + 1)}{12}$$

using the notation of the Wilcoxon−Mann−Whitney test. The values of m, n and N need to be obtained from previous studies.

For example, suppose an investigator wishes to detect a difference of 1 in the median condition scores of the two groups of ponies on the north and south ends of Assateague Island (i.e., the hypothesis is two-tailed); and $\alpha = 0.05$ and $\beta = 0.20$. First, a value of σ^2 is required, and this is known from the data in *Table 14.3b*:

$m = 20,$
$n = 24,$
$N = 44.$

Thus:

$$\sigma^2 = \frac{20 \times 24(44 + 1)}{12}$$

$$= 1800,$$

and:

$$\sigma = 42.3.$$

The value of u is specified as 1.
From Appendix XII:

$M_{\alpha/2} = 1.96,$
$M_{\beta} = 0.84.$

Thus:

$\sqrt{T} = 42.3(1.96 + 0.84)/1$
$= (42.3 \times 2.8)/1,$
$= 118.44.$

Therefore:

$T = 14\,028.$

Thus, approximately 7000 ponies are required in each group. Note the very large and probably unrealistic sample size required in order to have the sensitivity to

detect such a small difference between the median scores of the two groups. This illustrates that detection of small differences is generally impracticable when the variance is large.

If the hypothesis is one-tailed, $M_{\alpha/2}$ is again replaced by M_{α}.

The formula can be applied to related samples by replacing the large-sample variance of the Wilcoxon−Mann−Whitney statistic by the large-sample ($N > 15$) variance of the sum of the ranks computed in the Wilcoxon signed ranks test:

$$\frac{N(N + 1)(2N + 1)}{24}$$

using the notation of the signed ranks test. A value of N again is obtained from previous data.

Nominal data: comparing proportions

Counts of nominal data are the basis of comparison of proportions and are commonly encountered in observational studies. Some general methods are outlined in this chapter. Additional techniques, particularly relevant to observational studies, are described in the next chapter.

Hypothesis testing

Independent samples: the χ^2 test of association

The results of an investigation of physiological urinary incontinence (PUI) in bitches are recorded in *Table 14.6*. The question being asked was 'Does an association exist between the development of PUI and spaying?' The

Table 14.6 Cumulative incidence of physiological urinary incontinence (excluding congenital incontinence) in a sample of spayed and entire bitches six months of age and older (period of observation = 7 years; the numbers in each cell reflect the proportions of continent and incontinent animals, and spayed and entire animals, in the population from which the sample was drawn). (Hypothetical data.)

	Urinary incontinence present	*Urinary incontinence absent*	*Totals*
Spayed	34 (*a*)	757 (*b*)	791 (*a+b*)
Entire	7 (*c*)	2427 (*d*)	2434 (*c+d*)
Totals	41 (*a+c*)	3184 (*b+d*)	3225 (*n*)

investigators categorized dogs into those with PUI that were spayed, those with PUI that were not spayed, those without PUI that were spayed and those without PUI that were not spayed. These four permutations allow the construction of a two-way table with four 'cells' in it, called a 2×2 contingency table.

The values in the table need to be assessed. A simple method of assessment would be to express the values in each row as percentages of the total of each row. If each row showed similar percentages, this would imply that the row classification did not affect the column classification — that there was no association between the two classifications. This reasoning is sound, but requires large numbers, otherwise sampling variation could affect the result. Taking the data in *Table 14.6*, the percentage of these animals that were spayed and have PUI is 4.3% (34/791); the percentage of those that were not spayed and have PUI is 0.3% (7/2434). This difference could be significant, but it could also merely result from the variation induced by selection of a relatively small sample of the total population at risk.

A common way of conducting a test on these data is to calculate a non-parametric test statistic for independent samples called χ^2 (χ is the Greek letter chi). The distribution followed by this statistic is known as the χ^2-distribution. This statistic indicates the extent to which the observed values in the cells diverge from the values that would be expected if there were no association between row and column categories. A table of the χ^2-distribution is then consulted to decide whether the observed χ^2 value is larger than that which would be expected, based on a null hypothesis postulating no association.

This example involves only a 2×2 contingency table, and the χ^2 equation below is simplified to refer only to this type of table. The test can also be performed on contingency tables with several rows and columns, that is, with several categories (Bailey, 1981).

The χ^2 statistic is given by:

$$\chi^2 = \frac{n(|ad-bc| - n/2)^2}{(a+b)(c+d)(a+c)(b+d)}$$

where $n/2$ is a continuity correction for 2×2 contingency tables, to improve the approximation, because χ^2 is a continuous distribution, yet the data (numbers of animals), and therefore the test statistic, are discrete. The vertical bars, $|\ |$, are **moduli**. They indicate the absolute value of $ad-bc$; that is, the positive value of the difference is always used.

Using the values in *Table 14.6*:

$$\chi^2 = \frac{3225\,\{|82518 - 5299| - (3225/2)\}^2}{791 \times 2434 \times 41 \times 3184}$$

$$= 73.35.$$

Percentage points of the χ^2 distribution are given in Appendix XVII for various significance levels and degrees of freedom. As a rule, the degrees of freedom, v (upsilon), to be selected are given by:

$$v = (\text{number of rows} - 1) \times (\text{number of columns} - 1)$$

which, in this example, is:

$$(2 - 1) \times (2 - 1) = 1.$$

In a 2×2 table, where the row and column totals are all known, knowledge of **one** of the values in the four cells in the body of the table immediately implies knowledge of the values in the other three cells. Similarly, in a table with r rows and k columns, with the row and column totals all known, the knowledge of $(r - 1) \times (k - 1)$ of the values in the rk cells in the body of the table implies knowledge of the values in the other cells. This is the idea behind degrees of freedom in contingency tables; namely the freedom to choose the values in the body of a contingency table when the row and column totals are fixed.

Consulting row 1 (1 degree of freedom) of Appendix XVII, the observed value, 73.35, is greater than the tabulated statistic at the 5% level of significance (3.841) and so an association can be inferred between spaying and PUI. Note that, in this example, the result is also significant at the 1% and 0.1% levels. This corresponds to a two-tailed test.

Independent samples: Fisher's exact test

Sometimes sample sizes are limited, resulting in small numbers in some of the cells of a 2×2 contingency table. If, on the assumption that there is no difference between the groups being compared, one expected cell value is less than 5, the χ^2 test is not reliable, and a different test — **Fisher's exact test** — should be used. (Note that the χ^2 test can be applied when some observed values are less than 5, as long as all expected values exceed 5.)

Table 14.7 presents the same disease/factor relationship as that presented in *Table 14.6*, but with smaller numbers. The expected values are calculated, on the assumption that there is no difference between the two groups, by

Table 14.7 Cumulative incidence of physiological urinary incontinence (excluding congenital incontinence) in a sample of spayed and entire bitches six months of age and older (period of observation = 7 years). (Hypothetical data.)

	Urinary incontinence present	Urinary incontinence absent	Total
Spayed	7(a)	121(b)	128(a + b = r_1)
Entire	2(c)	642(d)	644(c + d = r_2)
Total	9(a + c = n_1)	763(b + d = n_2)	722(n)

considering the marginal totals. The proportion of animals with PUI is then:

$$(a+c)/n,$$

$$= \frac{9}{772}$$

$$= 0.0117.$$

This proportion can then be applied to each row separately to estimate the expected cell values. For spayed animals, the expected number of animals with PUI is $0.0117 \times 128 = 1.5$.

For entire animals, the expected number of animals with PUI is $0.0117 \times 644 = 7.5$.

The first expected value is less than 5, indicating that the χ^2 test is inappropriate and that Fisher's exact test should therefore be used.

Fisher's exact test calculates the P value associated with the observed contingency table on the hypothesis that there is no difference between the two population proportions. This is performed by summing the probability of occurrence of the observed table and of all tables that have the same marginal totals (r_1, r_2, n_1 and n_2), but are as extreme as, or more extreme than, it is. This is a one-tailed formulation.

First, choose the cell entry over which to sum to be the smallest of the four entries, c^*. In this example, $c^* = c = 2$. The formula for P is then:

$$\sum_{c=0}^{c^*} \left(\frac{r_1!r_2!n_1!n_2!}{n_1!a!b!c!d!} \right)$$

Similar expressions can be derived if a, b or d is the smallest entry.

As c^* varies from 0 to 2, the other values (a, b and d) vary also:

c^*	a	b	d
2	$a+c-2$	$b-c+2$	$c+d-2$
1	$a+c-1$	$b-c+2$	$c+d-1$
0	$a+c$	$b-c$	$c+d$

Thus, when $c^* = 2$, the contribution to P is:

$$\frac{(7+121)!(2+642)!(7+2)!(121+642)!}{772! \times 7! \times 121! \times 2! \times 642!}$$

Most pocket calculators will compute factorials up to about 70!, but, for larger values (as in this example), calculations are best performed using logarithms. Logarithms of factorials up to 999! are given in Appendix XVIII. From this appendix:

(log128! + log644! + log9! + log763!) − (log772! + log7! + log121! + log2! + log642!),

= (215.58 616 + 1531.04044 + 5.55976 + 1869.83994) − (1895.80816 + 3.70243 + 200.90818 + 0.30103 + 1525.42334),

= 3622.0263 − 3626.14314,

= −4.11684.

Thus, the contribution to P = antilog† −4.11684
= 0.000076.

When $c^* = 1$, the contribution to P is:

$$\frac{(7+121)!(2+642)!(7+2)!(121+642)!}{772! \times 8! \times 120! \times 1! \times 643!}$$

= 0.000 003 6.

†Antilogarithms can be obtained from a pocket calculator. Antilog$_{10} x = 10^x$. Most calculators have a '10^x' function key which therefore can be used to compute antilogarithms to the base 10. Thus, antilog$_{10} -4.116\,84 = 10^{-4.116\,84} = 1/10^{4.116\,84} = 0.000\,076\,41$.

When $c^* = 0$, the contribution to P is:

$$\frac{(7+121)!(2+642)!(7+2)!(121+642)!}{772! \times 9! \times 119! \times 0! \times 644!}$$

$$= 0.000\ 000\ 074.$$

The P value is therefore:

$$0.000\ 076 + 0.000\ 003\ 6 + 0.000\ 000\ 074$$
$$= 0.000\ 079\ 7.$$

The result is therefore significant at the 0.01% level ($P < 0.0001$), and again indicates that an association can be inferred between spaying and PUI.

There is also a two-tailed formulation of Fisher's exact test (Siegel and Castellan, 1988), but many authors advocate simply doubling the one-tailed P value (Armitage and Berry, 1987). The test can also be generalized to tables with more than two rows and columns (Mehta and Patel, 1983).

Related samples: McNemar's change test

A modification of the χ^2 test — **McNemar's change test** — can be applied to related samples. *Table 14.8* summarizes the possible results of two related samples, '+' denoting presence of a characteristic, and '−' its absence. This table could be generated, for example, by matching spayed (sample 1) and entire (sample 2) bitches with respect to breed and age, and then recording the cumulative incidence of PUI (the characteristic). The two samples would then comprise matched pairs of dogs.

The modified χ^2 formula uses only the values that are **not** in agreement between the two tests, that is, values from **discordant** pairs:

$$\chi^2 = \frac{(|s-t| - 1)^2}{s+t}$$

with one degree of freedom. The value of χ^2 obtained is interpreted by consulting Appendix XVII. This method is

Table 14.8 Possible outcomes of two related samples: (+) feature present, (−) feature absent.

Sample 1	Sample 2	Number of individuals
+	+	r
+	−	s
−	+	t
−	−	u
Total		n

based on a Normal approximation; an exact method should be used if $s+t < 10$ (Armitage and Berry, 1987).

Calculation of confidence intervals

Independent samples

Confidence intervals can be calculated for the difference between two unrelated proportions, and the interpretation is similar to that of confidence intervals for the difference between two means and two medians, which have already been described.

First, the standard error of the difference, SE_{diff}, is calculated:

$$SE_{diff} = \sqrt{\frac{\hat{p}_1(1 - \hat{p}_1)}{n_1} + \frac{\hat{p}_2(1 - \hat{p}_2)}{n_2}}$$

where:

$\hat{p}_1$ = estimated proportion of individuals with a feature in group 1;
$\hat{p}_2$ = estimated proportion of individuals with the feature in group 2;
n_1 = number of individuals in group 1;
n_2 = number of individuals in group 2.

Applying this formula to the data in *Table 4.7a* relating to the crude leptospiral seroprevalence in samples of dogs in Glasgow and Edinburgh:

$\hat{p}_1$ = proportion of seropositive dogs in Glasgow
= 69/251 = 0.275.
$\hat{p}_2$ = proportion of seropositive dogs in Edinburgh
= 61/260 = 0.235.
n_1 = 251.
n_2 = 260.

Thus:

$$\hat{p}_1 - \hat{p}_2 = 0.275 - 0.235 = 0.04;$$

and:

$$SE_{diff} = \sqrt{\frac{0.275(1 - 0.275)}{251} + \frac{0.235(1 - 0.235)}{260}}$$

$$= \sqrt{0.00079 + 0.00069}$$
$$= 0.038.$$

A 95% confidence interval can then be calculated:

$$(\hat{p}_1 - \hat{p}_2) \pm 1.96 \times SE_{diff}$$
$$= 0.04 \pm 1.96 \times 0.038$$

$= -0.034, 0.115.$

This confidence interval includes zero; thus a significant difference cannot be inferred at the 5% level.

This formula is based on the Normal approximation to the binomial distribution, and only gives approximate values when the sizes of each group are less than 30, and p is greater than 0.9 or less than 0.1. (For this reason, this formula should not, for example, be applied to the data in *Table 14.6*, where the two values of p are 0.043 and 0.003.) If exact confidence intervals are required, more complex methods should be used (Armitage and Berry, 1987).

Related samples

Confidence intervals can be calculated for related samples. Using the notation in *Table 14.8*:

proportion positive in the first sample,
$\hat{p}_1 = (r+s)/n;$

proportion positive in the second sample,
$\hat{p}_2 = (r+t)/n.$

The difference between $\hat{p}_1$ and $\hat{p}_2 = (s-t)/n.$
The standard error of this difference is then:

$$\mathrm{SE}_{\mathrm{diff}} = \frac{1}{n}\sqrt{s+t - \frac{(s-t)^2}{n}}$$

and the 95% confidence interval is $(\hat{p}_1 - \hat{p}_2) \pm 1.96 \times \mathrm{SE}_{\mathrm{diff}}.$

Exact methods should again be employed if sample sizes are small (Armitage and Berry, 1987).

What sample size should be selected?

The approximate sample size required to detect a difference between two proportions (i.e., a two-tailed test) is obtained from the formula:

$$n = \frac{\{M_{\alpha/2}\sqrt{2p(1-p)} + M_{\beta}\sqrt{p_1(1-p_1) + p_2(1-p_2)}\}^2}{(p_2-p_1)^2}$$

where:

n = sample size for each population;
p_1 = true proportion in population 1;
p_2 = true proportion in population 2;
p = $(p_1 + p_2)/2;$
$M_{\alpha/2}$ = multiplier associated with the required significance level, α;
M_{β} = multiplier associated with β, the probability of a Type II error.

A common one-tailed situation is demonstration that a specified group responds better than another; for example, when a vaccinated group is compared with an unvaccinated one. For instance, suppose that the annual prevalence of foot-rot in sheep is expected to be approximately 20%, and an investigator wishes to examine the performance of a new vaccine by demonstrating that it can reduce the prevalence by 5%. A flock of sheep is divided into two groups, one of which is vaccinated, and one of which is not vaccinated. Therefore, $p_1 = 0.20$ and $p_2 = 0.15$ (the value for the anticipated prevalence if there is a 5% reduction). If the level of significance is set at 5%, $\alpha = 0.05$ and, from Appendix XII, $M_\alpha = 1.64$ (because the hypothesis is one-tailed). If the investigator wishes to be 80% confident of detecting this difference, test power $(1 - \beta) = 0.80$, $\beta = 0.20$ and $M_\beta = 0.84.$

Therefore,

$$p = (0.20 + 0.15)/2 = 0.175;$$

and

$$n = \frac{\{1.64\sqrt{2\times0.175(1-0.175)} + 0.84\sqrt{0.20(1-0.20)+0.15(1-0.15)}\}^2}{(0.15-0.20)^2}$$

$$= \frac{(1.64\sqrt{0.289}+0.84\sqrt{0.16+0.128})^2}{-0.05^2}$$

$$= \frac{(0.882+0.451)^2}{0.0025}$$

$$= 710.8.$$

Thus, a total of 1422 animals is required: 711 in each group.

The sample size depends on the magnitude of the difference to be detected; the greater the magnitude, the smaller the sample size. Thus, the sample of 711 animals per group will detect a difference in annual prevalence of 5% or greater between the two groups.

This formula will slightly underestimate sample sizes for independent samples, and overestimate sample sizes for related samples.

χ^2 test for trend

Sometimes an hypothesized causal factor may have a **number** of ordered categories. For instance, herd size may be the factor under consideration, and herds may be divided into several categories according to their size. In such circumstances, the 'method of concomitant varia-

Table 14.9 Numbers of dairy herds affected by bovine spongiform encephalopathy according to herd size, Northern Ireland, 1988−90. (From Denny *et al.*, 1992. Crown copyright 1992. Produced by the Central Veterinary Laboratory.)

Herd size (number of adult cows)	Number of affected herds	Number of herds at risk	Percentage of affected herds
1−49	47	4802	1.0
50−99	49	1627	3.0
100−199	24	346	6.9
≥ 200	5	28	17.9
Total	125	6803	

tion' (see Chapter 3) can be used to infer an association, and an appropriate technique for assessing the statistical significance of the association is the χ^2 **test for trend** (Mantel, 1963). This test yields a χ^2 statistic on one degree of freedom, which tests for a linear trend over the ordered categories. The categories may be represented by **scores**, which can be numbers taken as the mid-point of each category (e.g., representing a herd size of 100−200 animals by '150'), by a variation of it, such as its logarithm, or by imprecisely defined, but ordered, arbitrary values, such as 0, 1, 2, ...

The test statistic is:

$$\chi^2 = \frac{T^2(T - 1)\{\Sigma x(a - E)\}^2}{M_1 M_0\{T\Sigma x^2 N - (\Sigma xN)^2\}}$$

where:

T = total number of individuals in all score categories,
x = score value,
a = observed number of affected individuals in each score category,
M_1 = total number of affected individuals,
M_0 = total number of unaffected individuals,
N = number of individuals in each score category,
E = expected number of affected individuals in each score category = NM_1/T.

Table 14.9 presents the results of a study of bovine spongiform encephalopathy (BSE) in Northern Ireland. The percentage of affected herds increases with herd size. The χ^2 test for trend can be applied to these results to assess the statistical significance of this apparent trend. (Note that in this example **herds**, not single animals, are the units of concern.)

The herd sizes 1−49, 50−99, 100−199 ($x_1 \ldots x_3$) are scored as their mid-point values, 25, 75 and 150,

respectively. The herd size, >200 (x_4), is arbitrarily scored as 250.

T = 6803,
M_1 = 125,
M_0 = 6803 − 125,
= 6678.

For x_1, the expected value of the number of affected individuals, E_1 = 4802 × 125/6803 = 88.23; and for x_2 . . . x_4, E_2 . . . E_4 = 29.90, 6.36, 0.52, respectively. Thus:

$$
\begin{aligned}
T^2(T-1) &= 6803^2 \times 6802, \\
&= 3.15 \times 10^{11}. \\
\{\Sigma x(a-E)\}^2 &= \{25(47 - 88.23) + 75(49 - 29.90) \\
&\quad + 150(24 - 6.36) + 250(5 - 0.52)\}^2 \\
&= (-1030.75 + 1432.50 + 2646.00 \\
&\quad + 1120.00)^2 \\
&= 4167.75^2 \\
&= 1.74 \times 10^7. \\
T\Sigma x^2 N &= 6803\{(25^2 \times 4802) + (75^2 \times 1627) \\
&\quad + (150^2 \times 346) + (250^2 \times 28)\} \\
&= 6803(3.00 \times 10^6 + 9.15 \times 10^6 \\
&\quad + 7.79 \times 10^6 + 1.75 \times 10^6) \\
&= 6803 \times 2.17 \times 10^7 \\
&= 1.48 \times 10^{11}. \\
(\Sigma xN)^2 &= \{(25 \times 4802) + (75 \times 1627) \\
&\quad + (150 \times 346) + (250 \times 28)\}^2 \\
&= (1.20 \times 10^5 + 1.22 \times 10^5 \\
&\quad + 5.19 \times 10^4 + 7000)^2 \\
&= (3.01 \times 10^5)^2 \\
&= 9.06 \times 10^{10}.
\end{aligned}
$$

Thus:

$$
\begin{aligned}
\chi^2 &= \frac{(3.15 \times 10^{11}) \times (1.74 \times 10^7)}{(125 \times 6678)(1.48 \times 10^{11} - 90.6 \times 10^{10})} \\
&= \frac{5.48 \times 10^{18}}{8.35 \times 10^5 \times 5.74 \times 10^{10}}
\end{aligned}
$$

$$= \frac{5.48 \times 10^{18}}{4.79 \times 10^{16}}$$

$$= 114.4.$$

Consulting Appendix XVII, row 1 (1 degree of freedom), the observed value, 114.4, is greater than the tabulated statistic at the 0.1% level of significance, and so a linear trend can be inferred between the proportion of affected herds and herd size. There is considerable evidence that BSE is transmitted in meat and bone meal (see Chapters 2, 3 and 4) and so the trend can be explained by the larger number of animals at risk in large herds and therefore the greater probability of purchasing a contaminated batch of food.

A continuity correction should be applied to this test if the x scores are one unit apart (e.g., scores of 0, 1, 2, etc.):

$\{\Sigma x(a-E)\}^2$ should be replaced by $\{\Sigma x(a-E) - 1/2\}^2$.

This test should be used with caution because a trend may be fitted and may be significant even if inspection of the data does not reveal a regular pattern over the ordered categories. The test therefore is appropriate only if there is a reasonable hypothesis of a linear relationship, as in the example above.

Correlation

Table 14.10 records the number of cases of lameness in cattle in relation to rainfall for a one-year period on a farm in south-west England. The question to be answered is: 'Does the amount of rainfall have an effect on the incidence of lameness?' This is a reasonable question; wet feet could be a causal factor. The values in *Table 14.10* are plotted graphically in *Figure 14.1*, each point being a lameness–rainfall pair. Lameness is measured on the horizontal (x) axis and rainfall on the vertical (y) axis.

If there were a positive association between increased rainfall (the explanatory variable) and incidence of lameness (the response variable), most entries would be concentrated in a line from the bottom left to the top right of the figure. If there were no association, the pairs would be randomly scattered over the figure. Visually, the results give a slight impression of concentrating along the diagonal, but it is necessary to know whether this clustering is significant.

A useful measure of correlation between x and y for data that fulfil parametric requirements, and successive

observations are **independent** of others, is the **correlation coefficient**, ρ (rho). This ranges from $+1$, representing a complete positive association, to -1, representing a complete negative association.

In this example, lameness incidence is assumed to be Normally distributed because lameness is fairly common. (If it were rare then it would more likely have a Poisson distribution.) Similarly, because there are many incidents of lameness, the data are considered to be continuous, although, technically, they are discrete. It is also assumed that the successive fortnightly observations of rainfall are independent, that is, the rainfall of one fortnight does not influence the rainfall of succeeding fortnights.

The correlation coefficient, ρ, refers to the total population; these measurements come from a sample and so can be used only to estimate the sample's correlation coefficient, r. Estimation involves calculating the means of the two variables and then estimating r, using the equation:

Table 14.10 The joint distribution of fortnightly lameness incidence and rainfall on a farm in south-west England for a one-year period (1977). (Data supplied by the Institute for Research on Animal Diseases, Compton, UK.)

Fortnight	Number of lameness incidents (x)	Fortnightly rainfall totals (mm) (y)
1	40	37.2
2	38	48.8
3	55	72.0
4	38	76.8
5	45	14.8
6	42	53.2
7	51	23.9
8	45	11.0
9	41	79.9
10	23	21.0
11	10	2.3
12	29	81.1
13	19	7.4
14	11	31.5
15	11	33.2
16	19	31.1
17	33	109.2
18	47	25.0
19	42	1.9
20	34	28.8
21	17	24.4
22	30	51.3
23	48	38.2
24	59	18.0
25	41	57.2
26	26	33.2

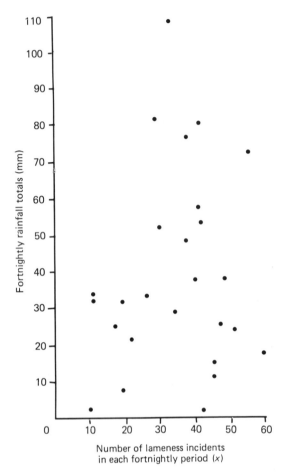

Figure 14.1 Plot of the joint distribution of fortnightly lameness incidence and rainfall on a farm in SW England for a one-year period (1977). (Data from *Table 14.10*)

$$\Sigma(x-\bar{x})(y-\bar{y})\sqrt{\{\Sigma(x-\bar{x})^2\Sigma(y-\bar{y})^2\}}.$$

This can be written alternatively in a form that is easier to handle during calculation:

$$r = \{\Sigma xy - (\Sigma x)(\Sigma y)/n\}\sqrt{([\Sigma x^2 - \{(\Sigma x^2)/n\}][\Sigma y^2 - \{(\Sigma y^2/n\}])}.$$

Using the data from *Table 14.10*:

$\Sigma x = 894$ $\Sigma y = 1012.4$
$\Sigma x^2 = 35\ 592$ $\Sigma y^2 = 57\ 880.04$
$\Sigma xy = 36\ 307.5$
$n = 26$
$\{\Sigma xy - (\Sigma x)(\Sigma y)/n\} = 36\ 307.5 - (894)(1012.4)/26$
$= 1496.52,$

$\{\Sigma x^2 - (\Sigma x)^2/n\}$ $= 35\ 592 - 894^2/26$
$= 4852.15,$
$\{\Sigma y^2 - (\Sigma y)^2/n\}$ $= 57\ 880.04 - 1012.4 = 2/26$
$= 18\ 458.742.$

Thus:

$$r = \frac{1496.52}{\sqrt{(4852.15 \times 18\ 458.742)}}$$

$$= \frac{1496.52}{9463.86}$$

$$= 0.158.$$

The significance of this value is obtained by consulting Appendix IXX. If the value is **greater** in absolute terms (i.e. ignoring sign) than the tabulated value, at a defined significance level, then a significant association is demonstrated. In this example, the value (0.158) is **less** than the tabulated value at the 5% level, which is 0.381. This value is chosen from the table by selecting the number of degrees of freedom, which is $n - 2 = 24$. This is one degree of freedom less than might be expected because the calculation of the correlation coefficient uses up one further degree of freedom. The most appropriate row therefore is 25 degrees of freedom. In this example, therefore, there is not a significant association between lameness incidence and rainfall ($P > 0.05$). Confidence intervals can also be calculated for ρ (Gardner and Altman, 1989).

If parametric assumptions are not met by data, an appropriate non-parametric measure of correlation can be calculated (*Table 14.2*).

Multivariate analysis

The analytical techniques that have been described concern the study of relationships between two variables. In some cases it is necessary to assess the relationship between a response variable and many explanatory variables. This requires statistical techniques that investigate multiple variables; these are therefore called **multivariate** techniques. They include cluster analysis, factor analysis, path analysis, discriminant analysis, analysis of principal components and multiple regression analysis. An introduction is provided in the next chapter, but most of these methods are beyond the scope of this book, and are described in detail elsewhere (e.g., Everitt and Dunn, 1991).

Statistical packages

There is now a wide range of applications software which performs statistical calculations including those of the mean, median, standard deviation and standard error, confidence limits, the tests of association, time series analysis, multivariate analyses and other statistical procedures relevant to epidemiology. Some of these packages are listed in Appendix III.

Such packages enable data to be managed and analysed efficiently and quickly. However, they can be dangerous. They facilitate easy analysis of data and so tend to encourage the collection of masses of data without a clear objective. It is also easy to try many of the different tests that are available without a knowledge of the tests' underlying principles and assumptions. These remarks are equally relevant to the use of those pocket calculators that have built-in programs for simple statistical tests.

Expert statistical advice therefore should always be sought if there is any doubt about the analytical technique that should be used in an investigation. This advice should be obtained **before** the investigation begins, not after it is completed, otherwise time may be spent collecting data, only to discover that they cannot be used to solve the problem that is being posed.

Further reading

Armitage, P. and Berry, G. (1987) *Statistical Methods in Medical Research*, 2nd edn. Blackwell Scientific Publications, Oxford

Bailey, N.T.J. (1981) *Statistical Methods in Biology*, 2nd edn. Hodder and Stoughton, London. (*An introduction to elementary statistics*)

Fleiss, J.L. (1981) *Statistical Methods for Rates and Proportions*, 2nd edn. John Wiley, New York

Leech, F.B. and Sellers, K.C. (1979) *Statistical Epidemiology in Veterinary Science*. Charles Griffin, London and High Wycombe

Siegel, S. and Castellan, N.J. (1988) *Nonparametric Statistics for the Behavioral Sciences*, 2nd edn. McGraw-Hill, New York

15 Observational studies

Observational studies are used to identify risk factors, and to estimate the quantitative effects of the various component causes that contribute to the occurrence of disease. The investigations are based on analysis of natural disease occurrence in populations by **comparing** groups of individuals* with respect to disease occurrence and exposure to hypothesized risk factors.

Observational studies differ from experimental studies. In the former the investigator is not free to randomly allocate factors (disease and hypothesized risk factors) to individuals, whereas in the latter the investigator is free to allocate factors to individuals at random.

Risk factors may be categorical (e.g., breed and sex) or quantitative continuous measurements (e.g. weight, age and rainfall). This chapter focuses on categorical data which are commonly the subject of observational studies. Continuous data can also be analysed using categorical methods by grouping the data into discrete categories (e.g., age intervals).

Types of observational study

Cohort, case–control and cross-sectional studies

There are three main types of observational study: **cohort**, **case–control** and **cross-sectional**. Each classifies animals into those with and without disease, and those exposed and unexposed to hypothesized risk factors. Therefore, they each generate a 2 × 2 contingency table for each disease/factor relationship (*Table 15.1*). However, the methods of generation differ between the types of study.

*Individuals are commonly, but not exclusively, the sampling units in observational studies. Herds, flocks, or other aggregates can also be studied.

Cohort studies

In a cohort study, a group (cohort) of animals exposed to a hypothesized risk factor, and a group not exposed to the factor are selected and observed to record development of disease in each group. For example, if spaying were considered to be a risk factor for physiological urinary incontinence (PUI) in bitches, a suitable cohort study would comprise a group of spayed ('exposed') puppies and a group of entire ('unexposed') puppies, each of which would be monitored for the development of PUI. Therefore, incidence is measured, and $a + b$ and $c + d$ in *Table 15.1* are predetermined.

Case–control studies

In a case–control study, a group of diseased animals (cases) and a group of non-diseased animals (controls) are selected and compared with respect to presence of the hypothesized risk factor. Thus, a case–control study of PUI would involve identification of cases of PUI and comparison of the sexual status (spayed versus entire) of these cases with a control group of bitches that were not incontinent. Therefore, $a + c$ and $b + d$ are predetermined. Case–control studies may be conducted with incident (new) cases or existing cases and therefore may utilize incidence or prevalence values.

Cross-sectional studies

The cross-sectional study involves the selection of a sample of n individuals from a larger population, and then the determination, for each individual, of the **simultaneous** presence or absence of disease and hypothesized risk factor; prevalence is therefore recorded. For example, in a cross-sectional study of PUI, a sample of bitches would be selected and classified according to sexual status and whether or not the animals were incontinent. At the beginning of a cross-sectional study only the total number

Table 15.1 The 2 × 2 contingency table constructed in observational studies.

	Diseased animals	Non-diseased animals	Total
Hypothesized risk factor present	a	b	$a+b$
Hypothesized risk factor absent	c	d	$c+d$
Total	$a+c$	$b+d$	$a+b+c+d = n$

In **cohort studies** $(a+b)$ and $(c+d)$ are predetermined.
In **case–control studies** $(a+c)$ and $(b+d)$ are predetermined.
In **cross-sectional studies** only n can be predetermined.

of animals (n in *Table 15.1*) is predetermined. The numbers of animals with and without disease, and possessing or not possessing the risk factor, are not known initially.

Nomenclature

A variety of alternative names have been applied to case–control and cohort studies. Both of these studies consider two events — exposure to an hypothesized causal factor or factors and development of disease — that are separated by a period of time. Because of this temporal separation of the two events, each of these studies is sometimes termed **longitudinal**.

The case–control study compares diseased animals (cases) with non-diseased animals (controls) and therefore has variously been called a **case-comparison**, **case-referent** or **case history** study. This study selects groups according to presence or absence of disease and **looks back** to possible causes; it has therefore sometimes been described as a **retrospective study** (looking back from effect to cause).

A cohort study selects groups according to presence or absence of exposure to hypothesized causal factors, and then **looks forward** to the development of disease. It has therefore sometimes been called a **prospective study** (looking forward from cause to effect). *Table 15.2* lists the types of observational study and their synonyms.

The groups may be selected as 'exposed' and 'unexposed' now, and then observed over a period of time to identify cases; such a cohort study is termed concurrent (*Figure 15.1*). Alternatively, if reliable records relating to exposure are available then groups may be selected according to presence or absence of previous exposure, and traced to the present to determine disease status; this constitutes a non-concurrent study.

Some investigators use 'retrospective' to refer to any study that records data from the past, and 'prospective' to refer to any study designed to collect future data. Therefore, a non-concurrent cohort (prospective, in the causal sense) study may alternatively be termed a retrospective (in the temporal sense) cohort study. Similarly, a concurrent cohort study can also be called a prospective (in the temporal sense) cohort study (*Figure 15.1*).

Some studies show characteristics of more than one of the three main types. The range of such 'hybrid' studies, and their nomenclature, are described by Kleinbaum *et al.* (1982).

Causal inference

The three types of study attempt to identify a cause by applying the first three of Evans' postulates (see Chapter 3; postulates 1 and 3, rephrased here, using 'prevalence' and 'incidence' in their definitions):

1. the prevalence of a disease should be significantly

Table 15.2 Nomenclature of observational studies.

Cross-sectional	Longitudinal	
	Case–control	Cohort
Synonym:	Synonyms:	Synonyms:
Prevalence	Retrospective	Prospective
	Case-referent	Incidence
	Case-comparison	Longitudinal
	Case-compeer	Follow-up
	Case history	
	Trohoc	

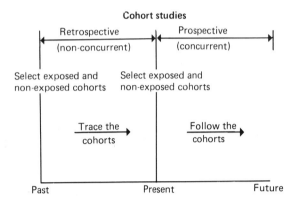

Fig. 15.1 The selection of cohorts in concurrent and non-concurrent cohort studies ('retrospective' and 'prospective' used in the temporal sense). (Modified from Lilienfeld and Lilienfeld, 1980.)

higher in individuals exposed to the supposed cause than in those who are not (evidence supplied by a cross-sectional study);

2. exposure to the supposed cause should be present more commonly in those with than those without the disease, when all other risk factors are held constant (evidence supplied by a case−control study);

3. the incidence of disease should be significantly higher in those exposed to the supposed cause than in those not so exposed (evidence supplied by a cohort study).

The credibility of cause is strengthened by fulfilling others of Evans' postulates. Thus, Jarrett's (1980) demonstration of an association between exposure to bracken and the development of intestinal cancer in cattle is more credible because a carcinogen has been isolated from bracken (Wang *et al.*, 1976) (Evans' postulate 10).

Causal inference is also strengthened if associations are detected in different circumstances (see Chapter 3) or in several studies, enabling results to be generalized more confidently. Thus, an association between spaying and PUI in bitches has been demonstrated in primary-care cases in Scotland and in referred cases in the south-west of England (Holt and Thrusfield, 1993); this strengthens the inference that the association holds in the general dog population. In contrast, a predisposition to valvular heart disease has been demonstrated in cocker spaniels in North America, but not in Scotland (see Chapter 5), suggesting that the breed predispostion may not be universal.

Comparison of the types of study

A comparison of cohort, case−control and cross-sectional studies is given in *Table 15.3*.

Case−control studies can be conducted relatively quickly and are a useful means of initially 'trawling' for risk factors. Cohort studies, in contrast, may have a long duration (particularly those of diseases with lengthy incubation and latent periods such as cancer) and often focus on a specific risk factor.

A logical requirement of demonstration of cause is that an animal is exposed to a causal factor **before** disease develops (see Chapter 3). The design of cohort studies, which resembles an experiment, ensures that this temporal sequence is detected. However, cross-sectional and case−control studies may not detect the sequence. For example, if the association between spaying and PUI in female dogs were being investigated using a cross-sectional study (spaying being the hypothesized risk factor), then spayed bitches with PUI may be identified; however, incontinence may have developed **before** spaying in some of the cases, in which instance spaying could not have been a component cause in those animals. For this reason, and the reason that a cohort study measures incidence, the cohort study therefore is a better technique for assessing risk and identifying causes than the other two types of study.

Ecological studies

In each of the three types of study just described it is necessary to know the exposure and disease status of all **individuals**. Sometimes this information is not available. Characteristics of **groups** may then be studied, although an inference may still be required at the level of the individual. Such studies are **ecological studies**.

For example, in The Netherlands, the highest human lung cancer mortality rate between 1969 and 1984 was found in the North Brabant region. Most pet bird keepers and bird clubs are also located in this region. Moreover, people who keep birds inhale allergens and dust particles which impair the function of lung macrophages, resulting in reduced protection of the bronchial epithelium (Voisin *et al.*, 1983). It is therefore tempting to speculate that bird-keeping is a risk factor for lung cancer, although the exposure and disease status of individuals is not known. This inference is logically defective because it is based on the erroneous assumption that group and individual characteristics are always the same; this logical error is termed the **ecological fallacy** (Robinson, 1950). The correlation between group (i.e., ecological) variables is often considerably different from the individual correlation in the same populations; although the lung cancer rate was highest in the region where bird-keeping was predominant, the cases may have occurred in people who

Table 15.3 Comparison of the advantages and disadvantages of cohort, case—control and cross-sectional studies. (Based on Schlesselman, 1982.)

	Advantages	*Disadvantages*
Cohort studies	1. Incidence in exposed and unexposed individuals can be calculated 2. Permit flexibility in choosing variables to be systematically recorded	1. Exposed and unexposed proportions in target population cannot be estimated 2. Large numbers of subjects are required to study rare diseases 3. Potentially long duration for follow-up 4. Relatively expensive to conduct 5. Maintaining follow-up is difficult 6. Control of extraneous variables may be incomplete
Case—control studies	1. Well-suited to the study of rare diseases or of those with long incubation periods 2. Relatively quick to mount and conduct 3. Relatively inexpensive 4. Require comparatively few subjects 5. Existing records occasionally can be used 6. No risk to subjects 7. Allow study of multiple potential causes of a disease	1. Exposed and unexposed proportions in target populations cannot be estimated 2. Rely on recall or records for information on past exposures 3. Validation of information is difficult or sometimes impossible 4. Control of extraneous variables may be incomplete 5. Selection of an appropriate comparison group may be difficult 6. Incidence in exposed and unexposed individuals cannot be estimated
Cross-sectional studies	1. When a random sample of the target population is selected, disease prevalence, and proportions exposed and unexposed in the target population can be estimated 2. Relatively quick to mount and conduct 3. Relatively inexpensive 4. Current records occasionally can be used 5. No risk to subjects 6. Allow study of multiple potential causes of disease	1. Unsuited to the study of rare diseases 2. Unsuited to the study of diseases of short duration 3. Control of extraneous variables may be incomplete 4. Incidence in exposed and unexposed individuals cannot be estimated 5. Temporal sequence of cause and effect cannot necessarily be determined

did not keep birds.

Ecological studies therefore should be interpreted with caution, but are useful preliminary indicators to causal hypotheses that should be tested more thoroughly. Thus, a subsequent case−control study demonstrated an association between bird-keeping and lung cancer (Holst *et al.*, 1988), supporting a causal hypothesis at the level of the individual.

Piantadosi *et al.* (1988) discuss the ecological fallacy in detail, and Kleinbaum *et al.* (1982) describe ways of strengthening causal inferences from ecological studies.

Measures of association

An hypothesis of association between disease and a factor can be tested using the χ^2 test (see Chapter 14). However, this test cannot be used to measure the **degree** of association. This is because χ^2 is a function of the proportions in the various cells and of the total sample size, whereas the degree of association is only really a function of the cell proportions; the sample size has a role to play in detecting significance but not in determining the extent of association. It is also desirable to provide a more informative **measure** of the impact of a factor on disease occurrence. This can be expressed by the absolute **difference** between disease occurrence in 'exposed' and 'unexposed' groups, estimated by determining the difference between the two proportions (see 'Attributable risk' below). Alternatively, the **ratio** of disease occurrence between the two groups can be caclulated. Ratios are relative measures, and two are widely used: the **relative risk** and **odds ratio**.

Relative risk

The **relative risk**, *RR*, is the ratio of the incidence of disease in exposed animals to the incidence in unexposed animals.* This is derived in *Table 15.4* using the notation of *Table 15.1*. An *RR* greater than 1 indicates a positive statistical association between factor and disease. Thus, an *RR* of 2 indicates that the incidence of disease in exposed animals is twice that in unexposed animals. An *RR* less than 1 indicates a negative statistical association: possession of the factor may be said to have a protective

---

*This is more fully termed the relative risk in **exposed** animals, RR_{exp}, to distinguish it from the less frequently derived **population** relative risk, $RR_{pop} = \{(a+c)/n\}/\{c/(c+d)\}$. (see footnote p. 225)

Table 15.4 Derivation of relative risk and odds ratio.

(a) Relative risk
*Cohort study**
$Incidence_{exposed} = a/(a+b)$
$Incidence_{unexposed} = c/(c+d)$
Relative risk $(RR) = \{a/(a+b)\}/\{c/(c+d)\}$

(b) Odds ratio
Case−control study
$Exposure\ odds_{cases} = a/c$
$Exposure\ odds_{controls} = b/d$
$Exposure\ odds\ ratio\ (\psi_c) = (a/c)/(b/d)$
$\qquad\qquad\qquad\qquad = ad/bc$

Cohort study
$Disease\ odds_{exposed} = a/b$
$Disease\ odds_{unexposed} = c/d$
$Disease\ odds\ ratio\ (\psi_d) = (a/b)/(c/d)$
$\qquad\qquad\qquad\qquad = ad/bc$

Cross-sectional study
Prevalence odds ratio $(\psi_p) = ad/bc$

---

*For a cross-sectional derivation of a relative 'risk', see footnote on p. 225.

---

effect against the disease. An *RR* of 1 suggests no association.

The *RR* can be derived from cumulative incidence, when it is also termed the **risk ratio**, and from incidence rates, when it is also called the **rate ratio**. (Some authorities use relative risk as a synonym only for risk ratio.) The *RR* is estimated directly in a cohort study.

Calculation of confidence intervals

The *RR* is estimated from a sample of the study population. Therefore, the significance of the result needs to be assessed. The hypothesis that the *RR* is significantly greater (or less) than 1 can be tested (Fleiss, 1981). Alternatively, confidence intervals can be estimated. The latter approach is usually adopted in this chapter because it also indicates the precision of the measure of association (see Chapter 14). However, care needs to be exercised because the relative risk statistic is not Normally distributed.

An approximate 95% confidence interval for the relative risk for large samples can be calculated, based on a transformation of the limits for the natural logarithm ($\log_e$) of the *RR* (Katz *et al.*, 1978).

Using the data in *Table 14.6* relating to PUI; first the sample (point) estimate of the *RR* is calculated:

$$\widehat{RR} = \{a/a+b)\}/\{c/c+d)\},$$

$$= (34/791)/(7/2434),$$
$$= 14.95.$$

The variance (var) of $\log_e \widehat{RR}$, based on cumulative incidence, is approximately equal to:

$$\{(b/a)/(a+b)\} + \{(d/c)/(c+d)\},$$
$$= \{(757/34)/(34+757)\} + \{(2427/7)/(7+2427)\},$$
$$= 0.028 + 0.142,$$
$$= 0.170.$$

The 95% confidence interval is:

$$\widehat{RR} \exp(-1.96\sqrt{\text{var}}), \ \widehat{RR} \exp(+1.96\sqrt{\text{var}}),$$
$$= 14.95 \exp(-0.8081), \ 14.95 \exp(0.8081),$$
$$= 14.95 \times 2.72^{-0.8081}, \ 14.95 \times 2.72^{0.8081},$$
$$= 14.95 \times 1/(2.72^{0.8081}), \ 14.95 \times 2.72^{0.8081},$$
$$= 14.95 \times 0.45, \ 14.95 \times 2.24,$$
$$= 6.73, \ 33.49.$$

Thus, the relative risk is significantly greater than 1 at the 5% level, suggesting an association between spaying (the risk factor) and PUI. Note that this result is in accord with the result of the χ^2 test conducted in Chapter 14, but also gives a **measure** of the association with defined **precision**.

The same formula can be used for calculation of a confidence interval for the relative 'risk' (prevalence ratio) in a cross-sectional study. However, the approximate variance of $\log_e \widehat{RR}$, based on incidence rates, is calculated differently:

$$\text{var} \log_e \widehat{RR} = 1/a + 1/c$$

Other confidence intervals can be constructed using appropriate multipliers (Appendix V). Exact intervals can also be calculated (Kleinbaum *et al.*, 1982; Rothman, 1986).

Relative risk estimations based on cumulative incidence are appropriate when individuals are observed throughout the period of study, but are inappropriate when the period of observation of individuals varies (e.g., when animals are enlisted to cohorts over a period of time and when there are many censored observations: see Chapter 4). In such circumstances, when the risk of disease can be assumed to be constant over the whole of the animal-time of experience, incidence rates should be used to calculate relative risk. Alternatively, survival methods can be used (Kleinbaum *et al.*, 1982; Kahn and Sempos, 1989).

Odds ratio

The **odds ratio (relative odds)**, ψ (psi) is another relative measure based on 'odds': the ratio of the probability of an event occurring to the probability of it not occurring (a ratio little used outside betting circles). Thus, the probability of throwing a head with a coin is 0.5 (1/2), whereas the odds are even', 1:1 ($0.5/\{1 - 0.5\}$). Similarly, the probability of throwing a specified number with a six-sided dice is 1/6 (0.167), whereas the odds is 1:5 ($0.167/\{1 - 0.167\}$).

In a cohort study, a disease odds ratio, ψ_d, is estimated; this is the ratio of the odds of disease in exposed individuals to the odds in those unexposed (*Table 15.4*). This simplifies to ad/bc, the **cross-product ratio**, which therefore is a synonym for the odds ratio.

In a case−control study, a different odds ratio, the exposure odds ratio, ψ_e, is determined. It is the ratio of the odds of exposure to the factor in cases to the odds of exposure in controls. Note, however, that this also simplifies to ad/bc.

A prevalence odds ratio, ψ_p, is derived in a cross-sectional study thus: ad/bc.

In a cohort study, when disease is rare, the incidence of disease in exposed animals approximately equals the odds of disease because a is small relative to b; thus $a/(a+b) \simeq a/b$. Similarly, $c/(c+d) \simeq c/d$. Thus, the values of the odds ratio and relative risk are similar. Moreover, since ψ_e, and ψ_d are equivalent (ad/bc), an odds ratio derived in a case−control study gives an indirect estimate of the relative risk (Cornfield, 1951) and, with appropriate sampling protocols, an estimate of the relative risk can be obtained without the assumption of rarity of disease (Rodrigues and Kirkwood, 1990). Similarly, ψ_p derived in a cross-sectional study gives an indirect estimate of the relative risk.*

The relative risk is the preferred parameter in a cohort study because, when the relative risk is greater than 1, the odds ratio will always overestimate it, particularly when disease is not rare.

---

*Strictly, cross-sectional studies and case−control studies based on prevalence values produce estimates of the relative 'risk' of *being* diseased, whereas cohort studies estimate the relative risk of *becoming* diseased. The former relative 'risk' is sometimes more properly termed the **prevalence ratio** (Kleinbaum *et al.*, 1982). This can also be calculated directly in a cross-sectional study, using the same formula as that for the relative risk. Cross-sectional studies also allow calculation of a *population* prevalence ratio, which is commonly termed the population relative 'risk', $RR_{pop} = \{(a+c)/n\}/\{c/(c+d)\}$. This adjusts the standard prevalence ratio (relative 'risk') for the prevalence of the factor in the population, and is therefore an indication of the relative impact of the factor in the population (Martin *et al.*, 1987). A *population* odds ratio, ψ_{pop}, can also be calculated in cross-sectional and case−control studies (if controls are representative of non-diseased animals in the study population) and is interpreted in the same way as RR_{pop}; $\psi_{pop} = \{d(a+c)\}/\{c(b+d)\}$ (Martin *et al.*, 1987).

Table 15.5 The relationship between type of ventilation system and porcine enzootic pneumonia. (Data from Willeberg, 1980b.)

(a) Crude relationships

	Cases* (No. of herds)	Controls** (No. of herds)	Total
Fan ventilation	91 (a)	73 (b)	164
No fan ventilation	25 (c)	60 (d)	85
Total	116	133	249

*Herds with a high prevalence of porcine enzootic pneumonia.
**Herds with a low prevalence of porcine enzootic pneumonia.

(b) Relationships according to herd size

	Herd size									
	≤ 200		$201-300$		$301-400$		$401-500$		>500	
	+	−	+	−	+	−	+	−	+	−
Fan ventilation	2	7	15	30	13	19	7	5	54	12
No fan ventilation	4	27	8	18	7	10	2	4	4	1

'+' = high prevalence of porcine enzootic pneumonia (disease 'present'); '−' = low prevalence of porcine enzootic pneumonia (disease 'absent').

$\hat{\psi}_i = 1.93$	$\hat{\psi}_i = 1.13$	$\hat{\psi}_i = 0.98$	$\hat{\psi}_i = 2.80$	$\hat{\psi}_i = 1.73$
$n_i = 40$	$n_i = 71$	$n_i = 49$	$n_i = 18$	$n_i = 71$
$w_i = 0.70$	$w_i = 3.38$	$w_i = 2.71$	$w_i = 0.56$	$w_i = 0.68$
$v_i = 0.93$	$v_i = 0.28$	$v_i = 0.37$	$v_i = 0.45$	$v_i = 1.35$
$w_i^2 = 0.49$	$wi^2 = 11.42$	$w_i^2 = 7.34$	$wi^2 = 0.31$	$w_i^2 = 0.46$
$w_i^2 v_i = 0.46$	$w_i^2 v_i = 3.20$	$w_i^2 v_i = 2.72$	$w_i^2 v_i = 0.14$	$w_i^2 v_i = 0.62$

Calculation of confidence intervals

An approximate 95% confidence interval for the odds ratio can be calculated, based on a transformation of the limits for the natural logarithm ($\log_e$) of $\hat{\psi}$ (Woolf, 1955).

The method is exemplified using the data in *Table 15.5a* relating to the association between type of ventilation and respiratory disease (specifically enzootic pneumonia) in pigs. In this example, herds — not individuals — are the sampling units. 'Cases' are herds with a high prevalence of pneumonia (a three-year average >5%), whereas 'controls' are herds with a low prevalence.

First, the sample estimate of ψ is calculated:

$$\hat{\psi} = ad/bc,$$
$$= (91 \times 60)/(25 \times 73),$$
$$= 2.99.$$

The variance (var) of $\log_e \hat{\psi}$ is approximately equal to:

$$(1/a + 1/b + 1/c + 1/d),$$
$$= 0.010\,99 + 0.013\,70 + 0.040\,00 + 0.016\,67,$$
$$= 0.081\,37.$$

The 95% confidence interval is:

$$\hat{\psi} \exp(-1.96\sqrt{\text{var}}), \hat{\psi} \exp(+1.96\sqrt{\text{var}}),$$
$$= 2.99 \exp(-0.5591), 2.99 \exp(0.5591),$$
$$= 2.99 \times 2.72^{-0.5591}, 2.99 \times 2.72^{0.5591},$$
$$= 2.99 \times 1/(2.72^{0.5591}), 2.99 \times 2.72^{0.5591},$$
$$= 2.99 \times 0.572, 2.99 \times 1.749,$$
$$= 1.71, 5.23.$$

The odds ratio is therefore significantly greater than 1 at the 5% level, suggesting an association between fan ventilation and pneumonia, based on these crude data.

A more precise method of estimating confidence intervals is described by Cornfield (1956), but in large studies the difference between this and Woolf's method is trivial. Exact confidence intervals can be calculated (Mehta *et al.*, 1985); the method requires an appropriate computer program.

An odds ratio cannot be calculated when a contingency table cell contains the value zero. This problem can be overcome by the addition of 1/2 to the values in each cell of the table before calculating the odds ratio and its associated confidence interval (Fleiss, 1981). However, if a study involves 2 × 2 tables with cell totals of zero, or with cell totals so small that adding 1/2 will substantially affect the calculation, then its precision is likely to be too low to contribute much to knowledge. Alternatively, if a cell has a zero value, the χ^2 test can be applied, or a confidence interval can be calculated for the difference between the two proportions (see Chapter 14).

Attributable risk

The terms 'attributable risk' and 'aetiological fraction' have been used to denote a number of different concepts, often with several inconsistently used synonyms (Last, 1988). The first describes absolute differences; whereas the second comprises relative measures. Each can relate either to animals exposed to the risk factor or to the total population.

Attributable risk (exposed)

Table 14.6 shows that although the incidence of urinary incontinence in spayed (exposed) dogs, $a/(a+b)$, is greater than the incidence in entire (unexposed) dogs, $c/(c+d)$, the spayed dogs are still susceptible to a 'background' risk, corresponding to $c/(c+d)$. Put another way, if some of the spayed dogs had not been neutered then they may still, as entire dogs, have developed urinary incontinence. The extent of the risk associated with spaying is the **attributable risk (risk difference** or **attributable rate)** in **exposed** animals, δ_{exp} (delta): the difference between the incidence of disease in exposed animals and the incidence in unexposed animals:

$$\delta_{exp} = \{a/(a+b)\} - \{c/(c+d)\}.$$

Thus, in this example:

$$\begin{aligned}\hat{\delta}_{exp} &= (34/791) - (7/2434) \\ &= 0.043 - 0.003 \\ &= 0.040.\end{aligned}$$

This represents an incidence of incontinence in spayed dogs, attributable to spaying, of 4.0 per 100 during the

period of observation. The attributable risk therefore indicates the extent to which the incidence of disease in exposed animals would be reduced if they had not been exposed to the risk factor, **assuming that the risk factor is causal**.

This attributable risk can be expressed in terms of the relative risk:

$$\begin{aligned}\delta_{exp} &= \{a/(a+b)\} - \{c/(c+d)\}, \\ &= [\{a/(a+b)\}/\{c/(c+d)\} - 1] \times \{c/(c+d)\}.\end{aligned}$$

Since $\{a/(a+b)\}/\{c/(c+d)\} = RR$, then $\delta_{exp} = (RR - 1) \times \{(c/c+d)\}$.

Note that the incidence in unexposed animals is required to calculate δ_{exp}.

An attributable risk, based on prevalence values, can also be estimated in a cross-sectional study because the prevalence in unexposed animals is known. However, this is not known in a case-control study, and so δ_{exp} cannot be determined in this type of study, unless information from other sources is available on the baseline prevalence.

It is clear that ratios $\{a/(a+b)\}/\{c/(c+d)\}$ of 0.02/0.01 and 0.0002/0.0001 give the same relative risk, even though they represent vastly different incidence ratios. The attributable risk, however, includes the baseline incidence, and therefore gives an indication of the magnitude of the effect of a causal factor in the population. Thus, the attributable risk gives a better indication than the relative risk of the effect of a preventive campaign that removes the factor (MacMahon and Pugh, 1970). However, the use of 'attributable' in the former term is dangerous because it implies a *causal* relationship, whereas the parameter is based only on *statistical associations*. Its practical application in reducing disease incidence therefore depends on strong evidence of a causal relationship between risk factor and disease which may need to be determined by other means (see Chapter 3).

The main advantage of the relative risk is the empirical finding that the relative risk for a particular disease/factor relationship is fairly consistent in a wide range of populations (Elwood, 1988) and, in contrast to the attributable risk, is therefore independent of the background incidence. This property of consistency makes the relative risk more valuable than the attributable risk in evaluating whether a relationship is likely to be causal. Moreover, the relative risk can be derived, either directly or indirectly, from any of the main types of study.

An approximate confidence interval for δ_{exp}, based on cumulative incidence or prevalence, can be calculated using the formula for the difference between two unrelated proportions (see Chapter 14).Rothman (1986) gives a formula based on incidence rates. (This author also argues a distinction between attributable risk and attributable rate, depending on whether cumulative incidence or incidence rate, respectively, are used.)

Population attributable risk

The **population attributable risk (population attributable rate)**, δ_{pop}, is the difference between the incidence of disease in the total population and the incidence of disease in the unexposed group:

$$\delta_{pop} = \{(a+c)/n\} - \{c/(c+d)\}$$
$$= \{(a+b)/n\} \times \delta_{exp}.$$

This gives a direct indication of the amount of disease in the total population attributable to the risk factor.

Using the data in *Table 14.6*:

$$\hat{\delta}_{pop} = (41/3225) - (7/2434)$$
$$= 0.013 - 0.003$$
$$= 0.010.$$

Thus, the incidence of incontinence in the population during the period of observation, attributable to spaying, is 1 per 100, and, if bitches were not spayed, the incidence in the population could be expected to be reduced by 1 per 100.

The population attributable risk can only be calculated when disease morbidity in the total population is known.

Again, a population attributable 'risk', based on prevalence values, can be estimated directly in a cross-sectional study.

Kahn and Sempos (1989) describe methods for calculating a confidence interval for δ_{pop}.

Aetiological fraction

Population aetiological fraction

The **population aetiological fraction**, λ_{pop}, (lambda: Schlesselman, 1982), also termed the **aetiological fraction** (Last, 1988), **population attributable proportion** (Elwood, 1988), **population attributable fraction** (Ouelett *et al.*, 1979, Martin *et al.*, 1987), **attributable risk** (Lilienfeld and Lilienfeld, 1980), **population attributable risk per cent** (Cole and MacMahon, 1971), **population attributable risk** (Kahn and Sempos, 1989), is the proportion of the incidence in the population attributable to exposure to a risk factor. Therefore, it represents the proportion by which incidence in the population would be reduced if exposure were eliminated.

$$\lambda_{pop} = \{(RR-1)/RR\} \times f,$$

where f is the proportion of diseased individuals exposed to the causal factor, $a/(a+c)$.

Using the figures in *Table 14.6*:

$$\widehat{RR} = 14.95$$
$$f = 34/41,$$
$$= 0.829.$$

Thus:

$$\hat{\lambda}_{pop} = \{(14.95-1)/14.95\} \times 0.829,$$
$$= 0.77.$$

Thus, if spaying is causal, 77% of cases of PUI in the population are attributable to spaying. The population aetiological fraction, like the population attributable risk, is therefore an indication of the impact that removal of a causal factor would have on reduction in incidence in the population.

Other formulae for calculating λ_{pop} are:

1. $\lambda_{pop} = (\text{incidence}_{pop} - \text{incidence}_{unexposed})/(\text{incidence}_{pop})$ (Leviton, 1973),
   $$= \{(a+c)/n - c/(c+d)\}/\{(a+c)/n\};$$
2. $\lambda_{pop} = \{p(RR-1)\}/\{p(RR-1)+1\}$, where $p = $ proportion of population exposed, $(a+b)/n$ (Elwood, 1988);
3. $\lambda_{pop} = \delta_{pop}/\{(a+c)/n\}$ (Martin *et al.*, 1987);
4. $\lambda_{pop} = (RR_{pop}-1)/RR_{pop}$ (Martin *et al.*, 1987).

The population aetiological fraction can only be calculated directly when disease morbidity in the total population is known. However, it can also be estimated in case–control studies (if controls are representative of the healthy population):

$$\lambda_{pop} = 1 - [\{c(b+d)\}/\{d(a+c)\}];$$

Again, a value for λ_{pop}, based on prevalence values, can be estimated directly in a cross-sectional study.

Aetiological fraction (exposed)

The **aetiological fraction (exposed)**, λ_{exp}, also termed the **attributable proportion (exposed)** (Elwood, 1988), **attributable fraction (exposed)** (Martin *et al.*, 1987), **attributable risk (exposed)** (Kahn and Sempos, 1989), **attributable risk per cent (exposed)** (Cole and MacMahon, 1971) is the proportion of incidence in exposed animals attributable to exposure to a risk factor.

$$\lambda_{exp} = (RR-1)/RR.$$

Using the data in *Table 14.6*:

$$\hat{\lambda}_{exp} = (14.95-1)/14.95,$$
$$= 0.93.$$

Thus, 93% of incontinence in spayed dogs is attributable to spaying.

Other formulae for calculating λ_{exp} are:

1. $\lambda_{exp} = (incidence_{exposed}$
   $- incidence_{unexposed})/(incidence_{exposed})$
   $= \{a/(a+b) - c/(c+d)\}/\{a/(a+b)\};$
2. $\lambda_{exp} = \delta_{exp}/\{a/a+b)\}.$

It is estimated directly in a cohort study, and can be estimated indirectly in case−control studies, using the odds ratio approximation to the relative risk:

$$\lambda_{exp} = (\psi - 1)/\psi.$$

A value for λ_{exp}, based on prevalence, can be estimated directly in cross-sectional studies.

The derivation of confidence intervals for λ_{pop} and λ_{exp} is described by Kahn and Sempos (1989).

Measuring interaction

Interaction was introduced in Chapter 5 as occurring between two or more factors when the frequency of disease is either in excess of or less than that expected from the combined effects of each factor. If there is a plausible biological mechanism for the interaction, then **synergism** is said to occur when the frequency is in excess of the anticipated value, and **antagonism** when the frequency is less than the anticipated value.

Two models of interaction were also introduced in Chapter 5: **additive** and **multiplicative** models. Generally, the additive model is most appropriate in indicating the impact of interaction on incidence (Kleinbaum et al., 1982). Therefore, an additive model will now be described (details of both types of model are given by Kleinbaum et al. (1982) and Schlesselman (1982)). The model is based on additivity of excess risks.

The additive model

Consider two factors, x and y. If p_{00} is the incidence rate when neither factor is present, p_{10} is the incidence rate when x alone is present, p_{01} is the incidence rate when y alone is present, and p_{11} is the incidence rate when both are present, then:

$p_{10} - p_{00}$ = risk attributable to x,
$p_{01} - p_{00}$ = risk attributable to y.

If the combined effect of x and y equals the sum of their individual effects, then:

$$(p_{11} - p_{00}) = (p_{10} - p_{00}) + (p_{01} - p_{00}),$$

and there is no interaction.

Lack of interaction can be expressed in terms of the excess relative risk, by dividing the formula above by p_{00}:

$$(p_{11}/p_{00} - 1) = (p_{10}/p_{00} - 1) + (p_{01}/p_{00} - 1).$$

The relative risk when both factors are present is denoted by $RR_{xy} = p_{11}/p_{00}$; the relative risks when x or y is present alone are denoted by $RR_x = p_{10}/p_{00}$ and $RR_y = p_{01}/p_{00}$, respectively. Thus:

$$(RR_{xy} - 1) = (RR_x - 1) + (RR_y - 1),$$

that is:

$$RR_{xy} = 1 + (RR_x - 1) + (RR_y - 1).$$

If more than two factors, j say, are being considered, then the combined relative risk, RR_m, for these is given by:

$$RR_m = 1 + \sum_{i=1}^{j} (RR_i - 1),$$

where $RR_1, \ldots, RR_j$ denote the individual relative risks.

Examples of positive interaction, based on an additive model, are given in *Table 15.7*, using the raw data in *Table 15.6* relating to the feline urological syndrome (Willeberg, 1976).

Hypothesized causal factors in males are feeding high levels of dry cat food, castration, and low levels of outdoor activity. The background risk, $(RR = 1)$, is therefore represented by entire male cats consuming low levels of dry cat food, and with high levels of outdoor activity.

Consider the two factors: low levels of outdoor activity and high levels of dry cat food intake. The estimated relative risk associated with low levels of outdoor activity and low levels of dry cat food intake in entire males is 3.43 (*a* in *Table 15.6*). The relative risk associated with high levels of dry cat food and high levels of outdoor activity is 4.36 (*b* in *Table 15.6*). Therefore, applying the additive model for these two factors (*Table 15.7*):

$$\widehat{RR}_m = 1 + (3.43 - 1) + (4.36 - 1),$$
$$= 6.79 \ (c \ in \ Table \ 15.7).$$

The estimated combined relative risk for these two factors is 6.00 (*d* in *Tables 15.6* and *15.7*).

Thus, there is no evidence for interaction between high levels of dry cat food and low levels of outdoor activity because the estimated combined relative risk (6.00) is similar to the expected combined relative risk, assuming no interaction (6.79). Similarly, there is no evidence of interaction between castration and low levels of outdoor

Table 15.6 Number of cases of the feline urological syndrome (FUS) and controls, and estimated relative risk values for combinations of categories within the factors, sex, diet and activity. (From Willeberg, 1976.)

Sex	Categories		No. of cats		Estimated relative risk ($\widehat{RR}$†)
	Level of dry cat food	Level of outdoor activity	Cases	Controls	
Entire male	Low	High	1	12	1
	Low	Low	2	7	3.43 (a)
	High	High	4	11	4.36 (b)
	High	Low	2	4	6.00 (d)
Castrated male	Low	High	5	12	5.00
	Low	Low	3	5	7.20
	High	High	14	5	33.60***
	High	Low	28	2	168.00***
Total no. of male cats			59	58	12.2**

**Significant at the 1% level; ***significant at the 0.1% level, by the χ^2 method.
†Odds ratio approximation, relative to unexposed group = entire cats with high levels of outdoor activity and receiving low levels of dry cat food.

Table 15.7 Comparison of estimated and expected relative risk values of the feline urological syndrome (FUS) for male cats for multiple excess risk category combinations based on an additive interaction model. (Adapted from Willeberg, 1976.)

Sexual status	Categories		Estimated relative risk ($\widehat{RR}$)	Expected relative risk based on additive model ($\widehat{RR}_m$)
	Level of dry cat food	Level of outdoor activity		
Entire	High	Low	6.00 (d)	6.79 (c)
Castrated	Low	Low	7.20	7.43
Castrated	High	High	33.60	8.36
Castrated	High	Low	168.00	10.67

activity. However, there is evidence of positive interaction between castration and high levels of dry cat food, and between castration, high levels of dry cat food and low levels of outdoor activity: in each case the estimated combined relative risk is greater than the expected combined relative risk, using the additive model.

A plausible biological mechanism for the interaction can be described, that is, synergism has occurred. Castration and high levels of dry cat food intake (usually associated with overfeeding) may both result in inactivity, thereby reducing blood flow to the kidneys, impairing kidney function, and therefore possibly promoting changes in the urine that are conducive to the formation of uroliths; this consititutes a possible common causal pathway.

Bias

Observational studies are subject to **bias** (see Chapter 9). Although many types of bias can occur in observational studies (Sackett, 1979), three are particularly pertinent to observational studies:

1. selection bias;
2. misclassification;
3. confounding.

Selection bias

Selection bias results from systematic differences between characteristics of the study population and the target population from which it was drawn. Most observational

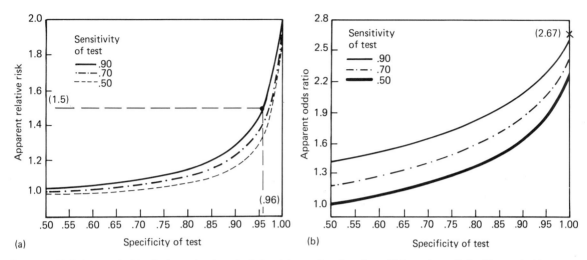

Fig. 15.2 (a) Cohort study: bias in the estimation of relative risk as a function of sensitivity and specificity. Disease incidence (cumulative) in exposed and unexposed cohorts is 0.10 and 0.05 respectively. True relative risk (exposed and unexposed) equals 2.0. (b) Case–control study: bias in the estimation of odds ratio as a function of sensitivity and specificity. Exposure in cases and controls 40% and 20% respectively. True odds ratio equals 2.67. (From Copeland *et al.*, 1977.)

studies use data gathered from convenient populations such as veterinary clinics, abattoirs and particular farms. Willeberg's investigation of the feline urological syndrome in Denmark (Willeberg, 1977), for instance, utilized data collected at a veterinary school's clinic. Ideally, a sample should be selected from the target population (all cats in Denmark in this example), but this is rarely possible. It was stated in Chapter 13 that the inferences from investigations that might be biased by selection need to be made with care if they are to be extrapolated to the target population. Consideration should be given to the likelihood of the study population being biased with respect to the disease and factors that are being investigated. Selection bias is unlikely if:

1. exposure to a factor does not increase the likelihood of an animal being present in the study population;
2. the likelihood of inclusion of cases and controls in the study population is the same.

For example, Darke *et al.* (1985) investigated the association between the presence of an entire tail (the hypothesized causal factor) and tail injuries (the disease) in a veterinary clinic population to determine whether docking reduces the risk of tail damage. It is improbable that docking or otherwise affects attendance at a veterinary clinic and so selection bias was unlikely in this study.

Misclassification

Misclassification is a type of measurement bias; it occurs when either diseased animals are classified as non-

diseased, or animals without a particular disease are classified as possessing it. The likelihood of misclassification depends on the frequency of disease, the frequency of exposure to the hypothesized causal factor and the sensitivity and specificity of the diagnostic criteria used in the study (see *Table 9.1* and *Figure 9.5*). For example, Thrusfield *et al.* (1985) studied the association between breed, sex and degenerative heart valve disease in dogs. Animals were classified as being diseased if they had either audible cardiac murmurs or signs of congestive cardiac failure. However, murmurs and cardiac failure can be produced by lesions other than heart valve incompetence — cardiomyopathy and anaemia are examples. Therefore, in order to prevent dogs with the latter two lesions being incorrectly classified as having heart valve incompetence (in which case they would constitute 'false positives'), their case records were scrutinized in detail to ascertain the exact nature of their murmurs. Similarly, early degenerative heart valve disease may not produce audible murmurs, and clinicians may miss the murmurs, in which case animals would be classified incorrectly as disease-free (i.e., 'false negatives').

Two types of misclassification can occur: **non-differential** and **differential**. The former occurs if the magnitude and direction of misclassification is similar in the two groups that are being compared (i.e., either cases and controls, or exposed and unexposed individuals). Non-differential misclassification produces a shift in the estimated relative risk and odds ratio towards zero (Copeland *et al.*, 1977) depicted in *Figure 15.2a* and

15.2b, respectively. *Figure 15.2a* illustrates that specificity is more important than sensitivity in determining bias in the estimate of relative risk. Even when sensitivity and specificity are seemingly acceptable (90% and 96% respectively, exemplified in *Figure 15.2a*), the relative risk can be severely biased. However, sensitivity plays a more important part as a source of bias in estimation of the odds ratio (*Figure 15.2b*).

Differential misclassification occurs when the magnitude or direction of misclassification is different between the two groups that are being compared. In this case, the odds ratio and relative risk may be biased in either direction (see Copeland *et al.*, 1977 for numerical examples). Therefore, misclassification can not only weaken an apparent association but also strengthen it.

If a simple, valid (i.e., highly specific and sensitive) test is not available, there can be difficulty in defining a case in the absence of a rigorous definition. For example, in an investigation of the relationship between enzootic bovine leukosis (EBL) and human leukaemia (Donham *et al.*, 1980), cattle were defined as being exposed to EBL virus when post-mortem examination revealed alimentary lymphosarcoma, even though this lesion may develop without exposure to the virus, and exposure to the virus may not produce alimentary tumours.

Similarly, it may be difficult to define and quantify an hypothesized causal factor to which an animal is exposed. For example, if 'inadequate feeding' is the factor, then the investigator may have to rely on an opinion based on owners' descriptions of diet, rather than using the more rigorous results of an examination by a nutritionist.

Confounding

Confounding was introduced in Chapter 3 where its effect on the inferring of causal associations was exemplified. In reiteration, a confounding variable (confounder) is any factor that is either positively or negatively correlated with both the disease and hypothesized causal factors that are being considered. For example, size of herd is a confounding variable in relation to porcine respiratory disease (see *Figure 3.7b*). If fan ventilation were being considered as the factor under study, then the results would be confounded (biased, confused, rendered unrepresentative) if the herds that were fan ventilated and that had respiratory disease comprised all large herds (which are likely to develop the disease), and the herds that were not fan ventilated and were non-diseased comprised all small herds (which are much less likely to develop the disease). The uneven proportion of large and small herds in each group therefore will confound the association between fan ventilation and disease, therefore distorting

the estimation of the odds ratio and relative risk.

Confounding is particularly important in case–control studies because animals are chosen according to presence and absence of disease: therefore cases may have a whole range of factors in common, some of which may be causal and some of which may be statistically significant but non-causal, because of an association with a confounder.

Confounding is not an 'all-or-none' event, but occurs to varying degrees, and can be accompanied by interaction, from which it should be distinguished. A pictorial representation of confounding is given by Rothman (1975). Identification of confounding and interaction are discussed by Breslow and Day (1980), Kleinbaum *et al.* (1982) and Schlesselman (1982), and described briefly below (see 'The Mantel–Haenszel procedure').

These three causes of bias (selection bias, misclassification and confounding) should not be considered in isolation but as an interconnected complex that can distort results.

Controlling bias

Selection bias

It is often not possible to control selection bias; this bias results from inherent characteristics of the study population, and a less biased study population may not be available.

Control can be attempted during either the design or analysis of the investigation. The former essentially involves avoiding the bias by selecting animals from a population that will not produce the bias. This may be impractical and obviously depends on the investigator being aware of the potential bias.

Control during analysis requires a knowledge of the probability of selection in the study population and the target population. Kleinbaum *et al.* (1982) provide formulae for this correction.

Misclassification

The control of non-differential and differential misclassification is described by Barron (1977) and Greenland and Kleinbaum (1983), respectively. Essentially, control is effected by algebraic manipulation during analysis, although this is never as satisfactory as using a highly sensitive and specific test to determine diseased and non-diseased cases.

Confounding

There are two simple methods of dealing with confounding:

1. by **adjusting** for the confounding variable in the analysis; for example, by using adjusted rates specific to the confounder (see Chapter 4), or by producing a summary odds ratio for the combined odds ratios of each level of confounder (Mantel and Haenszel, 1959);
2. by '**matching**' the two groups during the design of the study.

Additionally, more complex multivariate methods may be employed (see below). The control of confounding is discussed mainly in the context of case−control studies in this chapter. Breslow and Day (1987) discuss control in cohort studies.

The Mantel−Haenszel procedure: This technique produces a summary odds ratio which is the weighted average of individual odds ratios derived by stratifying data with respect to potential confounders. This approach is exemplified using the data in *Table 15.5*. The crude estimate of the odds ratio has already been calculated (2.99). The 95% confidence interval is 1.71, 5.23, suggesting an association between fan ventilation and pneumonia. However, herd size is also known to be associated with the prevalence of pneumonia **and** type of ventilation (Aalund *et al.*, 1976). Thus, herd size could be confounding the association between fan ventilation and pneumonia that was identified in the crude data (*Table 15.5a*). The first step in adjusting for this potential confounding is construction of a series of sub-tables, according to herd size (*Table 15.5b*). The stratum-specific odds ratios *differ* from the crude estimate of the odds ratio; this is indicative of confounding.

The Mantel−Haenszel summary odds ratio, ψ_{mh}, is given by:

$$\psi_{mh} = \{\Sigma(a_i d_i / n_i)\}/\{\Sigma(b_i c_i / n_i)\},$$

where a, b, c, d and n follow the same notation as *Table 15.1*.

$\Sigma(a_i d_i / n_i)$ and $\Sigma(b_i c_i / n_i)$ are calculated by summing the values of ad/n and bc/n, respectively, for each stratum. Thus, for the 'herd size ≤ 200' stratum, $a_i d_i / n_i = (2 \times 27)/40 = 1.35$, and $b_i c_i / n_i = (7 \times 4)/40 = 0.70$, and the stratum-specific odds ratio, ψ_i, is 1.93, and so on.

Thus:

$$\hat{\psi}_{mh} = (1.35 + 3.80 + 2.65 + 1.56 + 0.76)/$$
$$0.70 + 3.38 + 2.71 + 0.56 + 0.68),$$
$$= 10.12/8.03,$$
$$= 1.26.$$

An approximate 95% confidence interval is given by:

$$\hat{\psi}_{mh} \exp(-1.96\sqrt{\text{var}}), \ \hat{\psi}_{mh} \exp(+1.96\sqrt{\text{var}}),$$

where var = the variance of $\log_e \hat{\psi}_{mh}$

$$= \Sigma(w_i^2 v_i)/(\Sigma w_i)^2,$$

where $w_i = b_i c_i / n_i$,

and $\quad v_i = (a_i + c_i)/a_i c_i + (b_i + d_i)/b_i d_i.$

Thus, for the 'herd size ≤ 200' stratum:

$$w_i = (7 \times 4)/40,$$
$$= 0.70$$

and

$$v_i = (2 + 4)/(2 \times 4) + (7 + 27)/(7 \times 27),$$
$$= 0.75 + 0.180,$$
$$= 0.93,$$

and so on.

$$\Sigma(w_i^2 v_i) = 0.46 + 3.20 + 2.72 + 0.14 + 0.62,$$
$$= 7.14.$$

$$(\Sigma w_i)^2 = (0.49 + 11.42 + 7.34 + 0.31 + 0.46)^2,$$
$$= 20.02^2,$$
$$= 400.8.$$

Thus var $\log_e \hat{\psi}_{mh} = 7.14/400.8,$
$$= 0.018.$$

Therefore:

$$\hat{\psi}_{mh} \exp(-1.96\sqrt{\text{var}}), \ \hat{\psi}_{mh} \exp(+1.96\sqrt{\text{var}}),$$
$$= 1.26 \exp(-0.2630), \ 1.26 \exp(0.2630),$$
$$= 1.26 \times 0.769, \ 1.26 \times 1.301,$$
$$= 0.97, \ 1.64.$$

The adjusted odds ratio, 1.26, is much less than the crude odds ratio, 2.99, and its confidence interval includes 1, indicating that there is not a significant association between fan ventilation and pneumonia when the confounding effect of herd size has been removed.

Guidelines for the degree of stratification practised in the Mantel−Haenszel procedure are given by Breslow and Day (1980).

The Mantel−Haenszel procedure is applicable to estimation of summary odds ratios for all three types of study, and there is also a modification for summary relative risk estimation in cohort studies based on incidence rates (Kahn and Sempos, 1989).

The calculation of a summary, adjusted odds ratio implies that this adequately describes the data; that is, that the odds ratios in the different strata are *similar*. Tests are available that compare stratum-specific values with the summary value, distinguishing stratum-specific odds ratios that are genuinely different from those that are due to sampling variation, and testing the hypothesis that the summary estimate applies to all strata (Kahn and Sempos, 1989).

If there are major discrepancies in the stratum-specific values, either in the same or the opposite direction (i.e., some values being greater than 1, and others clearly less than 1), then the Mantel–Haenszel procedure should **not** be used. The summary statistic may disguise important real variation, and such results suggest that interaction is present; that is, the effect of the hypothesized causal factor is modified by the potential confounder.* This may indicate a biological mechanism for the interaction (i.e., synergism; see the example above relating to the feline urological syndrome) and so should be identified, quantified, reported and explained; multivariate techniques (see below) are appropriate. Confounding, in contrast, represents a source of bias which should be prevented or removed.

Matching: Matching is the process of making the groups that are being compared comparable with respect to a potential confounder. It can be undertaken in case–control and cohort studies, and can be performed in two ways:

1. **frequency matching**, in which the groups to be sampled are divided so as to contain the same proportion of the potentially confounding variable; for example, if there are four times as many males as females in the case group, then the control group also should be selected to contain four times as many males as females; this technique, therefore, is a form of stratification (see Chapter 13);
2. **individual matching**, a more precise form of matching in which each case is matched with a control with respect to the variable; for example, a 6-year-old dog with bladder cancer is paired with a 6-year-old dog without bladder cancer (matching for age).

Matching is useful when potential confounders are complex and difficult to measure or define (e.g., farm environments). Additionally, it can ensure comparability in terms of the information that is collected. However, it is cumbersome to match for many possible confounding variables. It is usual to match for the main possible ones: age, sex and breed (i.e., common determinants: see Chapter 5). As a general rule, if the confounding variable is unevenly distributed in the population (e.g., age in relation to chronic nephritis), then it is better to match cases or controls when the study is designed, rather than

correct for them in the analysis (all young control animals would, in a sense, be wasted when considering chronic nephritis). Unnecessary matching ('overmatching') should be avoided (Miettinen, 1970). If the effect of a factor is in doubt, then it is best not to match but to control it in subsequent analysis; **when a factor is matched, it cannot be studied separately**.

Matching is used to prevent confounding in cohort studies. However, in case–control studies the main value of matching is the enhanced efficiency in controlling confounding in subsequent stratified analysis (Rothman, 1986). (Matching can itself be a source of confounding in case–control studies, notably when the matched factor is correlated with the exposure factor but not with disease.)

Matched studies should be analysed as such. The simplest matched study involves 1:1 matching, where one matched control is chosen for each case (*Table 15.8*).

Table 15.8 Format for a 1:1 matched case–control study: numbers of pairs

	Controls exposed	Controls unexposed
Cases exposed	r	s
Cases unexposed	t	u

Matching results in the two groups being **related**; thus, McNemar's change test (see Chapter 14), rather than the χ^2 test, can be used to assess the significance of observed differences between exposure status in cases and controls. The formula for the odds ratio uses just discordant pairs:

$$\hat{\psi} = s/t.$$

The variance (var) of $\log_e \hat{\psi}$ is approximately equal to $(1/s + 1/t)$, and an approximate 95% confidence interval for large samples is again:

$$\hat{\psi} \exp(-1.96\sqrt{\mathrm{var}}), \ \hat{\psi} \exp(+1.96\sqrt{\mathrm{var}}).$$

Calculation of exact intervals is described by Schlesselman (1982).

The analysis of studies where the matching ratio is not 1:1, and where further stratification is also practised during analysis, is more complex (Elwood, 1988).

What sample size should be selected?

Appropriate sample sizes can be determined for cohort and case–control studies. The principles relating to sample size determination, outlined in Chapter 14, are

---

Effect modification is therefore also sometimes used to describe this interaction between factors (Miettinen, 1974).

followed. The examples below are conservatively based on two-tailed tests.

Cohort studies

Four values should be specified to determine optimum sample size in a cohort study:

1. the desired level of significance (α: the probability of a Type I error — claiming that exposure to a factor is associated with a disease when, in fact, it is not);
2. the power of the test ($1 - \beta$: the probability of claiming correctly that exposure to a factor is associated with disease, where β is the probability of a Type II error);
3. the anticipated incidence of disease in unexposed animals in the target population;
4. an hypothesized relative risk that is considered important enough, from the point of view of the health of the animal population.

The formula for an unmatched study in which exposed and unexposed cohorts are of equal size is:

$$n = \frac{(p_1 q_1 + p_2 q_2) K}{(p_1 - p_2)^2},$$

where:

n = number required in **each** cohort;
p_1 = anticipated incidence in unexposed animals;
$q_1 = 1 - p_1$;
p_2 = minimum incidence to be detected in exposed animals;
$q_2 = 1 - p_2$;
$K = (M_{\alpha/2} + M_\beta)^2$, where $M_{\alpha/2}$ and M_β are the respective multipliers associated with α and β.

For example, if a relative risk of 3 or more is to be detected, the anticipated incidence in unexposed animals during the period of the study is 1 per 100, and significance level and test power are set at 0.05 and 0.80 ($\beta = 0.20$), respectively, then:

$p_1 = 0.01$,
$q_1 = 0.99$,
$p_2 = 0.03$ (because the relative risk is set at 3),
$q_2 = 0.97$.

From Appendix XII,

$M_{\alpha/2} = 1.96$,
$M_\beta = 0.84$.

Therefore:

$K = (1.96 + 0.84)^2$,
$= 7.84$.

Thus:

$$n = \frac{(0.01 \times 0.99 + 0.03 \times 0.97) \times 7.84}{(0.01 - 0.03)^2}$$

$$= \frac{0.306}{0.0004}$$

$$= 765.$$

Therefore, a total of 1530 animals are needed for the study.

If a disease is rare, a cohort study requires a considerable number of animals in the exposed and unexposed groups to detect a significant difference, especially when the relative risk is small.

If the cohort sizes are different, a matched study is conducted, or a confounding factor is to be addressed, modifications of this formula are used (Elwood, 1988; Breslow and Day, 1987).

Case–control studies

Four values should be specified to determine optimum sample size in a case–control study:

1. the desired level of significance;
2. the power of the test;
3. the proportion of controls exposed to the risk factor;
4. an hypothesized odds ratio that is considered important enough, from the point of view of the health of 'the animal population.

The formula used to determine cohort sample sizes is used, but p_1 = proportion of cases exposed to the risk factor; and p_2 = proportion of controls exposed to the risk factor.

The value of p_1 is estimated from p_2, given the specified odds ratio:

$$p_1 = \frac{p_2 \times \psi}{1 + p_2 (\psi - 1)}.$$

For example, if an odds ratio of 4 or more is to be detected, the anticipated proportion of controls exposed to the risk factor is 0.05 (5%), and significance and test power are set at 0.05 and 0.80, respectively, first estimate p_1:

$$p_1 = \frac{0.05 \times 4}{1 + 0.05(4 - 1)}$$

$$= \frac{0.2}{1.15}$$

$$= 0.174.$$

Again, $K = 7.84$. Thus:

$$n = \frac{(0.174 \times 0.826 + 0.05 \times 0.95) \times 7.84}{(0.174 - 0.05)^2}$$

$$= \frac{1.499}{0.015}$$

$$= 100.$$

Therefore, a total of 200 animals are needed for the study.

If exposure to the risk factor is rare in the target population, a case–control study requires a considerable number of animals in the case and control groups to detect a significant difference, especially when the odds ratio is small.

If the case and control group sizes are different, a matched study is conducted, or a confounder is to be addressed when the study is designed, modifications of this formula are used (Elwood, 1988). Matching criteria and stratum sizes are discussed by Greenland *et al.* (1981).

Tables of the smallest and largest detectable relative risks and odds ratios, for different values of specified parameters, are given by Walter (1977). A program for determining sample size, which can be used on pocket calculators, is provided by Rothman and Boice (1982). Sample size estimations that include cost functions are described by Pike and Casagrande (1979).

Calculating the power of a study

The number of animals available for inclusion in a study may be limited (e.g., by financial constraints, availability or time). Additionally, a study may not detect a significant association between a risk factor and disease. In such circumstances, the investigation may have had insufficient **power**, and it is clearly useful to know the value of the study's power in detecting various levels of increased risk.

First, the value of M_β appropriate to the study is calculated. For a case–control study with groups of equal size, and a two-tailed test:

$$M_\beta = \sqrt{\frac{(p_1 - p_2)^2 n}{(p_1 q_1 + p_2 q_2)}} - M_{\alpha/2}$$

where p_1, q_1, p_2 and q_2 follow the same notation as that used in the formula for calculation of sample sizes in case–control studies, and n = number of animals studied in each group.

For example, suppose that a case–control study was

conducted to investigate the association between urinary incontinence and spaying in bitches, and that only 50 dogs were studied in each group. If 40% of control dogs were spayed then $p_2 = 0.40$. If a twofold increase in risk in spayed bitches is to be detected, then $\psi = 2$, and:

$$p_1 = \frac{p_2 \times \psi}{1 + p_2 (\psi - 1)}$$

$$= \frac{0.40 \times 2}{1 + 0.40(2 - 1)}$$

$$= 0.57.$$

Thus:

$$q_1 = 1 - 0.57$$
$$= 0.43;$$
$$q_2 = 1 - 0.40$$
$$= 0.60;$$
$$n = 50.$$

If the level of significance is 0.05, $M_{\alpha/2} = 1.96$, and:

$$M_\beta = \sqrt{\frac{(0.57 - 0.40)^2 \times 50}{(0.57 \times 0.43) + (0.40 \times 0.60)}} - 1.96$$

$$= \sqrt{\frac{1.445}{0.481}} - 1.96$$

$$= 1.73 - 1.96$$

$$= -0.23.$$

Appendix XII is now consulted. Note, though, that the value of M_β is negative* in this example, but, for brevity, the Appendix only tabulates β for positive values of M_β. However, the Appendix can still be used because the value of β for a negative M_β is 1 minus the value of β for a positive M_β. Thus, when M_β is negative, using the Appendix as if M_β is positive directly provides the power. The value of β corresponding to $M_\beta = 0.23$ is 0.4090, and this is therefore the power of the study. Thus, if the odds ratio in the target population were 2, a study comprising 50 cases and 50 controls would only have a 41% chance of finding that the sample estimate will be significantly ($\alpha = 0.05$) greater than 1.

Schlesselman (1982) gives an appropriate formula for determining power when case and control groups are of unequal size.

A similar calculation of power can be made for cohort

*Negative values of M_β indicate a power of less than 50%, whereas positive values point to a value greater than 50%.

studies, with:

p_1 = anticipated incidence in unexposed animals;
p_2 = minimum incidence to be detected in exposed animals.

Elwood (1988) gives an appropriate formula for determining power when exposed and unexposed cohorts are of unequal size.

The formula can also be used for power calculations in clinical trials (see Chapter 16) when outcome is measured as a proportion, and efficacy is assessed relatively. Cohen (1988) and Lipsey (1990) describe power calculations for absolute differences between proportions and between means.

Multivariate techniques

In case−control studies, if stratification is practised to adjust for confounding, there may be many 2 × 2 contingency tables, for example, for different combinations of age, sex, breed and management practices. The number of animals in each cell may then be small (even zero), resulting in inestimable or large confidence intervals that are statistically insignificant. Similarly, if the odds ratio varies considerably between each contingency table, interaction is present and calculation of a summary adjusted odds ratio is inappropriate. These problems can be overcome by using multivariate techniques which can consider the individual and joint effects of many factors simultaneously. These techniques (which are essentially mathematical models) also provide 'smoothed' estimates of the effects of factors by depressing variation induced by unimportant variables. A common method uses a **logistic model** (Schlesselman, 1982). This model is applicable to cohort studies but has been applied to case−control studies in particular because it is easily interpretable in terms of the odds ratio, and is introduced below. It is, however, more complex than the analytical methods described above, and therefore requires more intense study. In practice, appropriate computer programs are usually needed to 'fit' the model to data. It is presented formally below. Detailed descriptions of model building, including identification of interaction and confounding, are given in texts cited at the end of this chapter.

The logistic model

The logistic model derives its name from its use of natural logarithms ($\log_e$). It is based on a mathematical function which can be used to describe several biological phenomena including growth curves (see *Figure 7.3*) and dose−response relationships in biological assays.

It may be thought that a linear regression model (see Chapter 8) could represent the relationship between the probability of disease and the presence or absence of one or more risk factors, either alone or in combination. However, such a model may predict values which are outside the permitted range of probability of 0 to 1. Also, when fitting a linear regression model, the variance of the response variable is assumed to be a constant, independent of the values of the explanatory variables. This is not the case with a binary response variable — presence or absence of disease in this context — where the variance is proportional to $P(1-P)$, where P is the true, but unknown, probability of disease.

These problems are overcome by using a **logistic transformation**.* Let P be the probability of disease occurrence ($0 < P < 1$). The logistic transformation of P is defined to be $\log_e\{P/(1-P)\}$ where $P/(1-P)$ is the odds of developing disease. Define the transformed variable to be y, say, so that $y = \log_e\{P/(1-P)\}$. This transformation can take values ranging from 'minus infinity' when $P = 0$, to 'plus infinity' when $P = 1$ (i.e., it is unrestricted). Linear regression techniques may then be applied to this transformed variable. The function $\log_e\{P/(1-P)\}$ is known as the **logit** of P. Once a value of y has been predicted, the corresponding value for $P = \exp(y)/\{1+\exp(y)\}$. (Note that this takes values in the range 0 to 1.)

Now consider the simple 2 × 2 contingency table (*Table 15.1*). Suppose, in a cohort study, that a proportion, p, of animals was exposed at the beginning of the study. Denote by P_0 the probability of an exposed animal developing disease, and by P_1 the corresponding probability for an unexposed animal. Let Q_0 and Q_1 be $1-P_0$ and $1-P_1$, respectively; and $q = 1-p$. The expected proportions of animals falling into each of the four cells of the contingency table are given in *Table 15.9*.

The odds ratio, ψ, = $(P_0 \times Q_1)/(P_1 \times Q_0)$.

The logarithm of the odds ratio, β, may be expressed as:

$$\beta = \log_e \psi,$$
$$= \text{logit } (P_0) - \text{logit } (P_1),$$

the difference between the two logits.

This formulation is in the context of cohort studies; however, the same model can be applied to case−control studies in which the interpretation of the parameters β_i is essentially the same.

*Other transformations that have been suggested are the **probit** transformation (Finney, 1971) and the **complementary log−log** transformation (Collett, 1991).

Table 15.9 The expected proportions of animals falling into each of the four cells of the 2×2 contingency table constructed in observational studies, given the probabilities P_0 (P_1) of exposed (unexposed) animals developing disease, and the proportion, p, of animals exposed at the beginning of the study.

	Diseased animals	Non-diseased animals	Total
Animals exposed to the risk factor	pP_0	pQ_0	p
Animals not exposed to the risk factor	qP_1	qQ_1	q
Total	$pP_0 + qP_1$	$pQ_0 + qQ_1$	1

An example of expansion of the logistic regression model: a case – control study of vaccinal efficacy against canine infectious tracheobronchitis (kennel cough)

Canine kennel cough is a multifactorial disease in which several infectious agents have been incriminated (*Table 15.10*). Vaccines are available for protection against *Bordetella bronchiseptica*, CPIV, CAV-1, CAV-2 and CDV. However, isolation of specific causal agents is rarely justified and frequently impractical in the field and so direct assessment of the efficacy of the individual vaccines is impossible. However, an indirect assessment can be made by comparing the probability of disease in dogs vaccinated with various combinations of vaccine with the probability in unvaccinated dogs. Thus, several explanatory variables (the vaccines) are being considered simultaneously.

A suitable approach would be to conduct a case – con-

Table 15.10 Microorganisms incriminated in kennel cough. (Modified from Thrusfield, 1992.)

Major microorganisms	Minor microorganisms
Bordetella bronchiseptica	*Bacillus* spp.
Canine parainfluenza virus	Canine adenoviruses
(CPIV)	Type 1 (CAV-1)
	Type 2 (CAV-2)
	Canine distemper virus (CDV)
	Corynebacterium pyogenes
	Mycoplasma spp.
	Pasteurella spp.
	Staphylococcus spp.
	Streptococcus spp.

trol study of cases using data collected from general practices by questionnaire (Thrusfield *et al.*, 1989a). In this instance, the *unvaccinated* state constitutes a risk factor for developing kennel cough, and vaccinal efficacy is therefore defined in relation to a **reduction** in the estimated odds ratio in vaccinated dogs relative to unvaccinated dogs.

Vaccinal status, x, is a dichotomous variable which needs to be coded '0' indicating absence of vaccination ('exposed'), and '1' indicating its presence ('unexposed'). This type of variable is called a 'dummy' or 'indicator' variable because it has no numerical significance.

The derivation of the logistic regression model in this context is eased by the use of slightly different notation.

Thus, let $P(x)$ be the probability of a dog developing kennel cough if its vaccinal status is x. Then:

$$P(1) = P_1,$$
$$P(0) = P_0.$$

Write:

$$r(x) = \frac{P(x)Q_0}{P_0 Q(x)}$$

Then $\log_e r(x) = \log_e \{P(x)/Q(x)\} - \log_e(P_0/Q_0)$

and $\text{logit}\{P(x)\} = \text{logit}(P_0) + \log_e\{r(x)\}$.

Let $\alpha = \text{logit}(P_0)$.

Then $\text{logit}\{P(x)\} = \alpha + \log_e\{r(x)\}$.

When $x = 0$, $\text{logit}\{P(x)\} = \text{logit}\{P(0)\} = \alpha$, by definition.

Thus, $\log_e\{r(0)\} = 0$.

Let $\beta = \log_e\{r(1)\}$.

Then $\text{logit}\{P(x)\}$ may be written in the linear form $\alpha + \beta x$, where x is a dummy variable taking the values 0 (exposed) and 1 (unexposed).

Thus:

$$\text{logit}\{P(x)\} = \alpha + \beta x,$$

and a simple linear logistic (log-linear) model has been derived. There is one explanatory variable which takes the values 0 (exposed, i.e. unvaccinated) or 1 (unexposed, i.e. vaccinated) to a specific vaccine.

The two parameters, α and β, in the model, and the two risks correspond perfectly such that:

$$P_1 = P(1)$$
$$= \exp(\alpha+\beta)/1\{1 + \exp(\alpha+\beta)\}$$

and:

$P_0 = \exp(\alpha)/\{1 + \exp(\alpha)\}$.

In this example, β will be less than zero. A negative value of β indicates that dogs that have not been vaccinated have a higher risk of developing kennel cough than those that have been vaccinated.

This formulation extends naturally to the situation where there are two vaccines. Define the dichotomous 'dummy' variable x_i to be 1 or 0 according to a dog's vaccinal status against vaccine i, where i may take the value 1 or 2, corresponding to the two possible vaccines. Thus, $x_1 = 1$ indicates that the dog was vaccinated with vaccine 1; $x_1 = 0$ indicates that the dog was not vaccinated with vaccine 1; $x_2 = 1$ indicates that the dog was vaccinated with vaccine 2; $x_2 = 0$ indicates that the dog was not vaccinated with vaccine 2; (x_1,x_2) indicates the dog's vaccinal status with vaccines 1 and 2.

Define $P(x_1,x_2)$ as the disease probability corresponding to vaccinal status (x_1,x_2), and $r(x_1,x_2)$ as the odds ratio of $P(x_1,x_2)$ relative to the exposed (unvaccinated) category $x_1 = x_2 = 0$. (This represents the inverse of the usual ratio in observational studies, where the relative risk and odds ratio are relative to the *unexposed* category because exposure is usually in terms of presence, rather than absence, of a factor. Recall that exposure is defined as *absence* of vaccination.) These odds ratios and, equivalently, the probabilities, may be expressed using the model:

$$\log_e\{r(x_1,x_2) = (\beta_1 x_1) + (\beta_2 x_2) + (\gamma x_1 x_2),$$

or

$$\text{logit}\{P(x_1,x_2)\} = \alpha + (\beta_1 x_1) + (\beta_2 x_2) + (\gamma x_1 x_2).$$
(Equation 1)

In this example, there are four parameters, α, β_1, β_2 and γ, to describe four probabilities, $P(0,0)$, $P(0,1)$, $P(1,0)$ and $P(1,1)$ (summarized as $P(x_1,x_2)$), and therefore the model is termed 'saturated'. The model makes no assumptions about the association between disease status and exposure status. The log odds ratios for the individual exposures are given by:

$$\beta_1 = \log_e\{r(1,0)\}$$
$$\beta_2 = \log_e\{r(0,1)\}$$
$$\gamma = \log_e[\{r(1,1)\}/\{r(1,0) \times r(0,1)\}]$$
$$= \text{logit}\{P(1,1)\} - \text{logit}\{P(1,0)\} - \text{logit}\{P(0,1)\}$$
$$+ \text{logit}\{P(0,0)\}.$$

The parameter γ is an **interaction** parameter, and the function, $\exp(\gamma)$, of γ is an indication of any statistical interaction between factors. In this model, interaction is *multiplicative* and represents the multiplicative factor by which the odds ratio for those animals vaccinated with

both vaccines differs from the product of the odds ratios for those receiving only one of the individual vaccines. If $\gamma > 0$, there is interaction and the reduction in risk of developing kennel cough for dogs that have received both vaccines is not as great as that predicted by simply multiplying the effects, as measured by the corresponding odds ratios, of giving each vaccine separately (and the converse if $\gamma < 0$). If $\gamma = 0$ (no interaction), then the reduction in the risk of developing kennel cough for dogs that have received both vaccines is that predicted simply by multiplying the effects of giving each vaccine separately.

It is possible to test the hypothesis that $\gamma = 0$ for a given data set and, if this hypothesis is not rejected, to fit the reduced model which excludes the interaction parameter:

$$\text{logit}\{P(x_1,x_2)\} = \alpha + (\beta_1 x_1) + (\beta_2 x_2). \text{ (Equation 2)}$$

In this circumstance, β_1 now represents the $\log_e \psi$ for vaccine 1 relative to not receiving vaccine 1, whether or not the dog has been vaccinated with vaccine 2. This is a different interpretation than that from the saturated model (Equation 1). In the saturated model, β_1 represents the $\log_e \psi$ for vaccine 1 at level 0 (not vaccinated) of vaccine 2 whereas, in the reduced model, β_1 represents the $\log_e \psi$ for vaccine 1 independent of the level of vaccine 2. Testing the hypothesis $\beta_1 = 0$ in the reduced model is equivalent to testing the hypothesis that vaccine 1 has no effect on risk, against the alternative hypothesis that there is an effect, but one that does not depend on vaccine 2.

This approach can be easily generalized to incorporate the effects of more than two vaccines. Thus, for five vaccines, the extension to the reduced model (Equation 2) is given by:

$$\text{logit}\{P(x_1,x_2,x_3,x_4,x_5) = \alpha + (\beta_1 x_1) + (\beta_2 x_2) + (\beta_3 x_3) + (\beta_4 x_4) + (\beta_5 x_5).$$

If a better fit is provided by a model that includes some interaction terms, it is important to assess the significance of the interaction.

The results of the case−control study are presented in *Table 15.11*. The background risk (equivalent to $\alpha = \text{logit}(P_0)$) is represented by dogs vaccinated against CDV because all dogs in the study were vaccinated against this virus. Efficacy of CDV vaccine therefore was not considered.

The model was fitted to these data using an appropriate statistical package (Generalised Linear Interactive Modelling, GLIM: Payne, 1986), the best fit being provided by one that included some interaction terms. The estimated values of the parameters for various vaccine combinations in the model, and their associated

Table 15.11 Estimates and their associated standard errors of the log odds ratio* in favour of a kennel cough case for each of five vaccines and their associated interactions relative to vaccination only with canine distemper virus vaccine. (From Thrusfield *et al.*, 1989a.)

Vaccine	Estimated log odds ratio $(log_e\hat{\psi})$	Standard error of $log_e\hat{\psi}$
B. bronchiseptica	-0.3	0.48
CPIV	-2.0	0.53
CAV-1 (inactivated)	-0.7	0.21
CAV-1 ('live')	-2.8	0.84
CAV-2	-0.2	0.26
B. bronchiseptica + CPIV	1.3	0.42
B. bronchiseptica + CAV-1 (inactivated)	0.8	0.55
B. bronchiseptica + CAV-1 ('live')	-2.2	0.78
CPIV + CAV-1 (inactivated)	2.7	0.69
CPIV + CAV-1 ('live')	3.8	0.99
B. bronchiseptica + CAV-2	-1.5	0.56
CPIV + CAV-2	1.1	0.57

*A reduction is indicated by a negative value, and an increase by a positive value.

Table 15.12 The relationship between 'dummy' variables and vaccinal status. (From Thrusfield *et al.*, 1989a.)

'Dummy' variable	Value of 'dummy' variable	Vaccinal status
x_1	1	*B. bronchiseptica* given
	0	*B. bronchiseptica* not given
x_2	1	CPIV given
	0	CPIV not given
x_3	1	CAV-1 (inactivated) given
	0	CAV-1 (inactivated) not given
x_4	1	CAV-1 ('live') given
	0	CAV-1 ('live') not given
x_5	1	CAV-2 given
	0	CAV-2 not given

standard errors, are given in *Table 15.11*. The model that was fitted is thus:

$$\text{logit}\{P(x_1,x_2,x_3,x_4,x_5) = -0.3x_1 - 2.0x_2 - 0.7x_3 - 2.8x_4 - 0.2x_5 + 1.3x_1x_2 - 0.8x_1x_3 - 2.2x_1x_4 + 2.7x_2x_3 + 3.8x_2x_4 - 1.5x_1x_5 + 1.1x_2x_5,$$

where $x_1, \ldots, x_5$ are defined in *Table 15.12*.

The model may be used to predict the effect of various vaccine combinations. For example, the $log_e\hat{\psi}$ for a dog vaccinated against CDV, *B. bronchiseptica* and CAV-2

(for which $x_1 = 1$, $x_2 = x_3 = x_4 = 0$, $x_5 = 1$) is calculated from the results in *Table 15.11* thus: $-0.3 - 0.2 - 1.5 = -2.0$. This computation includes the main effects of the individual vaccines (the first two numbers) and the interaction (the third number).

Table 15.13. presents the results for the usual combinations of vaccines. Interactions are present, for example, that between *B. bronchiseptica* and CPIV vaccines. This could be explained biologically by the potentiating effect of prior inapparent infection with *B. bronchiseptica* on CPIV infection (Wagener *et al.*, 1984). This could result in more CPIV infections being manifest clinically in dogs

Table 15.13 Estimates and their associated standard errors of the log odds ratio* in favour of a kennel cough case for common combinations of vaccine, relative to vaccination with canine distemper virus vaccine only. (From Thrusfield *et al.*, 1989a.)

Vaccine combination	Estimated log odds ratio ($log_e\psi$)	Standard error of $log_e\psi$
CDV + CAV-1 (inactivated) + *B. bronchiseptica*	− 1.8	0.33
CDV + CAV-1 (inactivated) + CPIV	− 0.1	0.50
CDV + CAV-1 (inactivated) + *B. bronchiseptica* + CPIV	0.1	0.61
CDV + CAV-1 ('live') + *B. bronchiseptica*	− 5.3	1.04
CDV + CAV-1 ('live') + CPIV	− 1.0	0.27
CDV + CAV-1 ('live') + *B. bronchiseptica* + CPIV	− 2.3	0.45
CDV + CAV-2 + *B. bronchiseptica*	− 2.0	0.32
CDV + CAV-2 + CPIV	− 1.2	0.24
CDV + CAV-2 + *B. bronchiseptica* + CPIV	− 1.7	0.85

*A reduction is indicated by a negative value, and an increase by a positive value.

with both infections, and would therefore explain why *B. bronchiseptica* vaccine could have a protective effect against CPIV-induced kennel cough. Equally, however, it could simply have resulted from combined vaccination with these two vaccines occurring in dogs that had an increased risk of infection (e.g., in dogs that were vaccinated electively against these two major microorganisms because they were being kennelled), in which circumstance the interaction is interpreted predictively.

The log odds ratio can be converted to the odds ratio by taking the antilog$_e$. Thus, for the combination of CDV, CAV-1 ('live') and *B. bronchiseptica* vaccines, the $log_e\psi$ is −5.3, and antilog$_e$ −5.3 = 0.005.

The associated standard error of the $log_e\psi$ is 1.04. An approximate 95% confidence interval for $log_e\psi$ can be constructed using the Normal approximation:

$$-5.3 \pm (1.96 \times 1.04),$$
$$= -5.3 \pm 2.04,$$
$$= -7.34, -3.26.$$

Thus, the 95% confidence interval for the odds ratio = $e^{-7.43}$, $e^{-3.26}$, = 0.00065, 0.038. This interval clearly excludes 1 and so the reduction in risk of kennel cough associated with this combination of vaccines is statistically significant at the 5% level. This multivariate model can therefore be used to identify which combinations of vaccines predict the greatest reduction in the risk of kennel cough in the field.

Comprehensive discussions of the application of multivariate methods to observational studies are presented by Breslow and Day (1980, 1987), Kleinbaum *et al.* (1982) and Schlesselman (1982).

Some examples of observational studies which include both simple and multivariate analyses are listed in *Table 15.14* (pp. 242−55).

Further reading

Breslow. N.E. and Day, N.E. (1980) *Statistical Methods in Cancer Research, Vol. 1: The Analysis of Case−Control Studies*. IARC Scientific Publications No. 32. International Agency on Cancer Research, Lyon

Breslow, N.E. and Day, N.E. (1987) *Statistical Methods in Cancer Research, Vol. 2: The Design and Analysis of Cohort Studies*. IARC Scientific Publications No. 82. International Agency on Cancer Research, Lyon

Collett, D. (1991) *Modelling Binary Data*. Chapman and Hall, London. (*Describes the application of the logistic model to observational studies*)

Elwood, J.M. (1988) *Causal Relationships in Medicine. A Practical System for Critical Appraisal*. Oxford University Press, Oxford

Fleiss, J.L. (1981) *Statistical Methods for Rates and Proportions*, 2nd edn. John Wiley, New York

Kelsey, J.L., Thompson, W.D. and Evans, A.S. (1986) *Methods in Observational Epidemiology*. Oxford University Press, New York and Oxford

Kleinbaum, D.G., Kupper, L.L. and Morganstern, H. (1982) *Epidemiologic Research. Principles and Quantitative Measures*. Lifetime Learning Publications, Belmont

Rothman, K.J. (1986) *Modern Epidemiology*. Little, Brown & Co., Boston and Toronto

Schlesselman, J.J. (1982) *Case−Control Studies: Design, Conduct, Analysis*. Oxford University Press, New York and Oxford

Table 15.14 Some veterinary observational studies.

Species	Disease*	Hypothesized risk factors	Source
Ox, horse, pig, dog, cat	Congenital defects	Species, institution, for dogs and horses: breed	Priester *et al.* (1970)
Ox, horse, pig, dog, cat	Congenital umbilical and inguinal hernias	Breed, sex	Hayes (1974a)
Ox, horse, dog, cat	Congenital ocular defects	Breed, sex	Priester (1972a)
Ox, horse, dog, cat	Nervous tissue tumours	Breed, sex, age	Hayes *et al.* (1975)
Ox, horse, dog, cat	Oral and pharyngeal cancer	For dogs: sex, age, size of urban area	Dorn and Priester (1976)
Ox, horse, dog, cat	Pancreatic carcinoma	For dogs: breed, sex, age	Priester (1974b)
Ox, horse, dog, cat	Skin tumours	Breed, sex, age, annual sunlight	Priester (1973)
Ox, horse, dog, cat	Various tumours	Breed, sex, age	Priester and Mantel (1971); Priester and McKay (1980)
Horse, dog, cat	Tumours of the nasal passages and paranasal sinuses	Age For dogs: breed	Madewell *et al.* (1976)
Dog, cat	Dermatophytosis	Breed, sex, age	Sparkes *et al.* (1993)
Dog, cat	Leukaemia – lymphoma	Breed, sex, age	Bäckgren (1965); Dorn *et al.* (1967); Priester (1967); Schneider (1983)
Dog, cat	Pleural and peritoneal effusions	Sex, age, other diseases	Steyn and Wittum (1993)
Dog, cat	Various tumours	Breed, sex, age	Dorn *et al.* (1968)
Badger	Mortality	Sex, age, infection with *Mycobacterium bovis*, ELISA test status to *M. bovis*	Wilesmith and Clifton-Hadley (1991)
Cat	*Cryptosporidium* spp. infection	Age, lifestyle (domestic versus feral)	Mtambo *et al.* (1991)
Cat	Cutaneous and oral squamous cell carcinoma	Sex, skin, colour, exposure to sunlight	Dorn *et al.* (1971)
Cat	Diabetes mellitus	Breed, sex, age, body weight	Panciera *et al.* (1990)
Cat	Feline immunodeficiency virus (serological)	Breed, sex, age, clinical signs	Sukura *et al.* (1992)
Cat	Feline infectious anaemia	Breed, sex, age, prior disease	Hayes and Priester (1973)
Cat	Feline leukaemia	Feline infectious anaemia	Priester and Hayes (1973)
Cat	Feline leukaemia and feline immunodeficiency virus-induced disease	Breed, sex, age	Hosie *et al.* (1989)
Cat	Fibrosarcoma	Feline leukaemia virus vaccination, rabies vaccination	Kass *et al.* (1993)

*In some studies, 'disease' is used loosely to describe the response variables.

Table 15.14 continued

Species	Disease	Hypothesized risk factors	Source
Cat	Hyperthyroidism	Breed, sex, age, other demographic characteristics, exposure to herbicides, pesticides and other potential trace agents, diet, medical history	Scarlett *et al.* (1988)
Cat	Urolithiasis	Breed, sex, age, neutering, season of year, diet, weight, level of activity, time of diagnosis	Willeberg (1975a, b, c, 1976, 1977, 1981); Willeberg and Priester (1976)
Dog	Bladder cancer	Breed, sex, location (areas of industrial activity) Passive smoking, environmental chemicals, insecticides, obesity	Hayes (1976); Hayes *et al.* (1981); Glickman *et al.* (1989)
Dog	Bone sarcoma	Body size	Tjalma (1966)
Dog	Carcinoma of nasal cavity and paranasal sinuses	Breed, sex, age, skull type	Hayes *et al.* (1982)
Dog	Cauda equine syndrome	Degenerative disk disease, lumbosacral transitional vertebrae	Morgan *et al.* (1993)
Dog	Chemodectomas	Breed, sex, age	Hayes (1975); Hayes and Fraumeni (1974)
Dog	Chronic liver disease	Breed, sex, age	Andersson and Sevelius (1991)
Dog	Chronic pulmonary disease	Breed, sex, age, environmental pollution	Reif and Cohen (1979)
Dog	Congenital heart disease	Breed, sex, other congenital defects	Mulvihill and Priester (1973)
Dog	Cranial cruciate ligament rupture	Age, sex, breed, body weight	Whitehair *et al.* (1993)
Dog	Cryptorchidism	Breed	Pendergrass and Hayes (1975)
Dog	Diabetes mellitus	Breed, sex, age, obesity	Krook *et al.* (1960); Marmor *et al.* (1982)
Dog	Ectopic ureter	Breed	Hayes (1974b, 1984)
Dog	Elbow arthrosis	History of the disease in parents	Grondalen and Lingaas (1991)
Dog	Elbow disease (mainly dysplasia)	Breed, sex	Hayes *et al.* (1979)
Dog	Eyelid neoplasms	Breed	Krehbiel and Langham (1975)
Dog	Haemangioma and haemangiosarcoma	Breed	Srebernik and Appleby (1991)
Dog	Heart valve incompetence	Breed, sex, age	Thrusfield *et al.* (1985); Häggström *et al.* (1992)
Dog	Heartworm infection	Breed, grouping (e.g., working, sporting, toy), sex, age	Selby *et al.* (1980)

Table 15.14   continued

Species	Disease	Hypothesized risk factors	Source
Dog	Hepatic angiosarcomas	Breed, sex, age	Priester (1976b)
Dog	Hip dysplasia	Breed, sex, size	Keller and Corley (1989); Priester and Mulvihill (1972)
		Season of birth	Hanssen (1991)
Dog	Hypospadias	Breed, sex	Hayes and Wilson (1986)
Dog	Infectious tracheobronchitis (kennel cough)	Vaccinal status against *Bordetella bronchiseptica*, canine parainfluenza virus and canine adenoviruses	Thrusfield *et al.* (1989a)
Dog	Intervertebral disc disease	Breed, sex, age, site of involvement	Goggin *et al.* (1970); Priester (1976a)
Dog	Lung cancer	Passive smoking	Reif *et al.* (1992)
Dog	Malignant neoplasms	Benign neoplasms	Bender *et al.* (1982)
Dog	Mammary neoplasia	Breed, sex, age	Frye *et al.* (1967); Moulton *et al.* (1970)
		Inbreeding	Dorn and Schneider (1976)
		Oestrus irregularity, pseudopregnancy, gestation history	Brodey *et al.* (1966)
		Body conformation, weight, diet	Sonnenschein *et al.* (1987, 1991)
Dog	Mastocytoma	Ancestry (breed grouping)	Peters (1969)
Dog	Mesothelioma	Domestic and owner's exposure to asbestos, urban residence, management, flea repellants	Glickman *et al.* (1983)
Dog	Multiple primary neoplasia (benign and malignant) involving the reproductive system	Sex, index tumours, for malignant neoplasms: benign neoplasms	Bender *et al.* (1984)
Dog	Obesity	Breed, sex, age	Krook *et al.* (1960); Edney and Smith (1986)
Dog	Oesophageal sarcoma	Infection with *Spirocerca lupi*	Ribelin and Bailey (1958)
Dog	Oral and pharyngeal neoplasms	Breed, sex, age	Cohen *et al.* (1964)
Dog	Osteochondritis dissecans	Breed, sex, age	Slater *et al.* (1991)
Dog	Perianal adenocarcinoma	Breed, neutering, age, weight	Vail *et al.* (1990)
Dog	Pancreatic islet cell tumours	Breed, sex, age	Priester (1974c)
Dog	Pancreatitis (acute)	Breed, sex, age	Cook *et al.* (1993)
Dog	Patellar dislocation	Breed, sex, size	Priester (1972b)
Dog	Patent ductus arteriosus	Breed, sex	Eyster *et al.* (1976)

Table 15.14 continued

Species	Disease	Hypothesized risk factors	Source
Dog	Progressive retinal atrophy	Breed, sex, age	Priester (1974a)
Dog	Prostatic hyperplasia (benign)	Age	Berry et al. (1986)
Dog	Pyometra	Breed	De Troyer and De Shepper (1989)
		Breed, age, obesity Oestrus irregularity, pseudopregnancy, gestation history	Krook et al. (1960) Fidler et al. (1966)
Dog	Renal tumours	Breed, sex, age	Hayes and Fraumeni (1977)
Dog	Respiratory tract neoplasms	Environment (urban versus rural)	Reif and Cohen (1971)
Dog	Salivary cyst	Breed, sex, age	Knecht and Phares (1971)
Dog	Splenic haemangiosarcoma and haematoma	Breed, sex, age	Prymak et al. (1988)
Dog	Tail injuries	Undocked tails	Darke et al. (1985)
Dog	Testicular neoplasia	Breed, sex, age, cryptorchidism	Hayes and Pendergrass (1976); Hayes et al. (1985); Reif and Brodey (1969); Reif et al. (1979); Thrusfield et al. (1989b); Weaver (1983)
Dog	Thyroid neoplasms	Breed, sex, age	Hayes and Fraumeni (1975)
Dog	Transmissible venereal tumour	Breed, sex, age, management, other integumentary and genital diseases	Batamuzi et al. (1992)
Dog	Urethral cancer	Breed, sex, age	Wilson et al. (1979)
Dog	Urinary incontinence (female)	Breed, size, neutering, docking	Holt and Thrusfield (1993); Thrusfield (1985c)
Dog	Urinary tract infection (female)	Reproductive history, concurrent disease, drug administration, veterinary procedures	Freshman et al. (1989)
Dog	Urolithiasis	Breed, sex	Bovee and McGuire (1984); Brown et al. (1977); Case et al. (1993)
Dog	Various tumours	Breed, sex, age	Cohen et al. (1974); Howard and Nielsen (1965); Rahko (1968)
		Exposure to uranium mill tailings	Reif et al. (1983)
Dog	Vena cava syndrome (Dirofilaria-associated)	Sex, age, body size	Ganchi et al. (1992)
Hare	Various diseases	Climate	Rattenborg and Agger (1991)
Horse	Basal sesamoidean fractures	Breed	Parente et al. (1993)

Table 15.14 continued

Species	Disease	Hypothesized risk factors	Source
Horse	Chronic endometrial disease	Age, parity	Ricketts and Alonso (1991)
Horse	Colic	Breed, sex, age, weight, history, management	Morris *et al.* (1989); Pascoe *et al.* (1983); Proudman (1992); Reeves *et al.* (1989); Sembrat (1975); White and Lessard (1986)
Horse	Cryptorchidism	Breed	Hayes (1986)
Horse	Fever (associated with influenza)	Age, vaccinal history, track	Bendixen *et al.* (1993)
Horse	Impaired reproductive performance	Age, management	Meyers *et al.* (1991)
Horse	Influenza	Breed, sex, age, vaccinal status, antibody titre, type of barn	Nyaga (1975); Townsend *et al.* (1991)
		Vaccinal status	Estola and Neuvonen (1976)
Horse	Laminitis	Breed, sex, castration	Dorn *et al.* (1975)
Horse	Laryngeal hemiplegia	Breed, sex, age	Beard and Hayes (1993)
Horse	Leptospirosis (serological)	Age, sex, other diseases	Park *et al.* (1992)
Horse	Navicular disease	Breed, sex, age	Lowe (1974)
Horse	Osteochondrosis	Breed, sex, age, weight	Mohammed (1990a)
Horse	Perioperative fatality	Breed, sex, age, type, time and duration of surgery, anaesthetic	Johnston (1994)
Horse	Potomac fever	Age, sex, location, management, transportation	Kiper *et al.* (1992)
		Premises, husbandry, management, previous history of the syndrome on premises	Perry *et al.* (1984b, 1986)
Horse	Racing history and performance	Sex, age, gait, previous racing history	Physick-Sheard (1986a,b); Physick-Sheard and Russell (1986)
Horse	Racing and training injuries	Age, track type and condition, environmental conditions, length of race, racing history, season, training methods	Hill *et al.* (1986); Mohammed *et al.* (1991a); Robinson *et al.* (1988); Rooney (1982)
Horse	*Salmonella* spp. infection	Breed, sex, presenting complaint, emergency admission, pre-surgical status, procedures (e.g., anaesthesia, antibiotic administration)	Hird *et al.* (1984, 1986)
Horse	Sarcoids	Breed, sex, age	Angelos *et al.* (1988); Mohammed *et al.* (1992); Reid and Gettinby (1994)

Table 15.14 continued

Species	Disease	Hypothesized risk factors	Source
Horse	Strangles	Population size, number of mares served, location, fencing and feeder type, water source, vaccinal status	Jorm (1990)
Horse	Sweet itch	Breed, sex, age, coat colour, topographical location, rainfall	Braverman et al. (1983)
		Sex, geographical region, country of origin	Brostrom and Larrson (1987)
Horse	Upper respiratory tract disease	Age, sex management, immune status	Townsend et al. (1991)
Horse	Uveitis	Breed	Angelos et al. (1988)
Opossum	Tuberculosis	Climate, body condition, demographic variables	Pfeiffer et al. (1991)
Ox	Abortion	Management and husbandry, genital infection	Lemire et al. (1991)
Ox	Anaplasmosis	Management practices, herd location (vegetation)	Morley and Hugh-Jones (1989)
Ox	Antibiotic milk residues	Management	Kaneene and Willeberg (1988)
Ox	Bluetongue	Location, climate (relative humidity, temperature, rainfall)	Ward (1991)
Ox	Brucellosis	Breed, sex, age	McDermott et al. (1987)
		Herd size, stabling, registration status, history of previous reactors, time of exposure, vaccination level, farm density, herd type, insemination methods, other management factors	Kellar et al. (1976); Pfeiffer et al. (1988)
		Breed, sex, age lactation, source	Bedard et al. (1993)
Ox	Caesarian section	Age, gestation length, sex of calf, breed of sire, dry period, previous history of caesarian section	Barkema et al. (1991)
Ox	Campylobacter fetus infection (serological)	Breed, age, location, antibodies to other organisms	Akhtar et al. (1990)
Ox	Conception rate	Bovine virus diarrhoea virus infection	Houe et al. (1993)

Table 15.14 continued

Species	Disease	Hypothesized risk factors	Source
Ox	Contagious bovine pleuropneumonia	Breed, sex, age	McDermott *et al.* (1987)
Ox	Culling	Various diseases	Martin *et al.* (1982b); Milian-Suazo *et al.* (1988, 1989); Oltenacu *et al.* (1990)
		Parity, stage of lactation, production	Milian-Suazo *et al.* (1988, 1989)
Ox	Cystic ovaries	Breed, parity, season, previous history of the condition, twinning, milk yield	Emanuelson and Bendixen (1991)
Ox	Decreased milk production	*Campylobacter fetus* (serological)	Akhtar *et al.* (1993a)
		Ketosis (subclinical)	Miettinen and Setälä (1993)
Ox	Dermatitis interdigitalis (in dairy calves)	Breed, age, housing, sole haemorrhages, nutrition, management	Frankena *et al.* (1993)
Ox	Diarrhoea (in calves)	Age, season, management Rotavirus, coronavirus, *Cryptosporidium* spp., *Salmonella* spp., enterotoxigenic *Escherichia coli*	Waltner-Toews *et al.* (1986a,b) Reynolds *et al.* (1986); Snodgrass *et al.* (1986)
Ox	Digital haemorrhages (in dairy calves)	Breed, age, housing, dermatitis interdigitalis, nutrition, management	Frankena *et al.* (1992)
Ox	Displaced abomasum	Age, medical history Parity, retained placenta, stillbirth, ketonuria, aciduria, metritis, milk fever	Willeberg *et al.* (1982) Markusfeld (1986)
Ox	Dystokia	Breed, season, management, other diseases	Bendixen *et al.* (1986a,b)
		Breed, dimension of dam and calf	Schwabe and Hall (1989)
		Previous history of dystokia Management, environment	Rowlands *et al.* (1986) Mohammed *et al.* (1991b)
Ox	Endometritis	Previous history of other diseases	Rowlands *et al.* (1986)
Ox	*Escherichia coli* (verocytotoxigenic) infection	Age, management	Wilson *et al.* (1993)
Ox	Foot-and-mouth disease (vaccine-related)	Vaccine type	Nicod *et al.* (1991)

Table 15.14 continued

Species	Disease	Hypothesized risk factors	Source
Ox	High milk somatic cell counts	Age, year, season, herd size, stage of lactation	Bodoh et al. (1976)
		Management, environment	Bodoh et al. (1976); Erskine et al. (1987); Hueston et al. (1987); Hueston et al. (1990); Hutton et al. (1991); Lindstrom (1983); Moxley et al. (1978); Osteras and Lund (1988a,b)
Ox	Hypomagnesaemia	Body condition, feed quantity and quality, location	Harris et al. (1983)
Ox	Impaired production	Bovine leukaemia virus infection	Jacobs et al. (1991)
Ox	Inactive ovaries	High milk yield after calving, long dry period, low milk yield prior to calving, parity, primary metritis, retained placenta, serum glutamate oxaloacetate transaminase activity, stillbirth, twinning	Markusfeld (1987)
Ox	Infertility (female)	Exposure to high voltage transmission lines	Algers and Hennichs (1985)
		Lameness	Collick et al. (1989)
Ox	Intramammary infection with *Staphylococcus* spp.	Management, environment, hygiene	Bartlett et al. (1992); Bartlett and Miller (1993); Dargent-Molina et al. (1988); Hutton et al. (1991)
Ox	Intramammary infection with *Streptococcus* spp.	Management, environment	Dargent-Molina et al. (1988)
Ox	Ketosis	Metritis, low milk yield before calving, long dry period	Markusfield (1985)
		Breed, previous history of ketosis and other diseases	Bendixen et al. (1987c); Rowlands et al. (1986)
Ox	Lameness	Breed, parity, pedal lesions, stage of lactation, herd size, herd milk production	Frankena et al. (1991a)
		Previous history of lameness	Rowlands et al. (1986)
		Parity, herd size, housing, nutrition, bedding	Groehn et al. (1992)
		Physical hoof properties	Tranter et al. (1993)
		Body weight, condition score, pedal anatomy	Wells et al. (1993a)

Table 15.14 continued

Species	Disease	Hypothesized risk factors	Source
Ox	Lameness	Environmental and behavioural factors	Chesterton *et al.* (1989)
		Season, location, soil type, housing, nutrition, foot care, floor type	Faye and Lescourret (1989)
		Season, herd size, management, veterinary practice	Rowlands *et al.* (1983); Wells *et al.* (1993b)
Ox	Laminitis (in calves)	Breed, age, management, feeding, housing	Frankena *et al.* (1991b)
Ox	Leptospirosis (infection with *L. interrogans*, serovar *hardjo*)	Local geography (e.g., presence of rivers, number of arable hectares), presence of other species of livestock and bulls, management (including rodent control)	Pritchard *et al.* (1989)
Ox	Mammary lesions	Breed, parity, season, milk yield, other diseases	Bendixen *et al.* (1986a, 1988b)
		Management	Grohn *et al.* (1988)
Ox	Mastitis	Age, herd size, stage of lactation, stage of dry period, season, winter housing	Francis *et al.* (1986); Pearson *et al.* (1972); Rowlands and Booth (1989); Wilesmith *et al.* (1986)
		Breed, manure system, stall and bedding, type, lactation number, other diseases	Bendixen *et al.* (1988a); Oltenacu *et al.* (1988)
		Udder and teat characteristics	van den Geer *et al.* (1988)
		Previous history of mastitis	Rowlands *et al.* (1986)
		Management, environment	Agger *et al.* (1986); Bendixen *et al.* (1986a); Pearson *et al.* (1972)
		Retained placenta	Schukken *et al.* (1988)
		Teat disinfection	Blowey and Collis (1992)
Ox	Mastitis caused by mycoplasmata	Herd size, percentage culled, production	Thomas *et al.* (1981, 1982)
Ox	Mastitis caused by *Nocardia*	Breed, herd size, milking management, dry cow therapy, housing	Ferns *et al.* (1991); Stark and Anderson (1990)
Ox	Mastitis caused by *Streptococcus agalactiae*	Herd size, herd location, participation in a dairy herd improvement scheme	Thorburn *et al.* (1983)
Ox	Mastitis (somatic cell counts/subclinical)	Milking characteristics, teat structure	Slettbakk *et al.* (1990)
		Teat disinfection	Blowey and Collis (1992)
		Teat lesions (presence and position)	Agger and Willeberg (1986)
		Management	Osteras and Lund (1988a,b)

Table 15.14 continued

Species	Disease	Hypothesized risk factors	Source
Ox	Metritis	Diet	Barnouin and Chacornac (1992)
Ox	Mortality (in calves)	Management, husbandry (e.g., corn silage feeding, penning, vaccination)	Martin et al. (1982c)
		Herd size, environment, management	Lance et al. (1992)
Ox	Ocular squamous cell carcinoma	Corneoscleral pigmentation	Anderson (1963)
Ox	Parturient paresis (milk fever)	Age, season	Dohoo et al. (1984)
		Breed, age, nutrition	Harris (1981)
		Breed, age, parity, male calves, twinning, production, pasture feeding, housing system, previous history of parturient paresis, retained placenta	Bendixen et al. (1986a, 1987b); Ekesbo (1966)
		Diet (in the dry period)	Barnouin (1991)
		Breeding	Mohammed et al. (1991b)
		Calving season, production potential, exercise, prepartum nutrition, parity	Curtis et al. (1984); Rowlands et al. (1986)
		Prepartum grain feeding	Emery et al. (1969)
		Month, herd size, type of housing, milk recording	Saloniemi and Roine (1981)
		Previous milk production	Dohoo and Martin (1984)
Ox	Periparturient and reproductive traits	Serum cholesterol and non-esterified fatty acid levels	Kaneene et al. (1991)
		Previous history of traits	Markusfeld (1990)
Ox	Physical injuries	Season, cow characteristics, disease, production	Enevoldsen et al. (1990)
Ox	Pneumonia (in calves)	Age, season, management	Walter-Toews et al. (1986a,b)
Ox	Production efficiency	Antibodies to bluetongue virus and *Mycoplasma bovis*	Uhaa et al. (1990a)
Ox	Pruritus, pyrexia, haemorrhagic syndrome	Citrinin (in citrus pulp pellets)	Griffiths and Done (1991)
Ox	Reduced survival period (in calves)	Various diseases	Curtis et al. (1989)
Ox	Repeat breeder syndrome	Herd characteristics, environment, management, other diseases, milk production	Lafi and Kaneene (1992)
Ox	Reproductive disorders	Other diseases	Saloniemi et al. (1988)
		Parity, milk yield	Grohn et al. (1990)
Ox	Reproductive performance	Antibodies to bluetongue virus, *Mycoplasma bovis* and *Campylobacter fetus*	Emanuelson et al. (1992); Akhtar et al. (1993b); Uhaa et al. (1990b)

Table 15.14 continued

Species	Disease	Hypothesized risk factors	Source
Ox	Reproductive performance	Bovine leukaemia virus infection	Emanuelson *et al.* (1992)
		Retained placenta, metritis	Sandals *et al.* (1979)
		Various diseases	Borsberry and Dobson (1989); Oltenacu *et al.* (1990)
Ox	Respiratory disease	Immune status, antibody level to various infectious agents	Caldow *et al.* (1988); Pritchard *et al.* (1983)
Ox	Retained placenta	Breed, age, parity, other diseases, sex of calf, previous history of the disease	Bendixen *et al.* (1987a)
		Diet (in the dry period)	Barnouin and Chassagne (1990)
Ox	Salmonellosis	Management, environmental and production variables	Bendixen *et al.* (1986a); Vandegraaff (1980)
		Previous history of retained placenta	Rowlands *et al.* (1986)
Ox	Stillbirth and neonatal morbidity and mortality (in beef calves)	Sex, dystokia, twins, age of dam	Wittum *et al.* (1991)
Ox	Tail-tip necrosis	Management, behaviour	Drolia *et al.* (1990)
Ox	Trypanosomiasis	Several variables relating to host population size, vectors, climate and ecological zones	Habtermariam *et al.* (1986)
Ox	Tuberculosis	Breed, sex, age, location, source	Bedard *et al.* (1993)
		Husbandry, farm characteristics, environmental factors	Griffin *et al.* (1993)
Ox	Variations in oestrus and fertility	Exposure to high voltage transmission lines	Algers and Hultgren (1987)
Ox	Various diseases	Age, other diseases	Bigras-Poulin *et al.* (1990)
		Bovine leukaemia virus infection	Emanuelson *et al.* (1992)
Ox	Winter dysentery	Age, management, previous outbreaks of the disease	Jactel *et al.* (1990)
Pig	Atrophic rhinitis	Season, housing	Cowart *et al.* (1992)
Pig	Aujeszky's disease	Herd size and type, date of outbreak	Mousing *et al.* (1991)
		Husbandry, housing, herd size, clinical signs of pseudorabies and *Actinobacillus pleuro-pneumoniae* infection, feeding, time since quarantine	Anderson *et al.* (1990)

Table 15.14 continued

Species	Disease	Hypothesized risk factors	Source
Pig	Aujeszky's disease (test status)	Herd size and type, location	Cowen et al. (1991)
		Age, management, vaccination, geographical density of herds	Weigel et al. (1992)
		Management, husbandry	Austin et al. (1993)
Pig	Carcass condemnations	Herd size, management, environment	Tuovinen et al. (1992)
Pig	Culling	Management and environment	D'Allaire et al. (1989)
		Various diseases	Stein et al. (1990)
Pig	Enzootic pneumonia	Sex, age, clinical disease, ventilation, herd size, replacement policy, diarrhoea	Aaland et al. (1976); Pointon et al. (1985); Willeberg et al. (1978)
		Season, housing	Cowart et al. (1992)
Pig	Impaired growth	Respiratory disease, antibodies to Mycoplasma hyopneumoniae	Fourichon et al. (1990)
Pig	Intestinal lesions associated with Campylobacter spp.	Open drains, slatted floors, feed medication	Pointon (1989)
Pig	Leg and teat damage	Floor type	Edwards and Lightfoot (1986); Furniss et al. (1986)
Pig	Pale, soft and exudative pork	Pre-slaughter processing factors	Spangler et al. (1991)
Pig	Pleuritis	Sex, various infections, management	Mousing et al. (1990)
Pig	Pseudorabies (see Aujeszky's disease)		
Pig	Reproductive failure	Breed, management factors, previous reproductive performance, behaviour	Madec (1988)
		Antibodies to Leptospira interrogans subgroup Australis	Pritchard et al. (1985)
Pig	Respiratory disease	Housing, vermin control, husbandry, management	Elbers et al. (1992); Hurnik and Dohoo (1991); Vraa-Andersen (1991)
Pig	Trichinosis (serological)	Management (including access to cats and exposure to wildlife)	Cowen et al. (1990)
Pig	Various diseases	Breed, previous history of diseases	Lingaas (1991a)
		Season	Lingaas and Ronningen (1991)
		Herd size, management	Lingaas (1991b)
Pig	Various lesions (at slaughter)	Environment, management	Flesja et al. (1982)
		Rearing system, herd size	Flesja and Solberg (1981)

Table 15.14 continued

Species	Disease	Hypothesized risk factors	Source
Poultry	Coccidiosis	Several variables relating to host population density, parasite control, health and management of hosts, and environment	Stallbaumer and Skryznecki (1987)
Poultry	Hydropericardium syndrome	Location, management, broiler strain	Akhtar *et al.* (1992)
Poultry	*Mycoplasma gallisepticum* infection	Hygiene	Mohammed (1990b)
Poultry	Salmonellosis	Geographical region, type of ventilation, flock size, farm type, management and hygiene, source of feed	Graat *et al.* (1990)
Sheep	Abomasal bloat (in young lambs)	Geographical area, type of floor, diet	Lutnaes and Simensen (1983)
Sheep	Hepatic lesions (especially due to *Cysticercus tenuicollis*)	Spreading of pig slurry, access to grazing land by hunts, infrequent use of canine cestocides	Jepson and Hinton (1986)
Sheep	Infectious kerato-conjunctivitis	*Mycoplasma conjunctivae, Branhamella ovis, Escherichia coli, Staphylococcus aureus*	Egwu *et al.* (1989)
Sheep	Intestinal adenocarcinoma	Exposure to herbicides	Newell *et al.* (1984)
Sheep	Listeriosis	Housing, feeding of silage	Wilesmith and Gitter (1986)
Sheep	Maedi-visna	Breed, age, ewe/lamb relationship Husbandry, management	Houwers (1989) Campbell *et al.* (1991)
Sheep	Mastitis	Nonclinical intramammary infection	Bor *et al.* (1989)
Sheep	Mortality (during marine transportation)	Age, body condition, season	Higgs *et al.* (1991)
Sheep	Orf	Age, frequency of the disease, mammary lesions, infected pasture, animal density, nutritional deficiencies, lambing period	Ducrot and Cimarosti (1991)
Sheep	Poor body condition	Periodontal disease	Orr and Chalmers (1988)
Sheep	Preweaning lamb mortality	Breed, sex, litter size, birth weight, causes of death	Yapi *et al.* (1990)
Sheep	Toxoplasmosis (serological)	Cats (neutered versus intact), kittens' nutrition, pigs, management	Waltner-Toews *et al.* (1991)

Table 15.14 continued

Species	Disease	Hypothesized risk factors	Source
Turkey	Fowl cholera	Management, vaccinal status, previous history of disease, other diseases	Hird *et al.* (1991)
Water buffalo	Osteomalacia	Season, parity, stage of lactation, serum phosphorus level	Heuer *et al.* (1991)
Water buffalo	Redwater	Season, parity, stage of lactation, serum phosphorus level	Heuer *et al.* (1991)

16 Clinical trials

The effects of some treatments are so marked that they are obvious, for instance the intravenous administration of calcium to cases of acute bovine hypocalcaemia. However, this is not true for many prophylactic and therapeutic procedures, where, for example, the advantages of a new drug over an established one may be small. Moreover, the observations of individual veterinarians provide insufficient evidence for determining efficacy.* In the past, treatment was often based on beliefs that had never been scientifically assessed; and anecdotal or unattested cures entered the veterinary and medical literature. Indeed, it has been estimated that only about 20% of human medical procedures have been evaluated properly (Konner, 1993), and many veterinary procedures have also been poorly evaluated (Shott, 1985; Smith, 1988; Bording, 1990). Conclusive evidence of efficacy is provided by a **clinical trial**.

Clinical trials date back to the 18th century, when they provided clues to the cause of disease. The provision of citrus fruits to English sailors prevented scurvy, indicating that the cause (subsequently shown to be vitamin C deficiency) was nutritional (Lind, 1753). Similarly, at the beginning of this century, improvement in the diet of inmates of some American orphanages and asylums cured and prevented pellagra, and suggested a nutritional cause of the disease, which hitherto had been considered to be infectious (Goldberger et al., 1923).

---

*A distinction is sometimes made between *effectiveness* and *efficacy* (Last, 1988). The former is the extent to which a procedure does what it is intended to do when applied in the day-to-day routine of medical or veterinary practice. The latter is the extent to which a procedure produces beneficial results under ideal conditions. A procedure may be efficacious but relatively ineffective if it is not taken up widely (e.g., if owners' compliance with the advice of the veterinarian is low).

Definition of a clinical trial

A clinical trial is a systematic study in the species, or in particular categories of the species, for which a procedure is intended (the target species) in order to establish the procedure's **prophylactic** or **therapeutic** effects. In veterinary medicine, effects may include improvements in production as well as amelioration of clinical disease. The procedure may be a surgical technique, modification of management (e.g., diet), or prophylactic or therapeutic administration of a drug. If the latter is being assessed, a clinical trial would also include studies of its pattern of absorption, metabolism, distribution within the body and excretion of active substances. This chapter focuses on assessment of efficacy, and, for brevity, describes all types of procedure as 'treatment'.

Randomized controlled clinical trials

The clinical condition of sick animals can be compared before and after treatment. However, interpretation of such an **uncontrolled** trial may be difficult because any observed changes could result either from the treatment or from natural progression of the disease. An essential feature of a well-designed clinical trial therefore is a comparison between a group receiving the treatment with a **control** group not receiving it; this is a **controlled clinical trial**.

The control group may be selected at the same time as the group receiving the treatment (a **concurrent** control group) or generated using historical data (a **historical** control group). Early clinical trials, such as Lister's assessment of antiseptic surgery (Lister, 1870), utilized historical controls, but this approach is open to criticism because of the various factors, unrelated to treatment, that can produce observed differences over a period of time (e.g., improvements in husbandry, changes in diagnostic criteria, disease classification and selection of animals, alterations in virulence of infectious agents, and reduction in the severity of disease). The net result of these problems is that studies with historical controls tend to exaggerate the value of a new treatment (Pocock, 1983). Concurrent control groups are therefore usually advocated.*

The control group may receive another (standard) treatment with which the first treatment under trial is being compared (a 'positive' control group), no treatment (sometimes called a 'negative' control group), or a **placebo** (an inert substance that is visually similar to the treatment under trial, and therefore cannot be distinguished from the treatment by those administering and those receiving the treatment and placebo).†

Bias (see Chapter 9) can occur in a trial if there is preferential assignment of subjects to treatment or control groups, differential management of the groups, or differential assessment of the groups. For example, a veterinarian may allocate animals only with a good prognosis to the treatment group. A central tenet of a controlled clinical trial is that subjects are assigned to treatment and control groups randomly (see Chapter 13) so that the likelihood of bias due to preferential allocation is reduced. This process of **randomization** should also balance the distribution of other variables that may be outcome-related (e.g., age), and guarantees the validity of the statistical tests used in the analysis of the trial.

Randomized controlled clinical trials therefore adopt the experimental approach (see Chapter 2) and closely resemble cohort studies (see Chapter 15).‡

*A notable early example of the use of concurrent controls was Pasteur's trial of an anthrax vaccine in sheep (Descour, 1922).
†The first placebo-controlled clinical trial was probably undertaken by the English physician, John Haygarth, at the end of the 18th century (Haygarth, 1800). At that time, a popular treatment for many diseases was the application of metal rods, called 'Perkins' tractors', to the body to relieve symptoms by the supposed electromagnetic influence of the metal. Haygarth made wooden imitation tractors, and found that they were as efficacious as the metal ones. In so doing, he demonstrated the 'placebo effect': the expectation that a treatment will have an effect is sufficient to produce an improvement. A placebo was originally a substance with no known therapeutic effect which was administered in the hope that the power of suggestion, alone, would alleviate symptoms (Latin: *placebo* = I shall be pleasing).
‡In the UK, randomized controlled clinical trials were introduced in the mid-1940s by Bradford Hill: the first to test the efficacy of pertussis vaccine, and the second to test the efficacy of streptomycin in the treatment of pulmonary tuberculosis (Doll, 1992).

Field trials

The term **field trial** is also applied to some veterinary clinical trials. Two characteristics of field trials have been identified:

1. the trial is undertaken on subjects 'in the field', that is, under husbandry and management practices typical of those under which the procedure is intended to be used (operational conditions);
2. the trial is frequently prophylactic and therefore relies on natural challenge to the treatment that is being assessed (e.g., assessment of the efficacy of a bacterial pneumonia vaccine would rely on vaccinated animals being naturally exposed to infection with the relevant bacterium during the period of the trial).

However, these characteristics only represent related circumstances under which clinical trials may be conducted (2 is a logical consequence of 1), and so a distinction between clinical and field trials is not maintained in this chapter.

Community trials

A **community trial** is a trial in which the experimental unit (see below) is an entire community. Community trials have been undertaken in human medicine; for example, the fluoridation of the public water supply to prevent dental caries.

Design, conduct and analysis

The trial protocol

The goal and design of a clinical trial should be documented in a **trial protocol**. This is required by regulatory organizations which assess the value and validity of the proposed trial, and also provides background information to veterinarians and owners who are asked to participate in the trial. The main components of a protocol are listed in *Table 16.1*.

The primary hypothesis

The first step in writing a protocol for a clinical trial is determination of its **major objective**, so that a **primary hypothesis** can be formulated. Thus, a primary hypothesis could be 'evening primrose oil has a beneficial effect against canine atopy' (Scarff and Lloyd, 1992). Several principal criteria of response might be assessed, but it is helpful if one particular response variable can be identified as the main criterion for testing the primary

Table 16.1 Components of a protocol for a clinical trial. (Modified from Noordhuizen *et al.*, 1993.)

General information
  Title of trial
  Names and addresses of investigators
  Name and address of sponsor(s)
  Identity of trial site(s)

Justification and objectives
  Reason for execution of the trial
  Primary hypothesis to be tested;
    Primary end point
  Secondary hypotheses to be tested

Design
  Response variables:
    Nature of response variables (level of measurement)
    Scoring system (for ordinal variables)
    Definition of efficacy (magnitude of the difference to be detected between treatment and control groups)

  Duration:
    Date of beginning
    Date of end
    Duration of disease under study
    Period for recruitment of cases
    Duration of treatment
    Drug withdrawal period (for food-producing animals)
    Decision rules for terminating a trial

  Experimental population:*
    The experimental unit
    Composition (e.g., age, sex, breed)
    Inclusion/exclusion criteria
    Post-admission withdrawal criteria
    Definition of cases/diagnostic criteria
    Case identification
    Selection of controls
    Sample size determination
    Owners' informed consent

  Therapeutic or prophylactic procedure:
    Dosage
    Product formulation and identification
    Placebo/standard treatment formulation and identification
    Method of administration
    Operators' safety
    Definition of stage at which administration stops
    Blinding technique
    Compliance monitoring
    Type of trial:
      Randomization
      Stratification variables
      Implementation of allocation process

Table 16.1 Continued

  Data collection:
    Data to be collected
    Frequency of data collection
    Method for recording adverse drug reactions
    Identification of experimental units
    Training/standardization of data collection and recording
    Confidentiality
    Communication between participants

  Data analysis:
    Technique for 'unblinding'
    Description of statistical methods
    Interpretation of significance levels/confidence intervals
    Approach to withdrawals and animals 'lost to follow up'

* Some authorities refer to the experimental population as the study population. The latter term is not used, to avoid confusion with study population defined as the population from which a **sample** of animals is drawn (see Chapter 13).

hypothesis; this is the **primary end point**. The following topics must be addressed in determining this end point:

1. which end points are the most *clinically* and *economically* important?
2. which of these can be measured in a reasonable manner?
3. what practical constraints (e.g., budgetary limits) exist?

Thus, the primary end point in the evening primrose oil trial might be the level of pruritus. Other end points could include the levels of oedema and erythema; these constitute **secondary end points**.

The response variables that are used to measure the end points should adequately represent the effect that is being studied in the trial, and therefore address the primary hypothesis (**construct validity**). Thus, there is a relationship between plasma essential fatty acid levels and the inflammatory response (Horrobin, 1990), and so changes in plasma phospholipid levels could be monitored, but these are less clinically relevant than the actual clinical signs which may, therefore, be more appropriate response variables for ensuring construct validity. However, clinical signs are often measured subjectively on an ordinal or visual analogue scale (see Chapter 9), whereas fatty acid levels can be measured on the ratio scale. Thus,

Table 16.2 Response variables assessed in clinical trials.

Response variable		Efficacy	
Level of measurement	*Examples*	*Definition*	*Description of method and sample size determination*
Nominal	Mortality Incidence Prevalence	Difference between two proportions Relative risk	Chapter 14 Chapter 15
Ordinal	Scores of clinical severity Condition scores	Difference between two medians	Chapter 14
Interval and ratio and the visual analogue scale	Liveweight gain Milk cell counts Visual analogue assessment of clinical severity	Difference between means (if the variables are Normally distributed)	Chapter 14

Table 16.3 Efficacy of a *Bacteroides nodosus* vaccine against foot rot (84 days after vaccination). (Raw data derived from Hindmarsh *et al.*, 1989.)

	Foot rot present	Foot rot absent	Total
Non-vaccinated sheep	94	328	422
Vaccinated sheep	21	296	317

a compromise between strength of measurement and relevance (construct validity) may be necessary.

Defining efficacy

The primary end point defines the **outcome** that is assessed, and therefore the nature of the trial's response variables (*Table 16.2*), and efficacy is determined in terms of differences between treatment and control groups. The relative risk can be used as a *relative* measure of efficacy when outcome is expressed as a proportion.

A useful measure of **vaccinal efficacy** is the aetiological fraction (exposed) (see Chapter 15) in which unvaccinated animals are defined as 'exposed' to the risk factor. *Table 16.3* shows the results of a clinical trial of the efficacy of a *Bacteriodes nodosus* vaccine against foot rot in sheep. In this trial, prevalence figures are used instead of incidence figures; thus:

$$\lambda_{exp} = (prevalence_{exposed} - prevalence_{unexposed})/$$
$$(prevalence_{exposed})$$

$$= (94/422 - 21/317)/(94/422),$$
$$= 0.157/0.223,$$
$$= 0.704.$$

Therefore, 70.4% of foot rot in unvaccinated sheep is attributable to not being vaccinated; this is alternatively the percentage of disease prevented by the vaccine in vaccinated animals.

There is not always a fixed standard for acceptable therapeutic effect or efficacy. In the European Union, for example, the therapeutic effect of a veterinary medicinal product is generally understood by the relevant regulatory body to be the effect 'promised by the manufacturer' (Beechinor, 1993). European regulatory guidelines have attempted to define efficacy of ectoparasitic preparations (CVMP, 1993):

$$\% \text{ efficacy} = \frac{C - T}{C} \times 100,$$

where:

C = mean* number of ectoparasites/animal in the control group,

T = mean number of ectoparasites/animal in the treated group.

Target levels of efficacy include 'approximately 100%' for flea and louse infestations; '80−100% (preferably more than 90%)' for infestations with Diptera; and 'more than 90%' for tick infestations. Note, however, that the

*The mean may be the arithmetic mean, geometric mean, or other appropriate transformation (see chapters 12 and 17).

value of a therapeutic effect lies ultimately in its clinical and economic impact.

The experimental unit

The **experimental unit** is the smallest *independent* unit to which the treatment is randomly allocated. It may be elementary units (usually individual animals) or aggregates such as pens or herds. Most companion animal and human clinical trials involve allocation to individuals. Some trials in livestock, however, may involve allocation of treatments to groups (e.g., Gill, 1987). In contrast, the experimental unit may be the udder quarter when locally administered intramammary preparations are being assessed; the elementary unit is then the quarter, not the animal.

The experimental unit may be a group because events at the individual level cannot be measured, even though they are of interest. For instance, in trials of in-feed compounds likely to affect weight gain in poultry and pigs, either the amount eaten by, or the weight increase of, individuals within a house or pen is not recorded. This often arises because it is not practical to identify individual animals at weighing. Consequently, liveweight gain per house or pen is the response variable. Moreover, when animals are penned together, external factors (e.g., farm hygiene) may affect the group, and such 'group effects' cannot be separated from individual treatment effects; therefore the group must be identified as the experimental unit (Donner, 1993).

Thus, the efficacy of in-feed antibiotic medication in reducing the incidence of streptococcal meningitis in pigs could be assessed by dividing a herd into pens containing a specified number of animals (Johnston *et al.*, 1992). The treatment is then randomly allocated to the pens, and medicated and 'placebo' diets supplied to pigs in the respective treatment and control pens. In this circumstance, each pen only contributes the value 1 in sample size determination for the trial because variability can only be legitimately assessed between pens, rather than between individuals.

A particular problem arises with trials involving some infectious diseases. If the treatment could reduce excretion of infectious agents (e.g., vaccination in poultry houses or anthelmintic trials on farms) then treated and control animals should not be kept together because any reduction in infection 'pressure' will benefit treated and control animals; similarly, control animals constitute a source of infection to treated animals. This can lead to similar results in both categories (Thurber *et al.*, 1977), therefore reducing the likelihood of detecting beneficial

therapeutic effects. The practice of mixing animals in each group is therefore unacceptable when herd immunity or group immunity is being assessed. In these circumstances, an appropriate independent unit must be identified. Thus, separate houses could be used on an intensive poultry enterprise, or separate tanks on a fish farm. Dairy farms, in contrast, usually have a continuous production policy with mixing of animals, and so the herd may become the experimental unit.

The experimental population

The population in which a trial is conducted is the **experimental population**. This should be representative of the target population (see also Chapter 13). Differences between experimental and target populations may result in the trial not being generalizable (**externally valid**); that is, unbiased inferences regarding the **target population** cannot be made. For example, findings from a trial of an anaesthetic drug conducted only on thoroughbred horses may not be relevant to the general horse population because of differences in levels of fitness between thoroughbreds and other types of horse (Short, 1987). External validity (which is facilitated by conducting trials 'in the field') contrasts with **internal validity**, which indicates that observed differences between treatment and control groups in the experimental population can be legitimately attributed to the treatment. Internal validity is obtained by good trial design (e.g., randomization). The evaluation of external validity usually requires much more information than assessment of internal validity.

Prophylactic trials require selection of an experimental population that is at high risk of developing disease so that natural challenge can be anticipated during the period of the trial. Previous knowledge of disease on potential trial sites may be sufficient to identify candidate populations (Johnston *et al.*, 1992). However, the period of natural challenge may vary, reflecting complex patterns of infection. Many infections are seasonal (*Figure 8.13*); others may be poorly predictable (Clemens *et al.*, 1993).

Admission and exclusion criteria

Criteria for inclusion of animals in a trial (**admission criteria, elegibility criteria**) must be defined. These should be listed in the protocol, and include:

1. a precise **definition of the condition** on which the treatment is being assessed;
2. the **criteria for diagnosis** of the condition.

Table 16.4 Summary of the types of blinding to assignment of treatment.

Type of blinding	Knowledge of assignment of treatment	
	Owner	Investigator
None	Yes	Yes
Single	No	Yes
Double	No	No

For example, in the trial of the efficacy of evening primrose oil in the treatment of canine atopy, chronically pruritic dogs were included only if they conformed to a documented set of diagnostic criteria (Willemse, 1986) and reacted positively to the relevant intradermal skin tests. Similarly, specific types of mastitis may need to be defined in bovine mastitis trials; other admission criteria could include parity and stage of lactation.

Exclusion criteria are the corollaries of admission criteria. Thus, dogs with positive reactions to flea allergens were excluded from the trial of evening primrose oil. Cows might be excluded from a mastitis trial if they had been previously treated for mastitis during the relevant lactation, if they had multiple mammary infections, or if they also had other diseases which could affect treatment. Trials of non-steroidal anti-inflammatory drugs would require exclusion from the treatment group of animals to which corticosteroids were being administered. However, too many exclusion criteria should be avoided; otherwise external validity may be compromised. It may be prudent to accommodate factors either in the trial design by stratification, or during the analysis.

The objectives and general outline of a trial should be explained to owners of animals that are included in the trial, and then their willingness to participate documented. This is **informed consent**.

Blinding

Blinding (masking) is a means of reducing bias. In this technique, those responsible for measurements or clinical assessment are kept unaware of the treatment assigned to each group. The classification of blinding into **single** or **double** is based on whether the owner or attendant (patient in human medicine) or investigator is 'blinded' (*Table 16.4*). 'The investigator' can be more than one

category of person; for example, participating veterinary practitioners and the principal investigators that analyse the results (the term 'treble-blinding' has been advocated in this situation).

Blinding should be employed wherever possible, and is facilitated by the use of a placebo in the control group. However, there may be circumstances in which blinding is not feasible; for example, if two radically different treatments are being compared (e.g., a surgical and chemotherapeutic procedure) or if formulation of visually identical 'trial' and 'standard' drugs is impracticable.

Randomization

Simple randomization

Simple randomization is the most basic type of randomization. When there are only two treatments, tossing a coin is an elementary method. However, it is usually more convenient to randomize in advance using random numbers (Appendix VI), allocating units identified by odd numbers to one group, and evenly numbered units to the other. Randomization should be undertaken *after* eligible units have been identified.

When comparing a new treatment with an established one, and there is evidence that the new treatment is superior, it can be allocated to twice the number of units as the established one (Peto, 1978). This can increase the benefit to participating animals. For example, if a new treatment was expected to reduce mortality by 50%, 2:1 randomization would be expected to produce an equal number of deaths in the two groups. This randomization ratio can be obtained by using twice as many random numbers for allocation of the new treatment as those used to allocate the established one. There is no advantage in increasing the ratio further, because of the resultant loss of statistical power which can only be counteracted by increasing the total sample size.

Block randomization

Simple randomization can produce grossly uneven totals in each group if a small trial is undertaken. This problem can be overcome using **block (restricted) randomization**. This limits randomization to blocks of units, and ensures that within a block equal numbers are allocated to each treatment. For example, if randomization is restricted to units of four animals, receiving either treatment A or treatment B, the numbers 1−6 are attached to the six possible treatment allocations in a block: ABAB, AABB, BBAA, BAAB, ABBA and BABA. One of these numbers is then selected from a random number table for the next block of four individuals entering the trial, and gives its treatment allocation.

Stratification

Some factors (e.g., age, parity or severity of disease) may be known to affect the outcome of a trial and may bias results if they are unevenly distributed between the treatment and control groups. This can be taken into account during initial randomization by **stratifying** (i.e., matching) both groups according to these confounding factors. The experimental units are then allocated to treatment and control groups within the strata, using simple or block randomization. The most extreme case is individual matching (see Chapter 15), with subjects in the matched pairs being randomly allocated to the treatment and control groups.

Stratification leads to related samples and therefore decreases the number of units that are required to detect a specified difference between treatment and control groups (see Chapter 14).

These and other methods of randomization are described in detail by Zelen (1974).

Alternatives to randomization

Some alternatives to randomization include allocation according to date of entry (e.g., treatment on odd days, placebo on even days), clinic record number, wishes of the owner, and preceding results. An example of the last method is the 'play-the-winner' approach (Zelen, 1969): if a treatment is followed by success, the next unit receives the same treatment; if it is followed by failure, the next unit receives the alternative treatment. This limits the number of animals receiving an inferior treatment. All of these techniques have disadvantages and should never be considered as acceptable alternatives to randomization (Bulpitt, 1983).

Trial designs

There are three main trial designs:

1. standard;
2. cross-over;
3. sequential.

Standard trials

In the basic **standard trial**, experimental units are randomized to a single treatment group using either simple or block randomization, and each group receives a single treatment. A specified number of units enter the

trial and are followed for a predetermined period of time, after which the treatment is stopped. The basic design can be refined by stratification.

The analytical techniques employed in a standard trial involving two unstratified groups are listed in *Table 16.2*. Estimation of parameters with associated confidence intervals is preferred to hypothesis testing, for the reasons given in Chapter 14. Confidence intervals should also be quoted for negative results, in which circumstance it is also prudent to calculate the power of the trial.

Details of complex multivariate methods for stratified analyses are described by Meinert and Tonascia (1986) and Kleinbaum et al. (1982), but these are seldom used in veterinary product development.

Cross-over trials

In a **cross-over trial**, subjects are exposed to more than one treatment consecutively, each treatment regimen being selected randomly (Hills and Armitage, 1979). Experimental units therefore serve as their own controls, and treatment and control groups are therefore matched. This design is useful when treatments are intended to alleviate a condition, rather than effect a cure, so that after the first treatment is withdrawn the subject is in a position to receive a second. Examples are comparisons of anti-inflammatory drugs in arthritis, and hypoglycaemics in diabetes. Moreover, a comparison on the same individuals is likely to be more precise than a comparison between subjects because the responses are paired (see Chapter 14). The cross-over trial is therefore valuable if the number of experimental units is limited. However, analysis of results is complex if a treatment effect carries over into the next treatment period.

If treatment effects do not carry over into subsequent treatment periods, the techniques described in Chapter 14 for the analysis of related samples can be used. However, the absence of a carry-over effect may be difficult to prove. If there is any doubt, conclusions should be based only on the first period, using analyses of independent samples. Alternatively, more complex methods that identify interactions between treatment effect and period of treatment can be applied (Hills and Armitage, 1979).

Sequential trials

A sequential trial is one whose conduct at any stage depends on the results so far obtained (Armitage, 1975). Two treatments are usually compared, and experimental units (usually individuals) enter the trial in pairs; one individual being given one treatment, and one the other. Results are then analysed sequentially according to the outcome in the pairs, and boundaries are drawn to define

Table 16.5 Nominal significance level required for repeated two-tailed significance testing with an overall significance level $\alpha = 0.05$ or 0.01 and various values of N, the maximum number of tests. (From Pocock, 1977.)

N	$\alpha = 0.05$	$\alpha = 0.01$
2	0.0294	0.0056
3	0.0221	0.0041
4	0.0182	0.0033
5	0.0158	0.0028
6	0.0142	0.0025
7	0.0130	0.0023
8	0.0120	0.0021
9	0.0112	0.0019
10	0.0106	0.0018
15	0.0086	0.0015
20	0.0075	0.0013

levels at which specified differences are obtained at the desired level of statistical significance. The trial may be terminated when these levels are reached. If the desired level is not reached, the investigator may decide to increase the sample size indefinitely until the former is reached; this is an **open** trial. Alternatively, the trial may be terminated if a specified difference is not reached by a certain stage; this is a **closed** trial.

Sequential trials facilitate early detection of beneficial treatment effects and can require fewer experimental units. However, they may be difficult to plan because their duration is initially unknown. They are also unsuited to trials in which treatment response times are long because responses need to be analysed quickly so that a decision can be taken to enlist more subjects, if necessary.

A key feature of sequential trials therefore is that significance tests are conducted repeatedly on accumulating data. This tends to increase the overall significance level (Armitage *et al.*, 1969). For example, if five interim analyses are conducted, the chance of at least one analysis showing a treatment difference at the 5% level ($\alpha = 0.05$) increases to 0.23 (i.e., $1 - [1 - \alpha]^5$); if 20 interim analyses are undertaken, it increases to 0.64 ($1 - [1 - \alpha]^{20}$). The overall Type I error therefore increases if, for any single interim analysis, $\alpha = 0.05$ is used as the trial's stopping criterion. If data are analysed frequently enough, a value of $P < 0.05$ is likely, regardless of whether there is a treatment difference.

This problem can be overcome by choosing a more stringent *nominal* significance level for each repeated test, so that the overall significance level is kept at a reasonable value such as 0.05 or 0.01 (Pocock, 1983). *Table 16.5*

can be used for this purpose under two-tailed conditions. For example, if the overall significance level is set at $\alpha = 0.05$, and if a maximum of three analyses is anticipated, $P < 0.022$ is used as the stopping rule for a treatment difference at each analysis; similarly, if a maximum of five analyses is anticipated, $P < 0.016$ is used. Suitable values for one-sided tests are given by Demets and Ware (1980).

Sequential trials are considered in detail by Armitage (1975).

What sample size should be selected?

The number of experimental units in treatment and control groups should be determined using the techniques outlined in previous chapters (*Table 16.2*). In summary, the following parameters should be considered:

1. the acceptable level of Type I error, α (the probability of erroneously inferring a difference between treatment and control group);
2. test power, $1 - \beta$ (the probability of correctly inferring a difference between treatment and control group) where β = the probability of Type II error (the probability of erroneously missing a true difference between treatment and control group);
3. the magnitude of the treatment effect (i.e., the difference between proportions, medians or means);
4. the choice of alternative hypothesis: 'one-tailed' or 'two-tailed'.

There is no rule for defining parameters 1–3. Type I error is traditionally set at 0.05, but a value as low as 0.01 can be justified if a trial is unique and its findings are unlikely to be repeated in the future. Power can vary considerably (values between 0.50 and 0.95 have been quoted in human clinical trials; 0.80 is common when $\alpha = 0.05$, and 0.96 when $\alpha = 0.01$: see Chapter 14). The magnitude of the treatment effect depends on its clinical and economic relevance.

(In clinical trials in which treatment and control groups are matched the formulae for sample size determination listed in previous chapters will tend to overestimate the number of units required.)

If a placebo or no treatment has been administered to the control group, and there is therefore intuitive evidence that the treatment can cause only an improvement in comparison with the control group, a one-tailed test (see Chapter 14) is justifiable, and the sample size can be determined accordingly. However, the use of placebos or 'negative' control groups is now ethically debatable; consequently many contemporary clinical trials use a 'positive' control group and it is therefore prudent to assume two-tailed conditions (i.e., the treatment under test may be either better, or worse, than the standard treatment). Additionally, the magnitude of the difference between treatment and 'positive' control groups may be small; thus large sample sizes may be specified. These may be unattainable in practice. However, a knowledge of sample size determination is necessary to appreciate the inferential limitations that may be imposed by the number of experimental units included in a trial.

Sample size determination for cross-over trials is discussed by Senn (1993). Sample size determination for sequential trials is discussed by Armitage (1975); the estimated sample size for a given Type I and Type II error is smaller than for a non-sequential trial. General guidelines are provided by Shuster (1992). Hallstrom and Trobaugh (1985) provide formulae that incorporate diagnostic sensitivity and specificity (see Chapters 9 and 17).

Losses to 'follow-up'

The outcome of a trial may not be recorded in some experimental units because they are lost to 'follow-up'. For example, owners may move house or refuse to continue with the trial. The extent of this loss to follow-up needs to be assessed, and is frequently based on the experience of the investigator. The sample size then needs to be increased by multiplying the sample size by $1/(1-d)$, where d is the anticipated proportion of experimental units lost. For example, if $d = 10/100$, the sample size would need to be multiplied by 1.11 (1/0.9) to compensate. Losses to follow-up cannot be included in subsequent analyses.

Compliance

The success of a trial depends on participants acting in accordance with the instructions of the trial's designers; that is, **complying** with treatment. However, they may not comply; for example, they may decide to switch from the treatment under trial to an alternative treatment. Poor compliance will decrease the statistical power of the trial because the observed difference in outcome between treatment and control groups will be reduced, but it will not produce spurious differences between groups. Reasons for poor compliance include:

1. unclear instructions;
2. forgetfulness;
3. inconvenience of participation;

4. cost of participation;
5. preference for alternative procedures;
6. disappointment with results;
7. side effects.

Participants cannot be forced to comply, and so regular contact should be maintained with them, so that they can be encouraged to comply, and the degree of compliance regularly assessed. For example, if a treatment is formulated as a tablet, the number of tablets remaining can be counted regularly by the veterinarian. Assessment may be difficult (e.g., with in-feed medication) but should, nevertheless, be attempted. Other methods of improving compliance include:

1. enrolling motivated participants;
2. assessing the willingness of participants to comply;
3. providing incentives (e.g., free treatment);
4. supplying simple, unambiguous instructions;
5. limiting duration of the trial.

If non-compliance is substantial, the required sample size should again be modified in the same way as adjustment for loss to follow-up. If both losses to follow-up and non-compliance are anticipated, a composite value for d is required.

Terminating a trial

The number of experimental units entering a trial and the duration of treatment are specified during the design of a trial; therefore a trial will usually last as long as it takes to enlist the units and for the last unit to complete the trial. However, it may be necessary to terminate a trial (particularly a long-term one) prematurely if there are serious adverse side effects in the treatment group, and such a **decision rule** should be written into the trial's protocol. In sequential trials another decision rule may be that a trial will be terminated when the specified difference is detected at the predetermined level of significance (see above).

Decision rules, and the advantages of early and late termination of trials, are discussed in detail by Bulpitt (1983).

Further reading

Bulpitt, C.J. (1983) *Randomised Controlled Clinical Trials.* Martinus Nijhoff Publishers, The Hague
Chalmers, T.C., Smith, H., Blackburn, B., Silverman, B., Schroeder, B., Reitman, D. and Ambroz, A. (1981) A method

for assessing the quality of a randomized controlled trial. *Controlled Clinical Trials* **2**, 31−49

Code of Practice for the Conduct of Clinical Trials on Veterinary Medicinal Products in the European Community. Fédération Européenne de la Santé Animale (FEDESA), 1993. Rue Defacqz, 1/Bte 8, B-1050, Brussels. (*Guidelines for clinical trials*)

Conduct of Clinical Trials of Veterinary Medicinal Products (1990) Committee of Veterinary Medicinal Products, Commission of the European Communities, Brussels, Document III/3775/90. (*Guidelines for clinical trials*)

Dohoo, I.R. and Thomas, F.C. (Eds) (1989) Clinical trials in veterinary medicine. Special report. *Canadian Veterinary Journal*, **30**, 291−303. (*A series of short articles on the design and conduct of clinical trials with particular reference to respiratory vaccines for beef cattle*)

International Dairy Federation (1988) *Guidelines for Clinical Trials. Questionnaire 1088/A*. International Dairy Federation, Brussels. (*Guidelines with specific reference to mastitis*)

Meinert, C.L. and Tonascia, S. (1986) *Clinical Trials: Design, Conduct, and Analysis*. Oxford Univerity Press, New York

Noordhuizen, J.P.T.M., Frankena, K., Ploeger, H. and Nell, T. (Eds) (1993) *Field Trial & Error*. Proceedings of the international seminar with workshops on the design, conduct and interpretation of field trials, Berg en Dal, Netherlands, 27−28 April 1993. Epidecon, Wageningen

Peto, R., Pike, M.C., Armitage, P., Breslow, N.E., Cox, D.R., Howard, S.V., Mantel, N., McPherson, K., Peto, J. and Smith, P.G. (1976) Design and analysis of randomized clinical trials requiring prolonged observation of each patient. I. Introduction and design. *British Journal of Cancer*, **34**, 585−612. (*A clear and comprehensive introduction to the design of trials that study time to death*)

Peto, R., Pike, M.C., Armitage, P., Breslow, N.E., Cox, D.R., Howard, S.V., Mantel, N., McPherson, K., Peto, J. and Smith, P.G. (1977) Design and analysis of randomized clinical trials requiring prolonged observation of each patient. II. Analysis and examples. *British Journal of Cancer*, **35**, 1−39

Pocock, S.J. (1983) *Clinical Trials: A Practical Approach*. John Wiley, Chichester and New York

Proceedings of the First European Symposium on the Demonstration of Efficacy of Veterinary Medicinal Products. Toulouse, May 19−22 1992

Senn, S. (1993) *Cross-over Trials in Clinical Research*. John Wiley, Chichester and New York

Shuster, J.J. (1993) *Practical Handbook of Sample Size Guidelines for Clinical Trials*. CRC Press, Boca Raton (*Includes software*)

Note

Supplementary information on meta-analysis of clinical trials is provided in Appendix XXI.

17 Diagnostic testing

Infectious and non-infectious diseases may be diagnosed in the context of either an individual or a population. The latter is an important component of epidemiology — particularly when **screening** populations for the presence of infection, genetic defects or other abnormal conditions — and is the main subject of this chapter. Emphasis is placed on the diagnosis of infectious diseases using **serological** methods, but many of the principles and techniques can be extended to other diagnostic methods and conditions.

Serological epidemiology

Serological epidemiology is the investigation of disease and infection in populations by the measurement of variables present in serum. A range of constituents of serum can be measured, including minerals, trace elements, enzymes and hormones. One of the main constituents of serum that is frequently measured is the specific antibody activity of immunoglobulins. Alternative terms for antibody measurement are 'titration' and 'assay'. Antibodies provide evidence of current and previous exposure to infectious agents; their assay is commonly employed in veterinary medicine as a relatively efficient and cheap means of detecting this exposure in both individual animals and populations.

The statistical methods employed to analyse antibody levels are equally applicable to other serological tests, such as those that detect enzymes and minerals, in which case, however, results can be compared with normal reference ranges. These commonly include: (1) the mean ± 2 standard deviations for Normally distributed data, selected from a normal (i.e., reference) population; and (2) the middle 95% of values (i.e., from the 2.5th to 97.5th percentile: see Chapter 12) from a reference population for data that are not Normally distributed (Hutchison *et al.*, 1991). Although values for reference levels are available in published tables (e.g., Kaneko,

Table 17.1 Methods of diagnosing infectious disease.

Evidence of current infection
  Isolation of agent
  Identification of agent's genes
    (molecular epidemiology)
  Clinical signs
  Pathognomonic (characteristic) changes
  Biochemical changes
  Demonstration of an immune response:
    detection of antigens and antibodies
    (serological epidemiology)

Evidence of past infection
  Clinical history
  Pathognomonic changes
  Demonstration of an immune response:
    detection of antibodies

1989), each laboratory should establish its own norms. If the values are Normally distributed, or can be transformed to Normality, then a one-sample *t*-test (see *Table 14.1*) can be applied to compare a sample's values with those of a reference population; otherwise one-sample non-parametric methods may be appropriate (see *Table 14.2*).

The serological diagnosis of disease based on the detection of circulating antibodies is one of the techniques available for the identification of current and previous exposure to infectious agents. This and other methods are listed in *Table 17.1*. A range of tests to detect antigen/antibody reactions has been developed over the last 100 years and more are being added to the range. Descriptions of these techniques are found in standard immunology texts (e.g., Tizard, 1982; Roitt, 1988; Hudson and Hay, 1989; Paraf and Peltre, 1991), and a basic knowledge of them is assumed. Emphasis is now shifting towards the

Table 17.2 Antibody titres expressed as reciprocal dilutions (X) and coded titres ($\log_2 X$).

Reciprocal dilution (X)	Coded titre (log₂X)
1 (undiluted serum)	0
2	1
4	2
8	3
16	4
32	5
64	6

detection of antigens, rather than antibodies, in current infections.

Assaying antibodies

Methods of expressing amounts of antibody

The concentration of antibody is expressed as a **titre**. This is the highest dilution of serum that produces a test reaction. Thus, if the highest dilution that produces a test reaction is 1 in 32, then the titre is 1/32. Alternatively, the reciprocal, 32, can be quoted, indicating that the undiluted serum contains 32 times the antibody for the reaction. Animals with detectable antibody titres are **seropositive**; animals with no detectable antibodies are **seronegative**. Animals previously seronegative and now seropositive have **seroconverted**.

Logarithmic transformation of titres

Serum is usually diluted in a geometric series, that is, with a constant ratio between successive dilutions. The commonest ratio is 2. Thus, serum is diluted 1/2, 1/4, 1/8, 1/16, 1/32 and so on. This suggests that the titres should be measured on a logarithmic scale. There are two reasons for this measurement:

1. the frequency distribution of titres is often approximately lognormal (see *Figure 12.5*); statistical tests that assume Normality may therefore be applied;
2. geometric dilution series are equally spaced on a logarithmic scale; thus serum may be diluted geometrically 1/2, 1/4, 1/8, 1/16 and so on, corresponding to log transformation to base 2, the respective logs to base 2 of the reciprocals of the dilutions being 1, 2, 3, 4 and so on; the dilution can be coded as the value of these logarithms to base 2 (*Table 17.2*).

In some cases, high concentrations of serum that react non-specifically are avoided by initially diluting by $\log_{10}$, and then continuing in $\log_2$ dilutions, thus: 1/10, 1/20, 1/40, 1/80.

Mean titres

If several coded titres are recorded, their **arithmetic mean** can be calculated. This is simply the sum of the coded titres divided by the number of titres. For example, if five titres are 1/2, 1/4, 1/2, 1/8 and 1/4, then the coded titres are 1, 2, 1, 3 and 2 respectively. The arithmetic mean therefore is $(1+2+1+3+2)/5 = 1.8$.

The **geometric mean titre** (*GMT*) is the antilog₂ of the coded mean. This can be obtained from a pocket calculator with an 'x^y' function key on it. For example, if the arithmetic mean of several coded titres is 4.7, then $\log_2 GMT = 4.7$; thus $GMT = 2^{4.7} = 26$.

If an initial $\log_{10}$ dilution has been carried out, subsequently followed by $\log_2$ dilutions, values are divided by 10 before taking logarithms to base 2. For example, dilutions of 1/10, 1/20, 1/40, 1/80 would be coded as 0, 1, 2, 3 (1/10 is coded 0 because it is equivalent to undiluted serum), giving a mean of 1.5. Then: $GMT/10 = 2^{1.5} = 2.8$. Thus, $GMT = 28$.

The logarithm of zero cannot be expressed because it is 'minus infinity'. Therefore, when calculating means of coded titres, seronegative animals have to be excluded because their reciprocal titres are zero and therefore cannot be coded; *mean titres can be calculated only for seropositive animals*. Thus, when comparing coded antibody titres in populations, two parameters must be considered before inferences are made: the relative proportion of seropositive animals, irrespective of titre, and the *GMT*s of the seropositive populations. For instance, it might be found that in two dairy herds approximately 20% of cows in each herd were seropositive to *Leptospira*, serovar *pomona*, but that the *GMT* in one herd was 40 while in the other it was 640. Such circumstances might indicate a recent epidemic in the second herd and merely the persistence of antibodies in convalescent animals in the first. Conversely, a serological survey of workers in two different abattoirs might reveal similar *GMT*s of complement fixing antibodies to *Coxiella burnetti* in each group of seropositive workers, but at one abattoir 30% of workers may have titres, while at the other only 3% may be seropositive. Such results would indicate a much greater probability of infection at the first abattoir, although the *GMT*s of the groups were similar.

Table 17.3 Example of a 50% end-point titration (Spearman–Kärber method).

Serum dilution	Log_{10} dilution	Monolayers showing cytopathic effect	Intact monolayers	Proportion 'positive' (intact) P	1 − P
1/1	0.0	0	5	1.00	0.00
1/2	−0.3	0	5	1.00	0.00
1/4	−0.6	0	5	1.00	0.00
1/8	−0.9	1	4	0.80	0.20
1/16	−1.2	1	4	0.80	0.20
1/32	−1.5	3	2	0.40	0.60
1/64	−1.8	4	1	0.20	0.80
1/128	−2.1	5	0	0.00	1.00

Quantal assay

A quantal assay measures an 'all-or-none' response; for example, agglutination or no agglutination, infected or non-infected. Two systems are frequently used:

1. single serial dilution assay;
2. multiple serial dilution assay.

The first is the commoner. Both techniques utilize geometric (logarithmic) dilutions, the range of dilution depending on the sensitivity of the test. Sensitivity here refers to the ability of the system to detect amounts of antibody and antigen: the more sensitive the test, the smaller the amount of antibody and antigen it will detect. This is sometimes more fully termed **analytical sensitivity**, to avoid confusion with sensitivity as a validity parameter of a diagnostic test — more fully termed **diagnostic sensitivity** (Stites and Rodgers, 1991).

Single serial dilution assay

In a single serial dilution assay, each dilution is tested once. For instance, in a virus haemagglutination-inhibition test, the highest dilution that prevents agglutination of erythrocytes on a test plate is the antibody's haemagglutination-inhibition titre. This is a relatively weak form of measurement. If the titre is 1/32 it implies that 1/31 would not produce the effect. However, since 1/16 is the next lowest dilution that is tested, the actual titre could lie between 1/17 and 1/32. Thus, this type of titration, which tests only dilution intervals, actually divides the dilutions into blocks. The blocking is more marked when titres are expressed as 'greater than' or 'less than' (e.g. < 1/8 or > 1/256). The data therefore are essentially **ordinal** (see Chapter 9).

Multiple serial dilution assay

In a multiple serial dilution assay, each dilution is tested several (preferably at least five) times. The object is to achieve a 'strong' measure. The end point is the dilution

of a substance at which a specified number of members of a test group show a defined effect, such as death or disease. The most frequently used and statistically useful end point is 50% (Gaddum, 1933). Thus, in pharmacology, the toxicity of a drug can be expressed as an LD_{50} (lethal dose$_{50}$): the amount of drug that will kill 50% of test animals. An amount of drug therefore can be expressed in terms of the number of LD_{50}s that it contains.

Fifty per cent end-point titrations can also be used to estimate antibody concentrations, in which case antibody titres are expressed in terms of the dilution of serum that *prevents* an effect in 50% of members of a test group, the effect being produced by the infectious agent responsible for induction of the antibodies that are being titrated. For example, the dilution of serum that prevents infection of 50% of cell culture monolayers with a standard concentration of virus can be estimated: an 'effective dose$_{50}$' (ED_{50}). Several methods of calculating 50% end points are available, including the Reed–Muench and Spearman–Kärber methods, and moving averages. The Reed–Muench method is not recommended because precision cannot be assessed, there is no validity test, and the method is less efficient than some of the alternatives (Finney, 1978). The second method (Spearman, 1908; Kärber, 1931), which involves relatively simple calculations, is described below.

Example of a Spearman–Kärber titration

The antibody titre to a virus is required. The defined measured response is a cytopathic effect (CPE) in cell culture monolayers. The test serum is diluted (usually in twofold geometric increments). One-tenth of 1 ml of each dilution is inoculated into groups of five cell culture monolayers, each of which has been inoculated with a fixed, potentially lethal, dose of the virus. *Table 17.3* depicts the results. The 50% end point is the dilution of serum that prevents a CPE in 50% of the monolayers in a group, that is, in two and a half monolayers (note that this is a statistical estimation).

According to the Spearman−Kärber formula:

$$\log ED_{50} = L - d(\Sigma P - 0.5)$$

where

L = log highest dilution at which all monolayers survive intact;

d = log of the dilution factor (i.e., the difference between the log dilution intervals);

ΣP = sum of the proportion of 'positive' tests (i.e., intact monolayers), from the highest dilution showing a positive result to the highest dilution showing all results positive (i.e., $P = 1$).

From *Table 17.3*:

$$L = -0.6$$
$$d = \log_{10}2$$
$$ = 0.3$$
$$\Sigma P = 0.20 + 0.40 + 0.80 + 0.80 + 1.00$$
$$ = 3.2.$$

Thus:

$$\log_{10}ED_{50} = -0.6 - \{0.3(3.2-0.5)\}$$
$$= -0.6 - (0.3 \times 2.7)$$
$$= -0.6 - 0.8$$
$$= -1.4.$$

Therefore, ED_{50} = antilog (-1.4)
$$= 1/\text{antilog } 1.4$$
$$= 1/25.1.$$

Thus, 0.1 ml of serum contains 25.1 ED_{50}s, and 1 ml contains 251 ED_{50}s.

The estimated standard error (e.s.e.) is calculated using:

$$\text{e.s.e. } (\log_{10}ED_{50}) = d\sqrt{\Sigma\{P(1-P)\}/(n-1)}$$

where n = number of animals in each group.

Substituting the values from *Table 17.3*:

$$\log_{10}\text{e.s.e.} = \frac{0.3\sqrt{[\{(0.2\times0.8) + (0.4\times0.6) +}}{(0.8\times0.2) + (0.8\times0.2)\}/(5-1)]}$$

$$= 0.3\sqrt{(0.16+0.24+0.16+0.16)/4}$$
$$= 0.13.$$

Multiple serial dilution assays are now less common than previously because they are more expensive and slower than single serial dilution assays and titrations conducted on just a single dilution — notably the enzyme-linked immunosorbent assay (ELISA). However, they still have a role in measuring vaccinal potency.

Serological estimations and comparisons in populations

Antibody prevalence

The presence of detectable antibody indicates that an animal or its dam has been exposed to the antigen that stimulates the antibody's production. In the absence of further challenge, the antibody level will decline. The rate of decline, usually measured in terms of the antibody's **half-life** (the time taken for its level to halve), varies between antibodies. Titres to some antibodies persist because the antibodies have a long half-life or there is persistent infection or repeated challenge. The possession of a long half-life explains why some vaccines can produce lifelong immunity after a single course. The half-life of vaccinal antibodies is therefore an important aspect of vaccinal efficacy (see also Chapter 16) and of passively acquired immunity in young animals. The half-life of antibodies following natural infection, however, is rarely estimated.

If the amount of antibody in an animal population is to be estimated, without particular regard to the frequency distribution of antibody titres, animals are categorized as either 'positive' or 'negative', and the prevalence of antibodies in the population (i.e., seroprevalence), with its associated confidence interval, can be calculated using the methods described in Chapter 13. A titre cut-off point, below which animals are considered to be negative, and above which animals are categorized as positive, is often defined (see below).

The prevalence of detectable antibody depends on the rate of infection, the rate of antibody loss and the time at which these rates have been effective. A high prevalence therefore may reflect not a high rate of infection but a low rate of antibody loss; recall (see Chapter 4) that prevalence, P, is related to incidence rate, I, and duration, D:

$$P \propto I \times D.$$

It follows that not only the prevalence of detectable antibody in a population but also the titre in the individual is related to the half-life of the antibody.

If the frequency distribution of antibodies is required then, if the scale of measurement is 'strong' (e.g., an ED_{50}), the mean and standard deviation can be quoted, and confidence intervals can be calculated (Chapter 12).

Table 17.4 Age-specific seroprevalence and annual mean seroconversion rates for bovine leukosis virus reactors in a sample of Louisiana beef cattle, 1982–84. (Modified from Hugh-Jones and Hubbert, 1988.)

Age (years)	Number of cattle tested	Seroprevalence (P_y)	Annual mean seroconversion rates (p)
1	67	0.15	0.150
2	191	0.21	0.111
3	105	0.23	0.083
4	143	0.39	0.116
5	167	0.40	0.097
6	137	0.47	0.100
7	98	0.53	0.102
8	92	0.55	0.095
9	32	0.63	0.105
10	53	0.60	0.088
>10*	19	0.37	0.036

*Average age used in calculating $p = 12.5$.

The much more common single serial dilution assays, which define a titre as the highest dilution producing a test reaction, produce ordinal data; this is particularly evident when a large proportion of the titres are expressed as 'less than' or 'greater than' a particular dilution. If there are not any 'less than' or 'greater than' titres, and there is a reasonable spread of titres, then the log titres can be regarded as crude approximations to Normally distributed measurements, and the mean, standard deviation and confidence intervals can again be quoted. However, if these assumptions are not met, the median and semi-interquartile range should be quoted. Confidence intervals for the median can also be calculated (Gardner and Altman, 1989).

Rate of seroconversion

If a population is susceptible to infection at birth, the duration of antibodies following infection is lifelong, and mortality due to infection is negligible, a simple mathematical model can be used to describe the age distribution of antibodies for various rates of seroconversion (Lilienfeld and Lilienfeld, 1980).

If: p = probability of becoming infected in one year (i.e., rate of seroconversion); y = age in years; $(1-p)^y$ = probability of not having become infected by age y (i.e., in y years); P_y = proportion of population that have become infected by age y (i.e., seroprevalence at age y); then:

$$P_y = 1 - (1-p)^y.$$

It is also possible to estimate the rate of seroconversion from age-specific seroprevalence values by inversion of the formula:

$$\log(1-p) = \{\log(1-P_y)\}/y.$$

Therefore:

$$(1-p) = \text{antilog}[\{\log(1-P_y)\}/y],$$

and:

$$p = 1 - \text{antilog}[\{\log(1-P_y)\}/y].$$

A series of age-specific seroprevalence values can therefore produce estimates of rates of seroconversion, and changes in these can provide information on the patterns and effects of infection in a herd. *Table 17.4* lists the age-specific seroprevalence values for antibodies against bovine leukosis virus in a random sample of beef cattle. There is a slow increase in seroprevalence with age, up to and including 10 years. This infection produces chronic latent infections with persistent antibodies, and so the rate of seroconversion can be estimated.

Thus, for one-year-old animals ($y = 1$):

$$p = 1 - \text{antilog}[\{\log(1-0.15)\}/1]$$
$$= 1 - \text{antilog}(-0.0706/1)$$
$$= 1 - 0.850$$
$$= 0.150;$$

for two-year-old animals ($y = 2$):

$$p = 1 - \text{antilog}[\{\log(1-0.21)\}/2]$$
$$= 1 - \text{antilog}(-0.1024/2)$$
$$= 1 - 0.889$$
$$= 0.111;$$

and so on.

There is a steady estimated annual rate of seroconversion in animals up to 10 years of age, suggesting that the disease is having little impact on the herd: if diseased animals were being culled, a reduction in estimated seroconversion rates (because of the removal of seropositive animals) could be expected from about six years of age. The relatively high seroconversion rate in animals 12–23 months of age could (speculatively) be due to the curiosity of young heifers or persistent passive immunity. The low seroprevalence and estimated annual seroconversion rate in animals greater than 10 years suggests that preferential culling of affected animals is only taking place at that age.

More complex models, which can be applied to infections in which antibodies decline during life, are reviewed by Muench (1959).

Comparison of antibody levels

Comparison of two different populations

If a comparison of two different populations in terms of presence and absence of antibody (i.e., 'positive' or 'negative' animals) is required, then the χ^2 test can be used; alternatively, confidence intervals for differences between two proportions for independent samples can be calculated (see Chapter 14).

If the frequency distributions of antibodies in two populations are to be compared then, if the scale of measurement is 'strong', a parametric test can be used. Further, since antibodies are usually lognormally distributed, standard tests that assume Normality can be used.

An ED_{50}, calculated in multiple serial dilution assays, is a 'strong' measurement. The following example uses the data in *Table 17.5* relating to vaccination titres in two groups of five dogs, one group vaccinated with killed rabies virus of porcine origin, and the other with vaccine of feline origin. The comparison is between the titres in each group, 60 days after vaccination. Log titres are used; this transformation allows the assumption of Normality. Student's t-test for independent samples less than 30 can be used (see Chapter 14), assuming unknown variance. Using the same notation as that in Chapter 14:

$$n_1 = 5, \bar{x}_1 = 2.354, s_1 = 0.083,$$
$$n_2 = 5, \bar{x}_2 = 1.288, s_2 = 0.342.$$

The hypothesis to be tested is that there is no difference in 60-day antibody titres between the dogs vaccinated with killed rabies virus of porcine origin and dogs vaccinated with vaccine of feline origin.

Let μ_1 and μ_2 be the mean 60-day titres in the two groups, and let $\delta = \mu_1 - \mu_2$. The hypothesis may then be written as $\delta = 0$.

First it is necessary to check that s_1^2 and s_2^2 are estimates of a common population variance. This is done by calculating the ratio of the two variances, where the

Table 17.5 Serum antibody titres (SN_{50}: 'serum neutralizing dose$_{50}$') of dogs, for two types of rabies vaccine, before and 60 days after vaccination. (From Merry and Kolar, 1984.)

Vaccine	Dog number	Pre-vaccination titre		Titre 60 days after vaccination	
		Reciprocal	*log_{10}*	*Reciprocal*	*log_{10}*
Killed vaccine	A653	3	0.48	214	2.33
feline cell origin	A616	3	0.48	182	2.26
	2C10	2	0.30	280	2.45
	2B39	2	0.30	267	2.43
	2B47	2	0.30	198	2.30
Mean:		2.4	0.372	228	2.354

$\Sigma x_1 = 11.77; n_1 = 5; \Sigma x_1^2 = 27.7339; \bar{x}_1 = 2.354; s_1 = 0.083$

Killed vaccine	A603	3	0.48	10	1.00
porcine cell line	A654	2	0.30	51	1.71
origin	A618	2	0.30	9	0.95
	2C16	2	0.30	16	1.20
	2C3	2	0.30	38	1.58
Mean:		2.2	0.366	25	1.288

$\Sigma x_2 = 6.44; n_2 = 5; \Sigma x_2^2 = 8.763; \bar{x}_2 = 1.288; s_2 = 0.342$

numerator is the greater of the two. This ratio is then compared with the appropriate percentage points of an F distribution (Appendix XX) with a pair of degrees of freedom, the first being one less than the sample size used in calculating the variance in the numerator, and the second being one less than the sample size used in calculating the variance in the denominator. In this particular case:

$$s_2^2/s_1^2 = 17.0$$

with (4,4) degrees of freedom.

The 1% point of the corresponding F distribution is 16.0. The sample value of 17.0 is greater than this value. The sample value is therefore significant at the 1% level and there is strong evidence to suggest that the variances of the $\log_{10}$ of 60-day antibody titres differ between groups.

The test statistic in this situation is now:

$$t = (\bar{x}_1 - \bar{x}_2 - \delta)/\sqrt{(s_1^2/n_1) + (s_2^2/n_2)}$$

with approximate degrees of freedom v, given by:

$$v = (v_1 + v_2)^2/(v_1^2/\{n_1 - 1\} + v_2^2/\{n_2 - 1\})$$

where:

$$v_1 = s_1^2/n_1$$

and

$$v_2 = s_2^2/n_2$$

to take account of unequal variances (Snedecor and Cochran, 1980).

For this example:

$$
\begin{aligned}
t &= (2.354 - 1.288 - 0)/\sqrt{(0.083^2/5) + (0.342^2/5)} \\
&= 1.066/\sqrt{0.00138 + 0.02339} \\
&= 6.773
\end{aligned}
$$

Thus:

$$v = \frac{(0.001\ 37 + 0.023\ 41)^2}{(0.000\ 000\ 466 + 0.000\ 137)} = 4.47.$$

Rounding down to the nearest whole number, when using the t-table (Appendix IV) there are only 4 degrees of freedom because the variances differ significantly. From Appendix IV, the 5% value for 4 degrees of freedom is 2.776, which is less than 6.773. Therefore, the two groups of dogs have significantly different mean titres at the 5% level. Note that the result is also significant at the 2% level and the 1% level.

An alternative approach is estimation of confidence intervals for the difference between the means of two independent samples, noting that the variances (and therefore standard deviations) differ (see Chapter 14).

Single serial dilution assays present a more difficult choice of statistical test because the titres are ordinal. Again, if there are not any 'less than' or 'greater than' titres, and there is a reasonable spread of titres, then the log titres can be regarded as crude approximations to Normally distributed measurements, and a t-test for independent samples can be used; otherwise the non-parametric Wilcoxon−Mann−Whitney test should be applied; alternatively, confidence intervals can be calculated for the difference between two medians for independent samples (see Chapter 14).

Comparison of different estimates on the same population

If a population is sampled twice over a period of time, and animals are classified as positive or negative, then a suitable comparison can be made using McNemar's change test (see Chapter 14). If the frequency distribution of antibodies is to be compared then a t-test for related samples should be applied — again using log titres to assume Normality. The appropriate non-parametric equivalent is the Wilcoxon signed ranks test (see Chapter 14). Again, confidence intervals can be calculated for the difference between two means or two medians for related samples (see Chapter 14).

Interpreting serological tests

Refinement

Infectious agents have a variety of antigens on their surfaces and in their interiors. Additionally, non-structural antigens can be detected in the early stages of virus replication. Some of the antigens are shared by several groups of isolates and are the basis of division into broad categories. Other antigens are unique to a particular group of isolates. For instance, influenza type A viruses are distinguished from types B and C by their core nucleoproteins and matrix proteins. Influenza A viruses are divided into subtypes on the basis of their surface haemagglutinin and neuraminidase antigens. Similarly, subtypes are divided further into strains according to more refined differences in the antigenic composition of the haemagglutinins and neuraminidases (*Table 17.6*). This refinement in antigenic definition is also termed specificity. This is sometimes more fully termed **analytical specificity**, to avoid confusion with specificity as a validity parameter of a diagnostic test — more fully termed **diagnostic specificity** (Stites and Rodgers, 1991).

Table 17.6 The classification of some influenza A viruses. (Based on Murphy and Webster, 1990.)

Haemagglutinins (H) and neuraminidases (N)	Strains
H1 N1	PR/8/34
H1 N1	Sw/Ia/15/30
H2 N2	Sing/1/57
H3 N2	HK/1/68
H3 N2	Sw/Taiwan/70
H3 N8	Eq/Miami/1/63
H4 N6	Dk/Cz/56
H5 N3	Tern/S.A./61
H6 N2	Ty/Mass/3740/65
H7 N7	Eq/Prague/1/56

The epidemiological value of a serological test, for example, when tracing the spread or origin of a particular infection, increases in relation to the test's ability to detect more refined antigenic differences. The new molecular diagnostic techniques are particularly valuable in this respect (see Chapter 2).

Serological tests vary in their ability to detect subtle antigenic differences. *Table 17.7* illustrates varying refinement of serological tests for influenza A viruses. The complement fixation test (CFT), using virus extracted from chorioallantoic membranes as antigen, will detect antibody against virus nucleoprotein, and therefore is specific only to the level of virus type. However, the use of whole virus as antigen results in a CFT that is specific for subtypes because it will detect particular subtypes of haemagglutinins and neuraminidases. Identification of specific strains is possible if carefully selected reference strains are used as antigens; the titre of antibodies to haemagglutinins and neuraminidases is highest when the antibodies are directed against the strain-specific antigens. It should be emphasized that one type of test is not always more refined than another (e.g., radial immunodiffusion versus complement fixation) for all antigen/antibody reactions; the refinement also depends on the nature of the antigen that is used in the test.

Accuracy

In common with other diagnostic tests, 'false positives' and 'false negatives' can occur (see Chapter 9). *Table 17.8* lists the reasons for positive and negative results in serological tests.

Table 17.7 Summary of tests for influenza serology. (From Stuart-Harris and Schild, 1976.)

Test	Test antigens	Antibody detected	Recommended use[θ]	
			Serosurvey	Serodiagnosis
HI	Whole virus	HA[ζ]	++++	++++
NI	Whole virus	NA[ζ]	++++	
CF	CAM extract	NP		++
	Whole virus	HA, NA		+++
SRD	Whole virus*	HA, NA	+++	++++
	Disrupted virus*	NP, MP		+++
IDD	Disrupted virus*	HA, NA	+	++
	Disrupted virus*	NP, MP	+	++
N-IHA	NA	NA	++++	

HI = haemagglutination inhibition
NI = neuraminidase inhibition
CF = complement fixation
SRD = single radial immunodiffusion
IDD = immuno-double-diffusion
N-IHA= neuraminidase-indirect haemagglutination
HA = haemagglutinin
NA = neuraminidase
NP = nucleoprotein
MP = matrix protein
CAM = chorioallantoic membrane
[θ]The usefulness of the test for the indicated purpose is expressed on a scale of + (least useful) to ++++ (most useful).
[ζ]Serum containing high antibody titre to the second surface antigen (HA or NA) may at low dilutions and under certain conditions cause inhibition.
*Test refinement (specificity) achieved by selecting viruses or recombinant viruses with the required antigenic composition.

Table 17.8 Reasons for positive and negative results in serological tests. (From Stites *et al.*, 1982).

Positive results	
Actual infection	true +ve
Group cross-reactions	
Non-specific inhibitors	false +ve
Non-specific agglutinins	
Negative results	
Absence of infection	true −ve
Natural or induced tolerance	
Improper timing	
Improper selection of test	
Non-specific inhibitors e.g. anticomplementary serum; tissue culture toxic substances	false −ve
Antibiotic induced immunoglobulin suppression	
Incomplete or blocking antibody	
Insensitive tests	

Positive results

A true positive result derives from actual infection.

False positive results occur for a variety of reasons. **Group cross-reactions** can occur between an infectious agent and antibodies to different organisms with similar antigens. For example, infection with *Yersinia enterocolitica*, serotype 9, can produce antibodies that cross-react with *Brucella abortus* antigens.

Non-specific inhibitors present in serum may inhibit reactions that are normally associated with the action of intact antigens that are not specifically bound to antibody. These inhibitors therefore mimic the effects of antibody in the latter's absence. An example is non-specific inhibitors in haemagglutination tests against influenza viruses. Agglutination of antigen by **non-specific agglutinins** similarly mimics the effect of antibodies that are agglutinins.

Negative results

A true negative result indicates absence of infection.

Again, false negative results can occur for several reasons. Some animals show **natural** or **induced tolerance** to antigens and therefore do not produce antibodies when challenged with the agent. Thus, exposure of the bovine foetus to bovine virus diarrhoea in the first half of gestation results in offspring that do not produce detectable antibodies when challenged with the same strain of virus (Coria and McClurkin, 1978).

Improper timing may result in a test's failure to detect infection. For instance, sampling of some cows before abortion, using the CFT, may not detect *Br. abortus*

because detectable complement fixing antibodies may not appear until after abortion (e.g., Robertson, 1971).

Some tests may be unsuitable for detecting infection. Thus, infection by African swine fever virus cannot be detected using a serum neutralization test because infected pigs do not produce detectable levels of neutralizing antibodies (De Boer, 1967); an immunofluorescence test, however, will detect antibodies.

Some **non-specific inhibitors** will produce false negative results by their mode of action (cf. those above that produce false positive results). Some sera, notably contaminated and haemolysed specimens, are anticomplementary; thus complement cannot be fixed in the CFT and the test is therefore assumed to be negative although antibodies may be present. This can occur with CFTs for *Br. abortus* infections (Worthington, 1982). Similarly, substances that are toxic to tissue culture monolayers may mimic the effects of unneutralized virus, giving the impression that neutralizing antibodies are absent when they may be present.

Some antibodies are incomplete and so cannot take part in antigen/antibody test reactions. A common type of canine autoimmune haemolytic anaemia is characterized by incomplete antibodies on the surface of red blood cells, which can only be detected by an antiglobulin test (Halliwell, 1978). Occasionally **blocking antibodies** prevent antigen/antibody reactions occurring. This sometimes occurs when conducting CFTs for bovine *Br. abortus* infection (Plackett and Alton, 1975), as a result of excess IgG_1 blocking IgG_2 (the latter being responsible for complement fixation) at low concentrations: this is the 'prozone' effect.

Finally, a serological test may be too insensitive to detect antibody. Sensitivity in this context again refers to the ability of a test to detect amounts of antibody or antigen (i.e., analytical sensitivity). *Table 17.9* lists some common serological tests and their approximate sensitivities. Some of the the new molecular techniques (e.g., the polymerase chain reaction) are extremely analytically sensitive (Belák and Ballagi-Pordány, 1993) and therefore compare favourably with serological tests in detecting infection (Kitchin *et al.*, 1990).

Evaluation of diagnostic tests

Sensitivity and specificity

Diagnostic sensitivity and diagnostic specificity were introduced in Chapter 9 as indicators of the **validity** of diagnostic tests; and, for brevity, were just termed

Table 17.9 Relative analytical sensitivity of assays for antigens and antibodies. (From Stites and Rodgers, 1991.)

Technique	Approximate sensitivity (per dl)
Total serum proteins (by biuret or refractometry)	100 mg
Serum protein electrophoresis (zone electrophoresis)	100 mg
Analytical ultracentrifugation	100 mg
Immunoelectrophoresis	5–10 mg
Immunofixation	5–10 mg
Single radial diffusion	<1–2 mg
Double diffusion in agar (Ouchterlony)	<1 mg
Electroimmunodiffusion (rocket electrophoresis)	<0.5 mg
One-dimensional double electroimmunodiffusion (counterimmunoelectrophoresis)	<0.1 mg
Nephelometry	0.1 mg
Complement fixation	1 μg
Agglutination	1 μg
Enzyme immunoassay (ELISA)	<1 μg
Quantitative immunofluorescence	<1 pg
Radioimmunoassay	<1 pg

sensitivity and specificity; this convention will be followed in the remainder of this chapter. Although the discussion is in the context of serological investigations, it is equally relevant to other types of diagnostic test and their application (e.g., in genetic screening), and to the evaluation of questionnaires. To reiterate: the **sensitivity** of a diagnostic method is the proportion of true positives that are detected by the method; the **specificity** of the method is the proportion of true negatives that are detected.

Continuous and ordinal test variables

Sensitivity and specificity can be calculated for tests in which the variable that is measured is nominal and dichotomous; for example, presence or absence of tapeworms (*Table 9.1*). However, in many tests, the test variables are continuous (e.g., α-mannosidase levels: see Chapter 22), or are measured on the ordinal scale (e.g., single serial dilution antibody titres). Although methods for evaluating such tests are available (e.g., estimating the mean and standard deviation of the difference between the test measurement and a valid reference measurement: Bland and Altman, 1986), it is common practice to dichotomize measurements into 'positive' or 'negative'. This requires definition of a **cut-off point**.

When a cut-off point is identified, there is then clearly an inverse relationship between sensitivity and specificity in a particular test. This is illustrated in *Figure 17.1* in

which the upper graph represents the frequency distribution of a variable in a healthy population and the lower graph represents its frequency distribution in a diseased population. Individuals for whom the variable's value is to the right of the cut-off point, *C*, are classified as diseased; individuals for whom the variable's value is to the left of the cut-off point are classified as healthy. Animals with values to the right of the cut-off point in the upper graph are false positives; animals with values to the left of the cut-off point in the lower graph are false negatives. If the area under each curve represents 100% then the marked area to the right of the cut-off point corresponds to the test's sensitivity, whereas the marked area to the left of the cut-off point corresponds to the test's specificity. If fewer false positives are required, *C* is moved to the right: specificity increases and sensitivity decreases. However, if fewer false negatives are required, *C* is moved to the left: sensitivity increases and specificity decreases.

Table 17.10 also illustrates the inverse relationship between sensitivity and specificity in the ELISA for antibody to *Brucella abortus*. As the cut-off point (positive threshold) increases, sensitivity decreases and specificity increases.

Defining the cut-off point: Cut-off points have been determined in several ways. They have been arbitrarily defined as two (e.g., Coker-Vann *et al.*, 1984) or three (e.g., Gottstein, 1984) standard deviations greater than

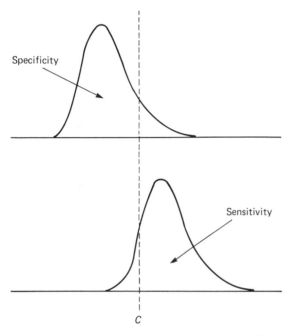

Fig. 17.1 The relationship between sensitivity and specificity for continuous test variables (see text for explanation). Upper graph = frequency distribution of a variable in a healthy population; lower graph = frequency distribution of the variable in a diseased population; C = cut-off point defining the boundary between healthy and diseased individuals.

the mean of the test values of the unaffected individuals. This approach fails to consider the frequency of disease and the distribution of test results in diseased individuals, and ignores the impact of false-positive and false-negative errors. Another approach is one that identifies 95% of individuals with disease as being test-positive (Weinstein and Fineberg, 1980). This ignores the distribution of test results in unaffected individuals, the prevalence of the disease, and all consequences except those that are due to false-negative error. Alternatively, the value that minimizes the total number (Cummings and Richard, 1988) or total cost (Anderson, 1958) of misdiagnoses can be selected. The optimum cut-off point also depends on the frequency distribution of the test variable in the healthy and diseased populations, which may be complicated. This topic is discussed in detail by Weinstein and Fineberg (1980) and Vizard et al. (1990).

When a large cross-section of a population is initially tested to detect disease (e.g., in screening) interpretation of the test is directed towards increased sensitivity at the expense of specificity. This is because initial tests are not usually intended to provide definitive diagnoses but are designed to detect as many cases as possible. Therefore, a high proportion of false positives (resulting from increased sensitivity) is not as critical as a high proportion of false negatives (resulting from increased specificity), and the cut-off point is shifted accordingly.

Ascertaining true status

Calculation of sensitivity and specificity requires an independent, valid criterion — also termed a '**gold standard**' — by which to define an animal's true disease status. Thus, when evaluating the centrifugation/flotation technique for diagnosing equine cestodiasis (*Table 9.1*), post-mortem examination of the intestinal tract was the gold standard. Similarly, in the evaluation of the ELISA for brucellosis, bacterial culture was used to define true positives, whereas true negative animals were selected from herds known to be *Brucella*-free (*Table 17.10*). A battery of alternative tests may also be used as a gold standard, animals being defined as true positives if they are simultaneously positive to several tests, and categorized as true negatives if they are simultaneously negative to the tests (Mateu-de-Antonio et al., 1993).

Additionally, the diseased and healthy animals to which the gold standard is applied should be representative of the population in which the test is to be applied. Thus, a screening test is conducted in the general population, and so the gold standard should be applied to a sample of diseased and healthy animals drawn from this population. In contrast, a clinical diagnostic test is run on animals for which there is usually already evidence of disease, and the test needs to distinguish between animals with the relevant condition (the 'diseased' animals) and those animals with diseases that are similar to the condition (these therefore constitute the 'healthy' animals). It follows that the sensitivity and specificity of a test may be different when it is applied as a screening test than when it is used as a diagnostic test in a veterinary clinic. Martin and Bonnett (1987) describe the derivation of sensitivity and specificity in a clinical setting.

Confidence intervals can be calculated for sensitivity and specificity using the formula for calculating disease prevalence for a simple random sample described in Chapter 13, because this is a general formula for estimating confidence intervals for proportions.

Estimating true prevalence

If the sensitivity and specificity of a test are known then a corrected estimate of the true prevalence, P, can be made by:

Table 17.10 Effect of various positive thresholds on the serodiagnostic interpretation of the enzyme immunoassay (ELISA) for the detection of bovine antibody to *Brucella abortus*. (From Agriculture Canada, 1984.)

Positive[a] threshold	Sensitivity[b]	Specificity[c] Non-vac	Vac[d]	Prevalence[e] of disease (%)	Predictive value +ve test Non-vac	Vac[e]	−ve test Either
≥0.220	0.960	0.990	0.852	10	0.92	0.42	1.00
				1	0.50	0.06	1.00
				0.1	0.09	0.01	1.00
≥0.260	0.943	0.995	0.930	10	0.95	0.60	0.99
				1	0.64	0.12	1.00
				0.1	0.15	0.01	1.00
≥0.300	0.937	0.998	0.948	10	0.98	0.67	0.99
				1	0.84	0.15	1.00
				0.1	0.34	0.02	1.00
≥0.340	0.920	0.999	0.969	10	0.99	0.77	0.99
				1	0.90	0.23	1.00
				0.1	0.48	0.03	1.00

[a] Minimum reactivity (expressed as Absorbence[414]) considered to be antibody positive.
[b] Sensitivity based on 175 sera from *Brucella* culture-positive cattle.
[c] Specificity (non-vaccinates) based on 1128 sera from *Brucella*-free herds; specificity (vaccinates) based on 1079 sera from field vaccinated cattle.
[d] *B. abortus* strain 19 vaccination status. [e] Theoretical disease prevalence.

$$P = \frac{P^T + \text{specificity} - 1}{\text{sensitivity} + \text{specificity} - 1}$$

where P^T is the test prevalence.

Confidence intervals for P also can be calculated by using the formula in Chapter 13. The numerator in P is extrapolated from the numerator in P^T, using the test's sensitivity and specificity.

Predictive value

When using either serological or other screening tests to determine the presence of disease in a population it is important to know the probability that an animal, 'positive' according to the test, is actually positive; alternatively that a test-negative animal is a true negative. These probabilities are the **predictive values** of the test. The parameter most often quoted as the predictive value of a test is the predictive value of a positive (as opposed to negative) test result.

The predictive value depends on specificity, sensitivity and prevalence. Sensitivity and specificity are innate characteristics of a test and (for a defined cut-off point) do

not vary, but the prevalence of a disease in a population being tested will affect the proportion of test positive animals, P^T, that are actually diseased.

There are two components to P_T:

1. the true positives;
2. the false positives.

The proportion of animals, P^T, is then:

$$P \times \text{sensitivity} + (1-P) \times (1-\text{specificity}).$$

For example, if $P = 0.01$ (1%), sensitivity = 0.99 (99%) and specificity = 0.99 (99%), then:

$$P^T = 0.01 \times 0.99 + (1-0.01) \times (1-0.99)$$
$$= 0.02.$$

This represents an overestimation of 100% (the actual prevalence is 0.01 and the estimated prevalence is 0.02). The smaller the prevalence, the larger the proportional overestimation, that is, the lower the predictive value (positive test result).

The predictive value (positive test result) is given by:

$$\frac{P \times \text{sensitivity}}{P \times \text{sensitivity} + (1-P) \times (1-\text{specificity})}$$

Table 17.11 Possible results of a diagnostic test.

Test status	True status		Totals
	Diseased	Not diseased	
Diseased	a	b	a + b
Not diseased	c	d	c + d
Totals	a + c	b + d	a + b + c + d

It can be expressed as a value between 0 and 1, but is commonly expressed as a percentage.

Alternatively, the calculation can be expressed more simply in terms of the values in *Table 17.11* which were exemplified originally in *Table 9.1*. The table categorizes animals into those that are 'true' and 'false' positives and negatives.

- Sensitivity = $a/(a+c)$.
- Specificity = $d/(b+d)$.
- The predictive value (positive test result) = $a/(a+b)$.
- The predictive value (negative test result) = $d/(c+d)$.

Again, confidence intervals can be calculated using the formula for calculating disease prevalence for a simple random sample (Chapter 13).

Five screening tests (or modifications of them) are available for brucellosis testing: the tube agglutination test (TAT), the CFT, the Brewer card test, the ELISA, and the milk ring test. Sufficient data are available to estimate the sensitivity and specificity of the first four (MAF, 1977; Agriculture Canada, 1984). These are summarized in *Table 17.12*.

Assume that the TAT will be applied to 100 000 cattle in three different areas in which the prevalence of brucellosis is 3%, 0.1% and 0.01% respectively. From these data, and the data in *Table 17.12*, the sensitivity, specificity and predictive value (of a positive test result) of the test can be calculated for the populations in each of

Table 17.12 Sensitivity and specificity of four screening tests for bovine brucellosis.

	Sensitivity (%)	Specificity (%)
Tube agglutination test	62.0	99.5
Complement fixation test	97.5	99.0
Brewer card test	95.2	98.5
ELISA*	96.0	99.0

*Positive threshold ≥ 0.220; specificity in non-vaccinated cattle (see *Table 17.9*).

the three areas. The results are given in *Table 17.13a, b* and *c*, respectively. As the prevalence of disease declines, so does the predictive value of the test, which could result in an increasing proportion of healthy animals being destroyed in a test and slaughter programme. This is also demonstrated in *Table 17.10*.

At low prevalence levels, even relatively 'good' tests (sensitivity = 99%; specificity = 99%) have a low predictive value (*Figure 17.2*). If a test with a sensitivity of 0.990 (99%) and a specificity of 0.999 (99.9%) were used in a disease eradication campaign then, if the prevalence were 0.1 (10%), a single test conducted on 10 million animals would record 990 000 true positives and 9000 false positives. The test therefore would be acceptable at the beginning of the campaign. However, as the campaign proceeded, the prevalence would fall. When the prevalence was reduced to 0.0001 (0.01%) the test would record 9900 true positives and 9990 false positives. *The number of false positives would be unchanged after the disease was eradicated.* Therefore, acceptable levels of sensitivity and specificity depend on the stage of a control or eradication campaign. Ideally, towards the end of an eradication campaign, a more sensitive and specific test is required if the campaign depends only upon a single serological test. In practice, other techniques are used, such as serial testing (see below), isolation of infected farms and maintenance of disease-free areas.

In some tests there are no false positives; for example, when identifying blood parasites by microscopic examination of blood films. Estimation of true prevalence in this circumstance is discussed by Waltner-Toews *et al.* (1986c).

Tests may also be applied to aggregates of animals (e.g., pens and herds) with the object of classifying the aggregate, rather than its individual members, as either diseased or healthy. If there is one biological sample (e.g., a bulk milk sample or a pooled faeces sample) from each aggregate, the formulae for sensitivity, specificity and predictive value, described above, may be applied. Assessment of the aggregate's status is also uncomplicated if the true status of test-positive animals can be ascertained quickly using a gold standard. However, if only a sample of animals is tested in each aggregate, sensitivity and specificity at the aggregate level are affected not only by the sensitivity and specificity at the individual level but also by the sample size. The overall effect is that, for a defined sensitivity and specificity at the individual level, aggregate-level sensitivity increases and aggregate-level specificity decreases as the sample size increases. Martin (1988), Martin *et al.* (1992) and Donald *et al.* (1994) discuss this topic in detail.

Table 17.13 Predictive value (positive test result) of the tube agglutination test for bovine brucellosis at three different prevalence levels (sensitivity = 62%; specificity = 99.5%).

Test status	True status		Total
	Brucellosis present	Brucellosis absent	
(a) Prevalence of brucellosis: 3%			
Brucellosis present	1860 (*a*)	480 (*b*)	2340
Brucellosis absent	1140 (*c*)	96 520 (*d*)	97 600
Total	3000	97 000	100 000

Predictive value (positive result) = *a*/(*a*+*b*) = 79.5%

(b) Prevalence of brucellosis: 0.1%			
Brucellosis present	62	500	562
Brucellosis absent	38	99 400	99 438
Total	100	99 900	100 000

Predictive value (positive result) = 11.0%

(c) Prevalence of brucellosis: 0.01%			
Brucellosis present	6	500	506
Brucellosis absent	4	99 490	99 494
Total	10	99 990	100 000

Predictive value (positive result) = 1.2%

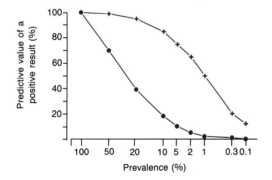

Fig. 17.2 The relationship between prevalence and predictive value of a positive test result. +: sensitivity = 99%; specificity = 99%. ●: sensitivity = 70%; specificity = 70%.

Further discussion of the predictive value of serological and other diagnostic tests is provided by Vecchio (1966), Galen and Gambino (1975) and Rogan and Gladen (1978), and Chapter 22 includes a discussion of diagnostic tests in relation to the risk of importation of diseases into a country.

Multiple testing

Multiple testing involves the use of more than one test, and is commonly encountered in clinical diagnosis and herd testing. Two main approaches can be adopted (Fletcher *et al.*, 1988): **parallel testing** and **serial testing**.

Parallel testing

Parallel testing involves conducting two or more tests on animals at the same time, and animals are considered to be affected if they are positive to *any* of the tests. For example, in the UK, cows that abort are tested routinely for brucellosis by means of bacterial culture from a vaginal swab, the Rose Bengal Test on serum and the milk ring test on milk, and animals are defined as affected if they are positive to any test. Parallel testing is often undertaken when animals are admitted to clinics, and an assessment is required quickly. In comparison with each

Table 17.14 The effect of parallel and serial testing on sensitivity, specificity and predictive value for two tests (A and B). (Modified from Fletcher *et al.*, 1988.)

Test	Sensitivity (%)	Specificity (%)	Predictive value (positive result)*	Predictive value (negative result)*
A	80	60	33	92
B	90	90	69	97
A and B (parallel)	98	54	35	99
A and B (serial)	72	96	82	93

*For 20% prevalence.

individual test, parallel testing increases sensitivity and therefore the predictive value of a negative test result, but reduces specificity and positive predictive value. A disease is therefore less likely to be missed; however, false positive diagnoses are more likely. Parallel testing effectively asks the animal to 'prove' that it is healthy.

Serial testing

In serial testing, tests are conducted sequentially (i.e., consecutively), based on the results of a previous test. Conventionally, only those animals that are positive to an initial test are tested again; therefore only animals that are positive to *all* tests are considered to be affected. Thus, *Serpulina hyodysenteriae* infection (see Chapter 5) is initially diagnosed by a fluorescent antibody test performed on faecal or gut mucosal smears; the status of positive animals is then confirmed by bacterial culture. Serial testing maximizes specificity and the predictive value of a positive test result, but lowers sensitivity and negative predictive value. More credence therefore can be attached to positive test results, but there is an increased risk that disease will be missed. Serial testing effectively asks the animal to 'prove' that it is affected by the condition that is being investigated. The test with the highest specificity should be used first to decrease the number of animals that are tested again.

Serial testing is an important part of disease eradication campaigns in which positive animals are culled from herds (see Chapter 22). Animals defined as diseased by an initial screening test are subjected to further tests to confirm their status, so that false positives are not unnecessarily removed.

The effects of serial and parallel testing on sensitivity, specificity and predictive value are shown in *Table 17.14*.

Negative-herd retesting

Testing can also be conducted only on animals that are negative to an initial test. This is usually applied at herd level, and involves periodically retesting animals in previously test-negative herds with the *same* test.

Negative-herd retesting is an important component of eradication campaigns. It improves aggregate-level sensitivity, that is, it increases the likelihood of detecting on a premises an infectious agent that eluded detection earlier (e.g., because antibodies had not yet been produced, or the infection was subsequently reintroduced). It therefore asks a herd to 'prove' that it is free from the condition that is being investigated. For instance, in tuberculosis eradication in the UK, using the comparative intradermal test, reactors are culled and negative or inconclusive reactors are retested every 60 days until two clear herd tests are achieved. Thereafter, a check test is conducted after 6 or 12 months, before returning the herd to a less stringent four-year testing cycle.

The important characteristics of multiple test strategies are listed in *Table 17.15*. Multiple testing is discussed in more detail by Smith (1991).

Agreement between tests: the *kappa* statistic

If a gold standard is not available, it is only possible to assess the agreement between different tests, without assuming that one test is the best. The logic of using this approach is that agreement between tests is evidence of validity, whereas disagreement suggests that the tests are untrustworthy.

Table 17.16 presents the results of an examination of pigs' heads to identify atrophic rhinitis using two techniques: cross-sectional and longitudinal examination.

The observed proportion agreement between the two tests, $OP = (a+d)/n$, where $n = (a+b+c+d)$. Substituting the values in *Table 17.16*:

$$OP = (8 + 223)/248$$
$$= 0.932.$$

Table 17.15 Characteristics of multiple test strategies. (Modified from Smith, 1991.)

Considerations	Test strategy		
	Parallel	*Serial*	*Negative-herd retesting*
Effect of strategy	Increase sensitivity	Increase specificity	Increase sensitivity at aggregate level
Greatest predictive value	Negative test result	Positive test result	Negative test result at aggregate level
Purpose	Rule out a disease	Rule in a disease	Rule out a disease
Application and setting	Rapid assessment of individual patients; emergencies	Diagnosis when time is not crucial; test and removal programmes	Test and removal programmes
Comments	Useful when there is an important penalty for missing a disease (i.e., false negative results)	Useful when there is an important penalty for false positive results	Useful when there is an important penalty for missing a disease (i.e., false negative results)

This comparison, however, does not consider agreement that could arise just by *chance*. A more rigorous comparison can be made by calculating a statistic, **kappa** (see *Table 14.2*), which takes account of chance agreement.

The expected proportion of agreement by chance, *EP*, is calculated thus:

$$EP = [\{(a+b)/n\} \times \{(a+c)/n\}] + [\{(c+d)/n\} \times \{(b+d)/n\}]$$

Substituting the values from *Table 17.16*:

$$EP = [\{(8+1)/248\} \times \{(8+16)/248\}]$$
$$+ [\{(16+223)/248\} \times \{(1+223)/248\}]$$
$$= (0.036 \times 0.097) + (0.964 \times 0.903)$$

Table 17.16 Number of pigs' heads showing turbinate atrophy determined by cross-sectional and longitudinal examination of 248 heads. (Data derived from Visser *et al.*, 1988.)

Longitudinal examination	Cross-sectional examination	
	Atrophy present	*Atrophy absent*
Atrophy present	8 (*a*)	1 (*b*)
Atrophy absent	16 (*c*)	223 (*d*)

$$= 0.0035 + 0.8705$$
$$= 0.874.$$

Observed agreement − expected agreement
$$= OP - EP$$
$$= 0.932 - 0.874$$
$$= 0.058.$$

The maximum possible agreement beyond chance = $1 - EP = 0.126$.

Kappa is the excess agreement over that expected by chance, divided by the potential excess; that is:

$$kappa = (OP - EP)/(1 - EP)$$
$$= 0.058/0.126$$
$$= 0.460.$$

Kappa ranges from 1 (complete agreement) to 0 (agreement is equal to that expected by chance), whereas negative values indicate agreement less than is expected by chance. Arbitrary 'benchmarks' for evaluating observed *kappa* values are >0.81: almost perfect agreement; 0.61−0.80: substantial agreement; 0.41−0.60: moderate agreement; 0.21−0.40: fair agreement; 0−0.20: slight agreement; 0: poor agreement (Everitt, 1989). Thus, the point estimate of *kappa*, 0.460, suggests moderate agreement between the two methods of examination of pigs' heads.

The same approach can be used to assess clinical agreement. An individual clinician's diagnoses made on the same animals on different occasions are likely to produce *kappa* values between 0.6 and 0.8. In contrast, lower *kappa* values (0.5−0.6) can be expected when comparing the results of the diagnosis made on the same animals by different clinicians.

Confidence intervals can be calculated for *kappa* (Everitt, 1989). The statistic can also be generalized to studies involving dichotomous nominal data with several ratings of subjects, and to nominal data with several categories (Fleiss, 1981). However, the statistic is not suitable for assessing agreement between tests based on grouped continuous or ordinal data, where other techniques are more appropriate (Bland and Altman, 1986; Maclure and Willett, 1987). *Kappa* may also be defined differently in the contexts of agreement and correlation (Bloch and Kraemer, 1989). Note, too, that the correlation coefficient (see Chapter 14) is *not* a valid indicator of agreement between two tests or measurement methods (Bland and Altman, 1986). Perfect correlation will exist between two methods if the points lie along any straight line; whereas perfect agreement is obtainable only if the points lie along the line of equality.

Repeatability of diagnostic tests

The value of a diagnostic test (or questionnaire) is also judged by its **repeatability**, which is an indication of its reliability (see Chapter 9). This can be determined for a dichotomous outcome (i.e., positive or negative) by assessing the agreement between results when the test is repeated two or more times on the same animals. If the test is conducted twice then McNemar's change test for related samples (see Chapter 14) can be used. If the test is repeated three or more times then an extension of

McNemar's change test, **Cochran's Q test** (see *Table 14.2*), should be applied.

Cochran's Q test

The test statistic, Q (Cochran, 1950), is given by:

$$Q = \frac{(k-1)\{k\Sigma G^2 - (\Sigma G)^2\}}{k\Sigma L_i - \Sigma L_i^2}$$

where:

k = number of runs,
G = total number of positive results in each run,
L_i = total number of positive results in each animal.

Applying the formula to the results in *Table 17.17*:

$(k-1) = 4.$
$\Sigma G^2 = 9+16+36+64+64,$
$\quad = 189.$
$(\Sigma G)^2 = 29^2,$
$\quad = 841.$
$\Sigma L_i = 29.$
$\Sigma L_i^2 = 107.$

Thus:

$$Q = \frac{4[(5 \times 189) - 841]}{(5 \times 29) - 107}$$

$$= \frac{416}{38}$$

$$= 10.95.$$

The sampling distribution of Q is approximated by the χ^2 distribution with $k - 1$ degrees of freedom. Thus, the

Table 17.17 Results of five runs of a diagnostic test on 10 animals. Positive results are classified '1'; negative results are classified '0'.

Animal	Run 1	Run 2	Run 3	Run 4	Run 5	Totals (L_i)	L_i^2
1	0	0	0	0	0	0	0
2	0	0	1	1	0	2	4
3	0	0	1	1	1	3	9
4	0	1	1	1	1	4	16
5	0	0	0	0	1	1	1
6	0	1	0	1	1	3	9
7	0	0	1	1	1	3	9
8	1	0	0	1	1	3	9
9	1	1	1	1	1	5	25
10	1	1	1	1	1	5	25
Total	$G_1=3$	$G_2=4$	$G_3=6$	$G_4=8$	$G_5=8$	$\Sigma L_i=29$	$\Sigma L_i^2=107$

probability that the proportion of positive (and therefore negative) results is the same in each run, except for chance differences, can be determined with reference to Appendix XVII. Consulting row 4 (4 degrees of freedom) of the table, the observed value, 10.95, is greater than the tabulated statistic at the 5% level of significance (9.488). The implication is that the proportions of positive and negative results differ significantly among the various runs, and therefore that the repeatability of the test may be low.

Note that the appropriate statistical test for assessing repeatability is based on related samples, and is selected with reference to the level of measurement used in the diagnostic test and the frequency distribution of the test variables (see Chapter 14). Thus, the Wilcoxon signed ranks test would be used if the level of measurement was ordinal (see *Table 14.2*) (e.g., single-serial dilution dilution titres).

Significance tests do not indicate the magnitude of differences between repeated tests, and therefore their practical importance. However, *measures* of reliability can also be calculated. *Kappa* is appropriate for nominal data. Everitt (1989) describes measures for continuous data.

Serological tests

The repeatability of serological tests depends on a variety of factors including the degree of standardization of test reagents and the expertise of the tester; different results might be produced by two different laboratory technicians conducting the same test on the same serum sample. Thus, a twofold difference in antibody titre between samples from the same animal, taken at different times, may reflect either a true change in titre or similar titres associated with low repeatability.

Generally, a geometric fourfold change in antibody titre (e.g., from 1/16 to 1/64) is assumed to reflect a real change; a twofold change is not considered to be significant. *Table 17.18* illustrates the reasoning behind this decision. The table shows typical results when sera from 100 individuals are tested twice. Each of the two readings should be identical for a single serum sample. However, the table shows that this is true only for 62 samples. Of the remaining 38 samples, 34 show a twofold shift and four show a fourfold shift. The shift is caused by the value of the test's repeatability not being 100%. Note also that the fourfold shift in titres occurs with high dilutions. If these titres are typical of the test then, when future samples are drawn from the study population, 4% of the animals might be expected to show a fourfold shift in titre which does not represent a true change. Since this shift can be caused by the second sample showing either a

Table 17.18 Typical titres of sera from 100 individuals tested twice. (From Paul and White, 1973.)

First reading (reciprocal titre)	Second reading (reciprocal titre)	Frequency
<8	<8	24
<8	8	2
8	16	2
16	8	2
16	32	3
32	16	3
32	32	8
32	64	6
64	32	4
64	64	16
64	128	1
128	64	3
128	128	6
128	256	2
128	512	2
256	128	4
256	256	6
256	1024	2
512	256	2
512	512	2

higher or a lower titre than the first, then, when evidence of a rising titre is required from two samples taken from the same animal at different times, 2% of the animals can be expected to show spurious fourfold increases in titre. This degree of error is generally acceptable.

Serum banks

A serum bank is 'a planned catalogued collection of serum forming a random sample that is as representative as possible of a population and that is stored to preserve its immunological and biochemical characteristics' (Moorhouse and Hugh-Jones, 1981, after Timbs, 1980).

Applications of serum banks

The general principles of serum banks are discussed in two World Health Organization Technical Reports (WHO, 1959, 1970), and by Moorhouse and Hugh-Jones (1981). Additionally, the last two authors describe a computerized database for storing serum bank information.

In the context of identifying and titrating antibodies, a serum bank can aid the following goals in relation to infectious diseases:

1. identification of major health problems;
2. establishment of vaccination priorities;

3. demarcation of the distribution of diseases;
4. investigation of newly discovered diseases;
5. determination of epidemic periodicity;
6. an increase in the knowledge of disease aetiology;
7. evaluation of vaccination campaigns;
8. assessment of economic losses due to disease.

Sources of serum

Table 17.19 lists the potential sources of serum and some of their characteristics. This indicates that each source has its own advantages and disadvantages. The validity of results obtained from a serum bank depends on:

1. the sensitivity and specificity of the test performed on the serum;
2. the quality of the survey design used in collecting the serum;
3. the degree of degradation that has occurred in the serum during storage.

The first component is an inherent characteristic of the tests that are employed. The third component is related directly to the means of storage.

Collection and storage of serum

Collection

Samples should be taken aseptically. Blood should be allowed to clot for $1-2$ hours at room temperature, stored horizontally overnight at 4 °C, and then the serum should be separated by centrifugation at $2000-3000$ rpm for $10-15$ min. Blood can also be collected on filter paper discs; the serum can then be eluted later, although the amount of serum that is stored is small and may only allow semi-quantitative investigations.

Storage

Two storage techniques are available: **deep freezing** and **lyophilization** (**freeze-drying**). Four options are available for the former:

1. liquid phase of liquid nitrogen: -196 °C;
2. vapour phase of liquid nitrogen: -110 °C;
3. ultra-deep freeze: -70 °C to -90 °C;
4. standard deep freeze: -20 °C to -40 °C.

Prolonged storage at -20 °C may allow deterioration of antibodies. Refrigeration at 4 °C is satisfactory for short-term storage. Lyophilization is a better technique than deep freezing, but is relatively expensive and technically complex. The following facts should be remembered in relation to freezing:

1. the degree of deterioration at -20 °C depends on the type and quantity of immunoglobulins; sera with high IgM levels may be expected to lose specific activity more rapidly than those with high IgG levels, due to fragmentation (Moorhouse and Hugh-Jones, 1983); this is particularly salient to chronic infections in which levels of IgM decline relative to IgG levels (Tizard, 1982);
2. repeated thawing and refreezing can be deleterious; this is apparently not due to the thawing/freezing process *per se* (Cecchini *et al.*, 1992), but may result from the bacterial and enzymatic contents of non-sterile samples (see '6' below); samples should therefore be refrozen as soon as possible;
3. the use of cryoprotectants and/or enzyme inhibitors will reduce or eliminate deterioration;
4. uninterrupted storage at -20 °C appears to be a satisfactory procedure with very little loss of specific activity for at least two years; however, precise indications of the longevity of whole serum stored

Table 17.19 Potential sources of samples for serum banks and some of their characteristics. (From Moorhouse and Hugh-Jones, 1981.)

Source	Potential no. of samples	Selection bias in study population	Cost to serum bank	Ease of collection	Standard of documentation
Ad hoc field visits	High	Low	High	Low	High
Other field visits	High	Low-high	Low	High	Moderate-high
Slaughter houses	High	High	Low	High	Low
Livestock marketing chain	High	High	Low-moderate	Moderate	Low
Veterinary diagnostic laboratories	Low	High	Low	High	Moderate-high
Private individuals	Low	High	Low	Moderate	Moderate-high
Existing collection	Low-high	Low-high	Low	High	Low-high

under serum bank conditions are not available;
5. rapid freezing of samples is required;
6. sterility is important;
7. samples should be tested immediately after being thawed;
8. delays will lead to increased rates of proteolysis.

Despite a recommendation, over 35 years ago, for the establishment of veterinary and medical serum banks (WHO, 1959) this recommendation has not been heeded widely in veterinary medicine. Established banks include one in Canada, using serum collected during the bovine brucellosis eradication campaign (Kellar, 1983), and others in New Zealand (Timbs, 1980) and in Louisiana, US (Moorhouse and Hugh-Jones, 1981; Hugh-Jones, 1986a). The last of these includes serum samples salvaged from previous studies which have provided information on diseases in domesticated and wild animals (leptospirosis in horses and leprosy in armadillos).

Further reading

Dunn, G. (1989) *Design and Analysis of Reliability Studies.* Oxford University Press, New York/Edward Arnold, London. (*A comprehensive description of assessment of reliability and validity*)

Fraser, C.G. (1986) *Interpretation of Clinical Chemistry Laboratory Data.* Blackwell Scientific, Oxford. (*Includes a concise discussion of reference values*)

Griner, P.F., Mayewski, R.J., Mushlin, A.I. and Greenland, P. (1981) Selection and interpretation of diagnostic tests and procedures. Principles and applications. *Annals of Internal Medicine*, **94**, 553−600. (*A comprehensive introduction to the use of diagnostic tests in screening and clinical practice*)

Martin, S.W. and Bonnett, B. (1987) Clinical epidemiology. *Canadian Veterinary Journal*, **28**, 318−325. (*A discussion of the application of diagnostic tests in clinical practice*)

Moorhouse, P.D. and Hugh-Jones, M.E. (1981). Serum banks. *Veterinary Bulletin*, **51**, 277−290

Paul, J.R. and White, C. (Eds) (1973) *Serological Epidemiology.* Academic Press, New York and London

Worthington, R.W. (1982) Serology as an aid to diagnosis: uses and abuses. *New Zealand Veterinary Journal*, **30**, 93−97

18 Comparative epidemiology

Investigations of disease in one species of animal can provide valuable insights into the cause and pathogenesis of disease in another, and are an important part of **comparative medicine**. These investigations often use animal diseases as **biological models** of diseases in man.

Types of biological model

There are four types of biological model (Frenkel, 1969):

1. experimental (induced);
2. negative (nonreactive);
3. orphan;
4. spontaneous (natural).

Experimental (induced) models

Many models are attempts to reproduce experimentally in one species of animal diseases, pathological conditions and impaired function that occur in other species and, notably, in man. For example, cigarette smoke has been administered via nasal catheters to donkeys to study the effects of long-term smoking on tracheobronchial mucociliary activity (Albert *et al.*, 1971), and pharmacological models have been developed to improve extrapolation from animals to man (Travis, 1987). This approach is particularly meaningful when causal factors can be manipulated easily, such as nutritional deficiencies and excesses, endocrine disorders, and some microbial diseases. However, if pathogenesis depends on several factors, or the causal effect is 'weak', results may differ between animal species and man. For instance, teratogenic defects may depend on maternal susceptibility to virus infection or absorption of chemicals during a brief but critical period of pregnancy, and many animal species may need to be tested before a suitable model is found.

Negative (nonreactive) models

A negative model represents the counterpart to an induced model, and can be useful in studying why disease does not occur. Thus, normal mink may be studied to discover why they are resistant to the pathogenic effects of the virus that causes disease in Aleutian mink. Such 'non-models' are relatively rare.

Orphan models

Orphan models are diseases in animals which currently have no known natural analogue in man, but which may subsequently prove to be valuable in changing thinking on human disease. An historical example is Rous sarcoma virus of chickens (see Chapter 1) which revolutionized thinking on the cause of cancer.

Spontaneous (natural) models

Spontaneous models utilize the natural occurrence of disease in animals in order to increase understanding of human diseases. For example, comparative radiological, histological and serological investigations of sheep with and without periodontitis have revealed features similar to those of rapidly destructive forms of human periodontal disease, suggesting that the disease in sheep may be a suitable model for similar diseases in man (Ismaiel *et al.*, 1989). Spontaneous models may also be based on epidemiological investigations (notably, observational studies of diseases of companion animals) and constitute **comparative epidemiology**, which is the subject of this chapter.

Spontaneous versus experimental models

Companion animal spontaneous disease models have several advantages over experimental models. First, companion animals share similar environments with man, rather than living in the 'protected' environment of the

Table 18.1 Crude estimated annual rates for all cancers in man, ox, horse, cat and dog, and lifespan-adjusted equivalents* (data from the US). (Simplified from Dorn and Priester, 1987.)

Species	Estimated rate of malignancy/100 000/year	
	Crude	Lifespan-adjusted
Man	287.3**	287.3**
Ox	177.2	53.2
Horse	256.3	117.9
Cat	257.4	72.1
Dog	828.3	165.7

*Method of adjustment outlined in *Table 18.5*.
**All cancers except those of skin (other than melanoma). Approximately 150 non-melanoma skin cancers/100 000 should be added to make comparison with other species more accurate.

laboratory. Secondly, their diseases occur in natural circumstances, where interactions between a variety of causal factors may occur; experimental induction of disease may not accommodate such interactions. Thirdly, companion animals are phylogenetically more closely related to man than are the species commonly used in the laboratory (rats, mice, etc.). Fourthly, companion animals are more likely than inbred laboratory animals to display the heterogeneity of response to some causal factors (e.g., toxic agents and carcinogens) that is characteristic of man (Calabrese, 1986). Finally, the ethical objection to animal experimentation cannot be levelled against studies of spontaneously occurring diseases.

The value of comparative epidemiological studies may be either the coincidental product of investigations directed mainly at improving the health of animals, or may stem directly from the use of animals as surrogates for man (Schwabe, 1984). Several areas of interest have developed, frequently using the surrogate approach.

Cancer

A major field of comparative epidemiology has been the study of cancer. Established veterinary databases, especially the Veterinary Medical Data Base (VMDB: see Chapter 11) and the California Animal Neoplasm Registry, have provided much of the data used in these studies, and the value of these databases to comparative studies was realized shortly after they were developed (Tjalma, 1968). The incidence of spontaneous tumours

(notably cancers) is sufficiently high, particularly in the dog, to compile a large series of cases for study (*Table 18.1*).

Monitoring environmental carcinogens

The ageing process in dogs and other animals is more rapid than in man (Kirkwood, 1985). Tumours in dogs are seen most frequently between the ages of 9 and 11 years (Dorn *et al.*, 1968) — much earlier than in man. Thus, it is possible to assess the affects of possible environmental carcinogens more quickly in dogs than in man. For example, the latent period of bladder cancer is as little as 4 years in the dog (Hayes, 1976) in contrast to at least 20 years in man (Hoover and Cole, 1973). There is an association between canine bladder cancer and exposure to insecticides (Glickman *et al.*, 1989). There is also a significant positive correlation between the overall level of industrial activity and both canine bladder cancer morbidity (*Figure 18.1a*) and human bladder cancer mortality (*Figure 18.1b*). These correlations suggest a causal relationship (reasoning by the 'method of concomitant variation'; see Chapter 3). Similarly, the proportion of canine oropharyngeal cancers that are tonsillar squamous cell carcinomas is much higher in polluted industrial locations than in non-industrial areas (Reif and Cohen, 1971; also *Table 18.2*). These results suggest that carcinogens, probably airborne, may be present in industrial areas, and that dogs and their tumours can act as **sentinels**, facilitating early identification of environmental carcinogens.

Negative findings can also be useful. For instance, increased incidence rates of neoplasia have not been

Fig. 18.1 (a) Proportional morbidity ratios (PMRs)* of bladder cancer among dogs living in a 25-mile radius of their veterinary clinic in the US, plotted against the percentage of men employed in manufacturing industries in the counties with the veterinary clinic. r = correlation coefficient (see Chapter 14). (b) Human age-adjusted mortality/100 000 for bladder cancer (1950–1969) in white men (WM) and white women (WF) living in the counties with the surveyed veterinary clinics, plotted against the percentage of men employed in manufacturing industries in 1970. r = correlation coefficient. (From Hayes et al., 1981.)

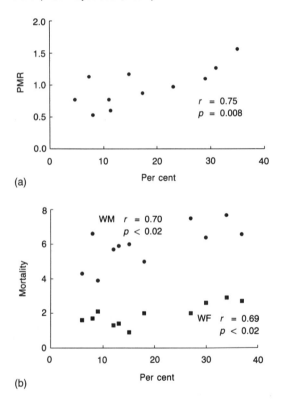

(a)

(b)

*Standardized ratios based on proportional morbidity rates (Hayes et al., 1981).

demonstrated in dogs environmentally exposed to uranium products following their use in the building industry (Reif et al., 1983). This provides evidence that uranium waste does not constitute a health hazard to dogs, and probably not to man either.

Identifying causes

Veterinary observational studies can provide clues to the causes of human cancer. For example, an association has

been found between canine mesothelioma and exposure to both asbestos (which is a risk factor for human mesothelioma) and to pesticides, notably flea preparations (Table 18.3). Some of the latter contain asbestos-like compounds, which could thus be risk factors for human mesothelioma and other tumours. Similar compounds are found in talc, and an association has been demonstrated between ovarian cancer in women and use of cosmetic talc (Cramer et al., 1982). The latent period of human mesothelioma following occupational exposure to asbestos is long, nearly always greater than 20 years, with most cases occurring after 30 years (Selikoff et al., 1979). In contrast, the greatest risk of development of canine mesothelioma is between 5 and 9 years of age. Thus, mesothelioma in dogs may be a useful sentinel for unrecognized human exposure to asbestos.

Comparison of site-specific cancer rates can also offer clues to aetiology. Human cancer rates are at least three times greater than canine and feline rates for six major cancer sites: the digestive, respiratory and urinary systems, and the uterus, ovary and prostate gland (Schneider, 1976). These disparities provide indirect evidence of possible causes. For instance, the high rate of human ovarian cancer may be related to the regular menstrual cycle. Female cats have a similar oestrus cycle to women (cats are seasonally polyoestrous, women are polyoestrous; each with cycles of three to four weeks) but a much lower rate of ovarian cancer, even with compensation for the proportion of neutered cats. However, pregnancy is much more frequent in cat than in woman. Thus, pregnancy may protect against the cancer, implying that hormonal status may be a determinant.

The age-specific incidence rates of mammary cancer in bitches and women are compared in Figure 18.2, after calculating a canine equivalent of human age (see 'Comparing ages' below). The rates are similar until the human menopause, when ovarian activity decreases and the human rate tends to stabilize, suggesting an hormonal determinant. This suggestion is supported by the demonstration of receptors for steroid hormones in the cytosol fractions from canine mammary carcinomas (Martin et al., 1984), and also by the reduction in their growth rate by the anti-oestrogen, tamoxifen, or by ovariectomy, after transplantation into nude mice (Pierrepoint et al., 1984).

Animals are not exposed to some factors which may act as confounders in human studies. Investigations in animal populations, therefore, can avoid these potential confounders. For instance, smoking is a risk factor for human mesothelioma. The significant association between canine mesothelioma and exposure to asbestos, described above,

Table 18.2 Proportions of canine oropharyngeal cancers that are tonsillar squamous cell carcinomas, by geographical location. (Modified from Bostock and Curtis, 1984.)

Location	Year	Proportion (%)	Number of cases	Totals (all malignant oropharyngeal neoplasms)
London	1950−53	46	35	76
US (non-industrial)	1959	6	8	124
	1964−74	7	31	469
Philadelphia	1952−58	22	29	130
South-east England	1978−81	13	19	152
Melbourne	1978−81	3	2	75

is demonstrated in the absence of active smoking, and therefore is not confounded by it.

Potential risk factors may also be easier to quantify accurately in animals than in man. The diet of dogs, for example, is relatively constant, particularly when proprietary foods are consumed. An investigation of the role of diet in the development of canine mammary cancer has not demonstrated an association between a high-fat diet and the disease, although similar human studies, with the attendant difficulties in estimating fat intake precisely, have produced conflicting results (Sonnenschein *et al.*, 1991).

Comparing ages

The lifespans of animals are different from that of man (*Figure 18.3*). Thus, as a calendar and a 'biological' year are the same for man, a correction should be made for the majority of species that have several 'biological' years during one calendar year, so that more meaningful comparisons of morbidity and mortality can be made.

Two techniques are used (Kirkwood, 1985). First, anatomical and physiological characteristics that correlate with age can be sought (e.g., adult brain weight, onset of puberty and reproductive senescence). Secondly, the survival pattern of different species can be compared mathematically using an equation based on Gompertz's law, which defines a relationship between probability of death and age. The two techniques are frequently combined (*Table 18.4*).

The lifespan-adjustment method of Lebeau (1953) also amalgamates these two approaches and is illustrated in *Figure 18.4*. Lebeau argued that once maturity is reached, ageing occurs at a constant rate in dogs and man. A 1-year-old dog is equivalent in age to a 15-year-old person; a 2-year-old dog to a 24-year-old person; and, above the age of 2 years, each one year of a dog's life is equivalent to four human years. Thus, a 10-year-old dog is equivalent to a 56-year-old person (24 years, plus four years for each canine year from 3 years old onwards). His technique for calculating human age equivalence is utilized in *Figure 18.2*. However, Reif (1983) emphasizes

Table 18.3 Odds ratios and associated 95% confidence intervals for two risk factors for canine mesothelioma. (Simplified from Glickman *et al.*, 1983.)

Risk factor	Estimated odds ratio $(\hat{\psi})$	95% confidence interval for ψ
Probable exposure of owner to asbestos by occupation or hobby	8.0	1.4, 10.6
Exposure to pesticide	11.0	1.5, 82.1

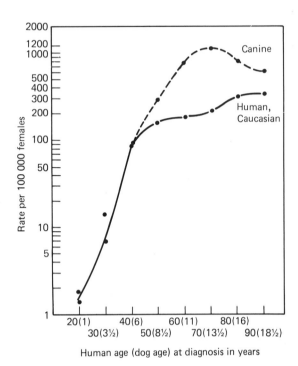

Fig. 18.2 Annual female human (Caucasian) and canine age-specific incidence rates for mammary cancer. (Modified from Schneider, 1970.)

the problems associated with such a conversion, because large breeds of dog tend to live shorter lives than small breeds.

Other criteria for age equivalence are based on the mean age of populations and correction factors related to recorded maximum lifespans such as those presented in *Figure 18.3*. Thus, using the correction factors in *Table 18.5*, the estimated bovine rate of malignancy in *Table*

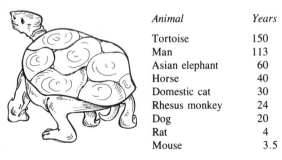

Animal	Years
Tortoise	150
Man	113
Asian elephant	60
Horse	40
Domestic cat	30
Rhesus monkey	24
Dog	20
Rat	4
Mouse	3.5

Fig. 18.3 The maximum verifiable lifespans of several animals.

18.1 (177.2/100 000/year) is lifespan-adjusted by multiplying the value by 0.30, giving a lifespan-adjusted value of 53.2/100 000/year.

Another correction, in addition to lifespan adjustment, should also be made when comparing human and companion animal populations because of the different proportions of individuals of various ages in each population. If canine populations (*Figure 5.4a* and *5.4b*) are compared with human populations it can be noted that the shape of the canine population pyramid is similar to that of human populations with high fecundity and a low proportion of individuals surviving to old age; for example, 19th century European and North American populations and contemporary populations in developing countries (*Figure 18.5a*). It contrasts with the pyramid of human populations with low fecundity and a high proportion of individuals surviving to old age; for example, in contemporary developed countries (*Figure 18.5b*). Most comparative studies are undertaken in developed countries, and so the lifespan-adjusted rates in the populations that are being compared should also be age-adjusted (see Chapter 4).

Figure 18.6 presents crude rates, and age- and lifespan-adjusted rates, for mammary cancer in bitches and women, indicating the difference between the crude rates and the rates with two levels of adjustment. The crude rates suggest that cancer incidence is greater in bitches than in women. However, the age- and lifespan-adjusted rates, which reflect the comparative incidence best, demonstrate that women are more prone to the cancer than either bitches or cats.

Some other diseases

Diseases with a major genetic component

Comparative studies also provide evidence for genetic causal mechanisms. Thus, there is evidence, derived from epidemiological and family studies, of the importance of genetic factors in the aetiology of human congenital heart disease. However, limited success has been achieved in identifying the anatomical defects that have significant genetic causal factors, and in determining the nature of the underlying genetic abnormality and the pathway from genetic defect to structural abnormality. However, studies on dogs have provided valuable insights into this type of disease. The inheritance of patent ductus arteriosus (PDA) in dogs is more complex than a simple autosomal dominant mode (Patterson *et al.*, 1971). There is evidence that inheritance of the condition is multifactorial (see

Table 18.4 Examples of comparative ages between humans, dogs and cats. (From Schneider, 1976.)

Human age (years)	Canine age equivalent (years)*	Feline age equivalent (years)*
24	2	1−1½
32−35	4	4
52−55	9	10
72−75	14	16
>91	>18	>21

*Based on the age when maturity is reached and on survival that excludes euthanasia of animals because of human-related reasons (e.g., if animals are unwanted).

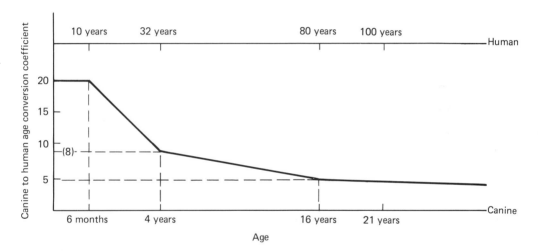

Fig. 18.4 Conversion of canine age to its human age equivalent (example: age of dog = 4 years, conversion coefficient = 8, thus human age equivalent = 4 × 8 = 32 years). (Modified from Lebeau, 1953.)

Table 18.5 Lifespan correction factors derived from the lifespan of several species. (From Dorn and Priester, 1987.)

Species	Recorded maximum lifespan (RML)	Correction factor (RML/100)
Man	100*	1
Ox	30	0.30
Horse	46	0.46
Pig	26	0.27
Sheep	20	0.20
Dog	20	0.20
Cat	28	0.28

*Arbitrary.

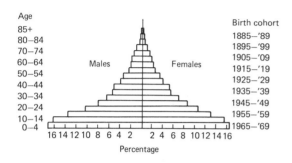

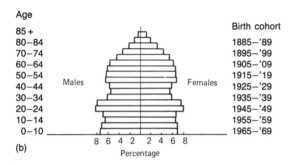

Fig. 18.5 Human population pyramids. (**a**) Mexico, 1970; (**b**) Sweden, 1970. (From Ewbank and Wray, 1980.)

Chapter 5), and that there are different thresholds for expression of the less severe ductus diverticulum and the fully-patent ductus arteriosus (*Figure 18.7*).

Histological studies on litters of poodles genetically predisposed to PDA subsequently demonstrated that PDA is the result of a genetically determined extension of the non-contractile wall of the aorta into the ductus arteriosus. The role of environmental factors (e.g., diet and

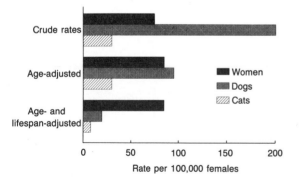

Fig. 18.6 Estimated annual incidence rates of mammary cancer in women, dogs and cats: crude rates and two levels of rate adjustment (data from the US). (From Dorn and Priester, 1987.)

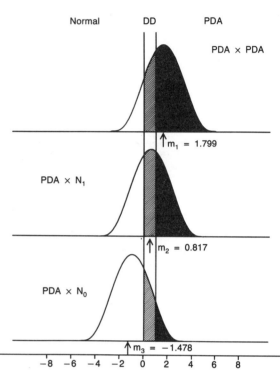

Fig. 18.7 Two-threshold model of hereditary patent ductus arteriosus (PDA) in dogs. PDA: patent ductus arteriosus; N_1: normal first-degree relatives; N_0: normal unrelated dogs; m: mean liability in offspring of crosses, expressed as standardized units for likely incidence of the condition (Falconer, 1989). Liability to defective ductal closure is depicted as a continuous variable, phenotypic discontinuities occurring at critical thresholds on the underlying scale. Below the lower threshold, the ductus closes throughout its length. Between the upper and the lower thresholds, the ductus closes at the end nearest the pulmonary artery, but remains open over the rest of its length, producing a ductus diverticulum. Beyond the upper threshold, the ductus remains open over its entire length, and PDA is present. The areas under the curves defined by the thresholds represent proportions of offspring observed in each phenotypic class. Mean liability of offspring from outcrosses of PDA-affected dogs to normal unrelated dogs (m_3) lies below, but overlaps, both thresholds. Mean liability in crosses between two dogs with PDA (m_1) lies above both thresholds. Crosses between PDA-affected dogs and normal first-degree relatives of PDA-affected dogs result in a distribution of offspring with a mean liability to defective ductal closure (m_2) approximately halfway between the other two matings. (Modified from Patterson *et al.*, 1971.)

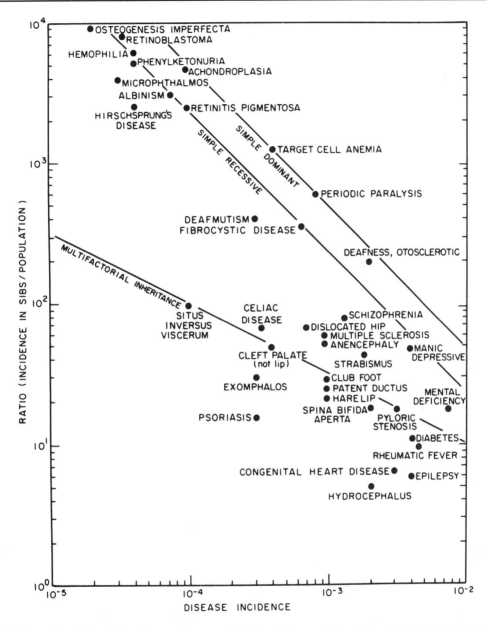

Fig. 18.8 Comparison of the risk in siblings of human patients for single-gene traits with the risk in siblings of patients for multifactorial traits. On a $\log_{10}$ scale, the incidence of each disease is plotted against the ratio of the incidence of the disease in siblings to the incidence in the general population. Single-gene and multifactorial conditions fall into two distinct clusters. The two-cluster effect is simply due to the reduced chance of individuals inheriting **all** necessary genes to show disease in multifactorial conditions. (From Newcombe, 1964.)

season) in the cause of this disease is unclear, but such factors are known to influence other threshold traits (e.g., cleft palate in laboratory animals). Epidemiological studies in man, based on comparison of disease rates in both siblings and offspring of affected individuals with rates in the general population (*Figure 18.8*), suggest a similar mode of inheritance to that in the dog (Zetterquist, 1972).

Other useful companion animal models of genetic diseases are discussed by Patterson *et al.* (1982); they include those of lysosomal storage diseases and disorders of the immune system.

Some non-infectious diseases

Congenital defects which may have known genetic determinants are common in man. Studies in companion animals can support or refute associated causal hypotheses. Hypospadias (a developmental abnormality of the urethral meatus) is relatively common in man but its cause is unclear. It occurs often with other developmental defects, is commoner in males than females, and has familial and seasonal associations. These characteristics suggest both genetic and environmental determinants. Using VMDB data, a breed predisposition has been demonstrated in Boston terriers (Hayes and Wilson, 1986), adding credence to genes as determinants.

Diseases associated with environmental pollution

Several environmental factors, including air pollution and occupational hazards, have been implicated as causes of various types of non-neoplastic chronic pulmonary disease (e.g., bronchitis and emphysema) in man. Chronic pulmonary lesions also occur in the dog. These include interstitial fibrosis and chronic inflammation, emphysema and pleural fibrosis — collectively termed 'chronic pulmonary disease' (CPD). The association between the prevalence of CPD, assessed radiographically, and age and environment (urban versus rural) has been studied in the US (Reif and Cohen, 1979). Results relating to Ithaca (rural) and Boston and Philadelphia (urban) showed a higher prevalence in dogs living in urban areas than in rural areas, but the difference was only identifd in dogs over seven years of age, indicating that, in the dog, this may be the latent period of the cumulative effects of environmental hazards. In Philadelphia, an urban/rural prevalence difference also has been identified (*Figure 18.9a*), and this correlated approximately with atmospheric air pollution (*Figure 18.9b*).

The effects of environmental toxic agents have also been first identified in animals (Buck, 1979). These include trichlorethylene (in cattle), chlorinated naphthalenes (in cattle), aflatoxins (in dogs, cattle and pigs) and organophosphorus nerve agents (in sheep).

Animals can also be effective sentinels of environmental toxins. For example, beef cattle are sentinels of chlorinated hydrocarbon insecticides (Salman *et al.*,

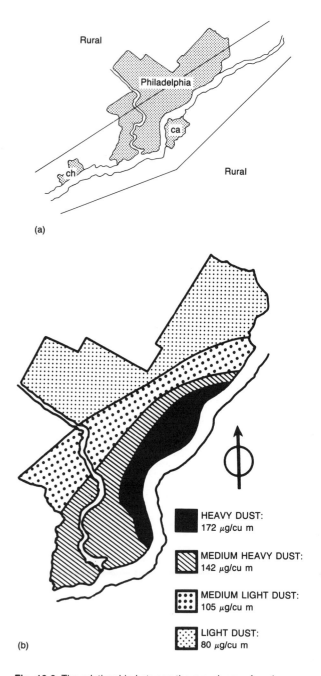

Fig. 18.9 The relationship between the prevalence of canine chronic pulmonary disease (CPD) and location, Philadelphia, US. (a) Relative prevalence of CPD in dogs 7–12 years of age: the prevalence is high in the area between the two lines, and low outside these lines. (b) Atmospheric dust concentration. (From Reif and Cohen, 1970.)

1990). Similarly, dogs scavenging on shorelines are sentinels of cyanobacterial toxins occurring in littoral bacterial scum (Codd *et al.*, 1992), possibly because they are attracted by the taste and odour of the bacteria.

Reasoning in comparative studies

Comparative studies involve reasoning by analogy, and the inferences can be wrong, exemplified by Snow's conclusion that cholera and yellow fever are transmitted by contaminated water because they both occur in insanitary conditions (see Chapter 3). Such conclusions should therefore be treated with caution.

Inferences also should be tempered by the knowledge that many diseases are multifactorial, either because several factors are required to induce a single disease, or because several factors cause disease manifestations that cannot be distinguished at present (MacMahon, 1972). For instance, canine epileptiform seizures appear to be genetically determined in some circumstances, but environmentally induced in others (Bielfelt *et al.*, 1971); and there is evidence that diabetes mellitus is caused by chemicals, autoimmune reactions and virus infection (Yoon *et al.*, 1987).

Inference is less reliable between species, because similar manifestations in different species may be the result of different pathological processes. For example, a variety of species are subject to epileptiform and experimental seizures (Biziere and Chambon, 1987), but the relationship of these conditions to human epilepsy is unclear. Part of the problem is taxonomic: diseases named by clinical signs (e.g., epilepsy) are more likely to be multifactorial than those named by a specific lesion, because the former may be produced by several lesions, each of which may have distinct sufficient causes (see *Figure 9.3*). Thus, the inferences drawn from comparative studies are strengthened when the studies are undertaken on specific structures with similar lesions (e.g., the studies of bladder cancer described above), on the plausible assumption that similar lesions in identical structures are likely to have similar causes.

An important criterion for producing a convincing model is its ability to work in more than one situation (Davidson *et al.*, 1987). There are similarities in the modes of inheritance of several genetic diseases (e.g., canine and human haemophilia), and there are close similarities between the causes and consequently treatment of tumours in animals and man. Such similarities *suggest* that animal models of human genetic and neoplastic diseases are sound, and that there is practical value in using them, particularly when the diseases are much more common in animals than in man (e.g., canine osteosarcoma: Brodey, 1979).

Further reading

Anon. (1991) *Animals as Sentinels of Environmental Health Hazards*. Committee on Animals as Monitors of Environmental Hazards, Board of Environmental Studies and Toxicology, Commission on Life Sciences, National Research Council. National Academy Press, Washington, DC

Bustad, L.K., Hegreberg, G.A. and Padgett, G.A. (1975) *Naturally Occurring Animal Models of Human Disease: A Bibliography*. Institute of Laboratory Animal Resources, National Academy of Sciences, Washington, DC

Brodey, R.S. (1979) The use of naturally occurring cancer in domestic animals for research into human cancer: general considerations and a review of canine skeletal osteosarcoma. *Yale Journal of Biology and Medicine*, **52**, 345–361

Dorn, C.R. and Priester, W.A. (1987) Epidemiology. In: *Veterinary Cancer Medicine*, 2nd edn. Eds Theilen, G.H. and Madewell, B.R., pp. 27–52. Lea and Febiger, Philadelphia. (*Includes a discussion of comparative oncology*)

Glickman, L.T. and Domanski, L.M. (1986) An alternative to laboratory animal experimentation for human health risk assessment: epidemiological studies of pet animals. *Alternatives to Laboratory Animals*, **13**, 267–285

Hayes, H.M. (1978) The comparative epidemiology of selected neoplasms between dogs, cats and humans. A review. *European Journal of Cancer*, **14**, 1299–1308

Reif, J.S. (1986) Animal models for environmental epidemiology. In: *Practices in Veterinary Public Health and Preventive Medicine in the United States*. Ed. Woods, G.T., pp. 273–290. Iowa State University Press, Ames

19 Modelling

Modelling is the representation of physical processes, designed to increase appreciation and understanding of them. Thus, two causal models were described in Chapter 3, and two models of interaction in Chapter 5. Similarly, the Normal distribution (see Chapter 12) is sometimes termed the Normal probability model. A more specific meaning of modelling is the representation of events in quantitative mathematical terms, so that predictions can be made about the events. Modelling, in this sense, is applied to many disciplines, including engineering, agriculture and medicine. In epidemiology, models are constructed to attempt to predict patterns of disease occurrence and what is likely to happen if various alternative control strategies are adopted. An introduction to this approach has already been given in Chapter 8 in which the Reed–Frost model of a propagating epidemic was described. Accurate models can be useful guides to choosing the most efficient disease control techniques as well as increasing understanding of the life-cycles of infectious agents. This chapter describes the main types of model, giving examples relating to infectious diseases.

Modelling dates back to the 18th century, when Daniel Bernoulli applied a simple life table to French smallpox data which indicated that variolation* was efficacious and conferred lifelong immunity (Bernoulli, 1766). Records of human deaths were maintained in parish registers in the UK, a notable example being those of the 1665–66 epidemic of plague in the village of Eyam in Derbyshire (Creighton, 1965). John Graunt (1662) published quantitative observations on London parish registers and 'Bills of Mortality'. Friendly Societies, founded early in the 19th century, recorded information on disease and deaths among their members (Ratcliffe, 1850). Thus, morbidity

and mortality data on diseases such as smallpox and plague were readily available by the middle of the 19th century, and mathematical models were proposed by medical statisticians to explain the observed mortality rates (Greenwood, 1943). William Farr fitted a Normal curve (see Chapter 12) to smallpox data in England and Wales (Farr, 1840), and predicted the course of the 1866 British rinderpest epidemic using a similar approach (Brownlee, 1915).

The early models, which founded general theory, described natural epidemics of human infectious diseases. Only within the last 30 years has significant attention been paid to the modelling of animal diseases. Since the early work, there has been a division into the theoretical approach, which is concerned with epidemic theory, and the practical approach, which attempts to be of direct value to disease control campaigns. Successive models have attempted to become more realistic, incorporating the effects of control techniques, such as vaccination and administration of anthelmintics, in order to evaluate alternative strategies for disease control. The effects of economic constraints and implications have, of necessity, been incorporated in the more recent formulations. Many techniques use computers to simulate situations, although they are not always necessary.

A model can be utilized effectively only if it is sound. This is not always easy to assess. Affirmative answers to three questions, however, will support the model's validity:

1. Have all the known determinants that influence occurrence of the disease been included?
2. Can the value of these determinants be estimated with accuracy?
3. Does the model make biological 'common sense'?

Additionally, the extent to which changes in values of an input parameter affect output parameters needs to be

---

*Variolation is the obsolete process of inoculating a susceptible person with material from the vesicle of a patient with smallpox.

assessed by **sensitivity analysis**. If minor changes in values of an input parameter induce major changes in output parameters then the model is highly sensitive to that input parameter. Conversely, if major changes in an input parameter induce only minor changes in output parameters then the model is relatively insensitive to the input parameter.

Models cannot stand alone in determining efficient control strategies, but should be used in conjunction with accurate field data and experimental techniques. They then provide a useful means of investigating diseases where experiments and field observations are impracticable. Thus, a model may be constructed to investigate the dissemination of foot-and-mouth disease virus in countries that are free from the infection.

Types of model

Density and prevalence models

Veterinary modelling has been directed towards infectious diseases, although non-infectious ones can also be modelled. Infectious agents can be classified into two groups according to their generation dynamics: **microparasites** (e.g., viruses and bacteria) and **macroparasites** (e.g., helminths and arthropods) (see Chapter 7), and the two different dynamic patterns lend themselves to two different types of modelling.

Density models consider the absolute number of infectious agents in each host and are commonly used in macroparasitic infections, where numbers of infectious agents can be estimated either in the host or in the environment. Enumeration of absolute numbers of microparasites is impracticable because of their rapid rate of replication, and so these cannot be readily modelled using density techniques. Microparasitic infections are frequently studied using **prevalence models** which consider the presence or absence of infection in various host cohorts; for example, young and mature, immune and susceptible. The density model is potentially the more refined of the two techniques because it attempts to enumerate the number of infectious agents with which a host is challenged.

Deterministic and stochastic models

In many models, the values of input parameters can be fixed, and the results obtained do not take account of uncertainty (i.e., random variation). Such mathematical descriptions are examples of **deterministic** models. In contrast, some models describe processes or events subject to random variation, so that the outcomes occur with a probability. These models are **stochastic**, the word being derived from the Greek *stochastikos*, meaning 'skilful in aiming at, able to guess'. Stochastic models often enable confidence intervals to be associated with the outputs.

It may not always be clear whether a model is deterministic or stochastic. For example, the basic Reed−Frost model (*see Table 8.1* and *Figures 8.5* and *8.6*) includes a probability of an animal infecting another, yet the predicted outcome has no measure of variation attached to it. This model is therefore deterministic.

Density and prevalence models can be formulated deterministically or stochastically using three approaches classifying models as:

1. models using differential calculus;
2. models using simulation;
3. models using matrices and networks.

Models using differential calculus

Differential calculus is a mathematical technique for finding small (theoretically infinitesimal) rates of change. Models based on this procedure generally establish equations in terms of the rate of change of either the number of parasites or the number of hosts, or subsets of these populations, with respect to time.

Deterministic models using differential calculus

Deterministic exponential decay paradigm

One of the earliest and simplest examples of a differential calculus model is that of **exponential decay**. The instantaneous rate at which susceptibles in a population become infectious individuals, denoted by dx/dt (where dx is the change in the population in the small time interval dt), is assumed to be directly proportional to x (the number of susceptibles in the population):

$$\frac{dx}{dt} = -\alpha x.$$

In the model, α is a positive number that remains constant and is therefore a parameter of the model. If an input condition is known, such as the number of susceptibles in the population at time 0, then solving the equation leads to:

$$x_t = Ne^{-\alpha t}$$

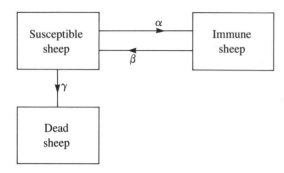

Fig. 19.1 Compartmental representation of a sheep vaccination model.

where x_t and N are the numbers of susceptibles in the population at times t and 0 respectively and e is the universal exponential constant, 2.718. If x_t is plotted for different values of t, a curve is obtained showing x_t decreasing rapidly for small values of t and thereafter more slowly.

Sheep vaccination paradigm

The following example demonstrates how immunity could be included in the simple exponential decay model. Suppose a flock of sheep is constantly under challenge from an infectious agent, infection with which usually causes death. The rate at which animals die is once again assumed to be in direct proportion to the number of animals that are under challenge and that are susceptible to infection. If a certain proportion of the animals show signs, and can be treated with a vaccine which provides temporary immunity, then these animals will not die. Once the protection of the vaccine ceases these immune animals become susceptible again and risk mortality. The system is illustrated by the two compartments shown in *Figure 19.1*.

The left-hand compartment represents the susceptibles under challenge. Animals in this compartment may either die at rate γ or be identified for vaccine treatment and so become transferred at rate α to the right-hand compartment, which represents the immune animals. When immunity ceases, these animals return to the susceptible group at rate β. The model consists of two equations, one for the rate of change of susceptible animals, dx/dt, and one for the rate of change of immune animals, dy/dt:

$$\frac{dx}{dt} = -\alpha x - \gamma x + \beta y,$$

and

$$\frac{dy}{dt} = \alpha x - \beta y.$$

Losses from the susceptible group due to mortality and vaccination are in proportion to the number in the group and are the terms $-\alpha x$ and $-\gamma x$ on the right-hand side of the equation for dx/dt. Animals returning to the susceptible group, however, lose immunity in proportion to the number in the immune group. This movement into the susceptible group is denoted by $+\beta y$. Similarly, the rate of change of animals in the immune group is the net result of the gain αx and loss $-\beta y$. Standard methods of solution enable expressions for x and y to be obtained in terms of t:

$$x = \frac{N}{(a-b)} \{ (\beta - b)e^{-bt} - (\beta - \alpha)e^{-at} \},$$

and

$$y = \frac{N\alpha}{(a-b)} (e^{-bt} - e^{-at}),$$

where:

$$a = \tfrac{1}{2}[(\alpha + \beta + \gamma) + \{(\alpha + \beta + \gamma)^2 - 4\gamma\beta\}^2],$$
$$b = \tfrac{1}{2}[(\alpha + \beta + \gamma) - \{(\alpha + \beta + \gamma)^2 - 4\gamma\beta\}2],$$

and N is the size of the flock at time 0. *Figure 19.2* shows the trends in the numbers of susceptible and immune animals. These are only general trends; the exact trend will depend on the values assigned to the parameters, α, β and γ. It can be seen that the numbers in the susceptible group decrease rapidly whereas the numbers in the immune group rise to a peak before falling. Eventually the numbers in both groups will be zero because all

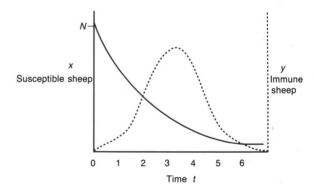

Fig. 19.2 Trends showing the changing number of sheep in the susceptible and immune groups in the sheep vaccination model paradigm.

animals will die unless some other control action is undertaken.

The early models of simple epidemics were based on the differential calculus approach, and usually contained simplistic assumptions, for example that no infectious individuals were removed from the population during the course of the epidemic. This assumption was incorporated into the Reed–Frost model, which formed the basis of many early models. Although this assumption may sometimes be valid in human epidemics, it is frequently untrue of animal epidemics: infectious animals are often removed by culling. Attempts have been made to model animal epidemics with regard to this difference (e.g., Takizawa *et al.*, 1977).

The early models assumed that a group was of a given size with homogeneous mixing and that a susceptible individual was infectious as soon as it was infected (i.e., the infection had no incubation or latent period). Most infectious diseases have latent periods and, in many situations, mixing is rarely homogeneous and individuals may become immune. Models have been produced which take account of these factors.

Additionally, only a few diseases are characterized by interepidemic periods when no cases of disease occur (e.g., rabies and food-and-mouth disease in the UK). Most diseases are endemic to a varying degree, and it is possible to have recurrent epidemics, requiring different models.

The earlier models considered epidemics as processes that occur in continuous time; these were **continuous time** models. **Discrete time** models have been designed which portray disease patterns in fixed intervals of time. For example, if an epidemic starts with a single individual or several simultaneously infected individuals, then new cases will occur in a series of stages separated by time intervals equal to the disease's incubation period. A further discrete time development has been of models that consider individuals as occurring in a variety of states (**multistate** models); for instance, susceptible, immune, infected and dead. Models that consider how individuals can move from one state to another are called **state-transition** models. These are frequently prevalence models.

Tuberculosis in badgers

Bovine tuberculosis continues to be a problem in the south-west of England because infected badgers are a source of infection to cattle. A possible method of disease control is to reduce the badger population density to a level below the threshold level (see Chapter 8) for maintenance of the infection.

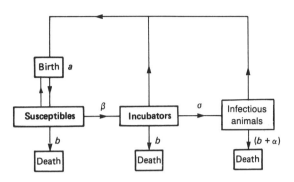

The flow of individual hosts between states is controlled by the rate parameters:

a	=	the per capita birth rate
b	=	the natural death rate
β	=	the disease transmission coefficient
σ	=	the rate at which incubating individuals become infectious
α	=	the disease induced death rate

Fig. 19.3 Flow chart of the deterministic model of bovine tuberculosis in badgers. The flow of individual hosts between states is controlled by the rate parameters: a = the per capita birth rate; b = the natural death rate; β = the disease transmission coefficient; σ = the rates at which incubating individuals become infectious; α = the disease induced death rate. (Modified from Trewhella and Anderson, 1983.)

The dynamics of bovine tuberculosis in badgers have been investigated using a deterministic, state-transition, differential calculus, prevalence model (Trewhella and Anderson, 1983) which includes three states: susceptible animals, animals incubating the disease, and infectious animals (*Figure 19.3*). There is no need to include an immune state because badgers show no immunity to bovine tuberculosis. Parameters include density-dependent regulation of the badger population, natural and disease-induced death rates, the incubation period of the infection, and the rate of transmission.

The model predicts that prevalence increases with badger density, the predicted values being supported by field observations, and that prevalence oscillations occur with a periodicity of 18 years. The model suggests that, in areas of high badger density, considerable effort would be required to control the infection.

Rabies in foxes

Foxes are hosts of rabies in North America and Europe, and constitute a serious obstacle to control of the disease. The infection became established in foxes in Poland towards the end of the Second World War. The epidemic has spread slowly westwards at a rate of about 30 km/ year. The standard method of control is slaughter of foxes, but results have been disappointing. A mathematical model (Macdonald and Bacon, 1980) suggests that control, other than by slaughter of foxes, may be more successful. The model has two components:

1. prediction of the course of the disease in fox populations;
2. evaluation of different control policies.

The model of the disease in fox populations makes plausible assumptions about the host and parasite. Foxes breed once a year in the autumn, and fox mortality is highest in the winter, resulting in an annual fluctuation in fox numbers. The virus has a long incubation period and can therefore survive in hosts of high, changing and low densities (see *Figure 6.4*); in the last circumstance it can exist for a long time in individuals.

If rabies enters a fox population, the future of the host and parasite will be affected by the number of healthy foxes that are infected by rabid foxes; expressed as a ratio, this is the **contact rate**. If the disease is modelled for various contact rates, there are different predicted outcomes; these are shown in *Figure 19.4a*. The upper lines of the graphs represent the total fox population, the lower lines the healthy foxes, and the shaded areas the number of rabid foxes. The horizontal lines represent the number of foxes which, theoretically, can be carried by the habitat. A contact rate of 0.5 (one rabid fox infecting half a healthy fox) will, according to Kendall's Threshold Theorem (see Chapter 8), be insufficient to allow the infection to become established; the model supports this. Higher contact rates result in fluctuation in the fox population and in the number of rabid foxes. A contact rate of 1.4 allows the disease to persist, oscillating annually. A contact rate of 1.9 produces epidemics every four years that are severe enough to reduce the population to a level that will not support infection. The infection again becomes epidemic when the fox population recovers. Field surveys have shown that this periodicity is demonstrated in European foxes. Higher contact rates would lead to extinction of the fox population.

The second component of the model considers three control techniques (*Figure 19.4b*):

1. slaughter;
2. temporary sterilization;
3. bait vaccination of foxes.

In case A, a single cull is instituted when rabies is at its earliest detectable level. Although slaughter initially decreases the prevalence of the disease, the latter soon

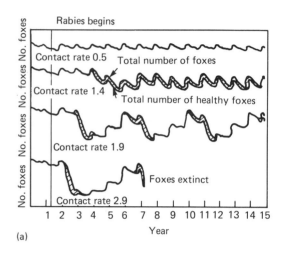

(a)

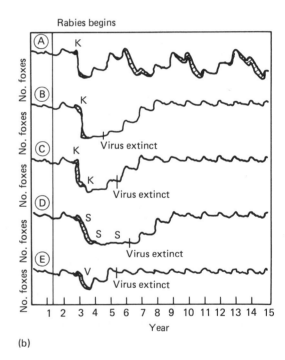

(b)

Control strategies:

K = controlled fox kill
S = temporary sterilization of foxes
V = bait vaccination of foxes

Fig. 19.4 (a) Merlewood model of rabies in foxes; (b) Merlewood model of alternative strategies for controlling rabies in foxes. In each graph the initial level of the fox population is the same. (From Macdonald and Bacon, 1980.)

increases again and then follows a pattern similar to that in the graph in *Figure 19.4a* depicting a contact rate of 1.9.

In case B, killing takes place later, probably when rabies is more likely to have been detected. Paradoxically, although initially there are more cases, the disease and the kill work together because more of the foxes that are not killed are incubating rabies and therefore will die. The virus thus becomes extinct as the fox population is dramatically reduced.

Case C represents two killings, separated by six months. Again, the virus becomes extinct, but the fox population is reduced below the levels in A and B.

Three applications of temporary sterilizing agent are illustrated in case D. The virus is again extinguished, but the fox population is reduced further.

Vaccination of foxes using vaccine-laiden bait, shown in case E, offers the best results: removing the virus from the population and maintaining the number of healthy foxes (with 60% of foxes assumed to be immunized).

This model therefore suggests a more efficient and ecologically acceptable way of controlling fox rabies than slaughter. This type of oral vaccination is being used successfully in Europe (Müller, 1991), where it can be complemented by the control of fox populations (Aubert, 1994). Oral vaccination is also being applied to other sylvatic hosts in North America.

A criticism of models based on differential calculus is the common assumption that parameters remain constant throughout the period of operation; for example, it may be assumed that the survival rate of helminth eggs does not change during a season, whereas, in reality, climatic variation may alter survival rates from day to day. Some models do have time-dependent parameters, but this may lead to a model for which a solution is unobtainable or may make the operation of the model clumsy. A major feature of such models is that they enable the long-term behaviour of the parasite population to be studied. The population may either become extinct, or increase indefinitely, or reach a **steady state**. It is often whether or not a steady state exists and the nature of the steady state that is of interest, although for many infections the initial progression may be of paramount importance if economic losses are to be minimized.

Stochastic models using differential calculus

The first epidemic models considered that *the course of an epidemic must depend on the number of susceptibles and the contact rate between susceptible and infectious individuals*; this is the basic assumption underlying deterministic models. In a deterministic model, the future state of an epidemic process can be predicted precisely if the initial number of susceptible and infectious individuals is known (e.g., *Figures 8.5* and *8.6*).

Later, it was realized that the deterministic approach was not always applicable: variation and choice (of contact between susceptible and infected individuals) should be considered as part of the epidemic process. **Stochastic** modelling, which includes the **probability of infection**, therefore evolved. This leads to results that have a probability distribution from which means, variances and confidence intervals can be derived. The deterministic and stochastic approaches produce a different result when modelling a simple epidemic (*Figure 19.5*); the deterministic curve represents the absolute point estimates. The stochastic curve represents the mean of all the values generated by the various probabilities.

Stochastic exponential decay paradigm

A stochastic analogue of the deterministic model for the changing number of susceptibles in a population, described above, can be formulated. As before, x_t denotes the number of susceptibles in the population at time t, and N the number at time 0. It is now assumed that x_t is a random variable and the probability of r susceptibles at time t is denoted by $p_r(t)$. A differential calculus approach, similar to that used in the deterministic model, can be applied to obtain an expression for the rate of change of $p_r(t)$. This rate of change, $dp_r(t)/dt$, will be influenced by flows in from the state $r+1$ and flows out from the state r. For state $r+1$ to have a flow in, there must be two events:

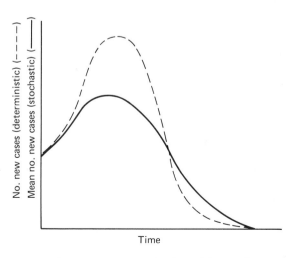

Fig. 19.5 Deterministic and stochastic model curves for a simple infectious epidemic. (After Bailey, 1975.)

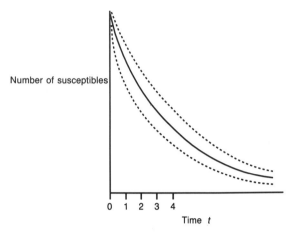

Number of susceptibles

0 1 2 3 4

Time t

Fig. 19.6 Mean (———) and 95% confidence interval (- - - - -) for the number of susceptibles in the stochastic exponential decay paradigm.

first, there must be $r+1$ susceptibles at time t; secondly, one of these susceptibles must leave. The probability of these two events is $\alpha(r+1)p_{r+1}(t)$. For state $\overset{*}{r}$ to have a flow out, there must be r susceptibles at time t and one susceptible must leave. The probability of these two events is $\alpha r p_r(t)$. The instantaneous rate of change of $p_r(t)$ is therefore:

$$\frac{dp_r(t)}{dt} = \alpha(r+1)p_{r+1}(t) - \alpha r p_r(t)$$

where α is a parameter.

The solution to such a differential equation may not be easily obtained but standard methods for solving are available. These methods lead to an expression for $p_r(t)$ in terms of t:

$$p_r(t) = {}^N C_r (1 - e^{-\alpha t})^{N-r} e^{-\alpha t r}$$

where ${}^N C_r$ is a mathematical shorthand notation for

$$\frac{N!}{r!(N-r)!}$$

The expression for $p_r(t)$ is known as the time-dependent binomial probability distribution, from which it can be deduced that x_t has mean value $Ne^{-\alpha t}$ and variance $Ne^{-\alpha t}(1 - e^{-\alpha t})$. Comparing these results with those of the deterministic model, it can be seen that the mean value of x_t is identical to the solution obtained before. This is often, but not always (*Figure 19.5*), true of deterministic and stochastic models. However, an important distinction between the deterministic and stochastic model is that the latter provides a variance, therefore the extent to which population susceptible numbers fluctuate at each point in time can be deduced. *Figure 19.6* illustrates this point,

where the mean number of susceptibles at each point is shown with a 95% confidence interval of plus and minus two standard deviations. The wider the confidence interval, the greater is the range of observed deviations from the mean number of susceptibles.

Models using simulation

The goal of these models is *simulation* of the performance of parasites or diseases in relation to conditions which change either deterministically or stochastically. Although simulation models do not always require a computer for implementation, their power and success have been closely linked to advances in computer technology. Many simulations undertaken today would have been impossible 50 years ago.

There are three main types of simulation model:

1. empirical models;
2. explanatory models;
3. Monte Carlo models.

Simulation can also be used to implement other types of model such as those based on differential calculus and network models (see below).

Successful empirical and explanatory models have the potential to *forecast* disease incidence accurately. These forecasts, like those possible using time series analysis (see Chapter 8), are of value in selecting suitable prophylactic procedures.

Empirical models using simulation

Empirical models utilize *indicators that are obtained by analysing the relationship between morbidity and any associated variables*. Frequently used variables are those relating to climate. These models are not strictly mathematical models because they do not attempt to analyse the dynamics of agents' life-cycles, but simply to quantify associated phenomena. They are sometimes referred to as 'black-box' models because the relationship between data that are fed into the model and the results that are generated cannot be satisfactorily explained.

Fascioliasis

Fascioliasis has been modelled empirically in Britain (Ollerenshaw and Rowlands, 1959; Ollerenshaw, 1966;

Table 19.1 Associations between ΣMt values* and losses owing to fascioliasis in England and Wales. (Data from Ollerenshaw, 1966.)

ΣMt		Losses
North-west England, south-east England and north Wales	Other parts of England and Wales	
<300	<400	No losses
300−450	400−450	Some losses
>450	>450	Heavy losses

*See text for explanation.

Gibson, 1978). The life-cycle of *Fasciola hepatica* is complex, involving stages inside a final and intermediate host, and on herbage. Two important meteorological factors in the development of the parasite are temperatures above 10 °C and the presence of free water. In the late 1950s Ollerenshaw suggested that development is therefore usually impossible during the winter (too cold) and that there may be insufficient water during some of the summer months (too dry). This is the basis of the 'Mt' forecasting system for fascioliasis. Mt is a monthly index of wetness given by:

$$(R - p + 5)n,$$

where, on a monthly basis:

R = rainfall in inches,
p = potential transpiration,
n = number of rain days.

Observations suggested that, because parasite development is also temperature-dependent, the rate of development is similar in June, July, August and September but is halved in May and October, when the Mt index should therefore be halved.

A seasonal summation of Mt indices (ΣMt) can be calculated by adding the Mt values for the six-month period May to October. This sum simulates the progression of the disease in relation to changing meteorological conditions and so can be used to predict losses owing to fascioliasis, so that suitable prophylactic measures can be undertaken (*Table 19.1*).

This prediction model is deterministic because no element of randomness is included in the formulation. Its simple approach enables its execution without a computer. The model has been adapted for use in France (Leimbacher, 1978) and Northern Ireland (Ross, 1978).

Nematodiriasis

The life-cycle of *Nematodiriasis* spp. is temperature-dependent. There is a correlation between soil temperature (taken 30 cm deep) and larval hatching dates. The mean soil temperature in March is used to predict the date of maximum larval count on the pasture. Additionally, there is a correlation between the estimated peak hatch date in north-east England and national disease severity which can be used to predict, semi-quantitatively, national prevalence (*Table 19.2*). Again, this is a deterministic model because no consideration is given to random variation.

Meteorological indices for the prediction of ostertagiasis have also been produced (Thomas and Starr, 1978; Thomas, 1978; Gettinby and Gardner, 1980).

Explanatory models using simulation

More recently, mathematical models that describe (i.e., explain) the dynamics of parasite and host populations have been formulated. These more refined techniques allow the course of a disease to be simulated. They include models for forecasting fluke morbidity (Hope-Cawdery *et al.*, 1978; Williamson and Wilson, 1978), the airborne spread of foot-and-mouth disease (Gibson and Smith, 1978a,b; Gloster *et al.*, 1981; Donaldson *et al.*, 1982) and the occurrence of clinical ostertagiasis.

Bovine ostertagiasis

The level of pasture contamination by infective *Ostertagia ostertagi* larvae can be predicted by simulating the course of events experienced by cohorts of parasite eggs deposited on pasture (Gettinby *et al.*, 1979). This involves estimating the proportion of eggs that proceed to the first, second and third larval stages using **development fractions** which quantify the rate of development of the parasite from one stage to the next according to the temperatures that it experiences. In addition, parameters associated with infectivity, fecundity and migratory behaviour of the larvae must be included.

Thus, suppose a calf commences grazing on contaminated grass on 1st April. The number of infective larvae, L, ingested on 1st April can be estimated from known pasture contamination levels and the daily herbage intake of the calf. Not all larvae become established. The number of adult worms, A, to be expected in the abomasum of the calf 21 days later on 22nd April is modelled using:

$$A = (K - A_0)(1 - e^{-\alpha L}) + A_0$$

Table 19.2 Estimated peak hatch dates of *Nematodirus* spp. eggs in north-east England in years of various national disease severities. (From Gibson and Smith, 1978a.)

Actual national disease severity	Year	Estimated peak hatch date in north-east England
Low	1957	11 April
	1961	11 April
Below average	1952	16 April
	1959	17 April
	1967	18 April
	1966	20 April
	1960	22 April
Above average	1953	21 April
	1964	28 April
	1968	29 April
	1956	30 April
High	1951	3 May
	1954	4 May
	1963	4 May
	1965	6 May
	1958	8 May
	1955	12 May
	1962	12 May

where A_0 is the number of adults already in the abomasum. The curve of A for different values of L is sigmoidal, reflecting the assumed density-dependent relationship between larval challenge and establishment of adult worms (see also *Figure 7.3*). The parameters K and α control the rate of establishment so that the proportion established is high for low levels of challenge and low for high levels of challenge. The adult worms will produce eggs on 1st April and thereafter. The number of eggs, E, produced on 22nd April is estimated from empirical data relating egg output to adult worm burden. These eggs undergo development. The time to the appearance of infective larvae is estimated by calculating from daily temperatures the fraction of development to take place each day and summing these fractions until all development has occurred n days later:

$$\frac{1}{D_1} + \frac{1}{D_2} + \ldots \frac{1}{D_n} = 1$$

where the Ds are the number of days that would be required to complete development under conditions of constant temperature. Adding n to 22nd April gives the earliest day on which the infective larvae can appear. Not all developing eggs and larvae survive and so the number of eggs that avoid mortality is the proportion, p^n, of the egg output on 22nd April. The parameter p is an estimate of the daily survival rate. If the values of n and p^n are determined for each day during which the calf grazes, then it is possible to estimate the expected totals of infective larvae on pasture and the number of adult worms infecting the calf. This type of simulation requires iterative calculations which can only be performed in a reasonable time by using a computer.

Figure 19.7 shows the results of such a simulation for calves that grazed on an experimental pasture from May to September 1975. Comparison of predicted and observed larval counts shows a high degree of correlation.

A prediction of herbage infective larval burdens using this type of simulation model can facilitate optimum use of anthelmintics, and movement of animals to safe pasture before challenge by large numbers of infective larvae, thereby preventing clinical ostertagiasis. A similar approach has been successfully applied to ovine ostertagiasis (Paton *et al.*, 1984) and tick infestations of sheep (Gardiner and Gettinby, 1983).

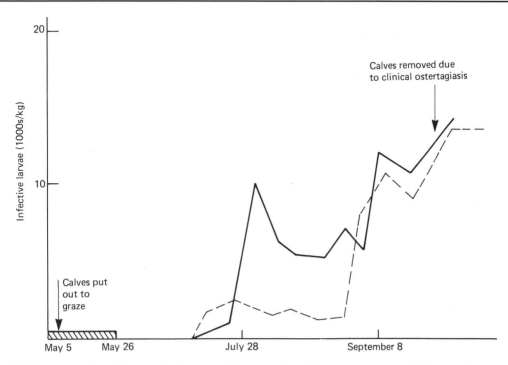

Fig. 19.7 Observed and predicted counts of infective *Ostertagia ostertagi* larvae on pasture in 1975. ——— Observed pasture count; − − − predicted pasture count; ⟨⟨⟨⟨⟨ overwintered infective larvae. (From Gettinby *et al.*, 1979.)

Monte Carlo methods

In many cases deterministic and stochastic models can be formulated for which no analytical solution is known. Alternatively, finding the solution may be extremely difficult or tedious. In such circumstances simulation methods can be undertaken. Since simulation studies attempt to mimic the physical process being modelled, they can be very informative and therefore are often preferred. In these methods, random processes are simulated using random numbers in order to decide whether or not an event takes place. This is somewhat akin to gambling; hence the term **Monte Carlo** simulation.

Sheep tick paradigm

Suppose a model is to be formulated for the outcome of adult ticks of the species *Ixodes ricinus* mating on the sheep host. In particular, a measure of the total number of female ticks is required so that future population numbers can be anticipated. Suppose a field study indicates that the total number of engorged ticks found on individual sheep is 0, 1, 2 or 3, and suppose that the respective probabilities are 0.4, 0.3, 0.2 and 0.1. The field study also suggests that male and female ticks are present in equal proportions. Using a fair ten-sided die with faces labelled 1 to 10, and a fair two-sided coin with faces labelled M for male and F for female, it is possible to simulate and obtain the number of mated female ticks on each sheep. The die is thrown and, depending on which of the sets $\{1,2,3,4\}$, $\{5,6,7\}$, $\{8,9\}$ and $\{10\}$ the outcome belongs to, the simulated number of adult engorged ticks on the sheep is taken to be 0, 1, 2 or 3, respectively. The above sets are chosen since the outcomes 0, 1, 2 and 3 will occur with probabilities 0.4, 0.3, 0.2 and 0.1, respectively, which is consistent with the results of the field study. Suppose the outcome of the throw of the die is a 10, the simulated number of adult engorged ticks on the sheep is then three. The coin is now tossed three times and the outcomes used to simulate the sex of the three adult engorged ticks. In the event of all three ticks having the same sex (i.e., outcomes MMM or FFF), there will be no mated females. All other outcomes will lead to at least one male and one female on a sheep and, assuming that one male mates only with one female, there will be only one mated female. *Table 19.3* shows the possible combinations of the outcomes of the throw of the die and the coin tossing.

The procedure can be repeated for each sheep to obtain a series of 0s and 1s reflecting the outcomes of the

Table 19.3 Possible number of mated female *Ixodes ricinus* on one sheep, resulting from simulated attachment and sex distribution of the tick population.

Outcome from one throw of a ten-sided die	Simulated number of engorged ticks on a sheep	Simulated sex distribution of engorged ticks from coin tosses	Number of mated females
{1,2,3,4}	0	—	0
{5,6,7}	1	M	0
		F	0
{8,9}	2	MM	0
		MF	1
		FF	0
		FM	1
{10}	3	MMM	0
		MMF	1
		MFM	1
		FMM	1
		FFF	0
		FMF	1
		MFF	1
		FFM	1

attachment and sex distribution of the tick population on the sheep flock. To summarize the results of the simulation: the proportion of the flock with 1 or 0 mated female ticks could be reported. When the simulation is carried out it is found that, on average, only 18 out of every 100 sheep are hosts to one mated female tick. A sensitivity analysis could also be undertaken to test the effects of different assumptions or parameter estimates on the outcomes. For instance, if the ratio of male to female ticks was no longer 1:1 but biased towards females, in the ratio 1:2, then the study could be repeated using a biased coin that would give an M outcome with probability 0.33 (1/3) and an F outcome with probability 0.67 (2/3) when tossed. The simulation then leads to an average of 15 out of every 100 sheep hosting one mated female tick. Comparison of the results suggests that the analysis is not very sensitive to changes in the sex distribution; consequently further field studies to accurately determine the sex ratio are not warranted. Similarly, if it was thought that male ticks could mate with several females, then the simulation could be repeated. If, for example, attachment led to the combination of one male and two female ticks on a sheep, then this would produce two, rather than one, mated females.

In modern simulation studies the computer takes over the role of the die and the coin. Thus, the results of these 'lotteries' are produced by replacing throws of a 10-sided die with an instruction to the computer to produce integer numbers from 1 to 10 in random order such that a large series of generated numbers would produce each of these numbers in equal proportions.

Sheep tick control

Monte Carlo simulation can be used to investigate the behaviour of a stochastic model for the incidence of tick mating which could be of value to control strategies (Plowright and Paloheimo, 1977). Field investigations (Milne, 1950) revealed that tick occurrence was patchy: a pasture may have a heavy burden whereas an adjacent field separated from the first only by a fence may have no ticks. This suggested that ticks have problems with effective dispersal. One reason may be that at low densities tick population growth is inhibited by a low rate of mating. The model proposed makes several assumptions: that each adult only mates if it encounters an individual of the opposite sex on the sheep to which it is attached; that each adult only mates once; that each tick has an equal probability of attaching to a sheep; that all ticks have an equal probability of encountering one another. The last two assumptions are dubious but do not affect the model appreciably.

The total number of matings at various sheep densities, and with varying numbers of ticks on each sheep, can be modelled by applying a Poisson distribution (see Chapter

Table 19.4 Comparison of the results of deterministic and stochastic models of incidence of mating in *Ixodes ricinus* for various parameter values. (From Plowright and Paloheimo, 1977.)

p	Number of ticks	Number of sheep	Total number of matings	
			Deterministic model	Stochastic model (mean of 600 replications)
0.05	40	10	3.3357	3.4400
0.05	40	20	4.7532	4.7833
0.05	40	40	5.1271	5.1533
0.05	40	80	3.9683	3.8395
0.05	40	160	2.2143	2.2117
0.05	80	10	8.9590	9.0883
0.05	80	20	13.2866	13.4567
0.05	80	40	15.3686	15.5733
0.05	80	80	12.6488	12.8450
0.05	80	160	7.9323	8.0050
0.01	40	10	0.3021	0.2933
0.01	40	20	0.5528	0.5567
0.01	40	40	0.9282	0.9017
0.01	40	80	1.3279	1.2733
0.01	40	160	1.4345	1.4633
0.01	80	10	1.0342	1.0017
0.01	80	20	1.8993	1.9483
0.01	80	40	3.2270	3.0550
0.01	80	80	4.7108	4.5867
0.01	80	160	5.2683	5.3367

p = probability of a tick attaching to a sheep.

12). *Table 19.4* lists the results and demonstrates the difference between the stochastic and deterministic output. By including a rate of survival in the model, it is possible to predict the growth rate of the tick population for different levels of tick population size and sheep density. When the sheep population is low, the rate of tick population increase is insensitive to changes in the size of the tick population, but highly sensitive to changes in the size of the sheep population. Conversely, when the tick population is low, the rate of tick population increase is relatively insensitive to changes in sheep numbers, but sensitive to changes in tick numbers. This supports the hypothesis that it is difficult for ticks to establish themselves in new pastures. It also suggests that a reduction in host density may not be an effective means of controlling tick infestation because the rate of tick population increase does not always depend on sheep density. The model also predicts that extinction of the tick population takes place over a narrow range of tick population sizes, corroborating field observations of patchy tick distribution.

Models using matrices and networks

Matrix and network methods are similar. The use of matrices to describe population changes became firmly established when Leslie (1945) published his Leslie matrix. In contrast, network models, although extensively exploited by control engineers, have been largely overlooked in the life sciences, with some exceptions (Lewis, 1977). Often the same problem can be formulated using a network and a matrix approach. The network formulation is particularly attractive when time delays are a feature of the life-cycle being modelled and when the output response of a biological system is to be measured for a given input. On the other hand, matrix formulations are attractive when the behaviour of several states of a population is of interest at successive points in time.

Matrix models

Matrices often take the form of a rectangular array containing numbers of hosts or parasites in a defined state or stage of development, known as the **state vector**, or containing reproduction and survival rates of hosts or parasites in different states or stages, known as the **transition matrix**. In this way it is possible to obtain the state of the system from one point in time to another.

Fascioliasis

The life-cycle of *Fasciola hepatica* can be used to illustrate the formulation of a simple matrix model. The parameters have been estimated from field studies. It is assumed that eggs from the adult fluke develop to miracidia after four weeks, that miracidia which penetrate the molluscan host, *Limnea truncatula*, develop, and emerge as metacercariae eight weeks later, and that the metacercariae can survive up to three weeks before desiccation. The weekly survival rates of the adult flukes, the developing eggs, the stages in the snail, and the metacercariae are 0.95, 0.3, 0.5 and 0.8, respectively. Each adult fluke is assumed to produce 2500 eggs weekly, and each miracidium is assumed to penetrate a snail with probability 0.005. The phases of development in the snail are simplified by labelling all of the asexual stages s. It is also assumed that reproduction occurs in the last intra-molluscan stage and the fecundity is 4.3. A further simplification is that each metacercaria in each week of development has probability 0.02 of becoming an adult worm.

Let a be the number of adult flukes and e_i, c_i and m_i be the number of eggs, cercariae and metacercariae, respectively in the ith week of development. The number of adult flukes from week t to week $t+1$ will be those adults in week t that survive plus those metacercariae that are ingested and become established:

$$a(t+1) = 0.95a(t) + 0.02m_1(t) + 0.02m_2(t) + 0.02m_3(t)$$

The number of eggs at time $t+1$ in the first week of development will be those produced by adults in the previous week:

$$e_1(t+1) = 2500a_1(t).$$

The number of eggs at time $t+1$ in the second week of development will be those surviving from the previous week:

$$e_2(t+1) = 0.3e_1(t).$$

The change from week to week of all the stages can be summarized in matrix form (see *Table 19.5*):

In shorthand notation, this is written:

$$\underline{x}_{t+1} = \underline{P}\,\underline{x}_t$$

where $\underline{x}_t$ and $\underline{x}_{t+1}$ are the state vectors and correspond to times t and $t+1$, and $\underline{P}$ is the transition matrix. Characters are underlined to denote a matrix. Note that to retrieve the first equation, the first element in the state vector (a_{t+1}) is equated with the sum, after the first row of the transition matrix has been turned on its side and each element of this row multiplied by the corresponding elements of the column state vector $\underline{x}_t$ at time $t+1$; that is:

$$\begin{aligned} a = &+ 0.95 \times a \\ &+ 0 \times e_1 \\ &+ 0 \end{aligned}$$

$$\begin{aligned} &0 \\ &0 \\ &. \\ &. \\ &. \\ &+ 0.02 \times m_3 \end{aligned}$$

Other relationships are similarly retrieved. For example, if the number of metacercariae in the first week of development at time $t+1$ is required, then the row transition matrix corresponding to this element is turned on its side and corresponding elements in $\underline{x}_t$ multiplied to give

$$m_1(t+1) = 4.3s_8(t).$$

The matrix model proposed for the life-cycle of *F. hepatica* is similar to that proposed by Leslie (1945) for populations in general. Leslie suggested that members of a population can be divided into exclusive age classes of fixed duration, so that every member of a class faces the same probability of surviving and the same probability of reproducing. If the vector containing the number in each class during a certain time interval is multiplied by the Leslie matrix describing the population dynamics, then the vector containing the number in each class during the following time interval is obtained. For example, if there are k age classes:

$$\begin{bmatrix} n_1 \\ n_1 \\ n_3 \\ . \\ . \\ . \\ n_{k-1} \\ n_k \end{bmatrix}_{t+1} = \begin{bmatrix} f_1 & f_2 & . & . & f_{k-1} & f_k \\ p_1 & 0 & . & . & 0 & 0 \\ 0 & p_2 & . & . & 0 & 0 \\ . & & & & & . \\ . & & & & & . \\ . & & & & . & . \\ 0 & 0 & . & . & p_{k-1} & 0 \end{bmatrix} \begin{bmatrix} n_1 \\ n_2 \\ n_3 \\ . \\ . \\ . \\ n_{k-1} \\ n_k \end{bmatrix}_{t}$$

Table 19.5 Matrix formulation of the life-cycle of *Fasciola hepatica*

$$\begin{bmatrix} a \\ e_1 \\ e_2 \\ e_3 \\ e_4 \\ s_1 \\ s_2 \\ s_3 \\ s_4 \\ s_5 \\ s_6 \\ s_7 \\ s_8 \\ m_1 \\ m_2 \\ m_3 \end{bmatrix}_{t+1} =$$

a	e₁	e₂	e₃	e₄	s₁	s₂	s₃	s₄	s₅	s₆	s₇	s₈	m₁	m₂	m₃
0.95	0	0	0	0	0	0	0	0	0	0	0	0	0.02	0.02	0.02
2500	0	0	0	0	0	0	0	0	0	0	0	0	0	0	0
0	0.3	0	.		.										0
.		0.3													
.			0.3												
				0.002											
					0.5										
						0.5									
							0.5								
								0.5							
									0.5						
										0.5					
											0.5				
												4.3			
.													0.8		
0	.	.												0.8	0

$$\begin{bmatrix} a \\ e_1 \\ e_2 \\ e_3 \\ e_4 \\ s_1 \\ s_2 \\ s_3 \\ s_4 \\ s_5 \\ s_6 \\ s_7 \\ s_8 \\ m_1 \\ m_2 \\ m_3 \end{bmatrix}$$

where $n_i(t+1)$ is the number in the ith class at time $t+1$, and f_i and p_i are respectively the fecundity and survival rates for age class i.

The advantage of the matrix approach is that once $\underline{P}$ and the numbers for the state vector at time 0 are known then the population size at any future time can be predicted. For example, the population numbers after four units of time could be obtained from the successive calculations:

$$\underline{x}_1 = \underline{P}\,\underline{x}_0$$
$$\underline{x}_2 = \underline{P}\,\underline{x}_1$$
$$\underline{x}_3 = \underline{P}\,\underline{x}_2$$
$$\underline{x}_4 = \underline{P}\,\underline{x}_3$$

The matrix equations described above have many interesting properties from which the salient features of the population can be investigated. Details of these are given by Leslie (1945).

A more realistic matrix representation of the life-cycle of *F. hepatica* is discussed by Gettinby and McClean (1979). This is a state-transition model with five states: mature flukes (in sheep), eggs (on grass), rediae (in snails), metacercariae (on grass), immature flukes (in sheep). A mortality rate is attached to all stages, and fecundity to the adult fluke and redia, which reproduce sexually and asexually respectively. The matrix includes probabilities of transition from one stage to the next, and fecundity, based upon available field data. The first part of the model describes the natural infection in sheep in Britain and Ireland. The second part investigates and compares various control strategies: the use of flukicides, molluscicides and land drainage. There are four conclusions. Molluscicides are most effective when applied in early spring. Flukicides eradicate the infection when given monthly and control it when given at two-monthly intervals. If dosing is only annual, then it is best given in August. Good drainage is an effective means of control. Again, the model only indicates possible outcomes, in the absence of accurate field data to support the values of the input parameters in the model.

Network models

The inability of many other models to cope with changing inputs during the period of operation of the model can be circumvented using a **network** representation of a parasite's life-cycle. Some elementary examples will demonstrate the symbolism used in this approach.

Protozoal paradigm

Consider a population of identical protozoa which reproduce by binary fission. A constant T units of time

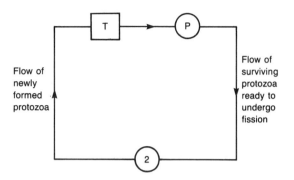

Fig. 19.8 Network representation in the protozoal paradigm.

occurs between successive fissions. The probability that any one protozoon survives this time is P. To construct the network shown in *Figure 19.8*, which represents the life-cycle, consider the flow of newly formed protozoa in the population. After a time delay, T, only a proportion, P, of these survives. This results in the flow after the time delay being scaled by a factor P. This is immediately succeeded by fission, which results in the flow doubling and so a further scaling by a factor 2 is required. The network convention is to denote time delays by squares and scaling parameters by circles. Since the products of fission are newly formed cells, this flow is connected back into the time delay. This is a very simple network and consists of one loop and no alternative paths.

Ostertagiasis

A network can be constructed for the life-cycle of *Ostertagia circumcincta*, an important parasite responsible for outbreaks of parasitic gastroenteritis in sheep (Paton and Gettinby, 1983). The network is shown in *Figure 19.9*. The unit of time is one week. Ewe and lamb egg inputs, $X(i)$ and $Z(i)$, voided out to the pasture in week i, undergo a time delay of Γ_1 (gamma) weeks before infective L_3 larvae appear. The proportion that survive is a. During the following week, these L_3 larvae, plus available over-wintered infective larvae $Y(i)$, either become ingested by the sheep to become adults at rate c, or accumulate on the pasture at rate $1 - c$. Those that accumulate are delayed for one week, during which their survival rate is b, before joining the flow of new infective larvae. The L_3 larvae that were ingested are delayed for Γ_2 weeks before reaching the adult egg-laying stage. Half of these adults will be females, which reproduce at a rate of e eggs per week. From successive egg cohorts, female adults will accumulate from week to week. To facilitate the accumulation, the existing females must enter a feedback loop in which the weekly survival rate is d, and

which connects them with the flow of new female adult worms in the sheep. The network therefore consists of a forward loop and two feedback loops.

When the model is operated, the effects of various anthelmintic strategies can be investigated by altering components of the network which will be affected by the particular strategy. For example, dosing of lambs will reduce the lamb egg input, and dosing of ewes will decrease the ewe egg input. The simulation suggests that regular dosing of lambs at four-weekly intervals for the first six months of life is very effective. Similarly, dosing lambs three times in July and August is effective. The single administration of an anthelmintic to ewes at lambing time is the least effective of the anthelmintic strategies.

Further veterinary applications of modelling

This chapter has introduced some modelling techniques, with examples from studies of infectious diseases (mainly helminth infections). 'Modelling' now has a broad remit, including the conceptual representation of any real event in mathematical terms. Models have been developed for the choice of disease control strategies; for example, for brucellosis in the UK (Hugh-Jones et al., 1976) and in the US (Dietrich et al., 1980). They have been used to investigate diseases of uncertain aetiology; for example, epizootic bovine abortion (Lehenbauer and Harman, 1982); to model genetic resistance (Barger, 1989) and antigenic drift (Hugh-Jones, 1986b); and to study resistance to anthelmintics and acaricides (Gettinby, 1989) and the value of identification and recording systems in the

control of contagious diseases (Saatkamp et al., 1994). Models that assess the cost of disease and its control have also been designed; some of these have been reviewed by Beal and McCallon (1983) and Dykhuizen (1993). Sørensen and Enevoldsen (1992) review models of herd health and production. Increasingly, models are being linked together to produce large-scale **systems models** (e.g., EpiMAN: see Chapter 11). A bibliography of veterinary models, including a discussion of model classification, is given by Hurd and Kaneene (1993).

Modelling is one component of the epidemiological approach. It cannot be used effectively without reliable field and experimentally derived data relating to diseases' natural history. The dangers of applying modelling in isolation from traditional field observation have been noted, both in human epidemiology — in the context of a reappraisal of Snow's classical investigation of cholera (Cameron and Jones, 1983) — and in veterinary epidemiology (Hugh-Jones, 1983). However, when used in association with diagnostic and experimental disciplines, modelling is a valuable aid to an increased understanding of disease.

Further reading

Ackerman, E., Elveback, L.R. and Fox, J.P. (1984) *Simulation of Infectious Disease Epidemics*. Charles C. Thomas, Springfield

Anderson, R.M. and May, R.M. (1991) *Infectious Diseases of Humans: Dynamics and Control*. Oxford University Press, Oxford. (*Includes a comprehensive description of the basic models*)

Anderson, R.M. and Nokes, D.J. (1991) Mathematical models of transmission and control. In: *Oxford Textbook of Public Health*, 2nd edn, Vol. 2. Eds Holland, W.W., Detels, R. and

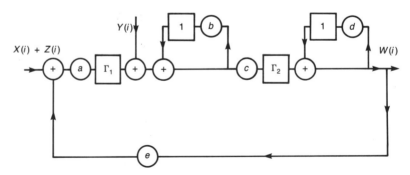

Fig. 19.9 Network representation of the life-cycle of *Ostertagia circumcincta* showing adult parasite output, *W*, derived from ewe egg input, *X*, lamb egg input, *Z*, and over-wintered infective larval input, *Y*. The constants *a*, *b*, *c*, *d* and *e* are parameters of survival, infectivity and fecundity; Γ_1 and Γ_2 are time-delays representing parasitic development times on the pasture and in the lamb, respectively. (Modified from Paton and Gettinby, 1985.)

Knox, G., pp. 225–252. Oxford University Press, Oxford. (*An introduction to mathematical modelling of infectious diseases and their control, with emphasis on human infections*)

Bailey, N.T.J. (1975) *The Mathematical Theory of Infectious Diseases and Its Applications*, 2nd edn. Charles Griffin, London

Becker, N.G. (1989) *Analysis of Infectious Disease Data*. Chapman and Hall, London. (*An introduction to models of infectious diseases*)

de Jong, M.C.M. (1994) Transmission of pathogenic agents: how can it be measured? In: Dutch Society for Veterinary Epidemiology and Economics, Proceedings (7), Utrecht, December 14 1994. Eds Shukken, Y.H. and Lam, T.J.G.M., pp. 23–38. (*A review of models of transmission of infectious agents*)

Hurd, H.S. and Kaneene, J.B. (1993) The application of simulation models and systems analysis in epidemiology: a review. *Preventive Veterinary Medicine*, **15**, 81–99

Manton, K.G. and Stallard, E. (1988) *Chronic Disease Modelling: Measurement and Evaluation of the Risks of Chronic Disease Processes*. Charles Griffin, London/Oxford University Press, New York. (*A comprehensive description of models of human chronic diseases and ageing*)

Nunn, M., Garner, G. and White, D. (Eds) (1993) Animal health. *Agricultural Systems and Information Technology*, **5**(1), 4–43. (*An overview of epidemiological modelling and examples of systems models*)

Proceedings of The Mathematical and Information Models for Veterinary Science Workshop, Wednesday, 22nd December 1993. Moredun Research Institute, Edinburgh, UK. Moredun Research Institute/University of Strathclyde/Scottish Agricultural Colleges Veterinary Services

Scott, M.E. and Smith, G. (Eds) (1994) *Parasitic and Infectious Diseases: Epidemiology and Ecology*. Academic Press, San Diego. (*An introduction to modelling, with case studies of infections in humans, livestock and wild animals*)

Squire, G.R. and Hamer, P.J.C. (Eds) (1990) *United Kingdom Register of Agricultural Models 1990*. AFRC Institute of Engineering Research, Wrest Park, Silsoe, Bedford. (*A list and summary of agricultural models, including some veterinary ones*)

Takizawa, T., Ito, T. and Kosuge, M. (1977) Prototype of simulation models for epizootics in domestic animals. *National Institute of Animal Health Quarterly*, **17**, 171–178

20 The economics of disease

The importance of financial evaluations in intensive livestock enterprises has been partly responsible for the increased application of economic techniques to animal disease control at farm, national and international levels since the late 1960s, when the principles were first broadly outlined (Morris, 1969) and 'veterinary economics' ('animal health economics') emerged as a specific area of interest in veterinary medicine. There has been a tendency to consider economic evaluations as separate, optional exercises, distinct from epidemiological investigations. However, this attitude is erroneous: economic assessments are integral parts of many epidemiological investigations (see *Figure 2.1*), providing a complementary perspective to that of biological (i.e., technical) studies with which the veterinarian is more familiar because of his professional training. This complementarity is explored by Howe (1989, 1992).

Other factors have also increased veterinary interest in economics (McInerney, 1988). First, in western countries, government veterinary services are increasingly required to justify budgets, as the role of the public sector diminishes. Secondly, as the importance of agricultural output declines in western countries, the economic justification for animal disease control is questioned more closely. Thirdly, diseases of farm livestock are barriers to international trade. This problem has become particularly acute with the harmonization of trade in the European Union (which requires free movement of commodities) and the global attempts to liberalize world trade through the General Agreement on Tariffs and Trade (GATT). Fourthly, rising incomes and changing social values focus attention on qualitative aspects of food production, the welfare of animals, and diseases of companion animals. This necessitates a widening of economic perspectives from the initial, relatively narrow, evaluation of disease in farm livestock.

This chapter introduces basic economic concepts and principles and outlines some economic techniques that are relevant to epidemiological investigations. Detailed analytical methods are not described because it is assumed that most veterinarians are not practising economists, and therefore do not need to apply the various methods for which some formal training in economics is recommended.

Economic concepts and principles

An economist's view of the world is based on a set of concepts and generalized abstractions about the nature of their interrelationship (i.e., a theory). The powerful simplicity of the theory means that it is applicable to a wide range of problems, including animal disease.

Economics is a science which illuminates how people exercise choice in the allocation of scarce resources for production, in the distribution and consumption of products, and in the consequences of those decisions for individual and social benefit (*Figure 20.1*). Animal disease therefore has economic, as well as biological, impacts because it affects the well-being of people.

Economic analysis is frequently concerned with identification of the optimum level of output in relation to total resource use, and the most efficient combination of resources within that total. The criteria for efficiency are both economic and technical.

Generally, disease in domesticated (and sometimes undomesticated) livestock populations reduces the quantity and/or quality of livestock products available for human consumption (i.e., benefit). Examples of such products range from meat and milk to pony rides and the companionship of pets. To be more precise, disease causes production from a given quantity of resources to be of lower quantity and/or quality than could be obtained in its absence.

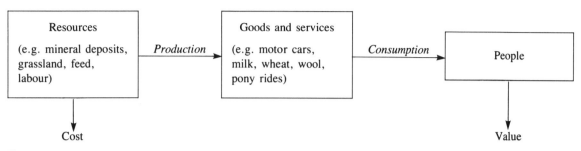

Fig. 20.1 The basic economic model.

Disease increases costs in two ways. First, because resources are being used inefficiently, the products actually obtained are for an unnecessarily high resource cost: in the absence of disease, the same (or more) output could be obtained for a smaller (or the same) expenditure of resources. Secondly, there is a cost to people, who are deprived because they have fewer, or lower quality, products to consume; that is, they obtain lower benefits. In summary, disease increases expenditures (production costs) and decreases output (consumer benefits).

Production functions

The relationship between the resources that provide the inputs to production and the goods and services that comprise the output is called a **production function** (*Figure 20.2*). The resources may be natural (e.g., land and mineral deposits) or man-made (e.g., buildings and machinery). Frequently, these undergo physical transformation (e.g., iron ore into steel, animal feed into body protein) or else facilitate a physical transformation process (e.g., manpower and managerial expertise). Empirical evidence shows that this relationship is typically non-linear because certain inputs are typically fixed,

and so beyond a certain point an increase in variable input* is associated with a less than proportionate increase in output — the 'law of diminishing returns' (Heady and Dillon, 1961; Dillon and Anderson, 1990).

Although the idea initially may seem unusual, technical and economic efficiency are seldom synonymous. Under normal circumstances of diminishing physical returns, they are the same only if inputs are costless. For example, it is efficient in an economic sense for a dairy farmer to aim for maximum milk yield per cow only when the cow's feed is free. If the farmer has to pay for the feed which, of course, is invariably the case, then it can be shown that optimum economic efficiency is obtained when the yield per cow is less than the maximum technical potential. Furthermore, the overall economic optimum (maximum profits) will change with variations in relative prices of both output and inputs and with methods of production. This observation is important in the context of animal disease, because the incidence of disease that is acceptable from an economic point of view may well change with relative prices and techniques of production.

Disease as an economic process

Livestock production is a specific example of a physical transformation process (*Figure 20.3*). Disease impairs this process (i.e., reduces output) and sometimes results in death. Thus, there is a loss of efficiency which poses both technical and economic problems. *Figure 20.4* depicts the technical efficiency loss as the difference between the production functions of 'healthy' and 'diseased' animals. Disease acts as a 'negative input', and the relationship between inputs and output is shifted downwards, reflecting lower output for given inputs in diseased animals compared with disease-free animals.

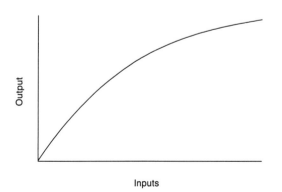

Fig. 20.2 The shape of a general production function, plotting inputs against output.

*A variable input is defined as an input whose use varies with the planned level of production.

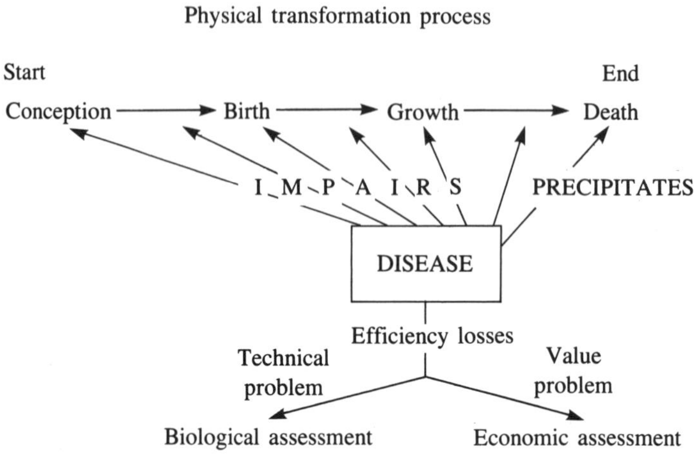

Physical transformation process

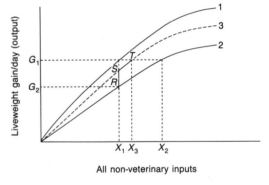

Fig. 20.3 The physical transformation process in relation to livestock production.

If restoration of technical efficiency is the goal, the corresponding economic objective is to find the least-cost method to restore health and productivity. The options are presented in *Figure 20.5*, in which only one output — liveweight gain per day — is considered. For an arbitrary quantity of non-veterinary variable inputs, say x_1, used with a fixed number of animals, point G_1 indicates the gain per day when they are 'healthy' animals (curve 1); G_2 identifies the liveweight gain if they are 'diseased' animals (curve 2). Thus, $G_1 - G_2$ is the loss in technical efficiency. One option is to control the disease exclusively by veterinary intervention, thus restoring G_2 to G_1. However, reduction of disease commonly does not depend *exclusively* on veterinary services and medicines. An economist regards these as just particular types of

Fig. 20.5 The recovery of planned output utilizing veterinary and non-veterinary inputs. (Based on Howe, 1985.)

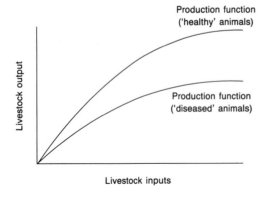

Fig. 20.4 General production function for 'healthy' and 'diseased' animals.

inputs that may have substitutes in the form of greater managerial expertise, use of more land to reduce stocking rate, and so on, all of which may reduce disease. Using $x_2 - x_1$ additional non-veterinary inputs also restores G_2 to G_1. In practice, the option most commonly adopted corresponds to a movement along some intermediate curve, say curve 3. Production is then lifted from G_2 to G_1 in two parts. The proportion of $G_1 - G_2$ given by RS is achieved by veterinary expenditures, while the remainder (climbing from S to T) is achieved by increasing non-veterinary inputs from x_1 to x_3. The main goal of economic evaluation is to identify the path corresponding to RST which enables G_1, rather than G_2, to be obtained most cheaply, that is, identifying the *combination* of veterinary and other inputs that will minimize the costs of recovery.

Assessing the economic costs of disease

The total economic cost of disease can be measured as the sum of **output losses** and **control expenditures**. A reduction in output is a loss because it is a benefit that is either taken away (e.g., when milk containing antibiotic residues is compulsorily discarded) or unrealized (e.g., decreased milk yield). Expenditures, in contrast, are increases in input, and are usually associated with disease control. Examples of control expenditures are veterinary intervention and increased use of agricultural labour, both of which may be used either therapeutically or prophylactically. Note, therefore, that economic costs are more than just the sum of financial outlays, and it is important not to confuse the two.

Optimum control strategies

Figures 20.4 and *20.5* have used the basic economic model of a production function to illustrate the implications of disease and its control for technical and economic efficiency. A related approach is to explore the general relationship between control expenditures and output losses as defined by a curve which again demonstrates the law of diminishing returns (*Figure 20.6*). Two control programmes, *A* and *B*, are identified in the figure. A change from programme *A* to programme *B* involves an increase in control expenditures of $\delta_E = E_B - E_A$, and a decrease in output losses of $\delta_L = L_A - L_B$. It

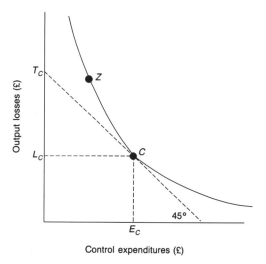

Fig. 20.7 Defining the economically optimum control programme. (From Schepers, 1990.)

is worth increasing the level of control expenditures by δ_E because δ_L is greater than δ_E. However, it becomes increasingly expensive to achieve incremental reductions in output losses.

The **optimum** control strategy is defined by point *C* in *Figure 20.7*. At this point, the total costs, $T_C = (L_C + E_C)$, are the lowest that can be attained (i.e., the avoidable costs = £0). To the left of *C*, £1 of control expenditures reduces output losses by more than £1; to the right of this point, £1 of control expenditures reduces output losses by less than £1. This is an illustration of **marginal analysis** and, specifically, the principle that resources should be used up to the point where the expenditure on the last unit of resource is just recouped by the additional returns.

An example of identifying an optimum control strategy: bovine subclinical mastitis in the UK (McInerney et al., 1992)

Bovine mastitis is considered to be the most important disease affecting dairy cattle in many developed countries. In the UK, a national mastitis survey conducted in 1977 provided detailed information on the prevalence of subclinical infection and control procedures practised in over 500 herds (Wilson and Richards 1980; Wilson *et al.*, 1983). The latter include:

1. teat dipping and spraying;
2. dry-cow therapy;
3. annual testing of milking machines.

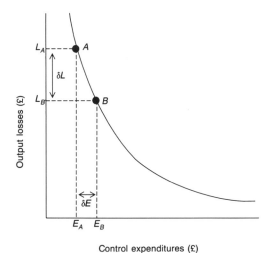

Fig. 20.6 The general relationship between output losses and control expenditures. (From Schepers, 1990.)

The losses due to subclinical mastitis include:

1. decreased milk yield;
2. changed milk composition;
3. decreased milk quality (e.g., antibiotic residues);
4. accelerated replacement of dairy cows.

Sometimes there are offsetting savings in some input expenditures such as decreased feed intake because of loss of appetite in affected cows.

Control expenditures relate to the three control techniques, and sufficient published information was available to attach financial values to these expenditures and the losses. The prevalence was expressed as the percentage of quarters that were subclinically infected per day, and annual incidence was estimated assuming that subclinical infection lasts an average of 0.6 years (Dodd and Neave, 1970).

Table 20.1 lists the predicted disease incidence and the economic costs associated with the various combinations of control strategy. The lowest costs that can be attained are associated with control strategy 1 (teat dipping throughout the year, administering dry-cow therapy to all eligible animals, and annual testing of milking machines), where the total cost is £3006 per 100 cows per year. The specific relationship between control expenditures and output losses is displayed in *Figure 20.8*, and is consistent with the general case (*Figure 20.7*). The curve identifies the 'best practical' options from a technical point of view, and so the corresponding economic optimum must be somewhere along its length.

If these results are extrapolated to the national herd, they suggest that if strategy 1 were implemented in all dairy herds, the overall cost of mastitis to the nation could be reduced from £172.7 million to £159.6 million, at which level the avoidable costs = £0. It is these costs that are relevant to decisions about resource allocation and disease control — not the costs measured from a base of zero which it may be impossible to reach with current control techniques. The costs cannot be reduced further unless investment is made in research into improved methods of mastitis control.

Cost − benefit analysis of disease control

The costs and benefits of disease control campaigns can be assessed using several methods including **gross margin analysis** and **partial budgeting** (Asby *et al.*, 1975). These are essentially straightforward accounting approaches, whereas **social cost − benefit analysis** (Pearce, 1971; Mishan, 1976; Sugden and Williams,

1978) is really the application of a specific technique which allows for the fact that costs and benefits are commonly distributed over time, and sometimes are more than simple financial values. If it is necessary only to compare the effectiveness of two alternative control strategies, without fully assessing benefits and costs, then a **cost-effective** study is undertaken. The remainder of this chapter introduces partial budgets and social cost − benefit analysis.

Partial farm budgets

Partial farm budgets have been used to assess the suitability of control strategies (notably against endemic diseases such as mastitis and internal parasitism) on individual farms. A partial budget is a simple description of the financial consequences of particular changes in farm management procedures, of which disease control programmes are a part. 'Partial' indicates that assessment is restricted to the factors that are likely to change as a result of the procedural changes.

There are four main components:

1. additional revenue realized from the change, r_1;
2. reduced costs stemming from the change, c_1;
3. increased costs as a result of the change, r_2;
4. cost of implementing the change, c_2.

If $(r_1 + c_1) > (r_2 + c_2)$, then the proposed change is justified.

For example (Erb, 1984), if a new programme to control subclinical mastitis comprised maintenance of milking machines, routine intramammary dry-cow therapy and teat dipping, then:

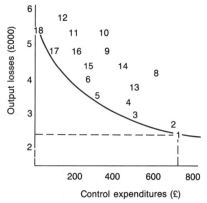

Fig. 20.8 Output losses and control expenditures of farms in the National Mastitis Survey. (Numbers refer to the control strategies listed in *Table 20.1*.) (From McInerney *et al.*, 1992.)

Table 20.1 Predicted mastitis incidence and economic costs associated with 18 different control strategies employed by dairy herds in the National Mastitis Survey, UK, 1977. (Modified from McInerney et al., 1992.)

Control method			Group no.	Effect on incidence		Loss/expenditure coordinates		
Teat dip/spray (period)	Dry-period therapy (cows)	Testing milk machine		Predicted incidence rate (/100 cows/year)	Decrease in incidence (relative to no control)	Control expenditures (£/100 cows/year) (E)	Output losses (£/100 cows/year) (L)	Total economic cost (C)
All year	All	Yes	1	18.5	24.8	710	2296	3006
		No	2	22.3	21.0	670	2770	3440
	Some	Yes	3	23.4	19.9	490	2899	3389
		No	4	27.2	16.1	450	3373	3823
	None	Yes	5	27.8	15.5	270	3446	3716
		No	6	31.6	11.7	230	3923	4153
Part of year	All	Yes	7	33.7	9.6	615	4148	4799
		No	8	37.6	5.7	575	4657	5232
	Some	Yes	9	38.6	4.7	395	4786	5181
		No	10	42.4	0.9	355	5260	5615
	None	Yes	11	43.0	0.3	175	5333	5508
		No	12	46.8	−3.5	135	5807	5942
Not used	All	Yes	13	30.3	13.0	480	3751	4231
		No	14	34.1	9.2	440	4225	4665
	Some	Yes	15	35.1	8.2	260	4354	4614
		No	16	38.9	4.4	220	4827	5047
	None	Yes	17	39.5	3.8	40	4900	4940
		No	18	43.3	0	0	5374	5374

- r_1 = sales due to increased milk production;
- c_1 = savings stemming from fewer cases of clinical mastitis to treat;
- r_2 = increased feed costs due to increased milk production;
- c_2 = costs of implementation (disinfectants, dry-cow intramammary preparations).

A one-year partial farm budget for this programme produced values of r_1 = £397, c_1 = £18, r_2 = £77, c_2 = £246. Thus:

$$r_1 + c_1 = £415,$$
$$r_2 + c_2 = £323,$$

and so there is a net benefit of £92, indicating that the farm will increase its annual profits by that amount if it invests in the control campaign.

Social cost – benefit analysis (CBA)

Social cost – benefit analysis developed as a means of assessing large-scale investment policies. It has been used widely in veterinary medicine to assess national animal disease control campaigns against epidemic and sporadic diseases; for example, swine fever eradication in Europe (Ellis *et al.*, 1977) and rinderpest control in Nigeria (Felton and Ellis, 1978).

Principles of CBA

Social cost – benefit analysis attempts to quantify the social advantages and disadvantages of a policy in terms of a common monetary unit.* For example, the building of a road will incur costs to society arising from the resources expended on construction and maintenance, the undesirable side-effects of pollution, increased noise levels and spoiling of the landscape. The benefits include savings in travelling time, reduced congestion and decreased noise levels in a town if the road is a bypass. Some of the costs or benefits (e.g., construction outlays — costs) are expressed easily in pecuniary values. Other costs or benefits (e.g., decreased noise level — a benefit), however, are much more difficult to translate into monetary terms; these are called **intangibles**. Only by using the common denominator of money is it possible to aggregate the gains and losses which ultimately interest society as the benefits and costs perceived in *real* terms, that is, as adding to or reducing people's sense of well-being. Consequently, it is important to quantify, in

*Remember, this is not the same as financial analysis (measuring actual money receipts and expenditures), which is really *accounting*, as opposed to true *economic analysis*.

monetary units, all important factors as comprehensively as possible, and to make the problem areas explicit, although the value of intangibles is often assessed somewhat subjectively.

If a disease control programme were initiated, costs would include those of manpower, drugs, vaccines, quarantine buildings, compensation for slaughter, transportation and training programmes. The benefits would include increased productivity, decreased animal and (in the case of zoonotic diseases) human suffering, increased trade and the psychological well-being accompanying the decreased disease incidence. The prefix 'social' to CBA is often dropped from the name but is important. It emphasizes that CBA is used by an organization to maximize the *net benefits to society*, rather than maximizing its own purely private benefits (Pearce and Sturmey, 1966).

'Internal' and 'external' costs and benefits

Internalities (private costs and benefits) are those that accrue directly to an investment project. Costs and benefits accruing to others are termed **externalities**. It is mainly the externalities that are not reflected in the price mechanism (which therefore becomes inadequate as a guide to correct investment decisions from the point of view of society). For example, a farm mastitis control campaign includes dry-cow antibiotic therapy (a cost) and increased milk yield (a benefit), both of which are part of the farm's budget and therefore internal. However, antibiotic residues in milk may have undesirable side-effects on unknowing consumers. If they were aware of the risks they would be prepared to pay less for the milk (if, indeed, they would buy it at all). To protect consumers, and to 'internalize' the external effects, legislation limiting the use of antibiotics and affected milk may be necessary, instead of reliance on a deficient price mechanism. Similarly, in a foot-and-mouth disease campaign in Britain, farmers' loss of slaughtered animals is an internal cost, whereas the inconvenience of restrictions on movement and access is an external cost.

Discounting

Control campaigns may operate over several years. The value of a sum of money now is greater than the same sum of money at a later date because it could be invested now to produce a larger sum in the future as interest accrues. If the interest rate is 5% per annum, then £100 now is worth £105 compound in one year's time, £110.25 in two years, and so on. If costs and benefits, spread over several years, are to be compared then they must be adjusted to calculate their value now. The process of adjustment, which is the opposite of compounding, is called **discounting**. The formulae for its calculation are described by Gittinger (1972) and Little and Mirrlees (1974). The calculation uses a rate of discount that is usually defined by governments, for example the World Bank Rate and, in Britain, the Treasury Rate. The latter is a target rate for public investments and is not the same as the Bank Rate. Cost-benefit analysis is performed in real terms which means that the rate of interest used in the calculations is adjusted to exclude the effects of price inflation.

Shadow prices

The social value of a benefit may not always be the market price. For example, a litre of milk is valued at its market price by the farmer. However, in the European Union, the value may be less because of a surplus of milk. A national disease control campaign that resulted in increased milk production would therefore use the value of the milk to the European Union, termed a **shadow price**, in economic evaluation.

Uncertainty

Any project is accompanied by uncertainty. The results of a control campaign cannot be known with certainty, but it is necessary to have an idea what the outcome might be. There are two approaches to dealing with uncertainty. First, if a model is constructed, the 'most probable outcome' can be defined; a sensitivity analysis (see Chapter 19) can then be conducted to determine whether changes in the model's parameters can produce major changes in the outcome. Alternatively, the likelihood of the various outcomes can be judged using probability theory (Reutlinger, 1970).

Criteria for selecting a control campaign

Three important measures of economic efficiency used as criteria for selecting a control campaign are:

1. net present value (*NPV*);
2. benefit:cost ratio (*B/C*);
3. internal rate of return (*IRR*).

The **net present value** (*NPV*) is the value of the stream of discounted benefits less costs over *n* time periods. It is given by:

$$NPV = \frac{B_0 - C_0}{(1 + r)^0} + \frac{B_1 - C_1}{(1 + r)^1} + \ldots + \frac{B_n - C_n}{(1 + r)^n}$$

$$= \sum_{t=0}^{n} \frac{B_t - C_t}{(1 + r)^t}$$

where:

C_t = value of costs incurred in time t,
B_t = value of benefits gained in time t,
r = discount rate,
n = life of project.

A project is considered to be viable if the *NPV* is positive.

The **benefit:cost ratio** (*B/C*) is the ratio of the present value of benefits to that of costs. It is given by:

$$B/C = \sum_{t=0}^{n} \{B_t/(1 + r)^t\}/\{C_t/(1 + r)^t\},$$

$$= \sum_{t=0}^{n} \frac{B_t}{C_t}$$

A project is viable if the ratio is greater than or equal to 1.

The **internal rate of return** (*IRR*) is the rate of discount that equates the present value of the costs with the present value of the benefits. It is given by solving for *r* such that:

$$NPV = \sum_{t=0}^{n} \frac{B_t - C_t}{(1 + r)^t} = 0.$$

If the internal rate of return of an investment project is greater than the actual interest rate, the project is economically worthwhile.

An example of CBA: alternative policies for the prevention, control and eradication of infestation with Chrysomyia bezziana in Australia (Cason and Geering, 1980)

Chrysomyia bezziana, the Old World screw-worm fly (SWF), causes serious economic losses in livestock in Africa, Asia and Papua New Guinea. Damage caused by burrowing larvae can result in a case fatality rate of up to 50% in young animals, and can cause loss of condition, occasional deaths and sterility (if genitalia are struck) in adults. The disease is not present in Australia, but if the fly entered Australia, potential losses have been estimated at around $100 million per annum. The most likely method of entry into Australia would be by movement of infested livestock across the Torres Strait islands from Papua New Guinea, although entry could also occur either by the direct flight of the flies or by transmission of the flies by migratory birds and aircraft.

Strategies to prevent the introduction and establishment of SWF in Australia include:

1. improved quarantine surveillance, including training of local inhabitants and education programmes;
2. better control of livestock in danger areas, possibly including total destocking of the Torres Strait islands — although this would probably be socially unacceptable to the islanders;
3. the development of an SWF monitoring system, facilitated by a specific chemical bait (Swormlure);
4. the construction of a clinic in the Torres Strait islands to neuter dogs and cats (potential hosts of SWF);
5. eradication of SWF from Papua New Guinea.

The major strategy to control and eradicate an outbreak of infestation with SWF in Australia is ground control of the fly, consisting of restriction of movement of livestock, dipping and spraying with insecticides, the use of a sterile insect release method, by which sterile male flies compete with fertile male flies for each mating female, and the use of a screw-worm adult suppression system (SWASS), in which poisoned baits are released by aeroplane over infested areas. The quickest response to an outbreak of

SWF infestation would be obtained if a sterile SWF facility were built in advance, but not opened until an outbreak occurred.

Table 20.2 shows the benefit:cost ratios for the various strategies over a 20-year period, assuming that infestation occurred after 1, 10 or 20 years. In all cases the benefit:cost ratios are greater than 1, indicating that all techniques are economically justifiable.

In the example the benefits do not derive from increased production, but from decreasing the risk of infestation. Although the benefit:cost ratios are high, they have to be weighed against the probability of infestation occurring when a particular policy either is or is not adopted. These and other considerations are discussed by the authors of the study.

Some problems associated with CBA

There are several general problems related to CBA. The technique assumes that the preferences and priorities of society are known; this may not always be true. The technique also applies current social preferences, rather than future ones. Additionally, as indicated earlier, the costs and benefits of externalities and intangibles may be difficult to assess.

There are specific problems relating to disease control policy formulation (Schepers, 1990). A CBA refers to

Table 20.2 Cost−benefit analysis of strategies for the prevention, control and eradication of infestation with *Chrysomyia bezziana* in Australia. (The analysis is in present values over a 20-year period, and assumes that the methods prevent Australia-wide losses commencing year 1, year 10, year 20; discounted at 9%). (Modified from Cason and Geering, 1980.)

Prevention method	*Year infestation prevented*					
	1		*10*		*20*	
	Benefit: $389m		*Benefit: $164m*		*Benefit: $69m*	
	Cost ($000)	*Benefit:cost ratio*	*Cost ($000)*	*Benefit:cost ratio*	*Cost ($000)*	*Benefit:cost ratio*
Strategic eradication from Papua New Guinea	2 962	131	11 734	14	16 123	4
Mothballed factory and maintenance colony	1 394	279	1 670	98	1 809	38
Ground control*	2 523	154	1 065	154	449	155
Destocking of Torres Strait islands	657	592	776	212	836	83
Improving quarantine	124	3 137	417	394	563	123
'Swormlure' trapping and myiasis monitoring	30	12 966	171	961	241	288
Training	26	14 961	69	2 383	91	763
Extension	13	29 923	83	1 980	119	583
Torres Strait clinic	7	55 571	40	4 110	56	1 239

*Includes the SWASS technique (*see* text).

only one combination of control expenditures and output losses. Thus, point *Z* in *Figure 20.7* represents a benefit:cost ratio greater than 1; that is, the reduction in output losses exceeds the control expenditures. Indeed, the combinations of expenditures and losses furthest to the left of the curve have the greatest benefit:cost ratios, and there may be the temptation to fallaciously conclude that the larger the benefit:cost ratio, the more economically efficient the control technique. However, the economically optimum control programme is indicated by point *C*; this will be identified by a CBA only if the CBA happens, by chance, to be concerned with evaluating a control policy corresponding to point *C*.

Moreover, CBA is a relatively sophisticated technique but may be applied in situations — especially in the developing countries — where accurate basic data are lacking (Grindle, 1980, 1986). For example, there may be inadequate information on livestock numbers, disease morbidity and the actual economic impact of disease. It may also be impossible to predict future market prices (e.g., of beef and milk) which need to be included in analyses. The sophistication of the economic techniques therefore needs to be balanced with the quality of the epidemiological data that are available. However, although CBA and other techniques of project evaluation are, at best, approximate (Gittinger, 1972), they play a useful role in economic evaluation. Despite its limitations, CBA is a rigorous approach to project evaluation, and its application can help towards better informed decisions regarding the efficient use of scarce resources in disease control programmes.

Further reading

Ansell, D.J. and Done, J.T. (1988) *Veterinary Research and Development: Cost – Benefit Studies on Products for the Control of Animal Diseases*. CAS Joint Publication No. 3, Centre for Agricultural Strategy, Reading/British Veterinary Association, London

Dykhuizen, A.A. (1993) Modelling animal health economics. In: Society for Veterinary Epidemiology and Preventive Medicine, Proceedings, Exeter, 31 March – 2 April 1993. Ed. Thrusfield, M.V., pp. ix – xx

Ellis, P.R. and James, A.D. (1979) The economics of animal health — (1) major disease control programmes. *Veterinary Record*, **105**, 504 – 506

Ellis, P.R. and James, A.D. (1979) The economics of animal health — (2) economics in farm practice. *Veterinary Record*, **105**, 523 – 526

Erb, H. (1984). Economics for veterinary farm practice. *In Practice*, **6**, 33 – 37

Hill, B. (1990) *Introduction to Economics for Students of Agriculture*, 2nd edn. Pergamon Press, Oxford. (*A general introduction to agricultural economics*)

Howe, K.S. and McInerney, J.P. (Eds) (1987) *Agriculture. Disease in Farm Livestock: Economics and Policy*. Proceedings of a symposium in the Community programme for coordination of agricultural research, 1 – 3 July 1987, Exeter. Report EUR 11285 EN. Commission of the European Communities, Luxembourg. (*A study of economic losses due to animal disease in the European Union, and methods for the economic assessment of disease control*)

Mather, E.C. and Kaneene, J.B. (Eds) (1986) *Economics of Animal Diseases*. Proceedings of a conference held at Michigan State University, 23 – 25 June 1986. Michigan State University, Michigan

McInerney, J.P., Howe, K.S. and Schepers, J.A. (1992) A framework for the economic analysis of disease in farm livestock. *Preventive Veterinary Medicine*, **13**, 137 – 154

Mishan, E.J. (1982) *Cost – Benefit Analysis: An Informal Introduction*, 3rd edn. Allen and Unwin, London

Ngategize, P.K. and Kaneene, J.B. (1985) Evaluation of the economic impact of animal diseases on production: a review. *Veterinary Bulletin*, **55**, 153 – 162. (*A review of some analytical techniques*)

Putt, S.N.H., Shaw, A.P.M., Woods, A.J., Tyler, L. and James, A.D. (1987) *Veterinary Epidemiology and Economics in Africa*. ILCA Manual No. 3, International Livestock Centre for Africa, Addis Ababa

21 Health schemes

Private health and productivity schemes

The traditional role of the veterinarian has been to attend individual sick animals when requested to do so by the owner: such attention has been called 'fire brigade' treatment. This approach was useful when most diseases, such as the classical epidemic infectious diseases, had a predominantly single cause and responded to a simple course of treatment. However, an appreciation during the 1960s of the multifactorial nature of many diseases, which coincided with intensification of animal industries in the developed countries, with a relative decrease in the value of animals, resulted in a change in attitude towards the management of diseases in individual livestock units (see Chapter 1). First, it became clear that diseases needed to be controlled by simultaneously manipulating all determinants: those associated with agent, host and environment. The veterinarian's objective should be to *prevent*, rather than to treat, disease. Secondly, it became necessary to consider disease in terms of its contribution to reduced performance (and therefore profitability) of a herd.*

The first change stimulated the development of **preventive medicine programmes** in the early 1960s. The second change resulted in the evolution of comprehensive **herd health and productivity schemes**, encompassing preventive medicine and the assessment of productivity. These schemes are concerned with problems that can be

*Performance-related diagnosis was introduced in Chapter 1, and an example of a multifactorial 'disease', defined in terms of a production shortfall in a population, was given in *Figure 5.2*. The concept of a 'sick' population is not confined to veterinary medicine, though. Medical epidemiologists also search for characteristics of 'sick' populations, for example to answer the questions 'Why is hypertension common in London but absent from Kenyans?' and 'Why is coronary heart disease common in Finland but rare in Japan?'

controlled by the stockowner on individual farms (e.g., bovine mastitis), and are run by general practitioners or bureaux; they are therefore **private** schemes.

Structure of private health and productivity schemes

Objectives

The goals of a health and productivity scheme are summarized by Blood (1976). They should:

1. identify disease problems on a farm;
2. rate the problems in order of importance, with reference to technical and economic criteria;
3. initiate suitable control techniques and measure their success, not only technically but also with regard to the economic efficiency of the utilization of resources at the national and individual farm level, thereby indicating which techniques should be increased and which reduced.

The scope of service offered by the veterinarian in a comprehensive health and productivity scheme (Grunsell *et al.*, 1969; Ribble, 1989) includes:

1. the diagnosis and prevention of the major epidemic diseases;
2. an emergency service for individual animals;
3. the supply of drugs;
4. advice on environmental determinants (nutrition, housing and management);
5. advice on production techniques and general policies of livestock farming.

This scope is broad and indicates that the veterinarian requires more than just a knowledge of the diagnosis and treatment of clinical disease. In many cases, the veterinarian may need to enlist further expert help from nutritionists, building advisors, and from management specialists who have some knowledge of farm economics.

Components

There are differences between the schemes applied to different species, but the principles are the same. The main components of a scheme are:

1. the recording of a **farm profile** comprising details of animal numbers, stocking density, nutrition, usual management practices, disease status and current levels of production;
2. identification of production shortfalls;
3. monitoring of all aspects of production;
4. identification of the major disease problems;
5. routine prophylaxis against the major disease risks;
6. definition of **production targets** that are suitable for the system of management operating on the particular livestock units and for the aims of the farmer;
7. advice on management and husbandry, to achieve the predetermined targets;
8. detection of unacceptable shortfalls in production (and therefore in profitability);
9. correction of the shortfalls by eliminating the defects associated with agent, host and environment, or revising the production targets in the light of experience.

Regular visits to farms are an important part of health schemes. An **action list** is drawn up containing details of procedures (e.g., vaccination) to be followed at certain times of the year.

Health and productivity schemes require accurate records to be kept. Early schemes used longhand records, but most contemporary systems store data on computers where the data can be analysed rapidly. The first computerized systems were run on mainframes and were organized by central advisory bureaux. Some systems are network-based (e.g., FAHRMX, 1984; Bartlett *et al.*, 1985), therefore combining the benefits of local data storage and retrieval with the advantages of a centralized facility for data analysis. There is now a trend towards complete decision support systems (see Chapter 11), mounted on microcomputers, which support farmers in herd management. For example, CHESS (*C*omputerized *H*erd *E*valuation *S*ystem for *S*ows) comprises a decision support system that assesses performance in pig breeding herds, and three expert systems that attempt to identify strengths and weaknesses in the enterprises in an

economic context (Huirne and Dijkhuizen, 1994). All of these systems are essentially microscale (see *Table 11.3*).

Targets

The variables that are used to determine production targets are described below in relation to the different species. Targets have usually been defined as measures of position (e.g., mean age of dry sows) or as upper or lower limits (e.g., maximum calving interval or minimum first service pregnancy rate in dairy cattle). Measures of location do not indicate the dispersion of values in a herd and can be misleading; measures of dispersion, such as the standard deviation (when a variable is Normally distributed) or the semi-interquartile range are more informative (see Chapter 12). Thus, if a farmer bred some cows very soon (less than 35 days) after calving then the measure of position would be reduced, but the measure of dispersion would be increased. This can eliminate the economic benefit that the owner thinks he is achieving because the economic benefit results from most cows calving with intervals close to 365 days (Morris, 1982); the benefit will not exist with a large dispersion.

Some variables that are used as production indices have frequency distributions that are skewed, in which case the mean may be far from the peak of the distribution. For example, the frequency distribution of calving to conception intervals is positively skewed; typically the median may be 10 days less than the mean. More appropriate measures of position and dispersion therefore would be the median and semi-interquartile range, respectively. Logarithmic transformation of values (see Chapter 12) may be undertaken because this may convert skewed distributions to Normal ones. Morant (1984) discusses the appropriateness of measures in relation to dairy fertility, giving examples.

No single set of production standards can be set as targets because satisfactory performance varies with type of farm and management practices (Kay, 1986). **Internal** standards can be set, using a farm's historical data (say, over the previous three years). Additionally, **external** standards, such as the mean performance (with the associated standard deviation) of similar herds, may be specified. In the Netherlands, for example, such standards are published for pig breeding herds (Baltussen *et al.*, 1988).

Measuring shortfalls in production

Shortfalls in production are defined by an **action level** (also termed an **interference level**). This is the level at which the recorded production variable ceases to be acceptable in relation to its target level. Action levels are often identified by experience, based on financial criteria;

Table 21.1   Suggested reproductive performance targets for a dairy herd in the UK. (Modified from Eddy, 1992.)

Index variable	Target	Interference level
Mean calving to conception interval	85 days	95 days
Mean calving to first service interval	65 days	70 days
Mean first service to conception interval	20 days	25 days
Pregnancy rate to first service (%)	60	50
Pregnancy rate to all services (%)	60	50
Overall culling rate (%)	<18	>23
Per cent served of cows calved	95	<90
Per cent conceived of cows calved	85	<80
Per cent conceived of cows served	95	<90
Per cent of interservice intervals 18−24 days	60	45
Per cent of interservice intervals <18 days	8	12
Submission rate* (%)	90	<75

*The number of cows or heifers served within a 21-day period, expressed as a percentage of the number of cows or heifers at or beyond their earliest service date at the start of the 21-day period.

and are defined as levels beyond which there is unacceptable financial loss. When the measurement of location of a variable (the mean has commonly been used), recorded over a period of time, is beyond the action level, corrective measures are undertaken. This method does not consider the effects of random variation. These can be accommodated by defining the action levels as statistical parameters of the target level; the standard error is a suitable parameter for Normally distributed data. Suitable techniques for continuous data are the construction of cusums and Shewhart charts (see Chapter 12).

Justification

A herd health and productivity scheme must be economically justifiable. The economic justification of these schemes is well documented (Williamson, 1980, 1987, 1993). Pharo *et al.* (1984) derived a benefit:cost ratio of approximately 3:1 for a computerized dairy herd health and productivity scheme in Britain over a five-year period, and a similar value has been estimated for a scheme in the US (Williamson, 1987).

Details of schemes for the various species given below are presented only as introductory examples and therefore are not comprehensive, definitive descriptions of the systems. Stein (1986) and Eddy (1992) give a concise summary of these schemes, and Radostits and others (1994) describe them in detail.

Dairy health and productivity schemes

Dairy health and productivity schemes were developed in the 1950s and since then have received considerable

attention (Lesch, 1981). The main object of a dairy scheme is to improve productivity by maximizing milk yield and quality under the particular system of management on the farm. Optimum milk yield and quality are achieved by:

1. efficient reproduction;
2. decreasing important diseases (especially mastitis);
3. optimum feeding.

Targets

Some suggested targets for efficient reproduction for a dairy enterprise in the UK are listed in *Table 21.1*. De Kruif (1978) cites European targets, and Woods and Howard (1980) give North American ones. A target mean calving to conception interval of 85 days is often recommended. This facilitates an annual reproductive cycle (because the cow's gestation period is approximately 280 days), with a calving interval (the interval between calving for an individual cow) of 365 days, and a calving index (the mean calving interval for all cows) with a similar value.

The index variables used in measuring reproductive performance are complex, and need to be interpreted with care (Eddy, 1992). Thus, the calving to conception interval is related to the calving to first service interval and to the first service to conception interval. The calving to first service interval, in turn, depends on restoration of ovarian function, uterine involution, oestrus detection, and farm policy on mating; whereas the first service to conception interval is affected by oestrus detection and the pregnancy rate. Moreover, no single index should be used as an indicator of reproductive effiency. Thus, the calving to conception interval and culling rate need to be considered jointly because they are inversely related: a reduced culling rate will result in an increased calving to conception interval, and vice versa (Eddy, 1992). Some authorities recommend assessing fertility performance in a single financial index (*Fertex*) which combines the calving interval, culling rate for failure to conceive, and pregnancy rate (Esslemont, 1993).

Routine visits

Regular farm visits are required to achieve reproductive targets. De Kruif (1980) recommends visits to cows:

1. that have calved during the previous three to six weeks and have abnormal histories of parturition and of the early post-partum period;
2. not seen in oestrus by 50–70 days post-partum;
3. with abnormal discharges or irregular oestrous cycles;
4. inseminated three or more times;
5. served 35–60 days earlier (for pregnancy diagnosis).

A reproductive examination schedule is also described by Morrow (1980). Additionally, farmers are advised on the control of important diseases and on nutrition during routine visits.

Decreasing important diseases

Mastitis is a major cause of loss of milk yield. A recommended control programme, recognizing the disease's various component causes (Kingwill *et al.*, 1970), includes:

1. the dipping of teats in a suitable disinfectant immediately after milking;
2. antibiotic therapy of chronic cases and of all cows at 'drying off';
3. culling of recurrent cases;
4. improved general husbandry, including milking machine maintenance.

Bramley *et al.* (1981), Blood *et al.* (1983), Jarrett (1984) and Anderson (1993) describe mastitis control in detail.

Pedal lameness is also an important cause of reduced production, especially when chronic. 'Lameness' is a disease definition based on presenting signs (see Chapter 9) which result from a range of lesions including hoof erosions, white line disease, sole trauma, sole ulceration, sandcrack, aseptic laminitis and interdigital hyperplasia. Component causes relate to host, agent and environment. Pododermatitis, for example, has a genetic component associated with sires (Peterse and Antonisse, 1981) and

therefore might be controlled partially by sire selection. Laminitis appears to be related to diet (excess feeding of carbohydrate and protein: Nilsson, 1978) and to have a heritable component. Control of lameness therefore depends on identification of the major lesions and manipulation of their component causes. The survey illustrated in Chapter 13 (*Figure 13.3*) was undertaken to identify the lesions associated with pedal lameness and their importance. Baggott (1982) describes hoof lameness in detail, and Edwards (1980) discusses its control.

Optimum feeding

The correct nutritional balance is important in maintaining optimum milk yield, milk quality and fertility. The likelihood of deficiencies arising can be estimated by feed analysis. Blood analysis can be of value in diagnosing chronic deficiencies (e.g., chronic hypomagnesaemia and hypocuprosis).

A popular means of assessing the nutritional balance in dairy herds is the **metabolic profile** (Payne *et al.*, 1970). This involves estimating the levels of blood constituents that are important components of metabolism related to milk yield. Such constituents include minerals, protein metabolites, glucose, butyrates and free fatty acids.

Much has been learned since the initial use of metabolic profiles in dairy cattle. It has become apparent that planning of blood sampling according to feed changes and calving patterns is necessary, and that care must be taken when selecting cows 'typical' of the herd. Useful and sensible interpretation of biochemical results can only be carried out with access to background information on the cows' level of performance, stage of lactation and diet. With these caveats, some authors conclude that practical information can be obtained on the important aspects of the nutritional status of animals (Whitaker *et al.*, 1983b; Kelly *et al.*, 1988). The usefulness of metabolic profiles is discussed by Lister and Gregory (1978) and MAFF/DAFS (1984).

Pig health and productivity schemes

Intensively reared pigs are housed in large units, sometimes with over 100 sows in a herd (*Table 1.9*).

There are four areas of concern:

1. reproduction in the dry sow;
2. production in the suckling sow;
3. performance of the growing pig;
4. performance of the boar.

Different constraints operate in each area. The dry sow's reproductive potential is governed by the service programme (the rate of reproduction), by the fertility of the sow (the sow's efficiency) and by disease. Productivity of the suckling sow is a function of the farrowing rate, the number of piglets born alive, piglet mortality, diseases of the sow, and the sucking piglets' growth rate. Performance of the growing pig is affected by the type of feed, feed costs, food conversion efficiency, disease and mortality. Boar performance, which affects the reproductive capacity of the sow, is affected by the age of the boar, the boar:sow ratio, frequency of mating, and the litter size and litter scatter* attributable to the boar.

Table 21.2 lists the basic variables that should be recorded to produce and regularly update a farm profile.

Targets

Table 21.3 lists target and interference levels (the latter based on experience) for dry sows, suckling sows, growing pigs and boars in an intensively reared pig herd. Stein (1988) discusses performance monitoring and target levels in detail.

Table 21.2 Recommended variables to be recorded monthly in a pig health and productivity scheme. (From Douglas, 1984.)

Stock numbers
 (1) Boars
 (2) Sows and served gilts
 (3) Maidens
 (4a) Culls/deaths—sows
 (4b) Culls/deaths—boars
Service area
 (5) Number of 1st services
 (6) Number of 2nd services
 (7) Number of 3rd services
Farrowing area
 (8) Number of farrowings
 (9) Number of pigs born alive
 (10) Number of pigs born dead
 (11) Number of sows weaned
 (12) Number of pigs weaned
 (13) Number of pigs transferred to finishing area
 (14a) Deaths—sucking
 (14b) Deaths—weaning
 (14c) Deaths—finishing
Finishing area
 (13) Number of pigs in
 (15) Number of pigs sold (including number of gilts retained for breeding)
Food (tonnes)
 (16) Amount of sow food used
 (17) Amount of pre-weaning (creep) food used
 (18) Amount of post-weaning food used

*Litter scatter is the percentage of litters of eight or less.

Routine visits

A schedule for regular visits to a pig herd is recommended by Muirhead (1980). *Table 21.4* lists components of monthly visits to a herd of 150−300 sows. Smaller herds may be seen less frequently. Visits comprise a standard procedure and discussion of special topics. The standard procedure involves:

1. pre-visit preparation, when previous reports, current investigations and clinical problems are studied;
2. a clinical examination of the reproductive and service areas, dry sows, the farrowing and weaning areas, and fattening pigs;
3. a discussion with the farmer.

Comprehensive examination of a pig herd is described by Goodwin (1971) and Muirhead (1978). Routine preventive measures are described by Douglas (1984).

Sheep health and productivity schemes

The major areas of concern in sheep health schemes, like schemes in other species, are reproductive efficiency, losses due to disease, and suboptimal production (which may be caused by subclinical disease).

Sheep schemes are designed primarily for lowland flocks. Examples include those developed in England (Hindson, 1982; Holland, 1984; Morgan and Tuppen, 1988; Clarkson and Faull, 1990), western Australia (Bell, 1980), south-west Australia (Morley *et al.*, 1983), New Zealand (McNeil *et al.*, 1984) and The Netherlands (Konig, 1985).

Initially, a farm profile should be produced, comprising details of the breeds of rams and ewes, the size and stocking density of the flock, current feeding, breeding, pasture management and disease control. *Table 21.5* illustrates a simple sheet for recording a farm profile.

Targets

Records of past performance of a flock enable the setting of suitable production targets. Examples of targets relating to a Scottish lowland flock are given in *Table 21.6*. In common with other health schemes, accurate records must be kept so that productivity can be assessed and corrective action taken if shortfalls are detected.

Routine visits

Advisory visits are made at important stages of sheep management. In Britain it is recommended (Holland, 1984) that visits should occur:

1. in mid to late summer (i.e., before tupping);

Table 21.3 Suggested targets and interference levels for an intensive pig unit in north-east England. (From Muirhead, 1978.)

Index variable	Target	Interference level	Index variable	Target	Interference level
(a) The dry sow			Piglet mortality (%):		
Average number of sows in herd	As determined	Fluctuation of 30% of target	Laid on	5	7
Average age	24 months	30 months	Congenital defects	0.5	1.5
Ratio of average number of maiden gilts:sows	1:15		Low viability	1.5	3
			Starvation	1	3
Service programme	As determined	>10% variation	Scour	0.5	2
			Miscellaneous	3	5
Weaning to service interval average	7 days	9 days	Pigs reared/sow/year	21	19
Normal repeat service (%)	5	8	Sow feed (tonnes/year)	1.1	1.2
Abnormal repeat service (%)	3	4	*(c) The growing pig*		
Abortions (%)	1	2.5	Mortality (%)	2.5	3.5
Sows infertile not in pig (%)	<2	5	Feed conversion from weaning:		
			Pork (60 kg)	2.7	2.9
Sow deaths (%)	2	3	Cutter (85 kg)	2.9	3.2
Sows culled due to disease (%)	<2	4	Bacon (90 kg)	2.9	3.2
			Heavy (115 kg)	3.6	3.8
Farrowing rate (%)	85–89	80	Feed cost/kg liveweight gain	Variable with feed costs	Comparative figures
*Litters/sow/year	2.25	2.0			
			(d) The boar		
(b) The farrowing/suckling sow			Average age	20 months	30 months
Number of piglets born alive/litter	10.9	10	Boar:sow ratio	1:20	1:30
			Matings/week	4	5
Number of piglets born dead (%)	5	7	Matings/sow	2	3
Number of mummified piglets (%)	0.5	1	Mating interval	12 hours (variable)	—
Number of piglets weaned/litter	9.6	9	Boar litter scatter (%)	15	25
			Litter size	9.8–10.8	Obtained by boar comparison
Deaths until weaning (%)	8–12	13			
**Litter scatter (%)	10	18	Conception to first service (%)	>90	85

*Assuming 5-week weaning
**Litter of 8 or less (*see* text for definition)

Table 21.4 A 12-monthly preventive medicine programme for a herd of 150–300 sows on monthly visits. (From Muirhead, 1980.)

Visit No.	Special topics
(1) Standard procedure*	Herd security
(2) Standard procedure	Stock introduction; methods of gene movement; herd replacement policies; gilt selection requirements
(3) Standard procedure	Economic losses in the herd; feed costs and utilization
(4) Standard procedure	External/internal parasites; vermin control; vaccination programme
(5) Standard procedure	Fertility; boar management
(6) Standard procedure	Herd security check; farrowing sow diseases; parturition, mastitis, etc.
(7) Standard procedure	Piglet problems
(8) Standard procedure	Diseases, mortality and management of the weaned and fattening pigs
(9) Standard procedure	Housing utilization; alterations; associated diseases
(10) Standard procedure	Man management, disease and productivity
(11) Standard procedure	Slaughter house monitoring; pathological tests
(12) Standard procedure	12-monthly appraisal and analysis

*See text for details.

2. during the pregnancy of the ewe;
3. at or around lambing;
4. after lambing.

During the first visit, culling of ewes, based on examination of condition score, udders, mouths, feet and legs, should be advised. The genitals of rams should also be examined. Advice should be given on management of the breeding flock at tupping. The second visit (when the ewe is pregnant) is primarily concerned with nutritional advice. Nutrition of pregnant ewes is important (Russel, 1985) and metabolic profiles, based on butyrate examination, are valuable. The third visit deals with problems at birth, and is used as a further opportunity for offering advice on nutrition and management. The fourth visit is timed to provide advice on the growing lamb.

Table 21.5 An information sheet recording a farm profile and illustrating some recorded variables in a lowland sheep flock health programme. (From Holland, 1984.)

INFORMATION SHEET

(1) RAMS Nos. Breed(s)
  – rams
  – ram lambs
(2) EWES Nos. Breed(s)
  – ewes
  – ewe lambs
(3) EWES TO TUP
  Nos. and date
(4) EWES LAMBED
(5) LAMBS BORN
  – alive
  –dead
(6) LAMB DEATHS BETWEEN BIRTH AND WEANING
(7) LAMBING COMMENCED – Date
(8) LAMBING COMPLETED – Date
(9) EWES HOUSED/HOUSED AT LAMBING/NOT HOUSED
(10) RATION
  (a) ewes
  (b) lamb creep
  (c) lamb fattener
(11) LAMB SALES
  (a) commenced
  (b) completed
(12) COMMENTS ON:
  (a) Results
  (b) Problem areas
(13) COMMENTS ON MASTITIS IN EWES
  (a) known cases this year
  (b) previous culling percentage
(14) CONDITION SCORING FULLY PRACTISED AND UNDERSTOOD?

Specific disease problems should be identified during visits. In Britain, problem diseases can include infection by orf, infectious abortion, mastitis, swayback, pregnancy toxaemia, mineral and trace element deficiencies, and ecto- and endoparasitism. Foot rot (Egerton, 1981) is a major problem in many sheep-producing countries. Infection by *Clostridium* spp., however, is now controlled effectively by routine vaccination. *Figure 21.1* illustrates an action list for British lowland flocks incorporating control strategies for the important diseases.

Beef health and productivity schemes

Beef cattle are managed less intensively than dairy cattle. There is also less contact between individual beef cattle than dairy cattle; therefore fewer records are kept.

Targets

Beef health and productivity schemes are designed to attain optimum reproductive efficiency and to reduce morbidity and mortality in the stock that are being fattened. Traditionally, the number of calves reared is the sole measure of production. The production target of beef rearing is to produce one calf per cow per year. This objective is somewhat optimistic, requiring a breeding season restricted to 42–63 days, a 95% pregnancy rate, and a 100% reared calf crop during each year, none of which usually occurs.

Table 21.7 lists some variables that are suggested as indices of reproduction and production, with target levels, for a North American feedlot enterprise.

Table 21.6 Performance targets for a Scottish lowland sheep flock (per 100 ewes put to the ram). (From Linklater and Speedy, 1980.)

Index variable	Target
Barren ewes	3%
Ewe deaths	2%
Productive ewes	95%
Total lambs born/ewe	1.81
Lambs born dead	4%
Perinatal lamb mortality	5%
Lambs surviving/ewe	1.72
Later lamb mortality	2%
Lambs weaned or sold/ewe	1.70
Lamb growth rate to 1 August	300 g/day
Target weight at 1 August	41 kg
Proportion sold fat at 1 August (remainder sold fat by 30 September)	50%

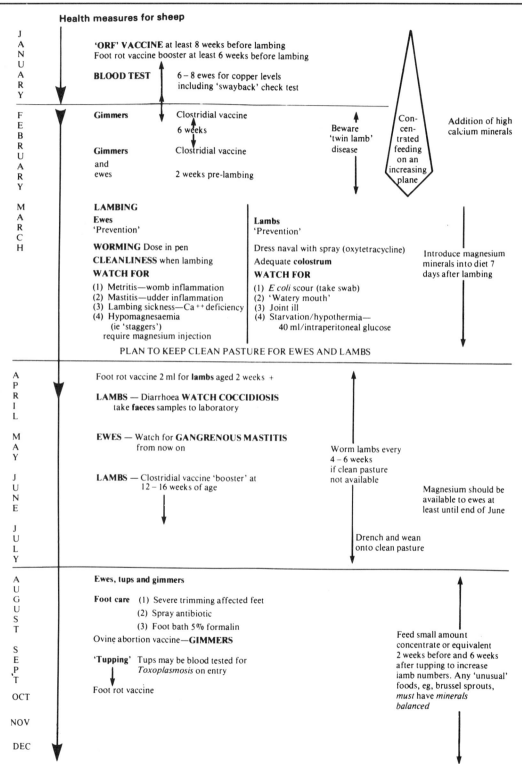

Fig. 21.1 An action list for a British health and productivity scheme for lowland sheep flocks. (From Hindson, 1982.)

Table 21.7 Suggested reproductive performance and production variables for a beef enterprise in the US. (From Rice, 1980a.)

Index variable	Target
Average weaning weight	500 lb
% Cows cycling during the first 21 days breeding	90%
First service conception rate	70%
% Cows pregnant	95%
Calf survival:	
$\dfrac{\text{Live calves at 24 hours}}{\text{Number pregnant cows released}}$	95%
Nursing survival:	
$\dfrac{\text{Calves weaned}}{\text{Calves alive at 24 hours}}$	85%
% Calf crop weaned:	
$\dfrac{\text{Calves weaned}}{\text{Total cows exposed to breeding during the previous season}}$	85%

Routine visits

Routine visits should coincide with major events. Rice (1980b) suggests that the reproductive year should be divided into six periods:

1. weaning;
2. weaning to calving (90−120 days);
3. calving (90 days);
4. pre-breeding (30 days);
5. breeding (60−90 days);
6. post-breeding to pre-weaning.

Relevant management procedures and prophylaxis are carried out and advice is given during each period. During the weaning period, calves are identified, weighed and vaccinated against blackleg, and their internal parasites are controlled; cows are examined for pregnancy, 'open', old and non-productive cows are culled and, if necessary, cows are vaccinated against leptospirosis and campylobacteriosis.

Beef health schemes are reviewed by Caldow (1984) and discussed in detail by Radostits (1983). Models of beef production systems in various developing countries are described by Levine and Hohenboken (1982) and models of breeding systems in developed countries by Congleton and Goodwill (1980).

National schemes

Some schemes operate at the national level and may be subject to legislation (Rees and Davies, 1992). They are frequently part of national control and eradication campaigns (see Chapter 22) directed at diseases that the farmer cannot control alone (e.g., tuberculosis and brucellosis) or at zoonotic infections that are of greater significance to human, than to animal, health (e.g., avian salmonellosis) (cf. private schemes).

Accredited/attested herds

Herds and flocks can be voluntarily certified free from *specified* diseases; they are then described as **accredited** or **attested** (Latin: *testis* = witness). Such schemes include rules for testing animals and maintaining disease-free status. For example, in the UK, the Deer Health Scheme provides a pool of deer herds of tuberculosis-attested health status (ADAS, 1989). Herds must pass three successive tuberculin tests before they are accredited (see *Table 17.15*), after which deer entering the herd must be isolated and tested. Disease status is monitored by regular periodic testing and the compulsory post-mortem examination of deer that die. Members of the scheme must identify all animals, maintain an approved herd record, and report all movements into the herd. Adequate security (e.g., boundary fences and walls) must also be maintained.

Accredited/attested herd schemes are frequently the initial component of eradication campaigns, and are generally followed by compulsory test-and-slaughter programmes (usually when the relevant disease has been voluntarily removed from 80−90% of herds). For example, the first attested herd scheme in the UK was introduced in 1935 as the initial stage of a national tuberculosis eradication campaign. Subsequently, a similar approach was adopted to eradicate brucellosis (MAFF, 1983). Incentives are frequently offered to increase participation (e.g., milk bonuses for participating dairy herds).

Health schemes

National health schemes establish a pool of herds or flocks of recognized health status. The schemes may be directed at one or more *specific* diseases that may be of economic importance to the livestock industry, but may not currently be suitable candidates for eradication. Alternatively, they may have the *general* aim of improving health and productivity. A consequence is enhancement of the market potential of animals for national and international trade. National health schemes are often run by government veterinary services in collaboration with private practitioners. The former provide field advice and

Table 21.8 General outline of a health scheme for dogs in the US. (Modified from Hoskins, 1988a.)

I. First office visit for the health programme (usually at 6 to 8 weeks of age)
    A. Perform a general physical examination and record the body weight
    B. Check for external parasites and dermatophytes, and initiate appropriate therapy for:
        1. Fleas, ticks and ear mites (*Otodectes cyanotis*)
        2. Mange mites, especially *Demodex canis* and *Sarcoptes scabiei*
        3. Dermatophytes, particularly *Microsporum* spp. and *Trichophyton mentagraphytes*
    C. Perform faecal examination (includes both direct smear and flotation)
    D. Initiate administration of heartworm programme
    E. Administer an anthelmintic, such as pyrantel pamoate for roundworms and praziquantel for tapeworms (if present)
    F. Vaccinate with canine distemper/infectious canine hepatitis/canine parainfluenza/leptospirosis/canine parvovirus vaccine and possibly against kennel cough
    G. Advise on nutrition and routine grooming
    H. Provide the owner with client education pamphlets on such topics as:
        1. Fleas, ticks and ear mite identification and their treatment and control
        2. Canine heartworm disease and the benefits of preventive management
        3. Management of normal and abnormal dog behaviours
        4. Grooming and nutrition
    I. Complete the dog's health record for the owner

II. Second office visit for the health programme (usually at 12 weeks of age)
    A. Perform a general physical examination and record the body weight
    B. Check for external parasites and dermatophytes and initiate appropriate therapy for:
        1. Fleas, ticks and ear mites (*Otodectes cyanotis*)
        2. Mange mites, especially *Demodex canis* and *Sarcoptes scabiei*
        3. Dermatophytes, particularly *Microsporum* spp. and *Trichophton mentagrophytes*
    C. Perform faecal examination (includes both direct smear and flotation)
    D. Adjust heartworm preventive dosage, especially for diethylcarbamazine products
    E. Administer an anthelmintic, such as pyrantel pamoate for hookworms and roundworms and praziquantel for tapeworms (if present)
    F. Vaccinate with canine distemper/infectious canine hepatitis/canine parainfluenza/leptospirosis/canine parvovirus and rabies vaccines
    G. Adjust the nutrition and grooming procedures
    H. Provide the owner with client education pamphlets to be taken home on such topics as:
        1. Fleas, ticks and ear mite identification and their treatment and control
        2. Canine heartworm disease and the benefits of preventive management
        3. Dental and ear care
        4. Grooming and nutrition
        5. Management of normal and abnormal dog behaviour
    I. Complete the dog's health record for the owner

diagnostic facilities, whereas the latter have the flexibility to cater for individual owners' requirements.

In Great Britain, four national schemes, comprising programmes for pigs, cattle, sheep and goats, and poultry, were introduced in 1987 (Rees and Davies, 1992). These were all modifications of earlier health schemes.

The Pig Health Scheme aims to improve the general health and productivity of herds, and membership is two-tiered. All participating herds are subjected to quarterly visits by government veterinarians and private practitioners and, in the 'higher' health status category, lungs and snouts are monitored at the abattoir to detect enzootic pneumonia and atrophic rhinitis, respectively. More recently, another category — the Pig Assurance Scheme — was added to give purchasers of pigs from registered herds assurances on aspects of medication, welfare and infection with *Salmonella* spp., and to assist producers in the production of food that is 'wholesome' and free from unwanted residues (Lomas, 1993).

In the Cattle Health Scheme, herds are tested for enzootic bovine leukosis (EBL), and may then become EBL-attested. The herds can also be monitored for infectious bovine rhinotracheitis. They can also participate in a *Leptospira hardjo* control programme, in which they may achieve a controlled, officially vaccinated or an

Table 21.8 Continued

III. Third office visit for the health programme (usually at 16 weeks of age)
    A.   Perform a general physical examination and record the body weight
    B.   Check for external parasites and dermatophytes and initiate appropriate therapy for:
        1.   Fleas, ticks and ear mites (*Otodectes cyanotis*)
        2.   Mange mites, especially *Demodex canis* and *Sarcoptes scabiei*
        3.   Dermatophytes, particularly *Microsporum* spp. and *Trichophyton mentagraphytes*
    C.   Perform faecal examination (faecal flotation)
    D.   Adjust heartworm preventive dosage, especially for diethylcarbamazine products
    E.   Administer an anthelmintic, such as pyrantel pamoate for hookworms and roundworms and praziquantel for tapeworms (if present)
    F.   Vaccinate with canine distemper/infectious canine hepatitis/canine parainfluenza/leptospirosis/canine parvovirus vaccine
    G.   Adjust the nutrition and grooming procedures
    H.   Provide the owner with client education pamphlets to be taken home on such topics as:
        1.   Fleas, ticks and ear mite identification and their treatment and control
        2.   Dental and ear care
        3.   Grooming and nutrition
        4.   Management of normal and abnormal dog behaviours
        5.   Recommendations for spaying and castration
    I.   Complete the dog's health record for the owner

IV. Subsequent visits for the health programme (usually annual visits)
    A.   Perform a general physical examination and record the body weight
    B.   Check for external parasites and dermatophytes and initiate appropriate therapy for:
        1.   Fleas, ticks and ear mites (*Otodectes cyanotis*)
        2.   Mange mites, especially *Demodex canis* and *Sarcoptes scabiei*
        3.   Dermatophytes, particularly *Microsporum* spp. and *Trichophyton mentagrophytes*
    C.   Perform faecal examination (flotation and a Knott's test and/or occult heartworm test for heartworm infection screen)
    D.   Adjust heartworm preventive dosage
    E.   Administer an anthelmintic according to faecal examination findings
    F.   Vaccinate with canine distemper/infectious canine hepatitis/canine parainfluenza/leptospirosis/canine parvovirus and rabies vaccines and possibly against kennel cough
    G.   Adjust the nutrition and grooming procedures
    H.   Provide the owner with client education pamphlets to be taken home on such topics as:
        1.   Fleas, ticks and ear mite identification and their treatment and control
        2.   Canine heartworm disease and the benefits of preventive management
        3.   Dental and ear care
        4.   Grooming and nutrition
        5.   Management of normal and abnormal dog behaviours
    I.   Complete the dog's health record for the owner

elite status, depending on what risk factors for the infection are identified in the herd.

The Sheep and Goat Health Scheme enables participating flocks and herds to qualify for accredited status in relation to maedi-visna and caprine arthritis-encephalitis. Additionally, the flocks and herds can be more generally monitored for enzootic abortion of ewes, jaagsiekte and scrapie.

The Poultry Health Scheme targets freedom from infection with *Salmonella pullorum* and *S. gallinarum*, and includes monitoring for other diseases. There are also guidelines to prevent contamination of eggs with *S. enterididis*.

Companion animal schemes

Companion animal health schemes are concerned with disease prevention in the individual animal, rather than in a group (although several individuals may be involved in kennels and stables). Production is not relevant to companion animal schemes. (The track performance of

Table 21.9 General outline of a health scheme for cats in the US. (Modified from Hoskins, 1988b.)

I. First office visit for the health programme (usually at 8 to 10 weeks of age)
  A. Perform a general physical examination and record the body weight
  B. Check for external parasites and dermatophytes and initiate appropriate therapy for:
   1. Fleas and ear mites (*Otodectes cyanotis*)
   2. Mange mites, especially *Notoedres cati*, *Demodex* spp. and *Cheyletiella* spp.
   3. Dermatophytes, particularly *Microsporum* spp. and *Trichophyton mentagrophytes*
  C. Perform faecal examination (includes both direct smear and flotation)
  D. Administer an anthelmintic, such as pyrantel pamoate for roundworms and hookworms and praziquantel for tapeworms (if present)
  E. Vaccinate with feline viral rhinotracheitis/feline calicivirus/feline panleukopenia vaccine and against *Chlamydia* infection and feline leukaemia virus (FeLV) (all cats should test FeLV negative before receiving the initial FeLV vaccination)*
  F. Advise on nutrition and routine grooming
  G. Provide the owner with client education pamphlets on such topics as:
   1. Fleas and ear mite identification and their treatment and control
   2. Feline leukaemia virus infection and the benefits of vaccination
   3. Management of normal and abnormal cat behaviour
   4. Grooming and nutrition
  H. Complete the cat's health record for the owner

II. Second office visit for the health programme (usually at 12 to 14 weeks of age)
  A. Perform a general physical examination and record the body weight
  B. Check for external parasites and dermatophytes and initiate appropriate therapy for:
   1. Fleas and ear mites (*Otodectes cyanotis*)
   2. Mange mites, especially *Notoedres cati*, *Demodex* spp. and *Cheyletiella* spp.
   3. Dermatophytes, particularly *Microsporum* spp. and *Trichophyton mentagrophytes*
  C. Perform faecal examination (includes both direct smear and flotation)
  D. Administer an anthelmintic, such as pyrantel pamoate for roundworms and hookworms and praziquantel for tapeworm (if present)
  E. Vaccinate with feline viral rhinotracheitis/feline calicivirus/feline panleukopenia vaccine and against *Chlamydia* infection, feline leukaemia virus and rabies
  F. Adjust the nutrition and grooming procedures
  G. Provide the owner with client education pamphlets on such topics as:
   1. Fleas and ear mite identification and their treatment and control
   2. Feline leukaemia virus infection and the benefits of vaccination
   3. Dental and ear care
   4. Management of normal and abnormal cat behaviour
   5. Exercise and its importance
   6. Recommendations for spaying, castrating and declawing
  H. Complete the cat's health record for the owner

racehorses and greyhounds is loosely described as 'production' but the animals are usually more commercial than companion.) Schemes involve:

1. routine examination of animals;
2. prophylaxis, such as vaccination;
3. routine therapy, including dosing with anthelmintics;
4. advice on management relating to diet and housing.

Table 21.8 outlines a health scheme for dogs in the US. This may require modification in other countries (e.g., heartworm prevention would be unnecessary in areas where the disease was absent). A preventive medicine scheme for commercial dog kennels in the US is given by Glickman (1980). It includes nutritional recommendations, vaccination, ecto- and endoparasite control, and the management of reproduction and common diseases. Systematic record keeping is advised, to provide a kennel profile, facilitating the detection of deviations from normal breeding performance and expected patterns of morbidity and mortality.

A health scheme for cats in the US is listed in *Table 21.9*. This should also be modified to suit local conditions

Table 21.9 Continued

III. Third office visit for the health programme (usually 2 to 4 months after the second office visit)
 A. Perform a general physical examination and record the body weight
 B. Check for external parasites and dermatophytes and initiate appropriate therapy for:
  1. Fleas and ear mites (*Otodectes cyanotis*)
  2. Mange mites, especially *Notoedres cati*, *Demodex* spp. and *Cheyletiella* spp.
  3. Dermatophytes, particularly *Microsporum* spp. and *Trichophyton mentagrophytes*
 C. Perform faecal examination (faecal flotation)
 D. Administer an anthelmintic, such as pyrantel pamoate for roundworms and hookworms and praziquantel for tapeworms (if present)
 E. Vaccinate with feline leukaemia virus vaccine
 F. Adjust the nutrition and grooming procedures
 G. Provide the owner with client education pamphlets on such topics as:
  1. Fleas and ear mite identification and their treatment and control
  2. Dental and ear care
  3. Management of normal and abnormal cat behaviour
  4. Exercise and its importance
  5. Recommendations for spaying, castration and declawing
 H. Complete the cat's health record for the owner

IV. Subsequent visits for the health programme (usually annual visits)
 A. Perform a general physical examination and record the body weight
 B. Check for external parasites and dermatophytes and initiate appropriate therapy for:
  1. Fleas and ear mites (*Otodectes cyanotis*)
  2. Mange mites, especially *Notoedres cati*, *Demodex* spp. and *Cheyletiella* spp.
  3. Dermatophytes, particularly *Microsporum* spp. and *Trichophyton mentagrophytes*
 C. Perform faecal examination (faecal flotation)
 D. Administer an anthelmintic according to faecal examination findings
 E. Vaccinate with feline viral rhinotracheitis/feline calicivirus/feline panleukopenia vaccine and against *Chlamydia* infection, FeLV and rabies (all cats should test FeLV negative before receiving the initial FeLV booster vaccination)*
 F. Adjust the nutrition and grooming procedures
 G. Provide the owner with client education pamphlets on such topics as:
  1. Fleas and ear mite identification and their treatment and control
  2. Feline leukaemia virus infection and the benefits of vaccination
  3. Dental and ear care
  4. Management of normal and abnormal cat behaviour
  5. Recommendations for spaying, castration and declawing
  6. Exercise and its importance
 H. Complete the cat's health record for the owner

*Cats should be tested for both FeLV antigen and feline T-lymphotropic lentivirus antibody before receiving the FeLV vaccine.

(e.g., omission of routine rabies vaccination in countries free from the disease).

Equine health schemes focus on vaccination, parasite control, care of the teeth and feet, and optimum nutrition (Anon., 1989; Pilliner, 1992). Stable hygiene is also important because infections can be readily spread by fomites such as water buckets, bits, trailers and clothing (Timoney, 1988). *Table 21.10* is an example of a health scheme in the US. Fraser (1969) and Owen (1985) describe equine schedules in the UK, and Verberne and Mirck (1976) list a programme for use in The Netherlands. Again, the programmes may need to be modified to suit local management practices and the preference of the veterinarian and owner.

Table 21.10 General outline of a health scheme for horses in the US. (Modified from Hoskins *et al.*, 1994.)

First Quarter: January to March

All horses

Deworm: minimum of every 8 weeks. Exercise care in choice of anthelmintics for mares in the third trimester. Begin deworming foals at 2 months of age

Trim feet: every 6 weeks: more frequently in foals requiring limb correction

Dentistry: check adults twice yearly and rasp (float) teeth as needed. Remove wolf teeth in 2-year-olds and retained caps in 2-, 3- and 4-year-olds. Immunize for respiratory diseases: influenza, strangles and rhinopneumonitis

Stallions

Perform complete breeding examination. Maintain stallions under lights if being used for early breeding

Pregnant mares

Immunize with tetanus toxoid and open sutured mares 30 days prepartum. Develop a colostrum bank. Ninth-day breeding only for mares with normal foaling history and normal reproductive tract. Wash udders of foaling mares

Non-pregnant mares

Maintain under lights if being used for early breeding. Use daily teasing. Perform reproductive tract examination during oestrus. Mares should not be too fat but improving in condition during breeding season

Newborn foals

Dip navel in disinfectant. Carefully give a cleansing enema at birth. Administer tetanus prophylaxis if indicated by antibody test

Second Quarter: April to June

All horses

Deworm: minimum of every 8 weeks

Trim feet: every 6 weeks

Dentistry: check teeth and remove or rasp teeth as needed

Immunize against equine encephalomyelitis. Administer appropriate vaccine boosters

Stallions

Maintain an exercise programme. Monitor the semen quality

Brood mares

Palpate at 21, 42 and 60 days after successful breeding

Foals

Creep feed the foals and provide free-choice minerals. Immunize at three months of age. Group the foals by sex and size when weaned

Table 21.10 Continued

Third Quarter: July to September

All horses
Deworm: minimum of every 8 weeks. Clip and sweep the pastures
Trim feet: every 6 weeks. Continue corrective trimming on foals
Dentistry: check teeth and remove or rasp teeth as needed

Stallions
Maintain an exercise programme

Brood mares
Administer rhinopneumonitis boosters to pregnant mares according to manufacturer's labelled directions. Administer appropriate vaccine boosters to foals and yearlings. Check condition of mare's udder at weaning and reduce the amount of feed given until milk flow is reduced

Foals
Administer all appropriate immunizations. Provide free-choice minerals. Maintain a protein supplement in creep feeders

Fourth Quarter: October to December

All horses
Deworm: minimum every 8 weeks. Select anthelmintics appropriate for season
Trim feet: every 6 weeks. Continue corrective trimming on foals
Dentistry: check teeth and remove or rasp teeth as needed

Stallions
Continue the exercise programme. Check immunizations. Perform breeding examination

Brood mares
Confirm pregnancy. Begin treating the non-pregnant mares. Check immunizations

Further reading

Esslemont, R.J., Bailie, J.H. and Cooper, M.J. (1985) *Fertility Management in Dairy Cattle*. Collins Professional and Technical Books, London

Hoskins, J.D., Seahorn, T.L. and Claxton-Gill, M.S. (1994) Preventive health programs. In: *Clinical Textbook for Veterinary Technicians*, 3rd edn. Ed. McCurnin, D.M., pp. 600–632. W.B. Saunders, Philadelphia

Moss, R. (Ed.) (1992) *Livestock Health and Welfare*. Longman Scientific and Technical, Harlow

Radostits, O.M., Leslie, K.E. and Fetrow, J. (1994) *Herd Health: Food Animal Production Medicine*, 2nd edn. W.B. Saunders, Philadelphia

22 The control and eradication of disease

The preceding chapters have outlined the scope of veterinary epidemiology. In reiteration: epidemiology is the study of disease and factors affecting its distribution in populations. This study involves the **description** and **analysis** of disease in groups of animals using three related techniques:

1. observation and recording of the natural occurrence of disease and its determinants, and presentation of the recorded observations;
2. statistical analysis of the observations;
3. modelling.

These three techniques are used in conjunction with experimental, clinical and pathological investigations to:

1. estimate disease morbidity and mortality;
2. elucidate the cause of disease;
3. understand the ecology of disease (transmission, maintenance and nidality);
4. investigate the efficiency of different techniques of disease control.

This final chapter outlines the ways in which the results of epidemiological investigations are applied to the **control** and **eradication** of disease.

Definition of 'control' and 'eradication'

Control

Control is the reduction of the morbidity and mortality from disease, and is a general term embracing all measures intended to interfere with the unrestrained occurrence of disease, whatever its cause (Done, 1985). It is an ongoing process (Last, 1988).

Control can be achieved by **treating** diseased animals, which therefore reduces disease prevalence, and by **preventing*** disease, which therefore reduces both incidence and prevalence. Veterinary medicine, like human medicine, developed as a healing art concerned with the treatment of sick individuals. This approach continues, with the improvement of medical and surgical skills. However, prevention is an increasingly important part of disease control, being better than cure on humanitarian and, frequently, economic grounds.

Eradication

The term 'eradication' was first applied in the 19th century to the regional elimination of *infectious* diseases of animals, notably Texas fever from cattle in the US, and pleuropneumonia, glanders and rabies from European animals. Since then, the term has been used in four different senses.

First, it has been used to mean the extinction of an infectious agent (Cockburn, 1963); eradication has not been completed if a single infectious agent survives anywhere in nature. According to this definition, very few diseases have been eradicated; human smallpox is an example (Fenner *et al.*, 1988).

Secondly, eradication has been defined as the reduction of infectious disease prevalence in a specified area to a level at which transmission does not occur (Andrews and Langmuir, 1963). For instance, in local areas in northern Nigeria trypanosomiasis can be 'eradicated' by clearing the vector (the tsetse fly) from riverine areas.

---

*Three types of prevention are sometimes distinguished (Caplan and Grunebaum, 1967): *primary*, which modifies determinants to prevent or postpone new cases of disease, and therefore reduces incidence; *secondary*, which detects and treats disease promptly to shorten disease duration or to prolong life; and *tertiary*, which treats long-term cases to reduce dysfunction or to prolong life (i.e., to make outcome less severe). In this book, prevention is synonymous with primary prevention, whereas treatment encompasses secondary and tertiary prevention.

Thirdly, eradication has been defined as the reduction of infectious disease prevalence to a level at which the disease ceases to be a major health problem, although some transmission may still take place (Maslakov, 1968).

Fourthly, and most commonly in veterinary medicine, eradication refers to the *regional* extinction of an infectious agent. For example, since the eradication of foot-and-mouth disease in the UK, no foot-and-mouth disease virus particles are believed to be present (apart from laboratory stocks).

Eradication involves a *time-limited* campaign (Yekutiel, 1980).

Elimination: The intermediate concept of elimination (Latin: *ex* = out of; *limen, liminis* = threshold) can also be identifed. This is reduction in the incidence of infectious disease below the level achieved by control, so that either very few or no cases occur, although the infectious agent may be allowed to persist (Payne, 1963; Spinu and Biberi-Moroianu, 1969).

Strategies of control and eradication

Doing nothing

In some circumstances, the natural history of a disease is such that the incidence of the disease is reduced by doing nothing. This is not strictly a technique of control but illustrates that the incidence of disease may be reduced by natural changes in host/parasite relationships without the intervention of man. Thus, bluetongue does not occur in Cyprus in winter because the vector (*Culicoides* spp.) of the causal virus cannot survive then. Similarly, the incidence of trypanosomiasis in the dry savannah regions of Nigeria is reduced during the dry season when the tsetse fly is absent.

Quarantine

Quarantine is the isolation of animals that are either infected or suspected of being so, or of non-infected animals that are at risk. Quarantine is an old method of disease control (see Chapter 1) that is still very valuable. It is used to isolate animals when they are imported from countries where exotic diseases are endemic; for example, the compulsory quarantine of dogs, cats and zoo animals when they are imported to some countries to prevent the introduction of rabies. It is also used to isolate animals suspected of being infected, until infection is either confirmed or discounted, such as cows suspected of being infected with *Brucella abortus*. Quarantine is commonly applied in human medicine during epidemics

to isolate infected from susceptible individuals. The period of quarantine depends on the incubation period of the agent, the time taken for the infection to be confirmed, and the time taken for an infected animal to become non-infectious (either with or without treatment).

Slaughter

The productivity of animals is usually decreased when they are chronically diseased. If a disease is infectious, affected animals can be a source of infection to others. In such circumstances it may be economically and technically expedient to slaughter the affected animals. For example, clinical bovine mastitis can produce a 15% drop in the milk yield of dairy cattle (Parsons, 1982); cows that have three or more bouts of mastitis per lactation therefore are often culled.

In eradication campaigns, infected or in-contact animals may be slaughtered to remove sources of infection. Thus, in some countries, all cloven-hoofed animals in infected herds are slaughtered during foot-and-mouth disease epidemics. Slaughter is usually accompanied by other procedures designed to reduce the risk of transmission (e.g., disinfection, and destruction of carcasses by burning or burial); this is termed 'stamping out' (see Appendix I).

Vaccination

Vaccines can confer immunity to many bacteria and viruses, and to some helminths. They are used routinely to prevent disease; for example, canine distemper vaccination. They may also be used in high risk situations (strategic vaccination). For example, dogs are compulsorily and regularly vaccinated against rabies in some countries in which the disease is endemic. 'Ring' vaccination is a type of strategic vaccination in which animals in an area surrounding an infected region are vaccinated to provide a barrier against spread of infection. For instance, in the 1950s and 1960s, rinderpest was endemic in the Karamoja region of north-eastern Uganda, but was absent from other parts of the country. A 20-mile deep ring of cattle around the region was vaccinated to prevent transmission to disease-free areas. Similarly, ring vaccination would be an option if an outbreak of foot-and-mouth disease occurred in the European Union (Donaldson and Doel, 1992).

Inactivated and live vaccines: Vaccines may be **inactivated**, in which the antigenic organisms such as bacteria are killed, and viruses are denatured. Alternatively, they may be **live**, and the organisms usually attenuated. Each type of vaccine has advantages and disadvantages. Inactivated vaccines are safer than live vaccines and can be produced more quickly when new agents are discovered. However, they cost more than live vaccines and stimulate mucosal and cell-mediated immunity less quickly and less effectively. On the other hand, there is a danger that the live immunizing agent might revert to a virulent form. Also, it may be difficult to differentiate between infections due to live vaccinal strains of agent and to natural 'field' strains.

Natural vaccination: When animals are exposed to a low level of challenge from agents in the environment, natural vaccination can occur. This mechanism has been enhanced in pigs by feeding faeces back to pregnant animals, a technique called 'feedback'. Immunity to pathogens, for example, porcine transmissible gastroenteritis virus and parvovirus (Stein *et al.*, 1982), thus may be increased and passed passively to the piglets via colostrum after birth. Although this may be of value when no other means of control is available, there are dangers (Porter, 1979): some agents, such as enteropathogenic *Escherichia coli*, can increase in virulence when passaged *in vivo*.

New vaccine technology: Modern biotechnology has facilitated new techniques for identifying immunologically active antigens and presenting antigens to the host (Biggs, 1993; Bourne, 1993; Wray and Woodward, 1990). The former include the cloning of T cells specific to small areas of stimulating antigens, and identification of parts of an infectious agent's proteins that are responsible for stimulation of the immune response (epitopes). The latter include attenuated mutants produced by deletion of genes responsible for pathogenicity (e.g., Aujeszky's disease vaccine produced by deletion of the thymidine kinase gene), and 'vectored vaccines': attenuated virus and bacterial vectors which also carry immunizing antigens derived from other infectious agents; vectors under development include vaccinia, fowl pox, adenoviruses, *Escherichia coli* and *Salmonella* spp. There are also potential alternatives to conventional whole inactivated vaccines, including synthetic epitopes (produced either chemically or in prokaryotic systems such as *E. coli*) and synthetic virus capsids.

The use of vaccination as a control strategy is discussed in detail by Biggs (1982). The potential and application of vaccination for the control of parasitic diseases are described by Urquhart (1980) and Willetts and Cobon (1993).

Therapeutic and prophylactic chemotherapy

Antibiotics, anthelmintics, other drugs and hyperimmune serum are used (therapeutically) to treat diseases, and are administered (prophylactically) at times of high risk to prevent disease and thus to increase productivity. Examples include the addition of antibiotics to livestock feed to promote growth, and the post-operative use of antibiotics to prevent bacterial infections. These procedures can have undesirable consequences, notably the selection of strains of bacteria that are resistant to the antibiotic to which they have been exposed. Furthermore, resistance can be spread by transfer to other bacteria by conjugation and by transducing phages (see Chapter 5).

Movement of hosts

Animals can be removed from 'high risk' areas where infections are endemic. This control strategy is implemented in tropical countries where hosts are seasonally migrated from areas in which biological vectors are active. The Fulani tribe in West Africa traditionally migrate, with their livestock, from the south to the north in the wet season to avoid the tsetse fly. Similarly, horses may be moved indoors at night, to prevent infection with African horse sickness virus which is transmitted by night-flying vectors of the genus *Culicoides* (Chalmers, 1968).

Mixed, alternate and sequential grazing

The level of infection with some nematodes can be reduced by mixed, alternate and sequential grazing (Brunsdon, 1980). The **mixed grazing** of susceptible animals with stock that are genetically or immunologically resistant to helminths reduces pasture contamination to an acceptable level. Thus, adult cattle (immune) can be grazed with calves (susceptible). Similarly, cattle (resistant to *Ostertagia circumcincta*) can be grazed with sheep (susceptible).

The **alternate grazing** of a pasture with different species of livestock again reduces pasture contamination. Thus, annual alternation of sheep and cattle in Norway has reduced to negligible levels the challenge to sheep from nematode species that overwinter (*Ostertagia* spp. and *Nematodirus* spp.: Helle, 1971).

The **sequential grazing** at different times of resistant and susceptible animals of the same species reduces pasture contamination. Thus, when clean grazing is not available in the late summer and autumn, trichostrongyle infections of calves (susceptible animals) can be reduced by transferring them to pastures that have been grazed by cows (resistant) (Burger, 1976).

Control of biological vectors

Infectious diseases transmitted by biological vectors can be controlled by removing the vectors. Insect vectors can be killed with insecticides. The habitat of the vectors can be destroyed, for example by draining land to remove snails that are intermediate hosts of *Fasciola hepatica*. Alternatively, an animal that competes with the vector can be introduced into the habitat, for example the exclusion of the molluscan vectors of schistosomiasis by a snail that is not a vector (see Chapter 7). Some infections of definitive hosts may be prevented by the elimination of infective material found at post-mortem meat inspection of intermediate hosts, for instance the inspection of cattle to condemn meat containing *Cysticercus bovis* cysts.

Control of mechanical vectors

Living organisms that mechanically transmit infectious agents can be controlled by destruction and disinfection. Biting fleas that transmit bacteria, for example, can be destroyed by insecticides. The veterinarian can also act as a mechanical vector and so must impose a strict procedure for personal disinfection when dealing with outbreaks of highly contagious infectious diseases such as foot-and-mouth disease.

Disinfection of fomites

Fomites (see Chapter 6) can be disinfected to prevent the transmission of infectious agents. Fomites include farm equipment, surgical instruments and sometimes drugs themselves, the last two being associated with iatrogenic transmission (see Chapter 6). Food is heat-treated (e.g., the pasteurization of milk) to destroy microbes and their heat-sensitive toxins, to prevent food-borne infection.

Niche filling

The presence of one organism within a niche can prevent its occupation by another organism. This is epidemiological interference (a particular case of competitive exclusion; see Chapter 7), and has been investigated experimentally in the poultry industry where suspensions of endogenous intestinal microbes have been fed to one-day-old chicks to prevent colonization of their digestive tract by virulent *Salmonella* spp. (Pivnick and Nurmi, 1982), *Campylobacter jejuni* and *Escherichia coli* (Nurmi, 1988). This technique of control has the advantage over prophylactic antibiotic chemotherapy that antibiotic resistance is not encouraged. In Sweden, it has been successful in restricting colonization by *Salmonella* spp. nationwide (Wierup *et al.*, 1988), but has not been exploited more widely.

Improvement in environment, husbandry and feeding

The diseases of intensively produced animals, particularly cattle and pigs, are major contemporary problems (e.g., Webster, 1982) which can be controlled only when epidemiological investigations have identified the determinants associated with inadequate management. Thus, the increase in Britain of bovine mastitis associated with *E. coli* and *Streptococcus uberis* ('environmental mastitis') has paralleled the increase in the number of cows that are housed loosely in cubicles. Poor hygiene has been incriminated as the most important environmental cause (Francis *et al.*, 1979). Recommendations to reduce this disease (Sumner, quoted by Webster, 1982) therefore include:

1. adjustment of head rails to minimize soiling of cubicles;
2. removal of faeces and soiled litter twice daily;
3. addition of clean litter daily;
4. scraping cubicle passages at least twice daily.

Genetic improvement

Many diseases of both agricultural and companion animals (Foley *et al.*, 1979) have a variable heritable component. The disease may be determined predominantly genetically, as in canine cyclic neutropaenia (the gray collie syndrome: Cheville, 1975) which is carried by a simple autosomal recessive lethal gene. Alternatively the disease may be determined by several factors, only one of which is genetic, as in canine hip dysplasia (Riser, 1974) whose determinants also include growth rate, body type, and pelvic muscle mass. The incidence of such diseases can be reduced by early detection; for example, by radiography in the case of hip dysplasia, followed by voluntary agreement of owners of affected animals not to breed from the animals.

A valuable aid to the identification of genetic diseases is **genetic screening** (Jolly *et al.*, 1981) to identify diseased animals by screening either the total population at risk or the part that is mainly responsible for the maintenance of a particular disease. The latter technique is commonly applied in veterinary medicine because animal populations tend to be very large, and most animals of 'superior' genetic potential are concentrated in pedigree 'nuclei' that are used for breeding. Human populations are screened to detect hereditary dietary deficiencies (e.g., aminoacidurias, so facilitating dietary control), and to identify serious genetic diseases prenatally so that elective abortion can be considered. In veterinary medicine the main value of screening is the reduction in defective gene frequency by identifying and removing normal and partially expressed carriers. The relatively short generation time of domestic animals, and artificial breeding techniques, help towards this objective.

Table 22.1 Cost−benefit analysis of a genetic screening programme for bovine mannosidosis in New Zealand, at different levels of heterozygote prevalence. (From Jolly and Townsley, 1980.)

Time horizon	Costs and benefits 10% discount rate	Prevalence of heterozygotes			
		10%	7.5%	5.0%	2.5%
Incurred first 8 years	Cumulative costs	$500 000	$500 000	$500 000	$500 000
	Discounted costs	$333 433	$333 433	$333 433	$333 433
20 years	Cumulative benefits	$3 471 600	$1 910 800	$874 300	$211 100
	Discounted benefits	$963 838	$530 850	$243 588	$58 576
	Benefit:cost ratio	2.89	1.59	0.73	0.18
Infinity	Discounted benefits	$1 381 527	$760 951	$348 951	$83 994
	Benefit:cost ratio	4.14	2.28	1.04	0.25
Break even time	Undiscounted benefits and costs	9 years	11 years	15 years	>20 years

Defects can be identified by clinical examination of animals (e.g,. canine progressive retinal atrophy: Black, 1972). However, the main benefit of screening is in the detection of heterozygotes where disease is either subclinical or is transmitted by healthy carriers. Techniques include test matings, cytogenetic studies (e.g., bovine Robertsonian translocations: Gustavsson, 1969), biochemical analyses (e.g., bovine mannosidosis: Jolly *et al.*, 1973), and, most recently, the identification of defective genes themselves using recombinant DNA techniques (Goldspink, 1993).

The requirements for a genetic screening programme are listed by Jolly *et al.* (1981):

1. the disease must occur in a defined population sufficiently frequently to make the disease of economic or social importance; the defined population may be a family, a herd, or a breed of animal within certain geographical boundaries;
2. a simple, relatively inexpensive test, capable of identifying heterozygotes with a high degree of accuracy, should be available; as most tests in biological systems do not have a sensitivity and specificity of 100%, there should be provision for follow-up testing, either with a more specific supplementary test or by replication of the original method;
3. control by culling of heterozygotes should neither have a deleterious effect on the overall genetic makeup of the population nor deplete breeding stock to an uneconomic or disadvantageous level;
4. the logistics of the programme should be acceptable to the breeders and be preceded by adequate educational and public relations programmes;
5. the logistics of the programme should satisfy the breeders but not encroach on other necessary disease prevention programmes; where possible, the programme should be integrated with other disease control schemes to simplify specimen collection;
6. there should be provision for adequate genetic counselling and either breed society or kennel club rules or legislation to ensure that control is instigated on the basis of information provided by the screening tests.

Table 22.1 illustrates the economic benefit of a screening programme for bovine mannosidosis. This disease causes a lethal nervous syndrome in Angus and Murray Gray cattle. It is inherited recessively; carriers can be detected biochemically because their blood α-mannosidase levels are approximately half of the normal. The cost−benefit analysis relates to New Zealand, where the prevalence of heterozygotes before the programme was 10%, and approximately one million Angus and Murray Gray calves are born each year, with a total estimated loss due to the disease of $281 000. Different values for the prevalence, number and value of susceptible cattle, cost of screening test and discount rate affect the results of such an analysis and therefore the economic viability of the control programme.

Other genetic diseases to which screening can be applied are bovine protoporphyria and canine inherited bleeding and eye defects (Jolly *et al.*, 1981), and fucosidosis, a lysosomal storage disease of English springer spaniels (Barker *et al.*, 1988).

The incidence of some infectious diseases can be reduced by **selective breeding** (Gogolin-Ewens *et al.*, 1990). For example, certain cattle are known to be tolerant to trypanosomiasis (so called 'trypanotolerant' cattle): Dolan, 1987). Other infectious diseases for which genetic resistance has been reported include foot-and-mouth disease and tuberculosis in cattle, jaagsiekte and scrapie in sheep, brucellosis and leptospirosis in pigs, and Newcastle disease, infectious bronchitis, Marek's disease and coccidiosis in poultry (Payne, 1982) and helminthiasis in sheep (Barger, 1989).

Modern **transgenic biology**, which involves the introduction of specific genes into the genome, now offers a means of changing the genome of the animal more rapidly than it has ever been changed by traditional selective breeding. The techniques are being directed at improved productivity (Ward *et al.*, 1990), but could also be used to introduce artificial genes that block amplification of pathogens, and to increase the rate of selective breeding programmes.

Minimal disease methods

Disease can be reduced in intensively reared livestock by disinfecting infected premises and by treating infected animals or removing them from the animal unit. Uninfected animals can be produced by caesarian section and by hatching uninfected eggs from poultry. These combined techniques are termed **minimal disease methods**. They have been applied commercially only in pig and poultry units. Successes include the eradication of enzootic pneumonia from some pig herds in the UK.

Techniques of control and eradication have developed gradually. Until the germ theory of infectious disease was adequately supported in the 19th century, only those people who believed in contagion could attempt to control infectious disease. Thus, Lancisi controlled rinderpest in Italy by a slaughter policy (see Chapter 1). Those who accepted the miasmatic theory of cause occasionally succeeded in controlling disease by applying basic sanitary principles such as disinfection and fumigation.

A combination of the various techniques that have been described is applied to the control and eradication of disease. An example is the use of vaccination, followed by mass testing of animals and slaughter of infected animals to control contagious bovine pleuropneumonia in Nigeria (David-West, 1980). The choice of technique involves assessing, technically and economically, the most efficient strategy for a particular disease and system of management (Sellers, 1982).

Table 22.2 lists some eradicable diseases in the UK and the methods chosen for eradication. Slaughter and quarantine campaigns against widespread epidemics and exotic diseases are usually conducted at the national level by government veterinary services. These campaigns are frequently supported by legislation.

Vaccination, treatment, alteration in environment and minimal disease techniques generally are carried out at the local level, and are often concerned with individual or herd problems, such as distemper in dogs (vaccination), and helminthiasis in herds of cattle and flocks of sheep (treatment and management practices). Vaccination may sometimes be carried out as part of a national government policy, for example against bovine brucellosis.

Table 22.2 Some eradicable diseases in the UK and chosen methods of eradication. (Adapted from Sellers, 1982.)

Method of eradication	Cattle	Sheep	Pigs	Poultry
Slaughter of infected and in-contact animals	Exotic infections, e.g. foot-and-mouth disease	Exotic infections, e.g. foot-and-mouth disease	Exotic infections, e.g. foot-and-mouth disease	Exotic infections, e.g. Newcastle disease
Identify infected animal and either destroy, treat or administer prophylactic vaccination or treatment	Tuberculosis, brucellosis, warble fly infection, leptospirosis, enzootic bovine leucosis, Johne's disease, infectious bovine rhinotracheitis (stud bulls), *Hypoderma bovis*	Sheep scab, Johne's disease	Tuberculosis	Pullorum disease, fowl typhoid, egg drop syndrome, fowl pox, duck hepatitis
Improvement of environment and management, and treatment	Streptococcal mastitis, coliform mastitis	Foot-rot, liver fluke	Streptococcal meningitis, mange	Chronic respiratory disease, *Mycoplasma meleagridis* infection
Minimal disease methods		Maedi-visna	Enzootic pneumonia, atrophic rhinitis	

Important factors in control and eradication programmes

Before either a control or an eradication campaign can be undertaken, several factors must be considered. These include:

1. the level of knowledge about the cause of the disease and, if infectious, also about its transmission and maintenance, including host range and the nature of the host/parasite relationship;
2. veterinary infrastructure;
3. diagnostic feasibility;
4. adequate surveillance;
5. availability of replacement stock;
6. producers' and society's views;
7. the disease's public health significance;
8. the existence of suitable legislation with provision for compensation;
9. the possible ecological consequences;
10. economic costs and the availability of funds for the programme.

Knowledge of the cause, maintenance and transmission of disease

A complete knowledge of the natural history of a disease, although not always necessary to control or eradicate the disease (recall Lancisi's eradication of rinderpest), is necessary to develop the *most effective* means of control. When the various disease determinants have been defined, often by epidemiological studies, a suitable control strategy can be selected; for example, improving ventilation to reduce respiratory disease in intensively reared pigs. If a disease is infectious then a knowledge of its incubation period and method of transmission, including the life-cycle and habitat of any vectors, assists in control. If the incubation period is long (e.g., tuberculosis) tests may have to be repeated several times to identify all infected animals. If the generation time (see Chapter 6) is short (e.g., foot-and-mouth disease) diagnosis and removal of affected animals must be rapid. If an infectious agent is aerially transmitted (e.g., Aujeszky's disease or foot-and-mouth disease) control necessitates visiting all herds that may infected (see EpiMAN: Chapter 11). In contrast, strictly contagious diseases (e.g., contagious bovine pleuropneumonia) can be controlled by simple quarantine of infected livestock. Careful disinfection of fomites is required when agents can survive outside the host (e.g., swine fever). A knowledge of the host range of an infectious agent and the host/parasite relationship (considered separately below) is also desirable.

Host range

An infectious agent that infects or can be transmitted by only one species of host is easier to control than an agent with a wide host range. The global eradication of human smallpox was possible because the virus infected only humans; control, by quarantine and vaccination, therefore needed to be directed towards only humans. Similarly, the British bovine brucellosis eradication programme required control of infection only in cattle because only cattle can transmit *Brucella abortus* significantly. On the other hand, the current obstacle to the control of bovine tuberculosis in England is the presence of the infection in badgers (Cheeseman *et al.*, 1989). Agents that are transmitted by arthropod vectors may be particularly difficult to control because of the problems associated with controlling infection in the arthropod.

Table 22.3 tabulates, for several infectious diseases, the factors that have been discussed.

Nature of the host/parasite relationship

Exogenous agents (see Chapter 5) have been (see *Table 1.1*) and still are the causes of the major animal plagues. Control is relatively straightforward and eradication is possible. Infected animals can be identified relatively easily using clinical and laboratory diagnosis, and can be removed by slaughter or quarantine.

The endogenous agents, by definition, however, are ubiquitous and their eradication is therefore impracticable because it would require elimination of the agent from most animals, including healthy ones in which no disease is present. Many infections of intensively reared animals are endogenous. Diseases in which endogenous agents are incriminated are best controlled by alteration of other determinants; for example, by improving hygiene to prevent mastitis involving *E. coli*.

Veterinary infrastructure

Veterinary services must be capable of implementing control and eradication campaigns. There are three main requirements:

1. a mobile field service, comprising adequately trained veterinarians and veterinary auxiliaries;
2. adequate diagnostic facilities;
3. adequate research facilities.

The first two requirements are important when controlling the infectious diseases such as the classic animal plagues whose causes are understood. The third requirement must be fulfilled to improve the techniques of controlling the diseases whose causes are not known, and

Table 22.3 Factors influencing the control of some infectious diseases. (Based on Rees and Davies, 1992.)

Disease	Incubation period		Host range			Method of transmission				
	Long[1]	Short[2]	Single	Limited	Wide	Contagious	Fomites	Vectors	Airborne	Vertical/milkborne
Foot-and-mouth disease		●		●*		●	●		●	
Classical swine fever		●	●*			●[3]	●[4]			●[5]
African swine fever		●	●*			●	●	●		
Swine vesicular disease		●	●			●	●			
Rinderpest/peste des petits ruminants		●	●*			●				
Vesicular stomatitis		●		●*		●		●		
Lumpy skin disease		●	●			?		?		
Rift valley fever		●		●*,†				●		
Bluetongue		●		●*				●		
Sheep/goat pox		●	●			●				
African horse sickness		●		●				●		
Teschen disease		●	●			●	●			
Tuberculosis	●				●*	●	●			
Brucellosis	●		●*			●	●			
Contagious bovine pleuropneumonia	●		●			●				
Maedi-visna	●		●							●
Scrapie	●		●							●

● Factor characteristic present.

[1] More than 4 weeks (average).
[2] Less than 4 weeks (average).
[3,4] Postnatal infections.
[5] Prenatal infections.
*The hosts include wildlife.
†The hosts include man.
? Factor characteristic suspected.

is also needed to elucidate the causes of new and emerging diseases, such as those of intensive animal production, so that the most appropriate control strategies can be selected.

Most developed countries possess the first two requirements, mainly because their veterinary services evolved at the beginning of this century to deal with the major plagues that were common then, such as foot-and-mouth disease, pleuropneumonia and rinderpest. The developing countries often lack the first two requirements. These countries have over half of the world's livestock units (see *Table 1.6*), but contain only 20% of the world's veterinary force. Disease control programmes in these countries therefore should include two stages (Mussman *et al.*, 1980):

1. a short-term programme that includes the development of diagnostic and field services, training of personnel to deal with the major exotic diseases, and associated control techniques, such as prevention of entry of diseases across borders;
2. a long-term programme, similar to those present in some developed countries, that includes disease reporting systems, facilities for field surveys, and economic and technical studies.

Diagnostic feasibility

Control and eradication can be carried out successfully only if a disease can be recognized. The main techniques of recognition are by:

1. clinical signs;
2. pathological changes;
3. isolation of causal agents;
4. demonstration of an immune, allergic or biochemical response, or novel nucleotide sequences;
5. epidemiological identification of changes of a variable in a population.

Presenting signs may be observed either in the individual sick animal or in its offspring (e.g., congenital abnormalities). The value of signs varies because they can be either pathognomonic or indicative of general lesions and causes (see *Figure 9.3*).

Identification of pathological changes may substantiate clinical impressions and may be of value when clinical signs are absent, but again the changes may have several causes.

Isolation of causal agents is the most valuable means of identification of disease, but agents may be missed in a specimen (i.e., there may be false negatives).

Identification of an immune reaction is frequently used in control programmes. It should be recalled that each serological test has its own inherent diagnostic sensitivity and specificity (see Chapter 17) whose acceptability for the control programme must be considered. Recall, too, that the predictive value of a test depends on the prevalence of the disease: the predictive value of a positive result decreases as control reduces prevalence because the proportion of false positives increases, and so appropriate test strategies must be identified (see *Table 17.15*).

Epidemiological diagnosis includes the detection of changes in production trends in populations, for example by constructing Shewhart charts and cusums (see Chapter 12).

Adequate surveillance

Control and eradication programmes require effective surveillance. Several surveillance and monitoring systems have been introduced in Chapter 11, where the principles of data collection were also described. They are therefore not discussed further. When new national or international disease control policies are formulated, the options for surveillance may need to be reassessed. Existing data-gathering procedures may be utilized; alternatively, new systems, based on active data collection (e.g., NAHMS: see Chapter 11) may be developed. Davies (1993) discusses the merits and disadvantages of these two approaches in the context of the European Union.

Availability of replacement stock

If a control or an eradication campaign involves the slaughter of many animals, sufficient replacement stock should be available in the livestock industry to minimize disruption to production. This consideration has not been critical hitherto, although it has been cited as a potential problem if a slaughter campaign were used to control or eradicate bovine tuberculosis in developing countries (FAO/WHO, 1967).

Producers' opinions and co-operation

The opinions of animal producers can affect the success of control and eradication campaigns. In Mexico in the 1940s a slaughter campaign to eradicate foot-and-mouth disease had to be abandoned because local farmers strongly disagreed with the technique. Producers' opinions and the degree of their co-operation are influenced by their understanding of the control campaign; an important preliminary step is a detailed explanation of its rationale to farmers. In developed countries, pamphlets and audio-visual presentations are useful, such as posters at ports of entry warning of the risk of bringing rabies into the UK. In developing countries, especially where illiteracy is widespread, these techniques may not be satisfactory and may need to be replaced or supplemented by more direct contact with farmers (Chain, 1980).

Public opinion

The opinion of society may be an important consideration in a possible control or eradication scheme. Bovine brucellosis and canine distemper have a similar natural history. Both are transmitted by a single host species: cattle in the case of brucellosis, dogs in the case of distemper (ferrets and mink are excluded because their contribution is minor). In situations where bovine brucellosis can be eradicated on economically justifiable grounds, a vaccination and slaughter campaign is socially acceptable in most countries (excepting Hindu countries for religious reasons). A slaughter campaign to control distemper, even though technically feasible, would not be acceptable in many Western countries because of social attitudes towards dogs. In other countries, slaughter of dogs may be acceptable to the public, for example to improve environmental hygiene in China (*The Times*, 1983). Again, education of the public plays an important part in influencing attitudes. The virtual eradication of echinococcosis from Iceland over the past century has been achieved by explaining to the public the dangers of keeping dogs unhygienically (Beard, 1973), beginning with the publication, in the 19th century, of a pamphlet that outlined precautions against infection (Krabbe, 1864).

Public health considerations

Over 70% of the known pathogens are infectious to both man and other animals. Many of these — the zoonoses — are naturally transmissible between man and animals. The control of zoonotic diseases is the main concern of veterinary public health authorities.

The public health significance of a disease may be a major factor in determining the need for control, usually when human infection is either fatal (e.g., rabies and, in the past, glanders), or when the infection can be clinically severe, such as occupationally-acquired leptospirosis in farmers and abattoir workers.

In many cases, however, prevention of human infection is secondary to control of the infection in animals. Routine prophylactic administration of anthelmintics to dogs, for instance, is practised primarily to prevent clinical and subclinical disease in dogs, although animal owners are sometimes made aware of the potential risk of human infection (e.g., Woodruff, 1976). The control of infectious disease in livestock is usually undertaken because of the financial impact of diseases; a decrease in the incidence of human infection is an added bonus, for example when controlling bovine brucellosis.

The requirement for legislation and compensation

Control and eradication programmes are more effective when supported by legislation, sometimes accompanied by penalties when the legislation is contravened. For example, in Australia, New Zealand, Papua New Guinea and other areas in which rabies is absent, there is legislation forbidding the entry, without quarantine, of animals from countries in which the disease is present. Severe fines are imposed (and the imported animals sometimes destroyed) if the legislation is ignored.

The benefits of disease control in agriculture are frequently realized by the consumer; thus, tuberculosis eradication results in uninfected milk. The culling of an infected cow, however, represents a financial loss to the farmer. An essential part of many control programmes therefore is the compensation of producers for the loss of infected animals as a result of the programme. Thus, from February 1990, farmers were awarded 100% of the value of affected cattle as part of the bovine spongiform encephalopathy control programme in the UK. In other cases, bonuses can be offered to increase co-operation of owners; for example, awarding a bonus to farmers whose cows' bulk milk cell count (which is an indirect measure of bovine mastitis) is below a defined level; farmers whose cows' bulk cell count is above the defined level are penalized.

Ecological consequences

It has been argued that control and, particularly, eradication of an infectious agent may disturb the 'balance of nature' in an ecosystem (see Yekutiel, 1980, for a detailed discussion). The elimination of an infectious agent may free a niche that could be occupied by a more virulent organism.

The use of insecticides to destroy arthropod vectors could kill other animals in the arthropods' ecosystems. These considerations have, so far, only been theoretical in relation to animal disease control, although the use of insecticides to control insect pests has resulted in the death of other animals, such as birds that have ingested the insecticides (Carson, 1963).

Similarly, anthelmintic residues might disturb the ecosystem. For example, concern has been expressed over the avermectin group of parasiticides which can be excreted unchanged, and so, through their effect on insects that breed in dung, might affect the rate of decomposition of dung pats with consequent local effects on soil composition and earthworm populations, and more widespread effects on pastureland ecology (Herd *et al.*, 1993). However, such adverse effects have not been unequivocally demonstrated (Herd *et al.*, 1993; Wratten *et al.*, 1993).

Financial support

Control and eradication campaigns require financial support. The control of companion animal diseases readily draws financial support from owners; canine, equine and feline vaccination programmes are examples.

Livestock disease control campaigns are ususally funded either totally or partially by the government, or by non-governmental sources (Parsons, 1982). Total government support is often given to the control of exotic infectious diseases of major economic importance. Diagnostic tests, vaccines, disinfection, compensation, quarantine facilities and veterinary staff are funded by the government. Examples of such diseases are foot-and-mouth disease and swine vesicular disease. There may be partial government support; for example, when a control scheme is initially voluntary (funded by the producer) and then compulsory (funded by the government). An example is the British bovine brucellosis scheme, which was initially financed by farmers, with incentives and compensation awarded for inclusion in the scheme, and which then became compulsory. Alternatively, costs may be shared by government and the livestock industry. For example, in Britain, before sheep scab was deregulated,

the disease was controlled by dipping: the dips were provided by farmers; veterinary supervision was funded by the government.

State financial support may also be provided indirectly; for example, through the state laboratory diagnostic services and participation in herd health schemes. Non-governmental financial support is supplied indirectly by the pharmaceutical industry in the development of therapeutic and prophylactic drugs and vaccines. In Israel, a part of farm insurance premiums is directed towards disease control. In Germany, compulsory levies on farm livestock are used to support control programmes. The extent of government support is reflected by current political and economic attitudes. Support may be reduced in circumstances when the government becomes less 'paternalistic' and when it supports private enterprise rather than state control.

In all cases of financial support, the cost of control has to be weighed against the cost of disease.

Control or eradication?

The ten factors discussed above are relevant to both disease control and eradication. However, in the livestock sector, governments usually need to decide on the final objective: control or eradication of a disease in national herds and flocks (Rees and Davies, 1992). Recall that the former is an ongoing process, requiring regular financial support, whereas the latter is time-limited. Eradication is therefore the more attractive option because its costs are limited to the duration of the programme, whereas its benefits are enduring. However, before an eradication campaign is undertaken, a government must be certain that:

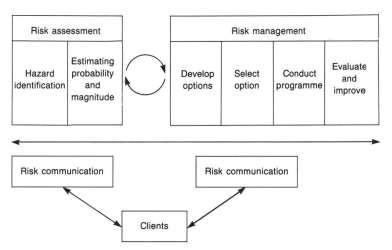

Fig. 22.1 The components of risk analysis. (From *OIE Scientific and Technical Review*, Vol. 12(4), December 1993.)

1. all technical resources (e.g., manpower) are available;
2. the agricultural community fully supports the policy to reduce the risk of illegal trade in infected animals;
3. state borders can be adequately 'policed';
4. adequate diagnostic facilities (see above) and other tools (e.g., effective vaccines) are available.

Moreover, eradication programmes should only begin when success is reasonably certain. During the initial and intermediate stages of a campaign, costs usually outweigh benefits; for example, in a programme to eradicate an infectious disease, based initially on vaccination and subsequently on a test-and-slaughter policy. If vaccination failed (e.g., because of movement of infected animals into cleared zones), there could be continuous high costs with few potential benefits.

National control schemes — without eradication — are becoming harder to justify because they need to demonstrate continuous long-term benefits in excess of costs. However, they have a role when the livestock industry is willing to support the control measures (e.g., tick-dipping to control East Coast fever), and when diseases are of public health significance (see above).

Risk analysis and animal disease control

Although diseases may occur at low levels and be adequately controlled (or eradicated), there may be a **risk** of importing them from other countries. Such a risk can only be removed completely if importation is totally prohibited. However, current political pressures in the world favour movement towards free trade, and the *unquantified* risk of introduction of a disease can now no longer be presented as a trade barrier. There is therefore a need to assess *objectively* the risks associated with particular diseases (rather than relying on the somewhat subjective judgements of individual scientists or individual parties),* and quantitative **risk analysis** has begun to be applied to animal health problems (Morley, 1993); this depends to a considerable extent on epidemiological principles and methods.

Risk assessment

The main components of risk analysis are presented in *Figure 22.1*. In risk assessment, **hazards** are identified, and then the **probability** and **magnitude** of the actual and predicted risk associated with the hazards are quantified by historical data analysis and modelling, respectively.

*However, there is also a role for subjective methods (Forbes *et al.*, 1994).

The results are often combined with subjective evaluation of risk, so that acceptable levels of risk can be determined. For example, in environmental policy making, qualitative judgements on the strength of evidence for the toxicity of agents can be linked to experimentally derived quantitative dose–response relationships (Russell and Gruber, 1987).

An assessment of the risk associated with the unrestricted importation of animals or animal products would consider the prevalence of pathogens in the source population, the probability of the pathogens surviving during importation, and the probability of the pathogens coming into contact with local livestock after importation. Examples include the risk of introducing maedi-visna, scrapie and anthrax into New Zealand (MacDiarmid, 1993). *Table 22.4* details the calculations for the last example, which are based on the binomial distribution (see Chapter 12). The estimated annual risk (the probability T) is less than one in a million. In reality, the risk is likely to be even lower because ante-mortem and post-mortem inspection at Australian abattoirs is effective in preventing anthrax cases from being processed for their hides and skins, and the probability of animals encountering anthrax on pasture is less than 1. Note that this is a deterministic model (see Chapter 19). Since most of the parameters are only estimates — and therefore the results of the assessment are debatable — the validity of the model could be improved by a stochastic formulation.

Risk management

Risk assessment is followed by evaluation of the options for diminishing or controlling the hazards (**risk management**), and communication of information about the hazards and risks between all interested parties (e.g., investigators and livestock owners).

Risk management includes a description, in a **scenario tree**, of all mutually exclusive outcomes that can occur (Miller *et al.*, 1993). For example, if the importation of an OIE List A disease (e.g., foot-and-mouth disease) were being considered, the scenario tree would include detection of infection in the exporting country (the 'planned scenario'); introduction of the disease when it is not detected in quarantine (a deviation from the planned scenario resulting in occurrence of the hazard); and detection of the infection in quarantine (a deviation from the planned scenario that does not result in occurrence of the hazard).

Risk management can usually be quantified more objectively than risk assessment. For example, knowledge of a test's sensitivity and specificity (see Chapter

Table 22.4   Risk assessment of the introduction into New Zealand of anthrax in unprocessed Australian hides and skins. (Based on MacDiarmid, 1993, with corrections.)

$$T = 1 - (1-p)^n$$

where:

T = annual probability of anthrax introduction in unprocessed hides,
p = probability that a hide contains anthrax spores,
n = number of occasions on which susceptible animals are exposed to the spores.

When $T < 0.001$, the formula simplifies to:

$$T = pn$$
$$p = ise$$

where:

i = probability that an Australian sheep or ox was infected with anthrax at slaughter = 9.94×10^{-7} (maximum annual incidence of anthrax estimated at 40 cases/year; 40.23 million cattle and sheep slaughtered annually; therefore, i = 40/4.023 $\times 10^{-7}$);
s = proportion of spore infectivity surviving pre-export handling = 0.9 (estimate based on the known resistance of anthrax spores);
e = annual proportion of unprocessed Australian hides among unprocessed New Zealand hides = 0.064 (13.5 million New Zealand hides produced; 0.92 million Australian hides imported; therefore, e = 0.92/{13.5 + 0.92}).

Thus:

$$p = 9.94 \times 10^{-7} \times 0.9 \times 0.064 = 5.7 \times 10^{-8}$$
$$n = gtvf$$

where:

g = number of approved tanneries in New Zealand = 23;
t = proportion of approved tanneries with a risk of contaminating pasture during flood periods = 0.2 (a guessed estimate);
v = average number of days per year on which flooding occurs downstream from tanneries = 25 (estimated from a range of 20−30 days);
f = probability of processing contaminated material during flood periods = 0.11 (average number of days flooding = 25; number of days worked/year = 235; therefore, f = 25/235).

Therefore:

$$n = 23 \times 0.2 \times 25 \times 0.11 = 12.65.$$

Thus:

$$T = 5.7 \times 10^{-8} \times 12.65$$
$$= 7.2 \times 10^{-7}.$$

17) enables predictions to be made about the likelihood of importing infected animals or products with various importation rules, and therefore can assist policy-making.

The probability of missing an infected individual using a given diagnostic test is (1-sensitivity); this probability would therefore be 0.05 if a test with a sensitivity of 0.95 (95%) were being applied. Recall, however (Chapter 17), that the predictive value of a diagnostic test also depends on disease prevalence. The probability of an animal that is negative to a test being actually infected, p_n, is:

$$\frac{P(1-Se)}{P(1-Se) + (1-P) \times Sp}$$

where P is the true prevalence, Se = sensitivity and Sp = specificity (Marchevsky et al., 1989).

If animals were being quarantined, exclusion of false positive animals is of little concern, and so specificity can be assumed to be 1. Table 22.5 lists the values of p_n for various values of P when a test with a sensitivity of 0.95 is used. The probability of any test-negative animal being infected *increases* when the prevalence in the source population increases.

Moreover, at a given prevalence, the probability of including even one test-negative infected animal in a group of imported animals, p_c, increases as the number of animals in the group increases (Marchevsky *et al.*, 1989):

$$p_c = 1 - \left\{ \frac{(1-P) \times Sp}{(1-P) \times Sp + P(1-Se)} \right\}^n,$$

where n is the group size.

If a policy dictates that a positive test result only disqualifies the *individual* animal that reacts positively, then the risks associated with such a policy are p_n (*Table 22.5*) and p_c (*Table 22.6*). Alternatively, it may be decided that a positive test result in any one animal will disqualify the entire *group* (e.g., tests for *OIE* List A diseases: see Chapter 11), in which circumstance the probability of disqualifying an infected *group* increases as the prevalence and/or group size increases. The probability of a test failing to detect at least one test-positive animal in an infected group, β, thus identifying the group as infected, can be calculated (MacDiarmid, 1987):

$$\beta = \{ 1 - (t \times Se)/n \}^{p_n},$$

where $t =$ the number of animals that are tested in the group.

Thus, the difference in risk between these two policies can be compared (*Table 22.7*). The risk of an infected animal being imported is considerably reduced when a single reactor disqualifies the entire group, rather than disqualifying only itself.

Further examples, and a detailed discussion of the application of risk analysis in veterinary medicine, are given by Morley (1993) and Waltner-Toews and McEwen (1994). Elementary (Ansell and Wharton, 1992; Stewart, 1992; Ansell, 1994) and more advanced (Report, 1983, 1992) general introductions to risk analysis may also be consulted.

Table 22.5 The probability that a test-negative animal is actually infected, when sensitivity = 0.95 and specificity = 1. (From MacDiarmid, 1991.)

Prevalence	Probability (p_n)
0.01	5.05×10^{-4}
0.05	2.63×10^{-3}
0.10	5.52×10^{-3}
0.20	1.23×10^{-2}

Table 22.6 The probability that a test-negative, infected animal will be included in a group destined for import when only reactor animals are excluded (prevalence = 0.01, sensitivity = 0.95 and specificity = 1). (From MacDiarmid, 1991.)

Group size	Probability (p_c)
10	5.04×10^{-3}
20	1.00×10^{-2}
30	1.50×10^{-2}
50	2.49×10^{-2}
100	4.92×10^{-2}
500	2.23×10^{-1}

Table 22.7 The probability that a test-negative, infected animal will be included in a group destined for import (prevalence = 0.01, sensitivity = 0.95 and specificity = 1; entire group tested). (Modified from *OIE Scientific and Technical Review*, Vol. 12(4), December 1993.)

Group size	Probability (if reactor animal only excluded) (p_c)	Probability (if a single reactor disqualifies **group**): probability of no test-positives (β)
100	4.92×10^{-2}	5.00×10^{-2}
200	9.61×10^{-2}	2.50×10^{-3}
300	1.41×10^{-1}	1.25×10^{-4}
400	1.83×10^{-1}	6.25×10^{-6}
500	2.23×10^{-1}	3.13×10^{-7}

Veterinary medicine towards the end of this century

Chapter 1 described how veterinary medicine coped with various challenges during its development. This final chapter ends with some thoughts on the future direction of the veterinary profession, highlighting the contribution that epidemiology will make. The topic is discussed in greater detail by Henderson (1982), Hugh-Jones (1983), Pritchard (1986, 1989) and Michell (1993).

Livestock medicine

Multifactorial diseases are the major problems in intensive livestock enterprises. Investigation of their cause does not involve the study of a simple infectious agent, but of several determinants associated with host, agent and environment. The environment is also recognized as important because of its significance to animal welfare (Ekesbo, 1992). Observational studies (see Chapter 15) provide a critical framework for identifying the many determinants of disease in intensive enterprises. Epidemiological principles and concepts are also applicable to welfare issues (McInerney, 1991; Willeberg, 1991).

Modelling of livestock units, using variables associated with disease and production, will continue to develop, facilitated by microcomputerized decision support systems (see Chapter 11). These also facilitate definition of the most suitable technical and economic production variables, and provide methods for assessing individual and herd performance (e.g., Huirne *et al.*, 1991, 1992; Huirne and Dijkhuizen, 1994).

In developing countries, there is a need for an improvement in the 'quality' of data. For example, the epidemic infectious diseases such as rinderpest still pose problems, and eradication campaigns require application of appropriate sampling techniques (see Chapter 13).

Methods of identifying infectious diseases are becoming more analytically sensitive and refined. Smaller quantities of antigen can be detected, and subtle differences between strains can be identified using ELISA tests, monoclonal antibodies and the newer molecular techniques (see Chapter 2). All of these techniques are now being applied to the diagnosis of bacterial, viral and parasitic diseases of animals (Ambrosio and de Waal, 1990; Knowles and Gorham, 1990; OIE, 1993). However, they have some disadvantages, and older techniques therefore still have an important role (Wilson, 1993). For example, the analytical sensitivity and specificity of DNA probe technology — which involves a whole new level of complexity — is similar to conventional microscopy in diagnosing human malaria. Similarly, the polymerase chain reaction can produce false positive results due to contamination (Kwok and Higuchi, 1989) and is relatively slow.

New techniques are producing vaccines that are safer than formerly. For example, sub-unit vaccines comprise only virus capsid antigens and lack nucleic acid, and therefore cannot be pathogenic. Vaccines against helminths (e.g., *Dictyocaulus viviparus*) are few but they have a considerable advantage over the current anthelmintics, with the latter's associated risk of resistance and short period of action. The breeding of resistant stock may be a more useful technique because techniques such as embryo cloning, superovulation and nuclear transplantation can accelerate this otherwise slow process.

Companion animal medicine

In developed countries, the number of pet-owning households is increasing (e.g., Singleton, 1993), and there is a concomitant increase in the proportion of veterinarians engaged in companion animal practice (e.g., *Figure 1.4*). The public's expectation of veterinary services will continue to rise, and this will be reflected in improvements in the quality of patient care, involving better surgical techniques and medical therapy. The latter are now subject to more critical evaluation than previously in properly designed clinical trials (see Chapter 16).

The aim of medical epidemiologists is to ensure that each person enjoys a long life with morbidity confined to a short period before death. This goal can be shared by veterinarians, and its achievement requires research on improved preventive techniques, such as vaccination, and on the determinants associated with chronic and refractory diseases, such as canine heart disease and dermatoses. Observational studies again provide a critical framework for such research. This research is still hampered by a lack of basic demographic and morbidity data from a wide cross-section of the companion animal population. However, the increasing availability of inexpensive microcomputers to veterinary practitioners (see Chapter 11), and the expansion of computer networks, should facilitate the gathering of these data, although attempts to pool data from companion animal practices have so far been limited (Thrusfield, 1991).

Epidemiology plays a central role in the continuing development and improvement of livestock and companion animal veterinary medicine. Its contemporary objectives have many similarities with those of ancient Greek medicine, described by Hippocrates, in the 'Second Constitution' of Book 1 of his *Epidemics*, as to:

'Declare the past, diagnose the present, foretell the future'

(Jones, 1923)

Further reading

Biggs, P.M. (1985) Infectious disease and its control. *Philosophical Transactions of the Royal Society of London, Series B*, **310**, 259–274

Bourne, F.J. (1993) Biotechnology and farm animal medicine. In: *The Advancement of Veterinary Science. The Bicentenary Symposium Series. Volume 1: Veterinary Medicine Beyond 2000*. Ed. Michell, A.R., pp. 41–57. CAB International, Wallingford. (*A discussion of the application of modern biotechnology to animal disease control*)

Hanson, R.P. and Hanson, M.G. (1983) *Animal Disease Control*. Iowa State University Press, Ames. (*A description of principles and techniques relating to regional control programmes in developed and developing countries*)

OIE (1994) Early methods of animal disease control. *Revue Scientifique et Technique, Office International des Epizooties*, **13**, 332–614

Peters, A.R. (Ed.) (1993) *Vaccines for Veterinary Applications*. Butterworth-Heinemann Ltd, Oxford

Rees, W.G.H. and Davies, G. (1992) Legislation for health. In: *Livestock Health and Welfare*. Ed. Moss, R., pp. 118–159. Longman Scientific & Technical, Harlow. (*A description of national and international control and eradication schemes*)

Report of a British Veterinary Association Trust Project on the Future of Animal Health Control (1982) *The Control of Infectious Diseases in Farm Animals*. British Veterinary Association, London

Schnurrenberger, P.R., Sharman, R.S. and Wise, G.H. (1987) *Attacking Animal Diseases: Concepts and Strategies for Control and Eradication*. Iowa State University Press, Ames. (*A general discussion of disease control, mainly with American examples*)

Woods, G.T. (Ed.) (1986) *Practices in Veterinary Public Health and Preventive Medicine in the United States*. Iowa State University Press, Ames. (*A general discussion of veterinary public health, including environmental health, and animal disease control in the United States*)

Yekutiel, P. (1980) *Eradication of Infectious Disease - A Critical Study*. Contributions to Epidemiology and Biostatistics Vol. 2. Karger, Basel

General reading

Books

Blaha, T. (Ed.) (1989) *Applied Veterinary Epidemiology.* Elsevier, Amsterdam

Campbell, R.S.F. (Ed.) (1983) *A Course Manual in Veterinary Epidemiology.* Australian Universities' International Development Program, Canberra

Elliot, R.E.W. and Tattersfield, J.G. (1979) *Investigating Animal Disease Status.* Ministry of Agriculture and Fisheries, Wellington, New Zealand

Halpin, B. (1975) *Patterns of Animal Disease.* Baillière Tindall, London

Leech, F.B. and Sellers, K.C. (1979) *Statistical Epidemiology in Veterinary Science.* Charles Griffin, London and High Wycombe

Lessard, P.R. and Perry, B.D. (Eds) (1988) Investigation of disease outbreaks and impaired productivity. *The Veterinary Clinics of North America: Food Animal Practice*, **4**(1)

Martin, S.W., Meek, A.H. and Willeberg, P. (1987) *Veterinary Epidemiology: Principles and Methods.* Iowa State University Press, Ames, IA

Meek, A.H. and Martin, S.W. (1991) Epidemiology of infectious disease. In: *Microbiology of Animals and Animal Products. World Animal Science, A6.* Ed. Woolcock, J.B., pp. 141–180. Elsevier, Amsterdam. (*Abridged adaptation of Martin et al., 1987*)

Putt, S.N.H., Shaw, A.P.M., Woods, A.J., Tyler, L. and James, A.D. (1987) *Veterinary Epidemiology and Economics in Africa*, ILCA Manual No. 3. International Livestock Centre for Africa, Addis Ababa

Schwabe, C.W. (1984) *Veterinary Medicine and Human Health*, 3rd edn. Williams and Wilkins, Baltimore and London

Schwabe, C.W., Riemann, H.P. and Franti, C.E. (1977) *Epidemiology in Veterinary Practice.* Lea and Febiger, Philadelphia

Waltner-Toews, D. (Ed.) (1991) *Veterinary Epidemiology in the Real World: a Canadian Potpourri.* Canadian Association of Veterinary Epidemiology and Preventive Medicine, Ontario Veterinary College, Guelph

Proceedings

Elbers, A.R.W. (Ed.) (1993) Dutch Society for Veterinary Epidemiology and Economics. Proceedings (**6**), Boxtel, 8 December 1993 (*in English*)

Ellis, P.R., Shaw, A.P.M. and Stephens, A.J. (1976) *New Techniques in Veterinary Epidemiology and Economics.* Proceedings of a symposium held at the University of Reading, 12–15 July 1976

Epidemiological Skills in Animal Health (1990) Refresher Course for Veterinarians. Proceedings 143, Sydney, 1–5 October 1990. Post Graduate Committee in Veterinary Science, University of Sydney

Epidemiology at Work (1990) Refresher Course for Veterinarians. Proceedings 144, North Head, 5–7 October 1990. Post Graduate Committee in Veterinary Science, University of Sydney

Epidemiology in Animal Health (1983) Proceedings of a symposium held at the British Veterinary Association's Centenary Congress, Reading, 22–25 September 1982. Society for Veterinary Epidemiology and Preventive Medicine

Frankena, K. (Ed.) (1990) Studievereniging voor Veterinaire Epidemiologie en Economie. Proceedings (**3**), Wageningen, 12 December 1990 (*in English*)

Frankena, K. and van der Hoofd, C.M. (Eds) (1992) Dutch Society for Veterinary Epidemiology and Economy. Proceedings (**5**), Wageningen, 9 December 1992 (*in English*)

Geering, W.A., Roe, R.T. and Chapman, L.A. (Eds) (1980) *Veterinary Epidemiology and Economics.* Proceedings of the 2nd International Symposium, Canberra, 7–11 May 1979. Australian Government Publishing Service, Canberra

Proceedings of the 6th International Symposium on Veterinary Epidemiology and Economics, Ottawa, 12–16 August 1991, Department of Population Medicine, Ontario Veterinary College, Guelph

Proceedings of the 3rd International Symposium on Veterinary Epidemiology and Economics (1983) Arlington, Virginia, 6–10 September 1982, Veterinary Medical Publishing, Edwardsville

Proceedings of the 4th International Symposium on Veterinary Epidemiology and Economics (1986) Singapore, 18–22 November 1985. Singapore Veterinary Association, Singapore

Rowlands, G.J. (Ed.) (1989) Society for Veterinary Epidemiology and Preventive Medicine, Proceedings, Exeter, 12–14 April 1989

Rowlands, G.J., Kyule, M.N. and Perry, B.D. (Eds) (1994) Proceedings of the 7th International Symposium on Veterinary Epidemiology and Economics, Nairobi, 15–19 August 1994, *The Kenya Veterinarian*, **18**(2), 1–597

Schukken, Y.H. and Lam, T.J.G.M. (Eds) (1994) Dutch Society for Veterinary Epidemiology and Economics. Proceedings (7), Utrecht, December 14 1994 (in English)

Thrusfield, M.V. (Ed.) (1983) Society for Veterinary Epidemiology and Preventive Medicine, Proceedings, Southampton, 12–13 April 1983

Thrusfield, M.V. (Ed.) (1984) Society for Veterinary Epidemiology and Preventive Medicine, Proceedings, Edinburgh, 10–11 April 1984

Thrusfield, M.V. (Ed.) (1985) Society for Veterinary Epidemiology and Preventive Medicine, Proceedings, Reading, 27–29 March 1985

Thrusfield, M.V. (Ed.) (1986) Society for Veterinary Epidemiology and Preventive Medicine, Proceedings, Edinburgh, 2–4 April 1986

Thrusfield, M.V. (Ed.) (1987) Society for Veterinary Epidemiology and Preventive Medicine, Proceedings, Solihull, 1–3 April 1987

Thrusfield, M.V. (Ed.) (1988) Society for Veterinary Epidemiology and Preventive Medicine, Proceedings, Edinburgh, 13–15 April 1988

Thrusfield, M.V. (Ed.) (1990) Society for Veterinary Epidemiology and Preventive Medicine, Proceedings, Belfast, 4–6 April 1990

Thrusfield, M.V. (Ed.) (1991) Society for Veterinary Epidemiology and Preventive Medicine, Proceedings, London, 17–19 April 1991

Thrusfield, M.V. (Ed.) (1992) Society for Veterinary Epidemiology and Preventive Medicine, Denary Proceedings, Edinburgh, 1–3 April 1992

Thrusfield, M.V. (Ed.) (1993) Society for Veterinary Epidemiology and Preventive Medicine, Proceedings, Exeter, 29 March–1 April 1993

Thrusfield, M.V. (Ed.) (1994) Society for Veterinary Epidemiology and Preventive Medicine, Proceedings, Belfast, 13–15 April 1994

Willeberg, P., Agger, J.F. and Riemann, H.P. (Eds) (1988) Proceedings of the 5th International Symposium on Veterinary Epidemiology and Economics, Copenhagen, 25–29 July 1988, *Acta Veterinaria Scandinavica*, **Supplementum 84**, 1–566

Journals

Papers on veterinary epidemiology are published in a wide range of journals. *Preventive Veterinary Medicine* is the main journal devoted to the subject. National veterinary journals such as *Acta Veterinaria Scandinavica*, the *American Journal of Veterinary Research*, the *Australian Veterinary Journal*, the *Canadian Veterinary Journal*, the *Journal of the American Veterinary Medical Association*, the *New Zealand Veterinary Journal* and the *Veterinary Record*; disciplinary journals such as *Cancer Research*, the *International Journal of Parasitology*, the *Journal of National Cancer Institute* and the *Journal of Pathology*; and journals specializing in particular species, such as the *Equine Veterinary Journal*, the *Journal of Small Animal Practice* and the *Journal of the American Animal Hospitals Association*, also publish epidemiological papers. *Epidemiology and Infection* (formerly the *Journal of Hygiene, Cambridge*) focuses on infectious diseases. The *Bulletin of the Pan American Health Organization*, *Bulletin of the World Health Organization*, *Revue Scientifique et Technique Office International des Epizooties*, *Tropical Animal Health and Production* and the *World Animal Review* (now defunct) contain material relevant to developing countries.

The *American Journal of Epidemiology* (formerly the *American Journal of Hygiene*) is primarily medical, but occasionally publishes veterinary material. It, *Epidemiology*, and the *International Journal of Epidemiology*, also contain papers on quantitative methods. These methods are also published in statistical journals such as *Applied Statistics*, *Biometrics*, the *Journal of the Royal Statistical Society (Series A and B)*, *Mathematical Biosciences* and *Statistics in Medicine*.

Appendices

Appendices IV, XVII, IXX and XX are taken from Tables III, IV, VII and V, respectively, in *Statistical Tables for Biological, Agricultural and Medical Research*, 6th edition (1974), edited by Fisher, R.A. and Yates, F. and published by Longman Group Limited (previously published by Oliver and Boyd Limited, Edinburgh), and are reproduced with the permission of the authors and publishers.

Appendix I

Glossary of terms

This glossary provides brief definitions of some common epidemiological terms that are used in this book. A more comprehensive guide is given in *A Dictionary of Epidemiology*, 2nd edition (edited by J.M. Last, Oxford University Press, New York, 1988),* from which some of the definitions below are derived.

Accuracy: the degree to which an individual measurement represents the true value of the attribute that is being measured: the greater the accuracy, the greater the degree.

Adjustment: a summarizing procedure for a parameter (e.g., incidence or mortality) in which the effects of differences in the composition of populations compared (e.g., different age distributions) are minimized. Two common techniques are **direct** and **indirect standardization**.

Antibody: a protein produced by an animal's immunological system in response to exposure to a foreign substance (an antigen; q.v.). Sometimes antibodies are produced against the individual's own proteins, causing autoimmune disease. Antibodies display specificity (q.v.) to particular antigens.

Antigen: a substance (usually a protein) that induces a specific immune response (e.g., circulating antibody production).

Association: the relationship between two variables (see Appendix II). The association is 'positive' when the variables occur together more frequently than is

expected by chance; the association is 'negative' when they occur less frequently than is expected by chance.

Bias: systematic (as opposed to random) departure from true values.

Binomial distribution: a probability distribution relating to two mutually exclusive and exhaustive outcomes (e.g., the birth of either male or female animals), where successive outcomes (e.g., births) are independent and occur with constant probability.

Carrier:
1. an animal that is infected with an infectious agent without displaying clinical signs, and that can be a source of infection to other animals;
2. **(genetic)** an animal that is heterozygous for a normal and an abnormal gene, the latter of which is not expressed but may be detected by tests.

Case: an animal in a population or study group identified as having a particular disease or other health related event that is being investigated.

Case–control study: an observational study (q.v.) in which a group of diseased animals (cases) is compared with a group of non-diseased animals (controls) with respect to exposure to an hypothesized cause.

Causality: the relating of causes to the effects that they produce.

Clinical trial: a systematic study in the species for which a prophylactic or therapeutic procedure is intended in order to establish the procedure's prophylactic or therapeutic effects. A 'field trial' is a clinical trial undertaken in the field, that is, under husbandry and management practices typical of those under which the procedure is intended to be used.

Cohort study: an observational study (q.v.) in which a group of animals exposed to an hypothesized cause is

---

*An English–French and French–English dictionary, based on the 1st edition (1983), is published (Fabia *et al.*, 1988). There is also a French glossary of veterinary epidemiology, with English/German/Spanish/Italian/Portuguese–French indices (Toma *et al.*, 1991).

compared with a group not so exposed, with respect to development of a disease.

Commensals: microbes found on the skin or within the body that do not usually cause disease (cf. pathogens).

Confidence interval: a range of values within which the value of a parameter (see Appendix II) lies with a specified level of confidence.

Confounding: the inseparability from a given data set of the effects of two possible causes of an observed result, because both occur together.

Continuous variable: a variable (see Appendix II) that may take any value in an interval; the interval may be finite or infinite.

Cost − benefit analysis: *see* Social cost − benefit analysis.

Cross-product ratio: *see* Odds ratio.

Cross-sectional study: an observational study (q.v.) in which animals are classified according to presence or absence of disease, and presence or absence of exposure to an hypothesized causal factor, at a particular point in time.

Cross-sectional survey: a survey (q.v.) undertaken at a particular point in time.

Database: a structured collection of data.

Determinant: a factor that affects the health of a population.

Discrete variable: a variable (see Appendix II) for which there is a definite distance from one value of the variable to the next possible value (e.g., numbers of cases of disease: 1, 2, 3 . . . where the distance is 1).

Endemic: an adjective describing:
1. the predictable level of occurrence of disease, infection, antibody, etc.;
2. the usual presence of disease, infection, antibody, etc.

Endogenous:
1. normally from within an animal;
2. (characteristic) an innate characteristic of an animal (e.g., breed).

Epidemic: an occurrence of disease in excess of its anticipated frequency (also used adjectivally).

Epidemic curve: a graph plotting the number of new cases against time of onset of disease; thus, an epidemic curve plots incidence.

Epidemiology (veterinary): the investigation of disease, other health-related events, and production in animal populations and the making of inferences from the investigation in an attempt to improve the health and productivity of the populations.

Exogenous:
1. normally from outside an animal;
2. (characteristic) a characteristic that is not innate, to

which an animal is exposed (e.g., climate, toxic substance and microbes).

Experimental study: a study (q.v.) in which the investigator can allocate animals to different categories; thus, the conditions of the study are controlled by the investigator.

Extrinsic factor: *see* Exogenous (2).

Extrinsic incubation period: the time between the entry of an infectious agent into an arthropod vector and the time at which the arthropod becomes infectious.

Field trial: *see* Clinical trial.

Fomites (singular: **fomes**): inanimate communicators of infection (cf. vector).

Health and productivity schemes: systems for recording disease and productivity in groups of animals (usually herds and flocks), their aim being to improve health and productivity of the groups.

Horizontal (lateral) transmission: transmission of an infection from an individual to any other individual in a population, but excluding vertical transmission (q.v.).

Hypothesis: a proposition that can be tested formally; after which the hypothesis may be either 'supported' or 'rejected'.

Inapparent infection: an infection that does not produce clinical signs.

Incidence: the number of new cases that occur over a specified period of time. It is usually expressed in relation to the population at risk and the time during which the population is observed.

Informatics: the supply of information through the medium of the computer.

Interaction:
1. (**biological**) the interdependent operation of two or more causes to produce an effect;
2. (**statistical**) in an epidemiological context, a quantitative interdependence between two or more factors, such that the frequency of disease when two or more factors are present is either in excess of that expected from the combined effects of each factor (positive interaction) or less than the combined effect (negative interaction).

Intrinsic factor: *see* Endogenous (2).

Longitudinal study:
1. a cohort study (q.v.);
2. a general description of both cohort and case − control studies (q.v.), so called because these studies investigate exposure to an hypothesized cause and development of disease (the effect) when cause and effect are separated temporally.

Longitudinal survey: a survey (q.v.) that records events over a period of time.

Misclassification: the incorrect allocation of individuals or features to categories to which they do not belong (e.g., the classification of a diseased animal as non-diseased).

Model:
1. (**biological**) a system that uses animals to study diseases, pathological conditions and impaired function; the model may be induced experimentally or may be constructed using naturally occurring conditions;
2. (**mathematical**) a representation of a system, process or relationship in mathematical form in which equations are used to simulate the behaviour of the system or process under study.

Monitoring: the routine collection of information on disease, productivity and other characteristics possibly related to them in a population.

Morbidity: the amount of disease in a population (commonly defined in terms of incidence or prevalence; q.v.).

Mortality: a measure of the number of deaths in a population.

Multifactorial disease: a disease that depends on the presence of several factors for its induction. Most diseases are multifactorial, although some may have one major component cause (e.g., foot-and-mouth disease virus in the cause of foot-and-mouth disease), in which case they are commonly termed 'unifactorial'.

Multivariate analysis: a set of statistical techniques used to study the variation in several variables simultaneously.

Necessary cause: a cause that must always be present for a disease to occur (e.g., *Mycobacterium tuberculosis* is the necessary cause of tuberculosis).

Nidality: the characteristic of an infectious agent to occur in distinct nidi (q.v.) associated with particular geographic, climatic and ecological conditions.

Nidus (plural: **nidi**): a focus of infection.

nm (nanometre): 10^{-9} m; equivalent to the obsolescent millimicron (μm).

Normal distribution: a probability distribution relating to continuous data and characterized by a symmetric, bell-shaped distribution with 'tails' extending to infinity.

Observational study: an epidemiological study (q.v.) in which the investigator has no freedom, or does not exercise his freedom, to allocate animals to different categories; disease is studied as it occurs 'naturally'.

Odds: the ratio (q.v.) of the probability of an event occurring to that of it not occurring.

Odds ratio: the ratio of two odds: a measure of association commonly used in observational studies

(q.v.). The odds are defined differently, depending on the type of study. Thus, in a cohort study (q.v.) a *disease-odds ratio* is estimated: this is the odds in favour of disease among exposed individuals divided by the odds in favour of disease among unexposed individuals. (See Chapter 15 for fuller details.) (*cf.* Relative risk.)

One-tailed test: a statistical significance test based on the assumption that the data have only one possible direction of variability.

Outbreak: an identified occurrence of disease involving one or more animals. The term generally implies that several animals are affected. Livestock in developed countries are usually kept as separated populations and so 'outbreak' can be applied unambiguously to an occurrence of disease on an individual farm. However, in developing countries, animal populations are frequently contiguous and so it may be difficult to define the limits of one outbreak. The *Office International des Epizooties* defines an outbreak as 'an occurrence of disease in an agricultural establishment, breeding establishment or premises, including all buildings as well as adjoining premises, where animals are present'.

Where it cannot be defined in this way, the outbreak shall have to be considered as occurring in the part of the territory in which, taking local conditions into account, it cannot be guaranteed that both susceptible and unsusceptible animals have had no direct contact with affected or susceptible cases in that area. For example, in the case of certain parts of Africa, an outbreak means the occurrence of the disease within a sixteenth square degree; the occurrence is still referred to as an outbreak even though the disease may occur in several places within the same sixteenth square degree. (Note that the area within a sixteenth square degree is not constant: it varies with latitude.)

Pandemic: a geographically widespread (sometimes global) epidemic (also used adjectivally).

Parameter: see Appendix II.

Pathogen: an organism that produces disease.

Pathogenicity: the ability of an infectious agent to cause disease.

Point (common) source epidemic: an epidemic resulting from exposure of animals to a single common cause.

Poisson distribution: a probability distribution relating to the distribution of events, independently, either throughout space (an area) or over time.

Population at risk: the population that is naturally susceptible to a disease.

Precision:
1. the reciprocal of the variance of an estimate;

2. the quality of being lucidly and clearly defined.

Prevalence: the number of occurrences of disease, infection, antibody presence, and so on in a population, usually relating to a particular point in time; it is commonly expressed as the proportion of the population at risk.

Predictive value:
1. of a positive test result: the probability that an animal with a 'positive' test is a true 'positive';
2. of a negative test result: the probability that an animal with a 'negative' test result is a true 'negative'.

Proportion: a ratio (q.v.) in which the numerator is part of the denominator.

Prospective study: a cohort study.

Rate: a ratio (q.v.) that indicates the change in one quantity with respect to one or more others over time. Thus, incidence rate is the number of new cases of disease occurring in a population observed for a defined period of time (e.g. 10 cases per 100 animal-years at risk).

Ratio: a value obtained by dividing one quantity (the numerator) by another (the denominator); for example, the number of males born per female birth. Proportions and rates are ratios.

Refinement: the quality of being sharply defined. Thus, a refined serological test will detect subtle antigenic differences between microbes, whereas a less refined test will only identify major antigenic groups.

Relative odds: *see* Odds ratio.

Relative risk: the ratio of disease incidence in individuals exposed to an hypothesized cause, to the incidence in those not so exposed. It is a measure of association commonly used in cohort studies (q.v.). (*cf.* Odds ratio.)

Reliability: the degree of stability exhibited when a measurement is repeated under identical conditions; reliability therefore may be demonstrated by repeating a measurement.

Reservoir: an animate or inanimate object on or in which an infectious agent usually lives, and which therefore is often a source of infection by the agent.

Retrospective study:
1. a case−control study (so-called because the study looks back from effect to cause);
2. any study that collects and utilizes historical data.

Sample: a selected part of a population.

Risk ratio: *see* Relative risk.

Screening: the presumptive identification of an unrecognized disease or defect using tests or other procedures that can be applied rapidly to a population or a selected subset.

Sensitivity (of a test):
1. **diagnostic:** the proportion of diseased animals that are detected by a test;
2. **analytical:** the ability of a test to detect amounts of antigen, enzyme, nucleic acid, and so on; a sensitive test will detect small amounts.

Social cost−benefit analysis: an economic technique used in epidemiology to assess the costs of disease and impaired productivity in relation to the benefits that accrue from their control.

Specificity:
1. degree of refinement; the greater the specificity, the greater the degree;
2. **diagnostic** (of a test): the proportion of non-diseased animals that are detected by a test;
3. **analytical** (of a test): degree of refinement in an infectious agent (e.g., antigenic type or nucleic acid composition) that can be detected by a test; the greater the specificity, the greater the degree.

Sporadic: an adjective describing the irregular, unpredictable occurrence of disease or infection.

Spreadsheet: a computer software package providing a representation of a large rectangular area upon which data tabulation may be displayed and a variety of calculations performed.

'Stamping-out policy': The *Office International des Epizooties* defines stamping out as the carrying out under the authority of the veterinary administration, on confirmation of a disease, of zoo-sanitary prophylactic measures, consisting of killing the animals that are affected and those suspected of being affected in the herd and, where appropriate, those in other herds that have been exposed to infection by direct animal-to-animal contact, or by indirect contact of any kind likely to cause transmission of the causal pathogen. All susceptible animals, vaccinated or unvaccinated, on an infected premises should be killed and the carcasses destroyed by burning or burial, or by any other method which will eliminate the spread of infection through the carcasses or products of the animals killed. This policy should be accompanied by approved cleansing and disinfection procedures.

A 'modified stamping-out policy' is any policy where the above zoo-sanitary measures are not implemented in full.

Study: an investigation that involves the testing of a causal hypothesis. A study may be either experimental (q.v.) or observational (q.v.).

Sufficient cause: the complex of component causes that induces a disease. Several different sufficient causes may induce the same disease.

Surveillance: an intensive form of monitoring (q.v.), designed so that action can be taken to improve the health status of a population, and therefore frequently used in disease control campaigns. Appropriate action to control disease thus follows surveillance.

Survey: an investigation involving the collection of information and in which a causal hypothesis usually is not tested (*cf.* Study). It may suggest aspects worthy of study.

Synergism: a positive statistical interaction (q.v.) where a causal pathway can be inferred (other authors may use the term differently).

Threshold level:

1. the spatial density of susceptible animals required to initiate an epidemic;
2. the minimum concentration of an infectious agent in a vertebrate host's circulation that allows successful transmission to an arthropod vector;
3. a critical level for the number and combination of genes above which a genetically determined disease occurs.

Two-tailed test: a statistical significance test based on the assumption that the data are distributed in both directions from some central value(s).

Validity: a term with a variety of meanings; in this book it is the degree to which a diagnostic test or survey produces, *on average*, an accurate result. It is therefore a long-run property of the test or survey.

Variable: see Appendix II.

Vector: a living organism (frequently an arthropod) that communicates an infectious agent from an infected to a susceptible animal.

Vertical transmission: transmission of an infection from one individual to its offspring.

Virulence: the disease-evoking power of an infectious agent in a particular host.

Zoonosis: an infection shared in nature by man and other vertebrates.

Appendix II

Basic mathematical notation and terms

Variables

There are properties of members of a population that vary between the members, for example, weights of cows or breed of pig; these properties are variables. Their values are denoted by Roman letters which usually take the lower case, x, y, z, etc. The letters often have subscripts (small-sized numbers to the right of, and slightly below, the letter), for example:

the weights x_1, x_2, x_3, of three calves
$x_1 = 230$ kg, $x_2 = 221$ kg, $x_3 = 155$ kg.,

Constants

There are two types of constant:

(1) **universal constants** have a single value, for example, $\pi = 3.141 \ldots$
(2) **parameters** are constants that are fixed for a particular study, but which may change from one study to another. Greek letters, λ, μ and so on, usually denote parameters. For example, the infectivity rate of a particular parasite could be denoted by λ, where λ may change from one isolate to another.

Logarithms

Logarithms are a class of arithmetical functions distinguished by a characteristic known as the **base**, such that the logarithm of a number is the power to which the base of the logarithm must be raised to give the number. Two bases are frequently used: base 10 and base e, where e = the universal exponential constant, $2.718281 \ldots$ Logarithms to base 10 are also called 'common' logarithms, whereas logarithms to the base e (abbreviated to 'log$_e$' or

'ln') are called 'natural' or Napierian logarithms. Additionally, logarithms to the base 2 are sometimes used.

Thus, $\log_{10} 100 = 2$ (i.e., $10^2 = 100$),
$\log_e 5 = 1.609$ (i.e., $2.718^{1.609} = 5$),
$\log_2 8 = 3$ (i.e., $2^3 = 8$).

The inverse of logarithmic transformation is anti-logarithmic transformation. Thus antilog$_{10}$ $2 = 10^2 = 100$.

Exponential function: exp(x)

The exponential function, $\exp(x)$, alternatively written e^x, is the particular case of antilogarithmic transformation which relates to natural logarithms. For example, if $x = 4$, $\exp(x) = 2.718^4 = 54.6$.

Summation notation: Σ

Σ is used to denote the sum of a set of data. For example:

$$\sum_{i=1}^{6} x_i = x_1 + x_2 + x_3 + x_4 + x_5 + x_6.$$

This means 'the sum of all the values of x from x_1 to x_6 inclusive'. This notation is of value if, for instance, one wanted to add x_3, x_4 and x_5 from the series of values, in which case one would write:

$$\sum_{i=3}^{5} x_i$$

In biological calculations it is usually necessary to add **all** of the values of x from x_1 to the last value of x, omitting none of the values in the series. It is therefore sufficient to write Σx, in which case it is assumed that all of the x values in the series are being added.

This system of notation can also be applied to powers. For example, Σx^2 means 'square all the individual values of x in the series and then add these square values together':

$$x_1 = 2, \; x_2 = 3, \; x_3 = 2,$$
$$\text{then} \;\; \Sigma x^2 = x_1^2 + x_2^2 + x_3^2 = 4 + 9 + 4 = 17.$$

$(\Sigma x)^2$ means 'add together all the values of x in the series and then square the result'. For example:

$$x_1 = 2, \; x_2 = 3, \; x_3 = 2,$$
$$\text{then} \;\; (\Sigma x)^2 = (x_1 + x_2 + x_3)^2 = (2 + 3 + 2)^2 = 49.$$

Order of calculation

Multiplication and division are conducted before addition and subtraction. Thus:

$$6 \times 3 + 1 = 18 + 1$$
$$= 19.$$

Brackets are used to indicate the order of calculation, taking precedence over multiplication and division when calculations would otherwise be ambiguous. Three types of brackets are commonly used: parentheses ( ), braces { }, and square brackets [ ], usually, but not always, in that order.

Thus: $3 \, [3 + \{6(4 + 2)\}]$

is calculated as

$$\begin{aligned}
& 4 + 2 = 6 \\
\text{then} \;\; & 6 \times 6 = 36 \\
\text{then} \;\; & 3 + 36 = 39 \\
\text{then} \;\; & 3 \times 39 = 117.
\end{aligned}$$

Similarly: $1 + 6 \times 3 = 19,$
but $(1 + 6) \times 3 = 21.$

Pocket calculators compute values following the order of calculation described above. Therefore, in circumstances in which brackets are required to avoid ambiguity, calculations must be undertaken in unambiguous stages. This is circumvented on some calculators by the presence of appropriate bracket keys on the keypad.

Magnitude notation

$>$ = greater than (e.g., $6 > 5$)
$<$ = less than (e.g., $5 < 6$)
$\geq$ = greater than or equal to
$\leq$ = less than or equal to

A vertical line through any of these symbols means 'not', for example $\ngtr$ means 'not greater than'.

Approximation notation

The symbol $\simeq$, read as 'approximately equal to', is used to indicate approximation. For example, the base of natural logarithms $e = 2.718281 \ldots$, and may be written as $e \simeq 2.72$.

Estimation notation

Parameters are frequently estimated from a **sample** of a population. The sample produces an **estimate** of the population parameter. An estimate is indicated either by $\hat{\;}$ (a 'hat') or by a single asterisk, $*$. Thus, a sample estimate of disease prevalence is presented as either $\hat{P}$ (P 'hat') or $P*$. The 'hat' notation is used in this book.

Factorial notation: x!

$x!$ is used to denote the successive multiplication of all positive integers (whole numbers) between x and 1. For example:

$$6! = 6 \times 5 \times 4 \times 3 \times 2 \times 1 = 720$$
$$2! = 2 \times 1 = 2$$
$$1! = 1.$$

Note that $0!$ conventionally equals 1.

Modulus notation: |x|

Vertical lines on each side of a numerical quantity, x, mean that the positive sign of the value of x should be used. The value thus obtained is known as the **absolute value** of x. For example, $|-2|$ is read as $+2$. Similarly $|-6+1|$ will simplify to $|-5|$ which is read as $+5$. Also, $-6 + 1 = -5$, but $|-6| + 1 = 7$.

Appendix III

Some computer software

This appendix lists some computer software packages that are of value to veterinary epidemiology. The list is not exhaustive; emphasis is placed on the simpler analytical packages, rather than on software suitable for multivariate analyses. The descriptions of the various packages also differ in the degree of detail and, for some packages, the list is hardly more than enumerative, but should be sufficient to allow potential users to identify appropriate software. Some of the packages are extracted from a more comprehensive list of epidemiological software, compiled by Kevin Sullivan and David Foster.* The specification of many general packages is listed in software guides (e.g., *The Good Software Guide**).

Relevant references are in square brackets, following the names of the packages (package manuals are not included).

Most of the packages run in the *MS DOS* environment on IBM 'desk-top' Personal Computers and similar 'clones'. Some of the packages are also produced for different environments (e.g., *MINITAB* is also available for Macintosh microcomputers, and *SAS* and *SPSS* are available as both microcomputer and mainframe versions). Some packages will interface with other software (e.g., files from the *PARADOX* relational database can be exported to the *LOTUS 1-2-3* spreadsheet), providing a comprehensive computing environment.

Potential users should ensure that their computers have sufficient memory (RAM) and disk space to run the packages efficiently. Additionally, appropriate hardware may be required to achieve maximum benefit (e.g., packages that include high-resolution graphics produce the best results on a laser printer).

The main addresses of suppliers are listed. Some suppliers also have local offices in various countries. To order software from the *Epidemiology Monitor*, write to: The Epidemiology Monitor, Software Inventory/Library, 2560 Whisper Wind Court, Roswell, GA 30076, USA.

---

*Available from Dr Kevin Sullivan, Division of Epidemiology, Emory School of Public Health, 1599 Clifton Road NE, Atlanta, GA 30329, USA.

**Absolute Research Ltd, Absolute House, 124 Leavesden Road, Watford, WD2 5EG, UK.

Package	Functions	Further information/Supplier
AGG [Donald *et al.*, 1994)	Aggregate-level sensitivity and specificity	A. Donald Department of Health Management, Atlantic Veterinary College, University of Prince Edward Island, Charlottetown, P.E.I. C1A 4P3, Canada
BIN20M [Guess *et al.*, 1987; Guess and Thomas, 1990]	Exact binomial confidence intervals for relative risks for stratified cohort studies (incidence rate data)	*Epidemiology Monitor*
BMDP	Comprehensive data analyses	BMDP Statistical Software, 1440 Sepulveda Blvd, Suite 316, Los Angeles, CA 90025, USA
CIA [Gardner and Altman, 1989]	Confidence interval calculation: means and their differences, proportions and their differences, regression and correlation, relative risks and odds ratios, standardized rates and ratios, survival analyses, medians and their differences	British Medical Association, Tavistock Square, London, WC1H 9JR, UK
dEPID	Stratified analyses and standardization	*Epidemiology Monitor*
EGRET	Descriptive statistics Contingency tables (relative risks and odds ratios), logistic regression, survival analysis	Statistics and Epidemiology Research Corporation, 909 Northeast 43rd Street, Suite 202, Seattle, WA 98105, USA
EISSTATS (requires *LOTUS 1-2-3* spreadsheet)	Sample size and power calculations Point and interval estimates of relative risks and odds ratios	*Epidemiology Monitor*
EPIDEMO	Descriptive statistics Diagnostic test parameters: point estimates, and graphical representation of sensitivity, specificity, predictive value, *kappa* Surveys: simple random and cluster sampling Sample size determination: surveys, proportions and their differences, differences between means Observational studies: relative risk, odds ratio, attributable risk, aetiological fraction Reed-Frost model (deterministic) Markov chain model Outbreak investigation	M. Beiboer Weibuorren 14b, 9247 BB Ureterp, The Netherlands

Package	Functions	Further information/Supplier
EPIDSIM [Foster and Sullivan, 1989a]	Reed—Frost model (stochastic)	*Epidemiology Monitor*

EPI INFO	Questionnaire design
	Descriptive statistics and graphics
	Surveys:
	    simple random, stratified
	    and cluster sampling
	Contingency tables:
	    point and interval estimates
	    of relative risks and odds ratios,
	    simple and stratified analyses,
	    χ^2 and Fisher's exact tests,
	    χ^2 test for trend
	Sample size determination:
	    surveys,
	    case—control, cohort and
	    cross-sectional studies
		USD Incorporated,
		2075-A West Park Place,
		Stone Mountain,
		GA 30087, USA

EPI PAK	Sample size and power calculations Exact confidence intervals for odds ratios and proportions, approximate confidence intervals for rates and population attributable risk	*Epidemiology Monitor*

EPISCOPE
(requires *SUPERCALC*
spreadsheet)
[Frankena *et al.*, 1990]
	Diagnostic test parameters:
	    Point and interval
	    estimates of sensitivity,
	    specificity, predictive
	    value, *kappa*
	Sample size determination:
	    detection of disease,
	    proportions and their
	    differences, differences
	    between means
	Observational studies:
	    simple, stratified and matched
	    case—control studies,
	    simple and stratified cohort
	    studies (cumulative incidence
	    and incidence rate data)
	Reed—Frost model (deterministic)
		K. Frankena,
		Department of Animal Husbandry,
		Wageningen Agricultural University,
		PO Box 338,
		6700 AH Wageningen,
		The Netherlands

EPISHEET
(requires *LOTUS 1-2-3* or
SUPERCALC spreadsheet)
[Gerstman, 1987]
	Sample size calculations:
	    case—control and cohort studies
	Observational studies:
	    simple, stratified and matched
	    case—control studies
	    simple and stratified cohort
	    studies (incidence rate data)
	Exact binomial confidence intervals
	for proportions
		Epidemiology Monitor

Package	Functions	Further information/Supplier
EPISTAT [Roberts and Cohen, 1985; Goldstein, 1988; Zeiger, 1990]	General statistical analyser for small or moderate-sized data sets: t-tests, contingency tables, Fisher's exact test, correlation and regression, rate adjustment, power analysis for rates	*Epidemiology Monitor*
EXACT [Martin and Austin, 1991]	Exact confidence limits for matched and unmatched odds ratios	*Epidemiology Monitor*
EXACTBIN	Exact binomial confidence intervals for proportions	*Epidemiology Monitor*
GLIM	Logistic regression	Numerical Algorithms Group, 7 Banbury Road, Oxford OX2 6NN, UK
IC2X2 [Thomas, 1975; Thomas and Gart, 1992]	Exact and approximate methods for odds ratios. Point and interval estimates of attributable risk	*Epidemiology Monitor*
IDR	Exact confidence intervals for relative risks	*Epidemiology Monitor*
KWIKSTAT [Elliott, 1988]	Descriptive statistics. Elementary analyses: t-tests, χ^2 test, Fisher's exact test, regression, life tables	*Epidemiology Monitor*
LOGRESS [McGee, 1986]	Logistic regression	*Epidemiology Monitor*
MHCHI	Calculation of variance of the Mantel–Haenszel odds ratio for matched and unmatched data, assessment of effect modification	*Epidemiology Monitor*
MINITAB	Data editing and sorting, arithmetic, data plotting, basic statistics, regression, analysis of variance, multivariate analysis, non-parametric analysis, tables, time series, exploratory data analysis	Minitab Inc., 3081 Enterprise Drive, State College, PA 16801-2756, USA
MLEPID [Foster and Sullivan, 1989b]	Exact methods for relative risk	*Epidemiology Monitor*
MULTLR [Campos Filho and Franco, 1989]	Logistic regression analysis of case–control data	*Epidemiology Monitor*

Package	Functions	Further information/Supplier
ORACLE	Relational database	Oracle Corporation, 20 Davis Drive, Belmont, CA 94002, USA
PANACEA	Data editing and sorting, data plotting, basic statistics, regression, analysis of variance	PAN Livestock Services Ltd, Department of Agriculture, University of Reading, PO Box 236, Reading G6 2AT, UK
PAR (requires *LOTUS 1-2-3* spreadsheet)	Estimation of population attributable risk	*Epidemiology Monitor*
PARADOX	Relational database	Borland International, 1800 Green Hills Road, PO Box 660001, Scotts Valley, CA 95067-0001, USA
PC-AGREE [Holman, 1984]	*Kappa* values and their standard errors	*Epidemiology Monitor*
POWERSIM	General simulation modelling	Powersim AS, Nygaten 3, Postboks 642, N-5001 Bergen, Norway
RISK (Requires *EXCEL* or *LOTUS 1-2-3* spreadsheet)	Quantitative risk analysis	Palisade Corporation, 31 Decker Road, Newfield, NY 14867, USA
SAS	Comprehensive statistical analyses	SAS Inc., SAS Campus Drive, Cary, NC 27513, USA
SPSS	Comprehensive statistical analyses	SPSS Inc., 444 N. Michegan Avenue, Chicago, IL 60611, USA
STATGRAPHICS	Data editing and sorting	STSC Inc., 2115 East Jefferson Street, Rockville, MD 20852, USA
STATISTICAL POWER ANALYSIS [Cohen, 1988]	Power calculations	LEA Associates, 365 Broadway, Hillsdale, NJ 07642, USA
STATXACT	Exact *p*-values for contingency tables and non-parametric tests	Cytel Software Corporation, 137 Erie Street, Cambridge, MA 02139, USA
XCLOR [Vollset and Hirji, 1991; Vollset *et al.*, 1991]	Exact and approximate tests and confidence intervals for odds ratios for a single and several 2×2 tables	S. Vollset Section for Medical Informatics and Statistics, University of Bergen, Armauer Hansens Hus, Haukeland sykehus, 5021 Bergen, Norway

Appendix IV

Student's *t*-distribution

Degrees of freedom	.9	.8	.7	.6	.5	.4	.3	.2	.1	.05	.02	.01	.001
1	.158	.325	.510	.727	1.000	1.376	1.963	3.078	6.314	12.706	31.821	63.657	636.619
2	.142	.289	.445	.617	.816	1.061	1.386	1.886	2.920	4.303	6.965	9.925	31.598
3	.137	.277	.424	.584	.765	.978	1.250	1.638	2.353	3.182	4.541	5.841	12.924
4	.134	.271	.414	.569	.741	.941	1.190	1.533	2.132	2.776	3.747	4.604	8.610
5	.132	.267	.408	.559	.727	.920	1.156	1.476	2.015	2.571	3.365	4.032	6.869
6	.131	.265	.404	.553	.718	.906	1.134	1.440	1.943	2.447	3.143	3.707	5.959
7	.130	.263	.402	.549	.711	.896	1.119	1.415	1.895	2.365	2.998	3.499	5.408
8	.130	.262	.399	.546	.706	.889	1.108	1.397	1.860	2.306	2.896	3.355	5.041
9	.129	.261	.398	.543	.703	.883	1.100	1.383	1.833	2.262	2.821	3.250	4.781
10	.129	.260	.397	.542	.700	.879	1.093	1.372	1.812	2.228	2.764	3.169	4.587
11	.129	.260	.396	.540	.697	.876	1.088	1.363	1.796	2.201	2.718	3.106	4.437
12	.128	.259	.395	.539	.695	.873	1.083	1.356	1.782	2.179	2.681	3.055	4.318
13	.128	.259	.394	.538	.694	.870	1.079	1.350	1.771	2.160	2.650	3.012	4.221
14	.128	.258	.393	.537	.692	.868	1.076	1.345	1.761	2.145	2.624	2.977	4.140
15	.128	.258	.393	.536	.691	.866	1.074	1.341	1.753	2.131	2.602	2.947	4.073
16	.128	.258	.392	.535	.690	.865	1.071	1.337	1.746	2.120	2.583	2.921	4.015
17	.128	.257	.392	.534	.689	.863	1.069	1.333	1.740	2.110	2.567	2.898	3.965
18	.127	.257	.392	.534	.688	.862	1.067	1.330	1.734	2.101	2.552	2.878	3.922
19	.127	.257	.391	.533	.688	.861	1.066	1.328	1.729	2.093	2.539	2.861	3.883
20	.127	.257	.391	.533	.687	.860	1.064	1.325	1.725	2.086	2.528	2.845	3.850
21	.127	.257	.391	.532	.686	.859	1.063	1.323	1.721	2.080	2.518	2.831	3.819
22	.127	.256	.390	.532	.686	.858	1.061	1.321	1.717	2.074	2.508	2.819	3.792
23	.127	.256	.390	.532	.685	.858	1.060	1.319	1.714	2.069	2.500	2.807	3.767
24	.127	.256	.390	.531	.685	.857	1.059	1.318	1.711	2.064	2.492	2.797	3.745
25	.127	.256	.390	.531	.684	.856	1.058	1.316	1.708	2.060	2.485	2.787	3.725
26	.127	.256	.390	.531	.684	.856	1.058	1.315	1.706	2.056	2.479	2.779	3.707
27	.127	.256	.389	.531	.684	.855	1.057	1.314	1.703	2.052	2.473	2.771	3.690
28	.127	.256	.389	.530	.683	.855	1.056	1.313	1.701	2.048	2.467	2.763	3.674
29	.127	.256	.389	.530	.683	.854	1.055	1.311	1.699	2.045	2.462	2.756	3.659
30	.127	.256	.389	.530	.683	.854	1.055	1.310	1.697	2.042	2.457	2.750	3.646
40	.126	.255	.388	.529	.681	.851	1.050	1.303	1.684	2.021	2.423	2.704	3.551
60	.126	.254	.387	.527	.679	.848	1.046	1.296	1.671	2.000	2.390	2.660	3.460
120	.126	.254	.386	.526	.677	.845	1.041	1.289	1.658	1.980	2.358	2.617	3.373
∞	.126	.253	.385	.524	.674	.842	1.036	1.282	1.645	1.960	2.326	2.576	3.291

Header spanning columns .9 to .001: *Probability*

The table gives the percentage points most frequently required for significance tests and confidence limits based on Student's *t*-distribution. Thus the probability of observing a value of *t*, with 10 degrees of freedom, greater in **absolute value** than 3.169 (i.e. < -3.169 or $> +3.169$) is exactly 0.01 or 1 per cent.

Appendix V

Multipliers used in the construction of confidence intervals based on the Normal distribution, for selected levels of confidence

These multipliers are based on two-tailed probabilities for
critical significance levels, extracted from Appendix XII.

Confidence interval	80%	90%	95%	99%	99.9%
Multiplier	1.282	1.645	1.960	2.576	3.291

Appendix VI

Technique for selecting a simple random sample

Example: An investigator requires a random sample of 10 animals from a population of 90.

Construct a sampling frame of all animals and label them consecutively from 1 to 90. The random numbers in the table overleaf are arranged in groups of two columns for visual convenience (other tables may have different numbers of columns grouped together).

(1) Select two columns arbitrarily, to correspond to tens and units — use columns 27 and 28 for visual convenience.
(2) Select a row arbitrarily — say row 7: number 89.
(3) Move down the columns: 89, 97, 32, 21, 60, 48, 10, 98, 23, 89, 08, 15, 44, 68 . . . . All numbers greater than 90 are ignored. The first 10 numbers are then: 89, 32, 21, 60, 48, 10, 23, 89, 08, 15.

(4) Number 89 has been selected twice. The second 89 should be rejected* and the next available number chosen: 44.

The sample size of 10 is then made up of animals labelled 89, 32, 21, 60, 48, 10, 23, 8, 15, 44.

If the table is used repeatedly, then the row and column starting point should be changed.

---

*Rejection of numbers that occur more than once is performed if animals are not returned to the selection pool after having been selected once: sampling 'without replacement'. If animals are returned to the pool after having been selected once, so that they can be selected again — sampling 'with replacement' — then a number corresponding to an animal can be selected more than once (number 89 in this example).

Table of random numbers.   (Extracted from Lindley and Scott, 1984.)

84 42	56 53	87 75	18 91	76 66	64 83	97 11	69 41	80 92	38 75
28 87	77 03	57 09	85 86	46 86	40 15	31 81	78 91	30 22	88 58
64 12	39 65	37 93	76 46	11 09	56 28	94 54	10 14	30 73	80 30
49 41	73 76	49 64	06 70	99 37	72 60	39 16	02 26	91 90	16 54
06 46	69 31	24 33	52 67	85 07	01 33	16 33	43 98	17 62	52 52
75 56	96 97	65 20	68 68	60 97	90 46	63 37	10 34	41 64	85 01
09 35	89 97	97 10	00 76	39 82	49 94	15 89	60 65	57 03	91 68
73 81	11 08	52 73	64 85	22 72	85 16	15 97	76 28	41 95	00 33
49 69	80 41	46 62	26 32	58 16	88 76	54 32	06 37	46 45	28 95
64 60	49 70	33 73	71 57	83 26	19 25	86 21	64 60	11 01	86 70
93 05	36 44	59 19	99 51	54 21	37 48	18 60	22 92	68 34	39 02
39 88	11 26	68 92	81 14	12 16	37 64	61 48	21 69	77 76	33 00
89 34	19 12	83 76	35 11	96 53	04 76	63 10	93 68	52 42	73 20
77 29	03 26	45 36	15 17	27 28	79 58	38 98	73 52	63 72	48 41
86 75	51 29	70 78	24 78	94 78	64 17	32 23	95 52	87 79	14 30
95 98	77 51	14 65	76 49	42 36	11 33	23 89	32 01	60 48	91 44
22 09	01 14	04 96	97 56	92 52	83 44	45 08	72 78	10 36	26 70
30 49	36 23	36 81	11 76	91 08	67 60	01 15	64 77	21 33	72 29
77 59	88 92	17 75	04 47	18 02	94 84	71 44	87 63	06 04	49 33
03 50	80 26	74 74	18 85	92 20	64 39	98 68	29 26	90 14	77 36
46 32	79 69	41 06	26 04	47 24	67 10	66 69	21 55	66 63	48 47
65 73	98 08	05 96	92 27	22 86	54 87	95 87	40 27	09 97	47 21
68 82	77 73	08 37	28 47	73 49	10 65	53 48	87 74	02 99	52 86
93 98	12 19	82 69	61 08	00 42	88 83	70 85	08 48	74 94	88 61
61 27	39 16	42 17	89 81	27 44	12 33	43 24	92 41	55 13	45 01
54 74	04 79	72 61	21 87	23 83	96 56	97 63	67 02	67 30	36 89
28 00	40 86	92 97	06 22	37 37	83 00	97 17	08 06	43 95	76 84
61 78	71 16	41 01	69 63	35 96	60 65	09 44	93 42	72 11	22 85
68 60	92 99	60 97	53 55	34 61	43 40	77 96	19 87	63 49	22 47
21 76	13 39	25 89	91 38	25 19	44 33	11 36	72 21	40 90	76 95
73 59	53 04	35 13	12 31	88 70	05 40	43 42	47 17	03 86	14 10
85 68	66 48	05 24	28 97	84 84	91 65	62 83	89 68	07 51	01 02
60 30	10 46	44 34	19 56	00 83	20 53	53 05	29 03	47 55	23 26
44 63	80 62	80 80	99 43	33 87	70 52	51 62	02 12	02 90	44 44
89 38	13 68	31 31	97 15	35 67	23 74	76 96	62 82	62 19	65 58
55 20	77 12	79 81	42 15	30 67	88 83	69 08	99 82	20 39	92 40
67 40	42 16	46 06	60 74	61 22	95 47	24 62	81 06	19 67	15 06
57 19	76 98	65 64	55 28	34 03	58 62	35 22	67 40	04 88	17 59
21 72	97 04	82 62	09 54	35 17	22 73	35 72	53 65	95 48	55 12
46 89	95 61	31 77	14 14	24 14	91 58	76 56	19 33	98 67	09 04
99 73	85 64	96 58	61 65	60 83	62 10	87 00	82 63	39 90	83 17
85 52	98 27	40 33	09 59	80 17	22 06	84 03	41 48	76 07	26 69
50 12	17 86	50 57	91 28	42 29	83 87	00 87	93 52	53 47	08 65
92 84	02 93	44 36	93 19	08 54	76 62	31 65	94 68	38 04	62 31
69 74	30 25	68 65	19 77	57 05	71 56	91 30	16 66	70 48	78 65
51 69	76 00	20 92	58 21	24 33	74 08	66 90	61 89	56 83	39 58
27 25	81 29	75 02	85 09	58 89	77 83	03 40	21 14	45 90	54 01
44 03	62 96	68 65	24 57	44 43	07 72	59 16	04 94	23 36	55 85
40 59	49 20	48 63	35 74	33 12	96 25	59 35	07 45	80 97	19 90
92 91	07 14	82 22	50 70	75 15	69 71	31 20	60 06	99 56	57 74

Appendix VII

Sample sizes

This Appendix comprises sample sizes required to attain a desired confidence interval around expected prevalence values of 5%, 10%, 20%, 30%, 40% and 50% (from WHO, 1973). For example, if the expected prevalence is 30%, consult *Figure 4*. A sample size of 200 will produce a 95% confidence interval of 24% to 36%. A sample size of 800 will produce a 95% confidence interval of 27% to 33%.

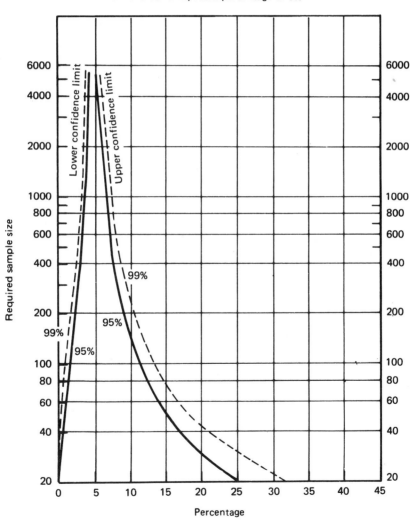

Sample size required to attain desired confidence interval around expected percentage of 5%

Figure 1

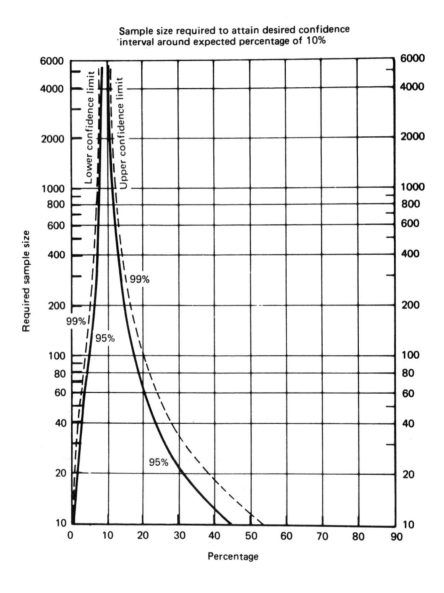

Sample size required to attain desired confidence interval around expected percentage of 10%

Figure 2

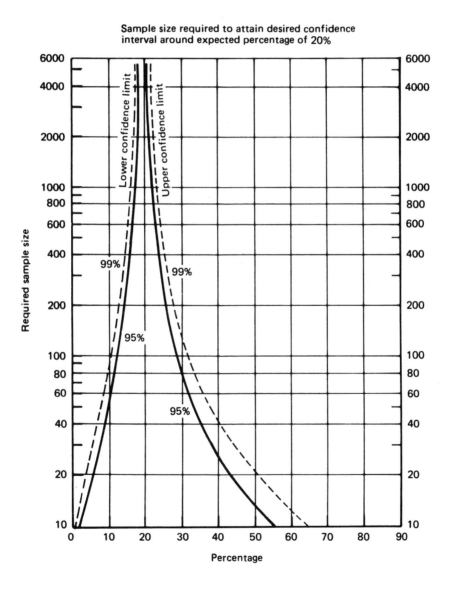

Sample size required to attain desired confidence interval around expected percentage of 20%

Figure 3

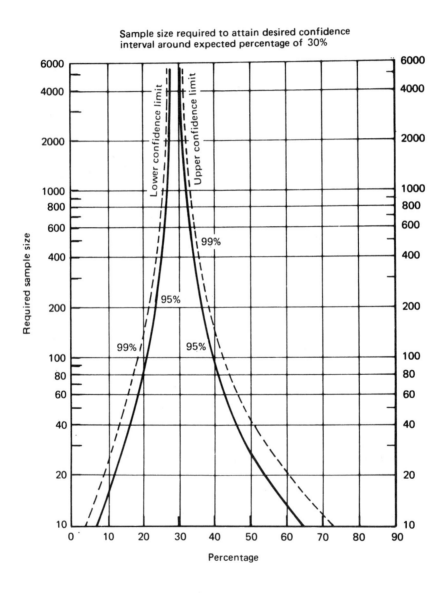

Sample size required to attain desired confidence interval around expected percentage of 30%

Figure 4

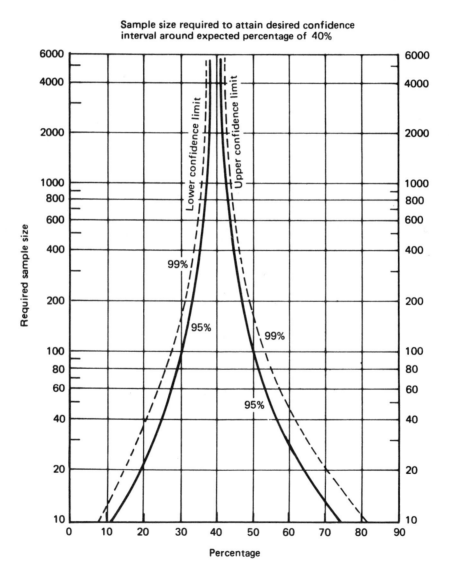

Sample size required to attain desired confidence interval around expected percentage of 40%

Figure 5

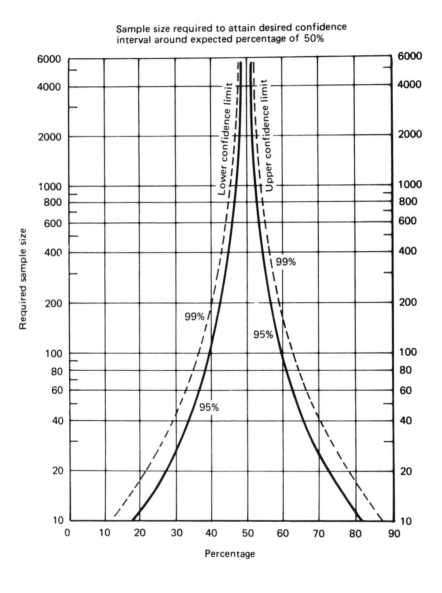

Sample size required to attain desired confidence interval around expected percentage of 50%

Figure 6

Appendix VIII

The probability of detecting a small number of cases in a population
(Modified from Cannon and Roe, 1982)

These tables give the probability of detecting at least one case for different sampling fractions and numbers of cases in the population.

Example: A 40% sample from a herd of 20 animals would have a 97.6% chance of including at least one positive if six were present in the herd.

20% Sampling

| Population size | Number sampled | Number of positives in the population | | | | | | | |
		1	2	3	4	5	6	7	8
10	2	0.200	0.378	0.533	0.667	0.778	0.867	0.933	0.978
20	4	0.200	0.368	0.509	0.624	0.718	0.793	0.852	0.898
30	6	0.200	0.366	0.501	0.612	0.702	0.773	0.830	0.874
40	8	0.200	0.364	0.498	0.607	0.694	0.764	0.819	0.863
50	10	0.200	0.363	0.498	0.603	0.689	0.758	0.813	0.857
60	12	0.200	0.363	0.495	0.601	0.686	0.755	0.809	0.853
70	14	0.200	0.362	0.494	0.599	0.684	0.752	0.807	0.850
80	16	0.200	0.362	0.493	0.598	0.683	0.751	0.804	0.847
90	18	0.200	0.362	0.492	0.597	0.682	0.749	0.803	0.846
100	20	0.200	0.362	0.492	0.597	0.681	0.748	0.802	0.844
∞	∞	0.200	0.360	0.486	0.590	0.672	0.738	0.790	0.832

30% Sampling

| Population size | Number sampled | Number of positives in the population | | | | | | | |
		1	2	3	4	5	6	7	8
10	3	0.300	0.533	0.708	0.833	0.917	0.967	0.992	1.000
20	6	0.300	0.521	0.681	0.793	0.871	0.923	0.956	0.976
30	9	0.300	0.517	0.672	0.782	0.857	0.909	0.943	0.965
40	12	0.300	0.515	0.668	0.776	0.851	0.902	0.936	0.960
50	15	0.300	0.514	0.666	0.773	0.847	0.898	0.933	0.956
60	18	0.300	0.514	0.665	0.770	0.844	0.895	0.930	0.954
70	21	0.300	0.513	0.663	0.769	0.842	0.893	0.928	0.952
80	24	0.300	0.513	0.663	0.768	0.841	0.892	0.927	0.951
90	27	0.300	0.512	0.662	0.767	0.840	0.891	0.926	0.950
100	30	0.300	0.512	0.661	0.766	0.839	0.890	0.925	0.949
∞	∞	0.300	0.510	0.657	0.760	0.832	0.882	0.918	0.942

40% Sampling

Population size	Number sampled	Number of positives in the population							
		1	2	3	4	5	6	7	8
10	4	0.400	0.667	0.833	0.929	0.976	0.995	1.000	1.000
20	8	0.400	0.653	0.807	0.898	0.949	0.976	0.990	0.996
30	12	0.400	0.648	0.799	0.888	0.940	0.969	0.984	0.993
40	16	0.400	0.646	0.795	0.884	0.935	0.965	0.981	0.990
50	20	0.400	0.645	0.793	0.881	0.933	0.963	0.980	0.989
60	24	0.400	0.644	0.791	0.879	0.931	0.961	0.978	0.988
70	28	0.400	0.643	0.790	0.878	0.930	0.960	0.977	0.987
80	32	0.400	0.643	0.789	0.877	0.929	0.959	0.977	0.987
90	36	0.400	0.643	0.789	0.876	0.928	0.959	0.976	0.987
100	40	0.400	0.642	0.788	0.876	0.927	0.958	0.976	0.986
∞	∞	0.400	0.640	0.784	0.870	0.922	0.953	0.972	0.983

50% Sampling

Population size	Number sampled	Number of positives in the population							
		1	2	3	4	5	6	7	8
10	5	0.500	0.778	0.917	0.976	0.996	1.000	1.000	1.000
20	10	0.500	0.763	0.895	0.957	0.984	0.995	0.998	0.994
30	15	0.500	0.759	0.888	0.950	0.979	0.992	0.997	0.999
40	20	0.500	0.756	0.885	0.947	0.976	0.990	0.996	0.998
50	25	0.500	0.755	0.883	0.945	0.975	0.989	0.995	0.998
60	30	0.500	0.754	0.881	0.944	0.974	0.988	0.995	0.998
70	35	0.500	0.754	0.880	0.943	0.973	0.988	0.994	0.998
80	40	0.500	0.753	0.880	0.942	0.973	0.987	0.994	0.997
90	45	0.500	0.753	0.879	0.942	0.972	0.987	0.994	0.997
100	50	0.500	0.753	0.879	0.941	0.972	0.987	0.994	0.997
∞	∞	0.500	0.750	0.875	0.937	0.969	0.984	0.992	0.996

60% Sampling

Population size	Number sampled	Number of positives in the population							
		1	2	3	4	5	6	7	8
10	6	0.600	0.867	0.967	0.994	1.000	1.000	1.000	1.000
20	12	0.600	0.853	0.951	0.986	0.994	0.997	1.000	1.000
30	18	0.600	0.848	0.946	0.982	0.994	0.997	1.000	1.000
40	24	0.600	0.846	0.943	0.980	0.993	0.997	0.999	1.000
50	30	0.600	0.845	0.942	0.979	0.993	0.997	0.999	1.000
60	36	0.600	0.844	0.941	0.978	0.992	0.997	0.999	1.000
70	42	0.600	0.843	0.940	0.978	0.992	0.997	0.999	1.000
80	48	0.600	0.843	0.940	0.977	0.992	0.997	0.999	1.000
90	54	0.600	0.843	0.939	0.977	0.991	0.997	0.999	1.000
100	60	0.600	0.842	0.939	0.977	0.991	0.997	0.999	1.000
∞	∞	0.600	0.840	0.936	0.974	0.990	0.996	0.998	1.000

Appendix IX

The probability of failure to detect cases in a population
(From Cannon and Roe, 1982)

The table gives the probability of failure to detect diseased animals from an 'infinite' population with the specified proportion of positives in the population.

Example: Tests of a series of random samples of 25 animals from a large population in which 10% of animals are positive would fail to detect any positives in 7.2% of such sample groups.

Prevalence	Number of animals in sample tested									
	5	*10*	*25*	*50*	*75*	*100*	*200*	*250*	*500*	*1000*
1%	0.951	0.904	0.778	0.605	0.471	0.366	0.134	0.081	0.007	0.000
2%	0.904	0.817	0.603	0.364	0.220	0.133	0.018	0.006	0.000	
3%	0.859	0.737	0.467	0.218	0.102	0.048	0.002	0.000		
4%	0.815	0.665	0.360	0.130	0.047	0.017	0.000			
5%	0.774	0.599	0.277	0.077	0.021	0.006	0.000			
6%	0.734	0.539	0.213	0.045	0.010	0.002	0.000			
7%	0.696	0.484	0.163	0.027	0.004	0.001	0.000			
8%	0.659	0.434	0.124	0.015	0.002	0.000				
9%	0.624	0.389	0.095	0.009	0.001	0.000				
10%	0.590	0.349	0.072	0.005	0.000					
12%	0.528	0.279	0.041	0.002	0.000					
14%	0.470	0.221	0.023	0.001	0.000					
16%	0.418	0.175	0.013	0.000						
18%	0.371	0.137	0.007	0.000						
20%	0.328	0.107	0.004	0.000						
24%	0.254	0.064	0.001	0.000						
28%	0.193	0.037	0.000							
32%	0.145	0.021	0.000							
36%	0.107	0.012	0.000							
40%	0.078	0.006	0.000							
50%	0.031	0.001	0.000							
60%	0.010	0.000								

Appendix X

Values of exact 95% confidence limits for proportions
(From Beyer, 1968)

These tables give exact confidence limits for a proportion, based on the binomial distribution. The first (x) column indicates the numerator in the proportion; the first $(n-x)$ row indicates the sample size; n, minus the numerator, x. For example, if 14 animals were sampled, of which 6 were diseased, then $x = 6$, $n = 14$, and $n-x = 8$. Thus, the point estimate of prevalence is $6/14 = 0.428$ (42.8%) and, from the table, the interval estimate $= 0.177, 0.711$ (17.7%, 71.1%).

| | | *Denominator minus numerator $(n-x)$* | | | | | | | | |
		1	*2*	*3*	*4*	*5*	*6*	*7*	*8*	*9*
	0	**975**	**842**	**708**	**602**	**522**	**459**	**410**	**369**	**336**
		000	000	000	000	000	000	000	000	000
	1	**987**	**906**	**806**	**716**	**641**	**579**	**527**	**483**	**445**
		013	008	006	005	004	004	003	003	003
	2	**992**	**932**	**853**	**777**	**710**	**651**	**600**	**556**	**518**
		094	068	053	043	037	032	028	025	023
	3	**994**	**947**	**882**	**816**	**755**	**701**	**652**	**610**	**572**
		194	147	118	099	085	075	067	060	055
	4	**995**	**957**	**901**	**843**	**788**	**738**	**692**	**651**	**614**
		284	223	184	157	137	122	109	099	091
	5	**996**	**968**	**915**	**863**	**813**	**766**	**723**	**684**	**649**
		359	290	245	212	187	167	151	139	128
	6	**996**	**968**	**925**	**878**	**833**	**789**	**749**	**711**	**677**
		421	349	299	262	234	211	192	177	163
	7	**997**	**972**	**933**	**891**	**849**	**808**	**770**	**734**	**701**
		473	400	348	308	277	251	230	213	198
	8	**997**	**975**	**940**	**901**	**861**	**823**	**787**	**753**	**722**
		517	444	390	349	316	289	266	247	230
	9	**997**	**977**	**945**	**909**	**872**	**837**	**802**	**770**	**740**
		555	482	428	386	351	323	299	278	260
	10	**998**	**979**	**950**	**916**	**882**	**848**	**816**	**785**	**756**
		587	516	462	419	384	354	329	308	289
	11	**998**	**981**	**953**	**922**	**890**	**858**	**827**	**797**	**769**
		615	546	492	449	413	383	357	335	315

Numerator of the proportion (x)

	Denominator minus numerator $(n-x)$								
	1	*2*	*3*	*4*	*5*	*6*	*7*	*8*	*9*
12	**998**	**982**	**957**	**927**	**897**	**867**	**837**	**809**	**782**
	640	572	519	476	440	410	384	361	340
13	**998**	**983**	**960**	**932**	**903**	**874**	**846**	**819**	**793**
	661	595	544	501	465	435	408	384	364
14	**998**	**984**	**962**	**936**	**909**	**881**	**854**	**828**	**803**
	681	617	566	524	488	457	430	407	385
15	**998**	**985**	**964**	**939**	**913**	**887**	**861**	**836**	**812**
	698	636	586	544	509	478	451	427	406
16	**999**	**986**	**966**	**943**	**918**	**893**	**868**	**844**	**820**
	713	653	604	563	529	498	471	447	425
17	**999**	**987**	**968**	**946**	**922**	**898**	**874**	**851**	**828**
	727	669	621	581	547	516	488	465	443
18	**999**	**988**	**970**	**948**	**925**	**902**	**879**	**857**	**835**
	740	683	637	597	564	533	506	482	460
19	**999**	**988**	**971**	**950**	**929**	**906**	**884**	**862**	**841**
	751	696	651	612	579	549	522	498	476
20	**999**	**989**	**972**	**953**	**932**	**910**	**889**	**868**	**847**
	762	708	664	626	593	564	537	513	492
22	**999**	**990**	**975**	**956**	**937**	**917**	**897**	**877**	**858**
	781	730	688	651	619	590	565	541	519
24	**999**	**991**	**976**	**960**	**942**	**923**	**904**	**885**	**867**
	797	749	708	673	642	614	589	566	545
26	**999**	**991**	**978**	**962**	**945**	**928**	**910**	**893**	**875**
	810	765	726	693	663	636	611	588	567
28	**999**	**992**	**980**	**965**	**949**	**932**	**916**	**899**	**882**
	822	779	743	710	681	655	631	609	588
30	**999**	**992**	**981**	**967**	**952**	**936**	**920**	**904**	**889**
	833	792	757	725	697	672	649	627	607
35	**999**	**993**	**983**	**971**	**958**	**944**	**930**	**916**	**902**
	855	818	786	758	732	708	686	666	647
40	**999**	**994**	**985**	**975**	**963**	**951**	**938**	**925**	**912**
	871	838	809	783	759	737	717	698	679
45	**999**	**995**	**987**	**977**	**967**	**956**	**944**	**933**	**921**
	885	855	828	804	782	761	742	724	707
50	**1000**	**995**	**988**	**979**	**970**	**960**	**949**	**939**	**928**
	896	868	843	821	800	781	763	746	730
60	**1000**	**996**	**990**	**983**	**975**	**966**	**957**	**948**	**939**
	912	888	867	848	830	813	797	782	767
80	**1000**	**997**	**992**	**987**	**981**	**974**	**967**	**960**	**953**
	933	915	898	882	868	855	842	820	816
100	**1000**	**998**	**994**	**989**	**984**	**979**	**973**	**967**	**962**
	946	931	917	904	892	881	870	859	849
200	**1000**	**999**	**997**	**995**	**992**	**989**	**986**	**983**	**980**
	973	965	957	951	944	938	932	926	920
500	**1000**	**1000**	**999**	**998**	**997**	**996**	**995**	**993**	**992**
	989	986	983	980	977	974	972	969	967
∞	**1000**	**1000**	**1000**	**1000**	**1000**	**1000**	**1000**	**1000**	**1000**
	1000	1000	1000	1000	1000	1000	1000	1000	1000

Numerator of the proportion (x)

	Denominator minus numerator $(n-x)$								
	10	11	12	13	14	15	16	17	18
0	**308**	**285**	**265**	**247**	**232**	**218**	**206**	**195**	**185**
	000	000	000	000	000	000	000	000	000
1	**413**	**385**	**360**	**339**	**319**	**302**	**287**	**273**	**260**
	002	002	002	002	002	002	001	001	001
2	**484**	**454**	**428**	**405**	**383**	**364**	**347**	**331**	**317**
	021	019	018	017	016	015	014	013	012
3	**538**	**508**	**481**	**456**	**434**	**414**	**396**	**379**	**363**
	050	047	043	040	038	036	034	032	030
4	**581**	**551**	**524**	**499**	**476**	**456**	**437**	**419**	**403**
	084	078	073	068	064	061	057	054	052
5	**616**	**587**	**560**	**535**	**512**	**491**	**471**	**453**	**436**
	118	110	103	097	091	087	082	078	075
6	**646**	**617**	**590**	**565**	**543**	**522**	**502**	**484**	**467**
	152	142	133	126	119	113	107	102	098
7	**671**	**643**	**616**	**592**	**570**	**549**	**529**	**512**	**494**
	184	173	163	154	146	139	132	126	121
8	**692**	**665**	**639**	**616**	**593**	**573**	**553**	**535**	**518**
	215	203	191	181	172	164	156	149	143
9	**711**	**685**	**660**	**636**	**615**	**594**	**575**	**557**	**540**
	244	231	218	207	197	188	180	172	165
10	**728**	**702**	**678**	**655**	**634**	**614**	**595**	**577**	**560**
	272	257	244	232	221	211	202	194	186
11	**743**	**718**	**694**	**672**	**651**	**631**	**612**	**594**	**578**
	298	282	268	256	244	234	224	215	207
12	**756**	**732**	**709**	**687**	**666**	**647**	**628**	**611**	**594**
	322	306	291	278	266	255	245	235	227
13	**768**	**744**	**722**	**701**	**680**	**661**	**643**	**626**	**609**
	345	328	313	299	287	275	264	255	245
14	**779**	**756**	**734**	**713**	**694**	**675**	**657**	**640**	**624**
	366	349	334	320	306	295	283	273	264
15	**789**	**766**	**745**	**725**	**705**	**687**	**669**	**653**	**637**
	386	369	353	339	325	313	302	291	281
16	**798**	**776**	**755**	**736**	**717**	**698**	**681**	**665**	**649**
	405	388	372	357	343	331	319	308	298
17	**806**	**785**	**765**	**745**	**727**	**709**	**692**	**676**	**660**
	423	406	389	374	360	347	335	324	314
18	**814**	**793**	**773**	**755**	**736**	**719**	**702**	**686**	**671**
	440	422	406	391	376	363	351	340	329
19	**821**	**801**	**782**	**763**	**745**	**728**	**712**	**696**	**681**
	456	439	422	406	392	379	366	355	344
20	**827**	**808**	**789**	**771**	**753**	**737**	**720**	**705**	**690**
	472	454	437	421	407	393	381	369	358
22	**839**	**820**	**803**	**785**	**768**	**752**	**737**	**722**	**707**
	500	481	465	449	434	421	408	396	385
24	**849**	**831**	**814**	**798**	**782**	**766**	**751**	**737**	**723**
	525	507	490	475	460	446	433	421	410
26	**858**	**841**	**825**	**809**	**794**	**779**	**764**	**750**	**736**
	548	530	513	497	483	469	456	444	432
28	**866**	**850**	**834**	**819**	**804**	**790**	**776**	**762**	**749**
	569	551	535	519	504	491	478	465	453

Numerator of the proportion (x)

		10	11	12	13	14	15	16	17	18
					Denominator minus numerator (n − x)					
Numerator of the proportion (x)	30	**873**	**858**	**843**	**828**	**814**	**800**	**786**	**773**	**760**
		588	571	554	539	524	510	498	485	473
	35	**888**	**874**	**860**	**847**	**834**	**821**	**809**	**797**	**785**
		628	612	596	581	567	554	541	529	517
	40	**900**	**887**	**875**	**862**	**850**	**838**	**827**	**815**	**804**
		662	646	631	616	602	590	578	566	555
	45	**909**	**898**	**886**	**875**	**864**	**853**	**842**	**831**	**821**
		690	675	661	647	633	621	609	598	587
	50	**917**	**906**	**896**	**885**	**875**	**865**	**854**	**844**	**835**
		714	700	686	673	660	648	636	625	614
	60	**929**	**920**	**911**	**902**	**893**	**884**	**874**	**866**	**857**
		752	740	727	715	703	692	681	670	660
	80	**945**	**938**	**931**	**923**	**916**	**909**	**901**	**894**	**887**
		804	793	783	773	763	753	744	734	726
	100	**955**	**949**	**943**	**937**	**931**	**925**	**919**	**913**	**907**
		838	829	820	811	802	794	786	778	770
	200	**977**	**974**	**970**	**967**	**964**	**961**	**957**	**954**	**950**
		914	909	903	898	893	888	883	878	873
	500	**991**	**989**	**988**	**986**	**985**	**984**	**982**	**981**	**979**
		964	962	960	957	955	953	950	948	946
	∞	**1000**	**1000**	**1000**	**1000**	**1000**	**1000**	**1000**	**1000**	**1000**
		1000	1000	1000	1000	1000	1000	1000	1000	1000

		19	20	22	Denominator minus numerator $(n-x)$ 24	26	28	30	35	40
	0	**176**	**168**	**154**	**142**	**132**	**123**	**116**	**100**	**088**
		000	000	000	000	000	000	000	000	000
	1	**249**	**238**	**219**	**203**	**190**	**178**	**167**	**145**	**129**
		001	001	001	001	001	001	001	001	001
	2	**304**	**292**	**270**	**251**	**235**	**221**	**208**	**182**	**162**
		012	011	010	009	009	008	008	007	006
	3	**349**	**336**	**312**	**292**	**274**	**257**	**243**	**214**	**191**
		029	028	025	024	022	020	019	017	015
	4	**388**	**374**	**349**	**327**	**307**	**290**	**275**	**242**	**217**
		050	047	044	040	038	035	033	029	025
	5	**421**	**407**	**381**	**358**	**337**	**319**	**303**	**268**	**241**
		071	068	063	058	055	051	048	042	037
	6	**451**	**436**	**410**	**386**	**364**	**345**	**328**	**292**	**263**
		094	090	083	077	072	068	064	056	049
	7	**478**	**463**	**435**	**411**	**389**	**369**	**351**	**314**	**283**
		116	111	103	096	090	084	080	070	062
	8	**502**	**487**	**459**	**434**	**412**	**391**	**373**	**334**	**302**
		138	132	123	115	107	101	096	084	075
	9	**524**	**508**	**481**	**455**	**433**	**412**	**393**	**353**	**321**
		159	153	142	133	125	118	111	098	088
Numerator of the proportion (x)	10	**544**	**528**	**500**	**475**	**452**	**431**	**412**	**372**	**338**
		179	173	161	151	142	134	127	112	100
	11	**561**	**546**	**519**	**493**	**470**	**449**	**429**	**388**	**354**
		199	192	180	169	159	150	142	126	113
	12	**578**	**563**	**535**	**510**	**487**	**465**	**446**	**404**	**369**
		218	211	197	186	175	166	157	140	125
	13	**594**	**579**	**551**	**525**	**503**	**481**	**461**	**419**	**384**
		237	229	215	202	191	181	172	153	138
	14	**608**	**593**	**566**	**540**	**517**	**496**	**476**	**433**	**398**
		255	247	232	218	206	196	186	166	150
	15	**621**	**607**	**579**	**554**	**531**	**509**	**490**	**446**	**410**
		272	263	248	234	221	210	200	179	162
	16	**634**	**619**	**592**	**567**	**544**	**522**	**502**	**459**	**422**
		288	280	263	249	236	224	214	191	173
	17	**645**	**631**	**604**	**579**	**556**	**535**	**515**	**471**	**434**
		304	295	278	263	250	238	227	203	185
	18	**656**	**642**	**615**	**590**	**568**	**547**	**527**	**483**	**445**
		319	310	293	277	264	251	240	215	196
	19	**666**	**652**	**626**	**601**	**578**	**557**	**538**	**494**	**456**
		334	324	307	291	277	264	252	227	207
	20	**676**	**662**	**636**	**612**	**589**	**568**	**548**	**504**	**467**
		348	338	320	304	289	276	264	238	217
	22	**693**	**680**	**654**	**631**	**614**	**588**	**568**	**524**	**487**
		374	364	346	329	314	300	287	260	237
	24	**709**	**696**	**671**	**648**	**626**	**605**	**586**	**543**	**505**
		399	388	369	352	337	322	309	281	257
	26	**723**	**711**	**686**	**663**	**642**	**622**	**603**	**559**	**522**
		422	411	386	374	358	343	330	300	276
	28	**736**	**724**	**700**	**678**	**657**	**637**	**618**	**575**	**538**
		443	432	412	395	378	363	349	319	294

		Denominator minus numerator (n − x)								
		_19_	_20_	_22_	_24_	_26_	_28_	_30_	_35_	_40_
	30	**748**	**736**	**713**	**691**	**670**	**651**	**632**	**590**	**552**
		462	452	432	414	397	382	368	337	311
	35	**773**	**762**	**740**	**719**	**700**	**681**	**663**	**622**	**586**
		506	496	476	457	441	425	410	378	351
	40	**793**	**783**	**763**	**743**	**724**	**706**	**689**	**649**	**614**
		544	533	513	495	478	462	448	414	386
	45	**811**	**801**	**781**	**763**	**745**	**728**	**711**	**673**	**639**
		576	566	548	528	511	495	480	447	419
	50	**825**	**816**	**797**	**780**	**763**	**746**	**731**	**694**	**660**
		604	594	575	557	540	525	510	476	447
	60	**848**	**840**	**823**	**807**	**792**	**777**	**763**	**728**	**697**
		650	641	622	605	589	574	559	526	497
	80	**880**	**874**	**860**	**846**	**833**	**820**	**808**	**778**	**750**
		717	708	692	676	662	647	634	603	575
	100	**901**	**895**	**883**	**872**	**860**	**847**	**838**	**812**	**787**
		762	755	740	726	713	700	687	658	632
	200	**947**	**943**	**937**	**930**	**923**	**917**	**910**	**894**	**878**
		868	863	854	845	836	828	819	799	780
	500	**978**	**976**	**973**	**970**	**967**	**964**	**961**	**954**	**947**
		944	941	937	933	928	924	920	910	901
	∞	**1000**	**1000**	**1000**	**1000**	**1000**	**1000**	**1000**	**1000**	**1000**
		1000	1000	1000	1000	1000	1000	1000	1000	1000

Numerator of the proportion (x)

	Denominator minus numerator $(n-x)$							
	45	50	60	80	100	200	500	∞
0	**079**	**071**	**060**	**045**	**036**	**018**	**007**	**000**
	000	000	000	000	000	000	000	000
1	**115**	**104**	**088**	**067**	**054**	**027**	**011**	**000**
	001	001	000	000	000	000	000	000
2	**145**	**132**	**112**	**085**	**069**	**035**	**014**	**000**
	005	005	004	003	002	001	000	000
3	**172**	**157**	**133**	**102**	**083**	**043**	**017**	**000**
	013	012	010	008	006	003	001	000
4	**196**	**179**	**152**	**118**	**096**	**049**	**020**	**000**
	023	021	017	013	011	005	002	000
5	**218**	**200**	**170**	**132**	**108**	**056**	**023**	**000**
	033	030	025	019	016	008	003	000
6	**239**	**219**	**187**	**145**	**119**	**062**	**026**	**000**
	044	040	034	026	021	011	004	000
7	**258**	**237**	**203**	**158**	**130**	**068**	**028**	**000**
	056	051	043	033	027	014	005	000
8	**276**	**254**	**218**	**171**	**141**	**074**	**031**	**000**
	067	061	052	040	033	017	007	000
9	**293**	**270**	**233**	**184**	**151**	**080**	**033**	**000**
	079	072	061	047	038	020	008	000
10	**310**	**286**	**248**	**196**	**162**	**086**	**036**	**000**
	091	083	071	055	045	023	009	000
11	**325**	**300**	**260**	**207**	**171**	**091**	**038**	**000**
	102	094	080	062	051	026	011	000
12	**339**	**314**	**273**	**217**	**180**	**097**	**040**	**000**
	114	104	089	069	057	030	012	000
13	**353**	**327**	**285**	**227**	**189**	**102**	**043**	**000**
	125	115	098	077	063	033	014	000
14	**367**	**340**	**297**	**237**	**198**	**107**	**045**	**000**
	136	125	107	084	069	036	015	000
15	**379**	**352**	**308**	**247**	**206**	**112**	**047**	**000**
	147	135	116	091	075	039	016	000
16	**391**	**364**	**319**	**256**	**214**	**117**	**050**	**000**
	158	146	126	099	081	043	018	000
17	**402**	**375**	**330**	**266**	**222**	**122**	**052**	**000**
	169	156	134	106	087	046	019	000
18	**413**	**386**	**340**	**274**	**230**	**127**	**054**	**000**
	179	165	143	113	093	050	021	000
19	**424**	**396**	**350**	**283**	**238**	**132**	**056**	**000**
	189	175	152	120	099	053	022	000
20	**434**	**406**	**359**	**292**	**245**	**137**	**059**	**000**
	199	184	160	126	105	057	024	000
22	**454**	**425**	**378**	**308**	**260**	**146**	**063**	**000**
	219	203	177	140	117	063	027	000
24	**472**	**443**	**395**	**324**	**274**	**155**	**067**	**000**
	237	220	193	154	128	070	030	000
26	**489**	**460**	**411**	**338**	**287**	**164**	**072**	**000**
	255	237	208	167	140	077	033	000
28	**505**	**475**	**426**	**353**	**300**	**172**	**076**	**000**
	272	254	223	180	153	083	036	000

Numerator of the proportion (x)

Numerator of the proportion (x)		Denominator minus numerator (n − x)							
		45	50	60	80	100	200	500	∞
30		**520**	**490**	**441**	**366**	**313**	**181**	**080**	**000**
		289	269	237	192	162	090	039	000
35		**553**	**524**	**474**	**397**	**342**	**201**	**090**	**000**
		327	306	272	222	188	106	046	000
40		**581**	**553**	**503**	**425**	**368**	**220**	**099**	**000**
		361	340	303	250	213	122	053	000
45		**607**	**579**	**529**	**451**	**392**	**238**	**109**	**000**
		393	370	332	276	236	137	061	000
50		**630**	**602**	**552**	**474**	**415**	**255**	**188**	**000**
		421	398	359	301	259	152	068	000
60		**668**	**641**	**593**	**515**	**455**	**287**	**136**	**000**
		471	448	407	345	300	181	083	000
80		**724**	**699**	**655**	**580**	**520**	**342**	**169**	**000**
		549	526	485	420	370	234	111	000
100		**764**	**741**	**700**	**630**	**571**	**395**	**199**	**000**
		608	585	545	480	429	280	138	000
200		**863**	**848**	**819**	**766**	**720**	**550**	**319**	**000**
		762	745	713	658	605	450	253	000
500		**939**	**932**	**917**	**889**	**862**	**747**	**531**	**000**
		891	882	864	831	801	681	469	000
∞		**1000**	**1000**	**1000**	**1000**	**1000**	**1000**	**1000**	—
		1000	1000	1000	1000	1000	1000	1000	—

Appendix XI

Values of exact 95% confidence limit factors for estimates of a Poisson-distributed variable
(From Haenszel *et al.*, 1962)

Example: If a random sample of 2000 dogs yielded two cases of osteosarcoma, then a prevalence of 100 per 100 000 can be extrapolated. To calculate 95% confidence limits, enter the table at $n = 2$ (the observed number of cases), with a lower limit factor (L) of 0.121, and an upper limit factor (U) of 3.61. These limits are converted to limits per 100 000 by multiplication by the estimated prevalence per 100 000, extrapolated from the original sample (100 in this example).

Thus:

lower limit = 100×0.121,
upper limit = 100×3.61,

and the 95% confidence interval for the prevalence of osteosarcoma is therefore 12.1, 361 cases per 100 000 dogs.

Observed number on which estimate is based (n)	Lower limit factor (L)	Upper limit factor (U)	Observed number on which estimate is based (n)	Lower limit factor (L)	Upper limit factor (U)	Observed number on which estimate is based (n)	Lower limit factor (L)	Upper limit factor (U)
1	0.0253	5.57	21	0.619	1.53	120	0.833	1.200
2	0.121	3.61	22	0.627	1.51	140	0.844	1.184
3	0.206	2.92	23	0.634	1.50	160	0.854	1.171
4	0.272	2.56	24	0.641	1.49	180	0.862	1.160
5	0.324	2.33	25	0.647	1.48	200	0.868	1.151
6	0.367	2.18	26	0.653	1.47	250	0.882	1.134
7	0.401	2.06	27	0.659	1.46	300	0.892	1.121
8	0.431	1.97	28	0.665	1.45	350	0.899	1.112
9	0.458	1.90	29	0.670	1.44	400	0.906	1.104
10	0.480	1.84	30	0.675	1.43	450	0.911	1.098
11	0.499	1.79	35	0.697	1.39	500	0.915	1.093
12	0.517	1.75	40	0.714	1.36	600	0.922	1.084
13	0.532	1.71	45	0.729	1.34	700	0.928	1.078
14	0.546	1.68	50	0.742	1.32	800	0.932	1.072
15	0.560	1.65	60	0.770	1.30	900	0.936	1.068
16	0.572	1.62	70	0.785	1.27	1000	0.939	1.064
17	0.583	1.60	80	0.789	1.25			
18	0.593	1.58	90	0.809	1.24			
19	0.602	1.56	100	0.818	1.22			
20	0.611	1.54						

Appendix XII

Probabilities associated with the upper tail of the Normal distribution

(Derived from Beyer, 1981)

The body of the table gives the one-tailed probability, P, under the null hypothesis, of a random value of the standardized Normal deviate, $z[(x-\mu)/\sigma]$, being greater than the value in the margin. For example, the one-tailed probability of $z \geq 0.22$ or ≤ -0.22 is 0.4129. The probability is doubled for a two-tailed test.

The table can also be used to calculate multipliers for confidence intervals based on the Normal distribution. For example, the multiplier for a 95% confidence interval is derived from a two-tailed significance level of 0.05, corresponding to a one-tailed level of 0.0250, for which $z = 1.96$: the value of the multiplier.

z	.00	.01	.02	.03	.04	.05	.06	.07	.08	.09
.0	.5000	.4960	.4920	.4880	.4840	.4801	.4761	.4721	.4681	.4641
.1	.4602	.4562	.4522	.4483	.4443	.4404	.4364	.4325	.4286	.4247
.2	.4207	.4168	.4129	.4090	.4052	.4013	.3974	.3936	.3897	.3859
.3	.3821	.3783	.3745	.3707	.3669	.3632	.3594	.3557	.3520	.3483
.4	.3446	.3409	.3372	.3336	.3300	.3264	.3228	.3192	.3156	.3121
.5	.3085	.3050	.3015	.2981	.2946	.2912	.2877	.2843	.2810	.2776
.6	.2743	.2709	.2676	.2643	.2611	.2578	.2546	.2514	.2483	.2451
.7	.2420	.2389	.2358	.2327	.2296	.2266	.2236	.2206	.2177	.2148
.8	.2119	.2090	.2061	.2033	.2005	.1977	.1949	.1922	.1894	.1867
.9	.1841	.1814	.1788	.1762	.1736	.1711	.1685	.1660	.1635	.1611
1.0	.1587	.1562	.1539	.1515	.1492	.1469	.1446	.1423	.1401	.1379
1.1	.1357	.1335	.1314	.1292	.1271	.1251	.1230	.1210	.1190	.1170
1.2	.1151	.1131	.1112	.1093	.1075	.1056	.1038	.1020	.1003	.0985
1.3	.0968	.0951	.0934	.0918	.0901	.0885	.0869	.0853	.0838	.0823
1.4	.0808	.0793	.0778	.0764	.0749	.0735	.0721	.0708	.0694	.0681
1.5	.0668	.0655	.0643	.0630	.0618	.0606	.0594	.0582	.0571	.0559
1.6	.0548	.0537	.0526	.0516	.0505	.0495	.0485	.0475	.0465	.0455
1.7	.0446	.0436	.0427	.0418	.0409	.0401	.0392	.0384	.0375	.0367
1.8	.0359	.0351	.0344	.0336	.0329	.0322	.0314	.0307	.0301	.0294
1.9	.0287	.0281	.0274	.0268	.0262	.0256	.0250	.0244	.0239	.0233
2.0	.0228	.0222	.0217	.0212	.0207	.0202	.0197	.0192	.0188	.0183
2.1	.0179	.0174	.0170	.0166	.0162	.0158	.0154	.0150	.0146	.0143
2.2	.0139	.0136	.0132	.0129	.0125	.0122	.0119	.0116	.0113	.0110
2.3	.0107	.0104	.0102	.0099	.0096	.0094	.0091	.0089	.0087	.0084
2.4	.0082	.0080	.0078	.0075	.0073	.0071	.0069	.0068	.0066	.0064
2.5	.0062	.0060	.0059	.0057	.0055	.0054	.0052	.0051	.0049	.0048
2.6	.0047	.0045	.0044	.0043	.0041	.0040	.0039	.0038	.0037	.0036
2.7	.0035	.0034	.0033	.0032	.0031	.0030	.0029	.0028	.0027	.0026
2.8	.0026	.0025	.0024	.0023	.0023	.0022	.0021	.0021	.0020	.0019
2.9	.0019	.0018	.0018	.0017	.0016	.0016	.0015	.0015	.0014	.0014
3.0	.0013	.0013	.0013	.0012	.0012	.0011	.0011	.0011	.0010	.0010
3.1	.0010	.0009	.0009	.0009	.0008	.0008	.0008	.0008	.0007	.0007
3.2	.0007									
3.3	.0005									
3.4	.0003									
3.5	.00023									
3.6	.00016									
3.7	.00011									
3.8	.00007									
3.9	.00005									
4.0	.00003									

Appendix XIII

Lower- and upper-tail probabilities for W_x, the Wilcoxon— Mann—Whitney rank-sum statistic
(From Siegel and Castellan, 1988)

The body of the table gives the one-tailed probability, P, of obtaining a value of $W_x \leq c_L$, and $W_x \geq c_U$ under the null hypothesis; W_x is the rank sum for the smaller group.

$m = 3$

c_L	$n=3$	c_U	$n=4$	c_U	$n=5$	c_U	$n=6$	c_U	$n=7$	c_U	$n=8$	c_U	$n=9$	c_U	$n=10$	c_U	$n=11$	c_U	$n=12$	c_U
6	.0500	15	.0286	18	.0179	21	.0119	24	.0083	27	.0061	30	.0045	33	.0035	36	.0027	39	.0022	42
7	.1000	14	.0571	17	.0357	20	.0238	23	.0167	26	.0121	29	.0091	32	.0070	35	.0055	38	.0044	41
8	.2000	13	.1143	16	.0714	19	.0476	22	.0333	25	.0242	28	.0182	31	.0140	34	.0110	37	.0088	40
9	.3500	12	.2000	15	.1250	18	.0833	21	.0583	24	.0424	27	.0318	30	.0245	33	.0192	36	.0154	39
10	.5000	11	.3143	14	.1964	17	.1310	20	.0917	23	.0667	26	.0500	29	.0385	32	.0302	35	.0242	38
11	.6500	10	.4286	13	.2857	16	.1905	19	.1333	22	.0970	25	.0727	28	.0559	31	.0440	34	.0352	37
12	.8000	9	.5714	12	.3929	15	.2738	18	.1917	21	.1394	24	.1045	27	.0804	30	.0632	33	.0505	36
13	.9000	8	.6857	11	.5000	14	.3571	17	.2583	20	.1879	23	.1409	26	.1084	29	.0852	32	.0681	35
14	.9500	7	.8000	10	.6071	13	.4524	16	.3333	19	.2485	22	.1864	25	.1434	28	.1126	31	.0901	34
15	1.0000	6	.8857	9	.7143	12	.5476	15	.4167	18	.3152	21	.2409	24	.1853	27	.1456	30	.1165	33
16			.9429	8	.8036	11	.6429	14	.5000	17	.3879	20	.3000	23	.2343	26	.1841	29	.1473	32
17			.9714	7	.8750	10	.7262	13	.5833	16	.4606	19	.3636	22	.2867	25	.2280	28	.1824	31
18			1.0000	6	.9286	9	.8095	12	.6667	15	.5394	18	.4318	21	.3462	24	.2775	27	.2242	30
19					.9643	8	.8690	11	.7417	14	.6121	17	.5000	20	.4056	23	.3297	26	.2681	29
20					.9821	7	.9167	10	.8083	13	.6848	16	.5682	19	.4685	22	.3846	25	.3165	28
21					1.0000	6	.9524	9	.8667	12	.7515	15	.6364	18	.5315	21	.4423	24	.3670	27
22							.9762	8	.9083	11	.8121	14	.7000	17	.5944	20	.5000	23	.4198	26
23							.9881	7	.9417	10	.8606	13	.7591	16	.6538	19	.5577	22	.4725	25
24							1.0000	6	.9667	9	.9030	12	.8136	15	.7133	18	.6154	21	.5275	24

$m = 4$

c_l	$n=4$	c_u	$n=5$	c_u	$n=6$	c_u	$n=7$	c_u	$n=8$	c_u	$n=9$	c_u	$n=10$	c_u	$n=11$	c_u	$n=12$	c_u
10	.0143	26	.0079	30	.0048	34	.0030	38	.0020	42	.0014	46	.0010	50	.0007	54	.0005	58
11	.0286	25	.0159	29	.0095	33	.0061	37	.0040	41	.0028	45	.0020	49	.0015	53	.0011	57
12	.0571	24	.0317	28	.0190	32	.0121	36	.0081	40	.0056	44	.0040	48	.0029	52	.0022	56
13	.1000	23	.0556	27	.0333	31	.0212	35	.0141	39	.0098	43	.0070	47	.0051	51	.0038	55
14	.1714	22	.0952	26	.0571	30	.0364	34	.0242	38	.0168	42	.0120	46	.0088	50	.0066	54
15	.2429	21	.1429	25	.0857	29	.0545	33	.0364	37	.0252	41	.0180	45	.0132	49	.0099	53
16	.3429	20	.2063	24	.1286	28	.0818	32	.0545	36	.0378	40	.0270	44	.0198	48	.0148	52
17	.4429	19	.2778	23	.1762	27	.1152	31	.0768	35	.0531	39	.0380	43	.0278	47	.0209	51
18	.5571	18	.3651	22	.2381	26	.1576	30	.1071	34	.0741	38	.0529	42	.0388	46	.0291	50
19	.6571	17	.4524	21	.3048	25	.2061	29	.1414	33	.0993	37	.0709	41	.0520	45	.0390	49
20	.7571	16	.5476	20	.3810	24	.2636	28	.1838	32	.1301	36	.0939	40	.0689	44	.0516	48
21	.8286	15	.6349	19	.4571	23	.3242	27	.2303	31	.1650	35	.1199	39	.0886	43	.0665	47
22	.9000	14	.7222	18	.5429	22	.3939	26	.2848	30	.2070	34	.1518	38	.1128	42	.0852	46
23	.9429	13	.7937	17	.6190	21	.4636	25	.3414	29	.2517	33	.1868	37	.1399	41	.1060	45
24	.9714	12	.8571	16	.6952	20	.5364	24	.4040	28	.3021	32	.2268	36	.1714	40	.1308	44
25	.9857	11	.9048	15	.7619	19	.6061	23	.4667	27	.3552	31	.2697	35	.2059	39	.1582	43
26	1.0000	10	.9444	14	.8238	18	.6758	22	.5333	26	.4126	30	.3177	34	.2447	38	.1896	42
27			.9683	13	.8714	17	.7364	21	.5960	25	.4699	29	.3666	33	.2857	37	.2231	41
28			.9841	12	.9143	16	.7939	20	.6586	24	.5301	28	.4196	32	.3304	36	.2604	40
29			.9921	11	.9429	15	.8424	19	.7152	23	.5874	27	.4725	31	.3766	35	.2995	39
30			1.0000	10	.9667	14	.8848	18	.7697	22	.6448	26	.5275	30	.4256	34	.3418	38
31					.9810	13	.9182	17	.8162	21	.6979	25	.5804	29	.4747	33	.3852	37
32					.9905	12	.9455	16	.8586	20	.7483	24	.6334	28	.5253	32	.4308	36
33					.9952	11	.9636	15	.8929	19	.7930	23	.6823	27	.5744	31	.4764	35
34					1.0000	10	.9788	14	.9232	18	.8350	22	.7303	26	.6234	30	.5236	34

						$m = 5$						
c_L	$n = 5$	c_U	$n = 6$	c_U	$n = 7$	c_U	$n = 8$	c_U	$n = 9$	c_U	$n = 10$	c_U
15	.0040	40	.0022	45	.0013	50	.0008	55	.0005	60	.0003	65
16	.0079	39	.0043	44	.0025	49	.0016	54	.0010	59	.0007	64
17	.0159	38	.0087	43	.0051	48	.0031	53	.0020	58	.0013	63
18	.0278	37	.0152	42	.0088	47	.0054	52	.0035	57	.0023	62
19	.0476	36	.0260	41	.0152	46	.0093	51	.0060	56	.0040	61
20	.0754	35	.0411	40	.0240	45	.0148	50	.0095	55	.0063	60
21	.1111	34	.0628	39	.0366	44	.0225	49	.0145	54	.0097	59
22	.1548	33	.0887	38	.0530	43	.0326	48	.0210	53	.0140	58
23	.2103	32	.1234	37	.0745	42	.0466	47	.0300	52	.0200	57
24	.2738	31	.1645	36	.1010	41	.0637	46	.0415	51	.0276	56
25	.3452	30	.2143	35	.1338	40	.0855	45	.0559	50	.0376	55
26	.4206	29	.2684	34	.1717	39	.1111	44	.0734	49	.0496	54
27	.5000	28	.3312	33	.2159	38	.1422	43	.0949	48	.0646	53
28	.5794	27	.3961	32	.2652	37	.1772	42	.1199	47	.0823	52
29	.6548	26	.4654	31	.3194	36	.2176	41	.1489	46	.1032	51
30	.7262	25	.5346	30	.3775	35	.2618	40	.1818	45	.1272	50
31	.7897	24	.6039	29	.4381	34	.3108	39	.2188	44	.1548	49
32	.8452	23	.6688	28	.5000	33	.3621	38	.2592	43	.1855	48
33	.8889	22	.7316	27	.5619	32	.4165	37	.3032	42	.2198	47
34	.9246	21	.7857	26	.6225	31	.4716	36	.3497	41	.2567	46
35	.9524	20	.8355	25	.6806	30	.5284	35	.3986	40	.2970	45
36	.9722	19	.8766	24	.7348	29	.5835	34	.4491	39	.3393	44
37	.9841	18	.9113	23	.7841	28	.6379	33	.5000	38	.3839	43
38	.9921	17	.9372	22	.8283	27	.6892	32	.5509	37	.4296	42
39	.9960	16	.9589	21	.8662	26	.7382	31	.6014	36	.4765	41
40	1.0000	15	.9740	20	.8990	25	.7824	30	.6503	35	.5235	40

| | | $m = 6$ | | | | | | | | |
| | | | | | | | | | | |
c_L	$n = 6$	c_U	$n = 7$	c_U	$n = 8$	c_U	$n = 9$	c_U	$n = 10$	c_U
21	.0011	57	.0006	63	.0003	69	.0002	75	.0001	81
22	.0022	56	.0012	62	.0007	68	.0004	74	.0002	80
23	.0043	55	.0023	61	.0013	67	.0008	73	.0005	79
24	.0076	54	.0041	60	.0023	66	.0014	72	.0009	78
25	.0130	53	.0070	59	.0040	65	.0024	71	.0015	77
26	.0206	52	.0111	58	.0063	64	.0038	70	.0024	76
27	.0325	51	.0175	57	.0100	63	.0060	69	.0037	75
28	.0465	50	.0256	56	.0147	62	.0088	68	.0055	74
29	.0660	49	.0367	55	.0213	61	.0128	67	.0080	73
30	.0898	48	.0507	54	.0296	60	.0180	66	.0112	72
31	.1201	47	.0688	53	.0406	59	.0248	65	.0156	71
32	.1548	46	.0903	52	.0539	58	.0332	64	.0210	70
33	.1970	45	.1171	51	.0709	57	.0440	63	.0280	69
34	.2424	44	.1474	50	.0906	56	.0567	62	.0363	68
35	.2944	43	.1830	49	.1142	55	.0723	61	.0467	67
36	.3496	42	.2226	48	.1412	54	.0905	60	.0589	66
37	.4091	41	.2669	47	.1725	53	.1119	59	.0736	65
38	.4686	40	.3141	46	.2068	52	.1361	58	.0903	64
39	.5314	39	.3654	45	.2454	51	.1638	57	.1099	63
40	.5909	38	.4178	44	.2864	50	.1942	56	.1317	62
41	.6504	37	.4726	43	.3310	49	.2280	55	.1566	61
42	.7056	36	.5274	42	.3773	48	.2643	54	.1838	60
43	.7576	35	.5822	41	.4259	47	.3035	53	.2139	59
44	.8030	34	.6346	40	.4749	46	.3445	52	.2461	58
45	.8452	33	.6859	39	.5251	45	.3878	51	.2811	57
46	.8799	32	.7331	38	.5741	44	.4320	50	.3177	56
47	.9102	31	.7774	37	.6227	43	.4773	49	.3564	55
48	.9340	30	.8170	36	.6690	42	.5227	48	.3962	54
49	.9535	29	.8526	35	.7136	41	.5680	47	.4374	53
50	.9675	28	.8829	34	.7546	40	.6122	46	.4789	52
51	.9794	27	.9097	33	.7932	39	.6555	45	.5211	51

				$m = 7$					
c_L	$n = 7$	c_U	$n = 8$	c_U	$n = 9$	c_U	$n = 10$	c_U
28	.0003	77	.0002	84	.0001	91	.0001	98
29	.0006	76	.0003	83	.0002	90	.0001	97
30	.0012	75	.0006	82	.0003	89	.0002	96
31	.0020	74	.0011	81	.0006	88	.0004	95
32	.0035	73	.0019	80	.0010	87	.0006	94
33	.0055	72	.0030	79	.0017	86	.0010	93
34	.0087	71	.0047	78	.0026	85	.0015	92
35	.0131	70	.0070	77	.0039	84	.0023	91
36	.0189	69	.0103	76	.0058	83	.0034	90
37	.0265	68	.0145	75	.0082	82	.0048	89
38	.0364	67	.0200	74	.0115	81	.0068	88
39	.0487	66	.0270	73	.0156	80	.0093	87
40	.0641	65	.0361	72	.0209	79	.0125	86
41	.0825	64	.0469	71	.0274	78	.0165	85
42	.1043	63	.0603	70	.0356	77	.0215	84
43	.1297	62	.0760	69	.0454	76	.0277	83
44	.1588	61	.0946	68	.0571	75	.0351	82
45	.1914	60	.1159	67	.0708	74	.0439	81
46	.2279	59	.1405	66	.0869	73	.0544	80
47	.2675	58	.1678	65	.1052	72	.0665	79
48	.3100	57	.1984	64	.1261	71	.0806	78
49	.3552	56	.2317	63	.1496	70	.0966	77
50	.4024	55	.2679	62	.1755	69	.1148	76
51	.4508	54	.3063	61	.2039	68	.1349	75
52	.5000	53	.3472	60	.2349	67	.1574	74
53	.5492	52	.3894	59	.2680	66	.1819	73
54	.5976	51	.4333	58	.3032	65	.2087	72
55	.6448	50	.4775	57	.3403	64	.2374	71
56	.6900	49	.5225	56	.3788	63	.2681	70
57	.7325	48	.5667	55	.4185	62	.3004	69
58	.7721	47	.6106	54	.4591	61	.3345	68
59	.8086	46	.6528	53	.5000	60	.3698	67
60	.8412	45	.6937	52	.5409	59	.4063	66
61	.8703	44	.7321	51	.5815	58	.4434	65
62	.8957	43	.7683	50	.6212	57	.4811	64
63	.9175	42	.8016	49	.6597	56	.5189	63

		$m = 8$			
c_L	$n = 8$	c_U	$n = 9$	c_U	$n = 10$	c_U
36	.0001	100	.0000	108	.0000	116
37	.0002	99	.0001	107	.0000	115
38	.0003	98	.0002	106	.0001	114
39	.0005	97	.0003	105	.0002	113
40	.0009	96	.0005	104	.0003	112
41	.0015	95	.0008	103	.0004	111
42	.0023	94	.0012	102	.0007	110
43	.0035	93	.0019	101	.0010	109
44	.0052	92	.0028	100	.0015	108
45	.0074	91	.0039	99	.0022	107
46	.0103	90	.0056	98	.0031	106
47	.0141	89	.0076	97	.0043	105
48	.0190	88	.0103	96	.0058	104
49	.0249	87	.0137	95	.0078	103
50	.0325	86	.0180	94	.0103	102
51	.0415	85	.0232	93	.0133	101
52	.0524	84	.0296	92	.0171	100
53	.0652	83	.0372	91	.0217	99
54	.0803	82	.0464	90	.0273	98
55	.0974	81	.0570	89	.0338	97
56	.1172	80	.0694	88	.0416	96
57	.1393	79	.0836	87	.0506	95
58	.1641	78	.0998	86	.0610	94
59	.1911	77	.1179	85	.0729	93
60	.2209	76	.1383	84	.0864	92
61	.2527	75	.1606	83	.1015	91
62	.2869	74	.1852	82	.1185	90
63	.3227	73	.2117	81	.1371	89
64	.3605	72	.2404	80	.1577	88
65	.3992	71	.2707	79	.1800	87
66	.4392	70	.3029	78	.2041	86
67	.4796	69	.3365	77	.2299	85
68	.5204	68	.3715	76	.2574	84
69	.5608	67	.4074	75	.2863	83
70	.6008	66	.4442	74	.3167	82
71	.6395	65	.4813	73	.3482	81
72	.6773	64	.5187	72	.3809	80
73	.7131	63	.5558	71	.4143	79
74	.7473	62	.5926	70	.4484	78
75	.7791	61	.6285	69	.4827	77
76	.8089	60	.6635	68	.5173	76

m = 9									
c_L	n = 9	c_U	n = 10	c_U	c_L	n = 9 (cont.)	c_U	n = 10 (cont.)	c_U
45	.0000	126	.0000	135	68	.0680	103	.0394	112
46	.0000	125	.0000	134	69	.0807	102	.0474	111
47	.0001	124	.0000	133	70	.0951	101	.0564	110
48	.0001	123	.0001	132	71	.1112	100	.0667	109
49	.0002	122	.0001	131	72	.1290	99	.0782	108
50	.0004	121	.0002	130	73	.1487	98	.0912	107
51	.0006	120	.0003	129	74	.1701	97	.1055	106
52	.0009	119	.0005	128	75	.1933	96	.1214	105
53	.0014	118	.0007	127	76	.2181	95	.1388	104
54	.0020	117	.0011	126	77	.2447	94	.1577	103
55	.0028	116	.0015	125	78	.2729	93	.1781	102
56	.0039	115	.0021	124	79	.3024	92	.2001	101
57	.0053	114	.0028	123	80	.3332	91	.2235	100
58	.0071	113	.0038	122	81	.3652	90	.2483	99
59	.0094	112	.0051	121	82	.3981	89	.2745	98
60	.0122	111	.0066	120	83	.4317	88	.3019	97
61	.0157	110	.0086	119	84	.4657	87	.3304	96
62	.0200	109	.0110	118	85	.5000	86	.3598	95
63	.0252	108	.0140	117	86	.5343	85	.3901	94
64	.0313	107	.0175	116	87	.5683	84	.4211	93
65	.0385	106	.0217	115	88	.6019	83	.4524	92
66	.0470	105	.0267	114	89	.6348	82	.4841	91
67	.0567	104	.0326	113	90	.6668	81	.5159	90

m = 10					
c_L	n = 10	c_U	c_L	n = 10 (cont.)	c_U
55	.0000	155	81	.0376	129
56	.0000	154	82	.0446	128
57	.0000	153	83	.0526	127
58	.0000	152	84	.0615	126
59	.0001	151	85	.0716	125
60	.0001	150	86	.0827	124
61	.0002	149	87	.0952	123
62	.0002	148	88	.1088	122
63	.0004	147	89	.1237	121
64	.0005	146	90	.1399	120
65	.0008	145	91	.1575	119
66	.0010	144	92	.1763	118
67	.0014	143	93	.1965	117
68	.0019	142	94	.2179	116
69	.0026	141	95	.2406	115
70	.0034	140	96	.2644	114
71	.0045	139	97	.2894	113
72	.0057	138	98	.3153	112
73	.0073	137	99	.3421	111
74	.0093	136	100	.3697	110
75	.0116	135	101	.3980	109
76	.0144	134	102	.4267	108
77	.0177	133	103	.4559	107
78	.0216	132	104	.4853	106
79	.0262	131	105	.5147	105
80	.0315	130			

Appendix XIV

Critical values of T^+ for the Wilcoxon signed ranks test
(From Siegel and Castellan, 1988)

The body of the table gives the one-tailed probability, P, under the null hypothesis, that $T^+ \geq c$, for N pairs of observations with non-zero differences.

			N									N				
c	3	4	5	6	7	8	9		c	3	4	5	6	7	8	9
3	.6250								24					.0547	.2305	.4551
4	.3750								25					.0391	.1914	.4102
5	.2500	.5625							26					.0234	.1563	.3672
6	.1250	.4375							27					.0156	.1250	.3262
7		.3125							28					.0078	.0977	.2852
8		.1875	.5000						29						.0742	.2480
9		.1250	.4063						30						.0547	.2129
10		.0625	.3125						31						.0391	.1797
11			.2188	.5000					32						.0273	.1504
12			.1563	.4219					33						.0195	.1250
13			.0938	.3438					34						.0117	.1016
14			.0625	.2813	.5313				35						.0078	.0820
15			.0313	.2188	.4688				36						.0039	.0645
16				.1563	.4063				37							.0488
17				.1094	.3438				38							.0371
18				.0781	.2891	.5273			39							.0273
19				.0469	.2344	.4727			40							.0195
20				.0313	.1875	.4219			41							.0137
21				.0156	.1484	.3711			42							.0098
22					.1094	.3203			43							.0059
23					.0781	.2734	.5000		44							.0039
									45							.0020

c	N 10	11	12	13	14	15
28	.5000					
29	.4609					
30	.4229					
31	.3848					
32	.3477					
33	.3125	.5171				
34	.2783	.4829				
35	.2461	.4492				
36	.2158	.4155				
37	.1875	.3823				
38	.1611	.3501				
39	.1377	.3188	.5151			
40	.1162	.2886	.4849			
41	.0967	.2598	.4548			
42	.0801	.2324	.4250			
43	.0654	.2065	.3955			
44	.0527	.1826	.3667			
45	.0420	.1602	.3386			
46	.0322	.1392	.3110	.5000		
47	.0244	.1201	.2847	.4730		
48	.0186	.1030	.2593	.4463		
49	.0137	.0874	.2349	.4197		
50	.0098	.0737	.2119	.3934		
51	.0068	.0615	.1902	.3677		
52	.0049	.0508	.1697	.3424		
53	.0029	.0415	.1506	.3177	.5000	
54	.0020	.0337	.1331	.2939	.4758	
55	.0010	.0269	.1167	.2709	.4516	
56		.0210	.1018	.2487	.4276	
57		.0161	.0881	.2274	.4039	
58		.0122	.0757	.2072	.3804	
59		.0093	.0647	.1879	.3574	
60		.0068	.0549	.1698	.3349	.5110
61		.0049	.0461	.1527	.3129	.4890
62		.0034	.0386	.1367	.2915	.4670
63		.0024	.0320	.1219	.2708	.4452
64		.0015	.0261	.1082	.2508	.4235
65		.0010	.0212	.0955	.2316	.4020
66		.0005	.0171	.0839	.2131	.3808
67			.0134	.0732	.1955	.3599
68			.0105	.0636	.1788	.3394
69			.0081	.0549	.1629	.3193
70			.0061	.0471	.1479	.2997
71			.0046	.0402	.1338	.2807
72			.0034	.0341	.1206	.2622
73			.0024	.0287	.1083	.2444
74			.0017	.0239	.0969	.2271
75			.0012	.0199	.0863	.2106
76			.0007	.0164	.0765	.1947
77			.0005	.0133	.0676	.1796
78			.0002	.0107	.0594	.1651

	N		
c	13	14	15
79	.0085	.0520	.1514
80	.0067	.0453	.1384
81	.0052	.0392	.1262
82	.0040	.0338	.1147
83	.0031	.0290	.1039
84	.0023	.0247	.0938
85	.0017	.0209	.0844
86	.0012	.0176	.0757
87	.0009	.0148	.0677
88	.0006	.0123	.0603
89	.0004	.0101	.0535
90	.0002	.0083	.0473
91	.0001	.0067	.0416
92		.0054	.0365
93		.0043	.0319
94		.0034	.0277
95		.0026	.0240
96		.0020	.0206
97		.0015	.0177
98		.0012	.0151
99		.0009	.0128
100		.0006	.0108
101		.0004	.0090
102		.0003	.0075
103		.0002	.0062
104		.0001	.0051
105		.0001	.0042
106			.0034
107			.0027
108			.0021
109			.0017
110			.0013
111			.0010
112			.0008
113			.0006
114			.0004
115			.0003
116			.0002
117			.0002
118			.0001
119			.0001
120			.0000+

Appendix XV

Values of *K* for calculating 95% confidence intervals for the difference between population medians for two independent samples
(From Gardner and Altman, 1989)

Sample sizes (n_1, n_2) Smaller	Larger	K	95% (approx) Exact level (%)	Sample sizes (n_1, n_2) Smaller	Larger	K	95% (approx) Exact level (%)
5	5	3	96·8	6	20	28	95·4
5	6	4	97·0	6	21	30	95·1
5	7	6	95·2	6	22	31	95·5
5	8	7	95·5	6	23	33	95·3
5	9	8	95·8	6	24	34	95·6
5	10	9	96·0	6	25	36	95·4
5	11	10	96·2	7	7	9	96·2
5	12	12	95·2	7	8	11	96·0
5	13	13	95·4	7	9	13	95·8
5	14	14	95·6	7	10	15	95·7
5	15	15	95·8	7	11	17	95·6
5	16	16	96·0	7	12	19	95·5
5	17	18	95·2	7	13	21	95·4
5	18	19	95·4	7	14	23	95·4
5	19	20	95·6	7	15	25	95·3
5	20	21	95·8	7	16	27	95·3
5	21	23	95·1	7	17	29	95·3
5	22	24	95·3	7	18	31	95·3
5	23	25	95·5	7	19	33	95·2
5	24	26	95·6	7	20	35	95·2
5	25	28	95·1	7	21	37	95·2
6	6	6	95·9	7	22	39	95·2
6	7	7	96·5	7	23	41	95·2
6	8	9	95·7	7	24	43	95·2
6	9	11	95·0	7	25	45	95·2
6	10	12	95·8	8	8	14	95·0
6	11	14	95·2	8	9	16	95·4
6	12	15	95·9	8	10	18	95·7
6	13	17	95·4	8	11	20	95·9
6	14	18	95·9	8	12	23	95·3
6	15	20	95·5	8	13	25	95·5
6	16	22	95·1	8	14	27	95·8
6	17	23	95·6	8	15	30	95·3
6	18	25	95·3	8	16	32	95·5
6	19	26	95·7	8	17	35	95·1
				8	18	37	95·3

Sample sizes (n_1, n_2)		Level of confidence 95% (approx)	
Smaller	Larger	K	Exact level (%)
8	19	39	95·5
8	20	42	95·1
8	21	44	95·3
8	22	46	95·5
8	23	49	95·2
8	24	51	95·4
8	25	54	95·1
9	9	18	96·0
9	10	21	95·7
9	11	24	95·4
9	12	27	95·1
9	13	29	95·7
9	14	32	95·4
9	15	35	95·2
9	16	38	95·1
9	17	40	95·5
9	18	43	95·4
9	19	46	95·2
9	20	49	95·1
9	21	51	95·5
9	22	54	95·4
9	23	57	95·3
9	24	60	95·1
9	25	63	95·0
10	10	24	95·7
10	11	27	95·7
10	12	30	95·7
10	13	34	95·1
10	14	37	95·2
10	15	40	95·2
10	16	43	95·3
10	17	46	95·4
10	18	49	95·5
10	19	53	95·0
10	20	56	95·1
10	21	59	95·2
10	22	62	95·3
10	23	65	95·3
10	24	68	95·4
10	25	72	95·0
11	11	31	95·3
11	12	34	95·6
11	13	38	95·3
11	14	41	95·6
11	15	45	95·3
11	16	48	95·6
11	17	52	95·3
11	18	56	95·1
11	19	59	95·3
11	20	63	95·1
11	21	66	95·4
11	22	70	95·2
11	23	74	95·0
11	24	77	95·3
11	25	81	95·1
12	12	38	95·5

Sample sizes (n_1, n_2)		Level of confidence 95% (approx)	
Smaller	Larger	K	Exact level (%)
12	13	42	95·4
12	14	46	95·4
12	15	50	95·3
12	16	54	95·3
12	17	58	95·2
12	18	62	95·2
12	19	66	95·2
12	20	70	95·2
12	21	74	95·2
12	22	78	95·2
12	23	82	95·1
12	24	86	95·1
12	25	90	95·1
13	13	46	95·6
13	14	51	95·2
13	15	55	95·4
13	16	60	95·0
13	17	64	95·2
13	18	68	95·4
13	19	73	95·1
13	20	77	95·2
13	21	81	95·4
13	22	86	95·1
13	23	90	95·3
13	24	95	95·1
13	25	99	95·2
14	14	56	95·0
14	15	60	95·4
14	16	65	95·3
14	17	70	95·2
14	18	75	95·1
14	19	79	95·4
14	20	84	95·3
14	21	89	95·2
14	22	94	95·1
14	23	99	95·1
14	24	103	95·3
14	25	108	95·3
15	15	65	95·5
15	16	71	95·1
15	17	76	95·1
15	18	81	95·2
15	19	86	95·3
15	20	91	95·4
15	21	97	95·1
15	22	102	95·1
15	23	107	95·2
15	24	112	95·3
15	25	118	95·0
16	16	76	95·3
16	17	82	95·1
16	18	87	95·4
16	19	93	95·2
16	20	99	95·1
16	21	104	95·3
16	22	110	95·2
16	23	116	95·0

Sample sizes (n_1, n_2)		Level of confidence 95% (approx)	
Smaller	Larger	K	Exact level (%)
16	24	121	95·2
16	25	127	95·1
17	17	88	95·1
17	18	94	95·1
17	19	100	95·1
17	20	106	95·2
17	21	112	95·2
17	22	118	95·2
17	23	124	95·2
17	24	130	95·2
17	25	136	95·2
18	18	100	95·3
18	19	107	95·1
18	20	113	95·2
18	21	120	95·1
18	22	126	95·2
18	23	133	95·0
18	24	139	95·2
18	25	146	95·0
19	19	114	95·0
19	20	120	95·3
19	21	127	95·3
19	22	134	95·2
19	23	141	95·2
19	24	148	95·2
19	25	155	95·1
20	20	128	95·1
20	21	135	95·2
20	22	142	95·3
20	23	150	95·1
20	24	157	95·2
20	25	164	95·3
21	21	143	95·1
21	22	151	95·0
21	23	158	95·2
21	24	166	95·2
21	25	174	95·1
22	22	159	95·1
22	23	167	95·1
22	24	175	95·2
22	25	183	95·2
23	23	176	95·0
23	24	184	95·2
23	25	193	95·1
24	24	193	95·2
24	25	202	95·2
25	25	212	95·1

Appendix XVI

Values of K^* for calculating 95% confidence intervals for the difference between population medians for two related samples
(From Gardner and Altman, 1989)

Sample size (n)	Level of confidence 95% (approx.)		Sample size (n)	Level of confidence 95% (approx.)	
	K^*	Exact level (%)		K^*	Exact level (%)
6	1	96.9	29	127	95.2
7	3	95.3	30	138	95.0
8	4	96.1	31	148	95.2
9	6	96.1	32	160	95.0
10	9	95.1	33	171	95.2
11	11	95.8	34	183	95.2
12	14	95.8	35	196	95.1
13	18	95.2	36	209	95.0
14	22	95.1	37	222	95.1
15	26	95.2	38	236	95.1
16	30	95.6	39	250	95.1
17	35	95.5	40	265	95.0
18	41	95.2	41	280	95.0
19	47	95.1	42	295	95.1
20	53	95.2	43	311	95.1
21	59	95.4	44	328	95.0
22	66	95.4	45	344	95.1
23	74	95.2	46	362	95.0
24	82	95.1	47	379	95.1
25	90	95.2	48	397	95.1
26	99	95.1	49	416	95.1
27	108	95.1	50	435	95.1
28	117	95.2			

Appendix XVII

The χ^2-distribution

Degrees of freedom	Value of P				
	0.99	0.95	0.05	0.01	0.001
1	0.000157	0.00393	3.841	6.635	10.83
2	0.0201	0.103	5.991	9.210	13.82
3	0.115	0.352	7.815	11.34	16.27
4	0.297	0.711	9.488	13.28	18.47
5	0.554	1.145	11.07	15.09	20.51
6	0.872	1.635	12.59	16.81	22.46
7	1.239	2.167	14.07	18.48	24.32
8	1.646	2.733	15.51	20.09	26.13
9	2.088	3.325	16.92	21.67	27.88
10	2.558	3.940	18.31	23.21	29.59
11	3.053	4.575	19.68	24.72	31.26
12	3.571	5.226	21.03	26.22	32.91
13	4.107	5.892	22.36	27.69	34.53
14	4.660	6.571	23.68	29.14	36.12
15	5.229	7.261	25.00	30.58	37.70
16	5.812	7.962	26.30	32.00	39.25
17	6.408	8.672	27.59	33.41	40.79
18	7.015	9.390	28.87	34.81	42.31
19	7.633	10.12	30.14	36.19	43.82
20	8.260	10.85	31.41	37.57	45.31
21	8.897	11.59	32.67	38.93	46.80
22	9.542	12.34	33.92	40.29	48.27
23	10.20	13.09	35.17	41.64	49.73
24	10.86	13.85	36.42	42.98	51.18
25	11.52	14.61	37.65	44.31	52.62
26	12.20	15.38	38.89	45.64	54.05
27	12.88	16.15	40.11	46.96	55.48
28	13.56	16.93	41.34	48.28	56.89
29	14.26	17.71	42.56	49.59	58.30
30	14.95	18.49	43.77	50.89	59.70

The table gives the percentage points most frequently required for significance tests based on χ^2. Thus the probability of observing a χ^2 with 5 degrees of freedom **greater** in value than 11.07 is 0.05 or 5 per cent. Again, the probability of observing a χ^2 with 5 degrees of freedom **smaller** in value than 0.554 is $1 - 0.99 = 0.01$ or 1 per cent.

Appendix XVIII

Common logarithms ($\log_{10}$) of factorials of the integers 1 – 999

(From Lentner, 1982)

n	0	1	2	3	4	5	6	7	8	9
0	0.00000	0.00000	0.30103	0.77815	1.38021	2.07918	2.85733	3.70243	4.60552	5.55976
10	6.55976	7.60116	8.68034	9.79428	10.94041	12.11650	13.32062	14.55107	15.80634	17.08509
20	18.38612	19.70834	21.05077	22.41249	23.79271	25.19065	26.60562	28.03698	29.48414	30.94654
30	32.42366	33.91502	35.42017	36.93869	38.47016	40.01423	41.57054	43.13874	44.71852	46.30959
40	47.91165	49.52443	51.14768	52.78115	54.42460	56.07781	57.74057	59.41267	61.09391	62.78410
50	64.48307	66.19064	67.90665	69.63092	71.36332	73.10368	74.85187	76.60774	78.37117	80.14202
60	81.92017	83.70550	85.49790	87.29724	89.10342	90.91633	92.73587	94.56195	96.39446	98.23331
70	100.07841	101.92966	103.78700	105.65032	107.51955	109.39461	111.27543	113.16192	115.05401	116.95164
80	118.85473	120.76321	122.67703	124.59610	126.52038	128.44980	130.38430	132.32382	134.26830	136.21769
90	138.17194	140.13098	142.09476	144.06325	146.03638	148.01410	149.99637	151.98314	153.97437	155.97000
100	157.97000	159.97433	161.98293	163.99576	166.01280	168.03398	170.05929	172.08867	174.12210	176.15952
110	178.20092	180.24624	182.29546	184.34854	186.40544	188.46614	190.53060	192.59878	194.67067	196.74621
120	198.82539	200.90818	202.99454	205.08444	207.17787	209.27478	211.37515	213.47895	215.58616	217.69675
130	219.81069	221.92797	224.04854	226.17239	228.29950	230.42983	232.56337	234.70009	236.83997	238.98298
140	241.12911	243.27833	245.43062	247.58595	249.74432	251.90568	254.07004	256.23735	258.40762	260.58080
150	262.75689	264.93587	267.11771	269.30240	271.48993	273.68026	275.87338	278.06928	280.26794	282.46933
160	284.67345	286.88028	289.08980	291.30198	293.51683	295.73431	297.95442	300.17713	302.40244	304.63033
170	306.86078	309.09378	311.32930	313.56735	315.80790	318.05094	320.29645	322.54442	324.79484	327.04770
180	329.30297	331.56065	333.82072	336.08317	338.34799	340.61516	342.88467	345.15651	347.43067	349.70713
190	351.98589	354.26692	356.55022	358.83578	361.12358	363.41362	365.70587	368.00034	370.29700	372.59586
200	374.89689	377.20008	379.50544	381.81293	384.12256	386.43432	388.74818	391.06415	393.38222	395.70236
210	398.02458	400.34887	402.67520	405.00358	407.33400	409.66643	412.00089	414.33735	416.67580	419.01625
220	421.35867	423.70306	426.04942	428.39772	430.74797	433.10015	435.45426	437.81029	440.16822	442.52806
230	444.88978	447.25340	449.61888	451.98624	454.35546	456.72652	459.09944	461.47418	463.85076	466.22916
240	468.60937	470.99139	473.37520	475.76081	478.14820	480.53737	482.92830	485.32100	487.71545	490.11165
250	492.50959	494.90926	497.31066	499.71378	502.11862	504.52516	506.93340	509.34333	511.75495	514.16825
260	516.58322	518.99986	521.41816	523.83812	526.25972	528.68297	531.10785	533.53436	535.96250	538.39225
270	540.82361	543.25658	545.69115	548.12731	550.56506	553.00439	555.44530	557.88778	560.33183	562.77743
280	565.22459	567.67330	570.12354	572.57533	575.02865	577.48349	579.93986	582.39774	584.85713	587.31803
290	589.78043	592.24432	594.70971	597.17657	599.64492	602.11474	604.58603	607.05879	609.53301	612.00868
300	614.48580	616.96436	619.44437	621.92581	624.40869	626.89299	629.37871	631.86585	634.35440	636.84436
310	639.33572	641.82848	644.32263	646.81818	649.31511	651.81342	654.31310	656.81416	659.31659	661.82038
320	664.32553	666.83204	669.33989	671.84910	674.35964	676.87152	679.38474	681.89929	684.41516	686.93236
330	689.45087	691.97070	694.49184	697.01428	699.53803	702.06307	704.58941	707.11704	709.64596	712.17616
340	714.70764	717.24039	719.77442	722.30971	724.84627	727.38409	729.92317	732.46350	735.00508	737.54790
350	740.09197	742.63728	745.18382	747.73160	750.28060	752.83083	755.38228	757.93495	760.48883	763.04392
360	765.60023	768.15773	770.71644	773.27635	775.83745	778.39974	780.96323	783.52789	786.09374	788.66077
370	791.22897	793.79834	796.36888	798.94059	801.51347	804.08750	806.66268	809.23903	811.81652	814.39516
380	816.97494	819.55587	822.13793	824.72113	827.30546	829.89092	832.47751	835.06522	837.65405	840.24400
390	842.83507	845.42724	848.02053	850.61492	853.21042	855.80701	858.40471	861.00350	863.60338	866.20436
400	868.80642	871.40956	874.01379	876.61909	879.22547	881.83293	884.44146	887.05105	889.66171	892.27343
410	894.88622	897.50006	900.11496	902.73091	905.34791	907.96595	910.58505	913.20518	915.82636	918.44857
420	921.07182	923.69611	926.32142	928.94776	931.57512	934.20351	936.83292	939.46335	942.09480	944.72725
430	947.36072	949.99520	952.63068	955.26717	957.90466	960.54315	963.18263	965.82312	968.46459	971.10705
440	973.75051	976.39495	979.04037	981.68677	984.33415	986.98251	989.63185	992.28216	994.93344	997.58568
450	1000.23889	1002.89307	1005.54821	1008.20431	1010.86136	1013.51937	1016.17834	1018.83825	1021.49912	1024.16093
460	1026.82369	1029.48739	1032.15203	1034.81761	1037.48413	1040.15158	1042.81997	1045.48929	1048.15953	1050.83071
470	1053.50280	1056.17582	1058.84977	1061.52463	1064.20041	1066.87710	1069.55471	1072.23322	1074.91265	1077.59299
480	1080.27423	1082.95637	1085.63942	1088.32337	1091.00821	1093.69395	1096.38059	1099.06812	1101.75654	1104.44585
490	1107.13604	1109.82712	1112.51909	1115.21194	1117.90566	1120.60027	1123.29575	1125.99211	1128.68934	1131.38744
500	1134.08641	1136.78624	1139.48695	1142.18851	1144.89094	1147.59424	1150.29839	1153.00339	1155.70926	1158.41598
510	1161.12355	1163.83197	1166.54124	1169.25135	1171.96232	1174.67412	1177.38677	1180.10026	1182.81459	1185.52976
520	1188.24576	1190.96260	1193.68027	1196.39877	1199.11810	1201.83826	1204.55925	1207.28106	1210.00369	1212.72715
530	1215.45142	1218.17652	1220.90243	1223.62916	1226.35670	1229.08505	1231.81422	1234.54419	1237.27497	1240.00656
540	1242.73896	1245.47215	1248.20615	1250.94095	1253.67655	1256.41295	1259.15014	1261.88813	1264.62691	1267.36648
550	1270.10684	1272.84799	1275.58993	1278.33266	1281.07617	1283.82046	1286.56554	1289.31139	1292.05803	1294.80544
560	1297.55363	1300.30259	1303.05232	1305.80283	1308.55411	1311.30616	1314.05898	1316.81256	1319.56691	1322.32202
570	1325.07790	1327.83453	1330.59193	1333.35008	1336.10899	1338.86866	1341.62908	1344.39026	1347.15219	1349.91487
580	1352.67829	1355.44247	1358.20739	1360.97306	1363.73948	1366.50663	1369.27453	1372.04317	1374.81254	1377.58266
590	1380.35351	1383.12510	1385.89742	1388.67048	1391.44426	1394.21878	1396.99403	1399.77000	1402.54670	1405.32413

n	0	1	2	3	4	5	6	7	8	9
600	1408.10228	1410.88115	1413.66075	1416.44107	1419.22210	1422.00386	1424.78633	1427.56952	1430.35343	1433.13804
610	1435.92337	1438.70941	1441.49617	1444.28363	1447.07179	1449.86067	1452.65025	1455.44054	1458.23152	1461.02322
620	1463.81561	1466.60870	1469.40249	1472.19698	1474.99216	1477.78804	1480.58462	1483.38188	1486.17984	1488.97849
630	1491.77784	1494.57787	1497.37858	1500.17999	1502.98208	1505.78485	1508.58831	1511.39245	1514.19727	1517.00277
640	1519.80895	1522.61581	1525.42334	1528.23155	1531.04044	1533.85000	1536.66023	1539.47114	1542.28271	1545.09496
650	1547.90787	1550.72145	1553.53570	1556.35061	1559.16619	1561.98243	1564.79933	1567.61690	1570.43513	1573.25401
660	1576.07356	1578.89376	1581.71461	1584.53613	1587.35830	1590.18112	1593.00459	1595.82872	1598.65350	1601.47892
670	1604.30500	1607.13172	1609.95909	1612.78710	1615.61576	1618.44507	1621.27501	1624.10560	1626.93683	1629.76870
680	1632.60121	1635.43436	1638.26814	1641.10256	1643.93762	1646.77331	1649.60964	1652.44659	1655.28418	1658.12240
690	1660.96125	1663.80073	1666.64083	1669.48157	1672.32293	1675.16491	1678.00752	1680.85075	1683.69461	1686.53909
700	1689.38418	1692.22990	1695.07624	1697.92320	1700.77077	1703.61896	1706.46776	1709.31718	1712.16721	1715.01786
710	1717.86912	1720.72099	1723.57347	1726.42656	1729.28026	1732.13456	1734.98948	1737.84500	1740.70112	1743.55785
720	1746.41518	1749.27312	1752.13165	1754.99079	1757.85053	1760.71087	1763.57181	1766.43334	1769.29547	1772.15820
730	1775.02152	1777.88544	1780.74995	1783.61505	1786.48075	1789.34704	1792.21391	1795.08138	1797.94944	1800.81808
740	1803.68731	1806.55713	1809.42754	1812.29853	1815.17010	1818.04225	1820.91499	1823.78831	1826.66222	1829.53670
750	1832.41176	1835.28740	1838.16362	1841.04041	1843.91778	1846.79573	1849.67425	1852.55335	1855.43302	1858.31326
760	1861.19407	1864.07546	1866.95741	1869.83994	1872.72303	1875.60669	1878.49092	1881.37571	1884.26108	1887.14700
770	1890.03349	1892.92055	1895.80816	1898.69634	1901.58508	1904.47439	1907.36425	1910.25467	1913.14565	1916.03718
780	1918.92928	1921.82193	1924.71514	1927.60890	1930.50321	1933.39808	1936.29351	1939.18948	1942.08601	1944.98308
790	1947.88071	1950.77889	1953.67761	1956.57689	1959.47671	1962.37707	1965.27799	1968.17944	1971.08145	1973.98399
800	1976.88708	1979.79072	1982.69489	1985.59961	1988.50486	1991.41066	1994.31699	1997.22387	2000.13128	2003.03922
810	2005.94771	2008.85673	2011.76629	2014.67638	2017.58700	2020.49816	2023.40985	2026.32207	2029.23482	2032.14811
820	2035.06192	2037.97626	2040.89114	2043.80654	2046.72246	2049.63892	2052.55590	2055.47340	2058.39143	2061.30999
830	2064.22906	2067.14867	2070.06879	2072.98943	2075.91060	2078.83229	2081.75449	2084.67722	2087.60046	2090.52422
840	2093.44850	2096.37330	2099.29861	2102.22444	2105.15078	2108.07764	2111.00501	2113.93289	2116.86129	2119.79019
850	2122.71961	2125.64954	2128.57998	2131.51093	2134.44239	2137.37435	2140.30683	2143.23981	2146.17330	2149.10729
860	2152.04179	2154.97679	2157.91230	2160.84831	2163.78482	2166.72184	2169.65936	2172.59737	2175.53589	2178.47491
870	2181.41443	2184.35445	2187.29497	2190.23598	2193.17749	2196.11950	2199.06200	2202.00500	2204.94850	2207.89249
880	2210.83697	2213.78195	2216.72741	2219.67338	2222.61983	2225.56677	2228.51420	2231.46213	2234.41054	2237.35944
890	2240.30883	2243.25871	2246.20908	2249.15993	2252.11126	2255.06309	2258.01540	2260.96819	2263.92146	2266.87522
900	2269.82947	2272.78419	2275.73940	2278.69509	2281.65125	2284.60790	2287.56503	2290.52264	2293.48072	2296.43929
910	2299.39833	2302.35785	2305.31784	2308.27831	2311.23926	2314.20068	2317.16258	2320.12495	2323.08779	2326.05111
920	2329.01489	2331.97915	2334.94388	2337.90909	2340.87476	2343.84090	2346.80751	2349.77459	2352.74214	2355.71015
930	2358.67864	2361.64759	2364.61700	2367.58688	2370.55723	2373.52804	2376.49932	2379.47106	2382.44326	2385.41593
940	2388.38906	2391.36265	2394.33670	2397.31121	2400.28618	2403.26161	2406.23750	2409.21385	2412.19066	2415.16793
950	2418.14565	2421.12383	2424.10247	2427.08156	2430.06111	2433.04112	2436.02157	2439.00249	2441.98385	2444.96567
960	2447.94794	2450.93066	2453.91384	2456.89747	2459.88154	2462.86607	2465.85105	2468.83647	2471.82235	2474.80867
970	2477.79545	2480.78266	2483.77033	2486.75844	2489.74700	2492.73601	2495.72546	2498.71535	2501.70569	2504.69647
980	2507.68770	2510.67937	2513.67148	2516.66403	2519.65703	2522.65047	2525.64434	2528.63866	2531.63342	2534.62861
990	2537.62425	2540.62032	2543.61683	2546.61378	2549.61117	2552.60899	2555.60725	2558.60595	2561.60508	2564.60464

Appendix XIX

The correlation coefficient

Degrees of freedom	Value of P				
	0.10	0.05	0.02	0.01	0.001
1	0.9877	0.99692	0.99951	0.99988	0.9999988
2	0.9000	0.9500	0.9800	0.9900	0.9990
3	0.805	0.878	0.9343	0.9587	0.9911
4	0.729	0.811	0.882	0.9172	0.9741
5	0.669	0.754	0.833	0.875	0.9509
6	0.621	0.707	0.789	0.834	0.9249
7	0.582	0.666	0.750	0.798	0.898
8	0.549	0.632	0.715	0.765	0.872
9	0.521	0.602	0.685	0.735	0.847
10	0.497	0.576	0.658	0.708	0.823
11	0.476	0.553	0.634	0.684	0.801
12	0.457	0.532	0.612	0.661	0.780
13	0.441	0.514	0.592	0.641	0.760
14	0.426	0.497	0.574	0.623	0.742
15	0.412	0.482	0.558	0.606	0.725
16	0.400	0.468	0.543	0.590	0.708
17	0.389	0.456	0.529	0.575	0.693
18	0.378	0.444	0.516	0.561	0.679
19	0.369	0.433	0.503	0.549	0.665
20	0.360	0.423	0.492	0.537	0.652
25	0.323	0.381	0.445	0.487	0.597
30	0.296	0.349	0.409	0.449	0.554
35	0.275	0.325	0.381	0.418	0.519
40	0.257	0.304	0.358	0.393	0.490
45	0.243	0.288	0.338	0.372	0.465
50	0.231	0.273	0.322	0.354	0.443
60	0.211	0.250	0.295	0.325	0.408
70	0.195	0.232	0.274	0.302	0.380
80	0.183	0.217	0.257	0.283	0.357
90	0.173	0.205	0.242	0.267	0.338
100	0.164	0.195	0.230	0.254	0.321

The table gives percentage points for the distribution of the estimated correlation coefficient r when the true value ϱ is zero. Thus when there are 10 degrees of freedom (i.e. in samples of 12) the probability of observing an r greater in **absolute value** than 0.576 (i.e. < -0.576 or $> +0.576$) is 0.05 or 5 per cent.

Appendix XX

The variance-ratio (*F*) distribution

5 per cent points

f_2	|	1	2	3	4	5	6	7	8	9	10	12	15	20	30	∞
	|								f_1							
1	|	161.4	199.5	215.7	224.6	230.2	234.0	236.8	238.9	240.5	241.9	143.9	245.9	248.0	250.1	254.3
2	|	18.51	19.00	19.16	19.25	19.30	19.33	19.35	19.37	19.38	19.40	19.41	19.43	19.45	19.46	19.50
3	|	10.13	9.55	9.28	9.12	9.01	8.94	8.89	8.85	8.81	8.79	8.74	8.70	8.66	8.62	8.53
4	|	7.71	6.94	6.59	6.39	6.26	6.16	6.09	6.04	6.00	5.96	5.91	5.86	5.80	5.75	5.63
5	|	6.61	5.79	5.41	5.19	5.05	4.95	4.88	4.82	4.77	4.74	4.68	4.62	4.56	4.50	4.36
6	|	5.99	5.14	4.76	4.53	4.39	4.28	4.21	4.15	4.10	4.06	4.00	3.94	3.87	3.81	3.67
7	|	5.59	4.74	4.35	4.12	3.97	3.87	3.79	3.73	3.68	3.64	3.57	3.51	3.44	3.38	3.23
8	|	5.32	4.45	4.07	3.84	3.69	3.58	3.50	3.44	3.39	3.35	3.28	3.22	3.15	3.08	2.93
9	|	5.12	4.26	3.86	3.63	3.48	3.37	3.29	3.23	3.18	3.14	3.07	3.01	2.94	2.86	2.71
10	|	4.96	4.10	3.71	3.48	3.33	3.22	3.14	3.07	3.02	2.98	2.91	2.85	2.77	2.70	2.54
11	|	4.84	3.98	3.59	3.36	3.20	3.09	3.01	2.95	2.90	2.85	2.79	2.72	2.65	2.57	2.40
12	|	4.75	3.89	3.49	3.26	3.11	3.00	2.91	2.85	2.80	2.75	2.69	2.62	2.54	2.47	2.30
13	|	4.67	3.81	3.41	3.18	3.03	2.92	2.83	2.77	2.71	2.67	2.60	2.53	2.46	2.38	2.21
14	|	4.60	3.74	3.34	3.11	2.96	2.85	2.76	2.70	2.65	2.60	2.53	2.46	2.39	2.31	2.13
15	|	4.54	3.68	3.29	3.06	2.90	2.79	2.71	2.64	2.59	2.54	2.48	2.40	2.33	2.25	2.07
16	|	4.49	3.63	3.24	3.01	2.85	2.74	2.66	2.59	2.54	2.49	2.42	2.35	2.28	2.19	2.01
17	|	4.45	3.59	3.20	2.96	2.81	2.70	2.61	2.55	2.49	2.45	2.38	2.31	2.23	2.15	1.96
18	|	4.41	3.55	3.16	2.93	2.77	2.66	2.58	2.51	2.46	2.41	2.34	2.27	2.19	2.11	1.92
19	|	4.38	3.52	3.13	2.90	2.74	2.63	2.54	2.48	2.42	2.38	2.31	2.23	2.16	2.07	1.88
20	|	4.35	3.49	3.10	2.87	2.71	2.60	2.51	2.45	2.39	2.35	2.28	2.20	2.12	2.04	1.84
21	|	4.32	3.47	3.07	2.84	2.68	2.57	2.49	2.42	2.37	2.32	2.25	2.18	2.10	2.01	1.81
22	|	4.30	3.44	3.05	2.82	2.66	2.55	2.46	2.40	2.34	2.30	2.23	2.15	2.07	1.98	1.78
23	|	4.28	3.42	3.03	2.80	2.64	2.53	2.44	2.37	2.32	2.27	2.20	2.13	2.05	1.96	1.76
24	|	4.26	3.40	3.01	2.78	2.62	2.51	2.42	2.36	2.30	2.25	2.18	2.11	2.03	1.94	1.73
25	|	4.24	3.39	2.99	2.76	2.60	2.49	2.40	2.34	2.28	2.24	2.16	2.09	2.01	1.92	1.71
26	|	4.23	3.37	2.98	2.74	2.59	2.47	2.39	2.32	2.27	2.22	2.15	2.07	1.99	1.90	1.69
27	|	4.21	3.35	2.96	2.73	2.57	2.46	2.37	2.31	2.25	2.20	2.13	2.06	1.97	1.88	1.67
28	|	4.20	3.34	2.95	2.71	2.56	2.45	2.36	2.29	2.24	2.19	2.12	2.04	1.96	1.87	1.65
29	|	4.18	3.33	2.93	2.70	2.55	2.43	2.35	2.28	2.22	2.18	2.10	2.03	1.94	1.85	1.64
30	|	4.17	3.32	2.92	2.69	2.53	2.42	2.33	2.27	2.21	2.16	2.09	2.01	1.93	1.84	1.62
40	|	4.08	3.23	2.84	2.61	2.45	2.34	2.25	2.18	1.12	2.08	2.00	1.92	1.84	1.74	1.51
60	|	4.00	3.15	2.76	2.53	2.37	2.25	2.17	2.10	2.04	1.99	1.92	1.84	1.75	1.65	1.39
120	|	3.92	3.07	2.68	2.45	2.29	2.17	2.09	2.02	1.96	1.91	1.83	1.75	1.66	1.55	1.25
∞	|	3.84	3.00	2.60	2.37	2.21	2.10	2.01	1.94	1.88	1.83	1.75	1.67	1.57	1.46	1.00

The table gives the 5 per cent points of the distribution of the variance-ratio, $F = s_1^2/s_2^2$, where the numerator and denominator have f_1 and f_2 degrees of freedom respectively. Thus if $f_1 = 7$ and $f_2 = 15$, the probability ..at the observed value of F is **greater** than 2.71 is exactly 0.05 or 5 per cent.

1 per cent points

f_2	f_1														
	1	*2*	*3*	*4*	*5*	*6*	*7*	*8*	*9*	*10*	*12*	*15*	*20*	*30*	*∞*
1	4052	4999	5403	5625	5764	5859	5928	5982	6022	6056	6106	6157	6209	6261	6366
2	98.50	99.00	99.17	99.25	99.30	99.33	99.36	99.37	99.39	99.40	99.42	99.43	99.45	99.47	99.50
3	34.12	30.82	29.46	28.71	28.24	27.91	27.67	27.49	27.35	27.23	27.05	26.87	26.69	26.50	26.13
4	21.20	18.00	16.69	15.98	15.52	15.21	14.98	14.80	14.66	14.55	14.37	14.20	14.02	13.84	13.46
5	16.26	13.27	12.06	11.39	10.97	10.67	10.46	10.29	10.16	10.05	9.89	9.72	9.55	9.38	9.02
6	13.75	10.92	9.78	9.15	8.75	8.47	8.26	8.10	7.98	7.87	7.72	7.56	7.40	7.23	6.88
7	12.25	9.55	8.45	7.85	7.46	7.19	6.99	6.84	6.72	6.62	6.47	6.31	6.16	5.99	5.65
8	11.26	8.65	7.59	7.01	6.63	6.37	6.18	6.03	5.91	5.81	5.67	5.52	5.36	5.20	4.86
9	10.56	8.02	6.99	6.42	6.06	5.80	5.61	5.47	5.35	5.26	5.11	4.96	4.81	4.65	4.31
10	10.04	7.56	6.55	5.99	5.64	5.39	5.20	5.06	4.94	4.85	4.71	4.56	4.41	4.25	3.91
11	9.65	7.21	6.22	5.67	5.32	5.07	4.89	4.74	4.63	4.54	4.40	4.25	4.10	3.94	3.60
12	9.33	6.93	5.95	5.41	5.06	4.82	4.64	4.50	4.39	4.30	4.16	4.01	3.86	3.70	3.36
13	9.07	6.70	5.74	5.21	4.86	4.62	4.44	4.30	4.19	4.10	3.96	3.82	3.66	3.51	3.17
14	8.86	6.51	5.56	5.04	4.69	4.46	4.28	4.14	4.03	3.94	3.80	3.66	3.51	3.35	3.00
15	8.68	6.36	5.42	4.89	4.56	4.32	4.14	4.00	3.89	3.80	3.67	3.52	3.37	3.21	2.87
16	8.53	6.23	5.29	4.77	4.44	4.20	4.03	3.89	3.78	3.69	3.55	3.41	3.26	3.10	2.75
17	8.40	6.11	5.18	4.67	4.34	4.10	3.93	3.79	3.68	3.59	3.46	3.31	3.16	3.00	2.65
18	8.29	6.01	5.09	4.58	4.25	4.01	3.84	3.71	3.60	3.51	3.37	3.23	3.08	2.92	2.57
19	8.18	5.93	5.01	4.50	4.17	3.94	3.77	3.63	3.52	3.43	3.30	3.15	3.00	2.84	2.49
20	8.10	5.85	4.94	4.43	4.10	3.87	3.70	3.56	3.46	3.37	3.23	3.09	2.94	2.78	2.42
21	8.02	5.78	4.87	4.37	4.04	3.81	3.64	3.51	3.40	3.31	3.17	3.03	2.88	2.72	2.36
22	7.95	5.72	4.82	4.31	3.99	3.76	3.59	3.45	3.35	3.26	3.12	2.98	2.83	2.67	2.31
23	7.88	5.66	4.76	4.26	3.94	3.71	3.54	3.41	3.30	3.21	3.07	2.93	2.78	2.62	2.26
24	7.82	5.61	4.72	4.22	3.90	3.67	3.50	3.36	3.26	3.17	3.03	2.89	2.74	2.58	2.21
25	7.77	5.57	4.68	4.18	3.85	3.63	3.46	3.32	3.22	3.13	2.99	2.85	2.70	2.54	2.17
26	7.72	5.53	4.64	4.14	3.82	3.59	3.42	3.29	3.18	3.09	2.96	2.81	2.66	2.50	2.13
27	7.68	5.49	4.60	4.11	3.78	3.56	3.39	3.26	3.15	3.06	2.93	2.78	2.63	2.47	2.10
28	7.64	5.45	4.57	4.07	3.75	3.53	3.36	3.23	3.12	3.03	2.90	2.75	2.60	2.44	2.06
29	7.60	5.42	4.54	4.04	3.73	3.50	3.33	3.20	3.09	3.00	2.87	2.73	2.57	2.41	2.03
30	7.56	5.39	4.51	4.02	3.70	3.47	3.30	3.17	3.07	2.98	2.84	2.70	2.55	2.39	2.01
40	7.31	5.18	4.31	3.83	3.51	3.29	3.12	2.99	2.89	2.80	2.66	2.52	2.37	2.20	1.80
60	7.08	4.98	4.13	3.65	3.34	3.12	2.95	2.82	2.72	2.63	2.50	2.35	2.20	2.03	1.60
120	6.85	4.79	3.95	3.48	3.17	2.96	2.79	2.66	2.56	2.47	2.34	2.19	2.03	1.86	1.38
∞	6.63	4.61	3.78	3.32	3.02	2.80	2.64	2.51	2.41	2.32	2.18	2.04	1.88	1.70	1.00

The table gives the 1 per cent points of the distribution of the variance-ratio, $F = s_1^2/s_2^2$, where the numerator and denominator have f_1 and f_2 degrees of freedom respectively. Thus if $f_1 = 7$ and $f_2 = 15$, the probability that the observed value of F is **greater** than 4.14 is exactly 0.01 or 1 per cent.

Appendix XXI

Meta-analysis of clinical trials
(Supplement to Chapter 16)

Meta-analysis is the statistical analysis of data pooled from several studies to integrate findings.* The technique has its origins in educational research (Glass, 1976) and has been widely applied in the social sciences, where key texts have been published (Wolf, 1986; Hunter and Schmidt, 1989).

Goals of meta-analysis in medicine

In medicine, meta-analysis has been applied in several areas, including the evaluation of diagnostic tests, observational studies, cost–benefit analysis of diagnostic techniques and treatments, and assessment of the magnitude of health problems. However, it has been used most extensively in the area of human clinical trials and, of late, is being adopted by veterinary researchers in this context (e.g., Willeberg's study of the relationship between treatment with bovine somatotropin and mastitis incidence: Willeberg, 1993) and in other fields (e.g. the evaluation of diagnostic tests: Greiner *et al.*, 1997).

The aims of meta-analysis (Sacks *et al.*, 1987; Dickersin and Berlin, 1992; Marubini and Valsecchi, 1995) are to:

1. increase statistical power for primary end points;
2. resolve uncertainty if there are conflicting results;
3. improve estimates of therapeutic effect, and their precision;†
4. answer questions not posed at the beginning of individual trials;

5. give a 'state-of-the-art' literature review;
6. facilitate analysis of subgroups when the power of individual analyses is low;
7. guide researchers in planning new trials;
8. offer rigorous support for generalization of a treatment (i.e. external validity);
9. balance 'overflow of enthusiasm' which might accompany introduction of a new procedure following a single beneficial report.

Correctly conducted meta-analyses therefore offer the strongest evidence for efficacy of treatment (*Table XXI.1*).

However, there are disadvantages, as well as advantages, to the technique (*Table XXI.2*). Perhaps the major disadvantage is the seductive notion that combination of several small trials is a substitute for a well-designed large one.‡

Table XXI.1 Hierarchy of strength of evidence concerning efficacy of treatment. (From Marubini and Valsecchi, 1995.)

---

1. Anecdotal case reports
2. Case series without controls
3. Series with literature controls
4. Analysis using computer databases
5. Case-control observational studies
6. Series based on historical control groups
7. Single randomized controlled clinical trials
8. Meta-analyses of randomized controlled clinical trials

The table lists the types of study used in medicine, suggested by Green and Byar (1984). The table can be considered as an eight-tiered pyramid. In the context of clinical trials, the base on which conclusions about efficacy can be built becomes broader as one moves downwards.

---

* The term is derived from the Greek preposition, $\mu\varepsilon\tau\alpha$- (*meta-*) = 'alongside', 'among', 'in connection with'. A subsidiary meaning is 'after'. Meta-analysis is therefore either one that is done alongside/in conjunction with the normal analysis, or one that is done after the normal analysis, that is, at a later stage in the process. An alternative term – 'overviews' of research – has also been suggested (Peto, 1987).

† This includes not only revealing beneficial effects that are not identified in isolated studies, but also identification of 'false-positive' effects in individual studies: meta-analysis is designed to produce *accurate* results – not necessarily positive ones.

‡ This may appear particularly attractive in the current academic climate, where financial support is in short supply and there is pressure to generate publications.

Table XXI.2 Advantages and disadvantages of meta-analysis. (Based on Meinert, 1989.)

Advantages:
Focuses attention on trials as an evaluation tool
Increases the impact of trials on clinical practice
Encourages good trial design and reporting

Disadvantages:
Current fashion for meta-analysis may discourage large definitive trials
Tendency to mix different trials unwittingly and ignore differences
Potential for tension between meta-analyst and conductors of original trials

In this section, the main issues associated with meta-analysis are outlined. For details of specific statistical procedures, the reader is directed to the standard texts mentioned above, and to the excellent reviews by Abramson (1991) and Dickersin and Berlin (1992).

Components

There are both **qualitative** and **quantitative** components to meta-analysis, listed in a scheme for meta-analysis of clinical trials (Naylor, 1989):

1. selection of trials according to inclusion and exclusion criteria;
2. evaluation of the quality of the trials;
3. abstraction of key trial characteristics and data;
4. analysis of similarity in design, execution and analysis, and exploration of differences between trials;
5. aggregation of data, testing various combinations and interpretations;
6. drawing of careful conclusions.

Note that the conventional, qualitative review article has traditionally been accepted as the means of summarizing research data – usually by listing the individual results of several studies – and lacks objective rigorous analysis. A properly designed meta-analysis, in contrast, goes further and uses quantitative analytical procedures to combine results from several sources, where possible, to produce an overall conclusion.

Sources of data

Data for meta-analyses are usually obtained from published material, most of which is presented in refereed journals. This has the advantage of guaranteeing (at least theoretically) minimum standards with respect to the design, conduct and analysis of the component studies.

However, there is a tendency for positive findings (beneficial treatment effects) to be more readily accepted for publication than results that either do not show significant effects or reveal only minor effects (Easterbrook *et al.*, 1991); this constitutes **publication bias**. This is a complex matter, though, and unpublished results can show larger effects than published ones (Detsky *et al.*, 1987). Assessment of the quality of *all* potential data is therefore desirable, so that useful material does not escape the analyst.

Various methods have been recommended for handling publication bias. A simple approach (Rosenthal, 1979) calculates an overall *P* value from the *P* values of the component studies, and then calculates a 'fail-safe *N*': the number of statistically non-significant studies that, if added, would increase the *P* value to a critical threshold level (say, 0.05).

Comparability of sources

A key feature of component trials is the **variability (heterogeneity)** in their results. The latter may actually be contradictory, but this is generally due to differences in the design, conduct or analysis of the studies (Horwitz, 1987). Additionally, different trials may be measuring different response variables on different scales (e.g., median values or visual analogue measurements). Differences between old and recent studies may be ascribed to underlying health trends unrelated to the therapy in question – somewhat akin to the use of historical controls. If a meta-analysis intends to address general policy or efficacy of a class of drugs, then incorporation of trials with obvious differences can be condoned. However, a specific question will require selection of a relatively homogeneous set of trials.

Differences between the different studies that are included in an analysis prevent interpretation of pooled estimates as being precise,* and 99% intervals may therefore be more prudent than the conventional 95% limits.

Data analysis

Analytical techniques treat each incorporated clinical trial as a **stratum**. The single treatment effects are estimated within each trial, and are then combined to

---

* The confidence limit is strictly a limit on the expected results, based on what was done in the studies rather than on future trials.

produce a suitable summary, weighted by treatment effect. Methods of weighting, and addressing variability in study results, vary. However, the tendency simply to pool the results of the trials and compute an average effect is avoided. This could be dangerously misleading; for example, a mean mortality rate computed from a series of separate mortality rates does not address differences in sample sizes between trials, and therefore the different precision of each trial's estimate.

A common approach for categorical data is to provide a weighted estimate, for example, of the relative risk or odds ratio. Standard methods include the Mantel-Haenszel procedure (see Chapter 15). More sophisticated procedures allow pooling of parameters that have been adjusted for confounding (Greenland, 1987).

Continuous explanatory variables require different procedures. A commonly used measure is the **effect size**. This is the difference between the mean values of the treatment and control groups divided by the standard deviation in the control group (or in both groups combined) (Glass *et al.*, 1981). This can be interpreted with reference to tables of probabilities associated with the upper tail of the normal distribution (Appendix XII). For example, an effect size of 2.9 means that 99.8% of controls have values below the mean value of treated individuals. Consulting Appendix XII, this percentage is obtained by identifying the one-tailed probability, P, in the body of the table for which the effect size equals z. The percentage then equals $(1 - P) \times 100$. Thus, if the effect size = 2.9, $P = 0.0019$, and $(1 - P) \times 100 = (1 - 0.0019) \times 100 = 99.81\%$. Similarly, for an effect size of 1.0, the corresponding percentage is 84% ($\{1 - 0.1587\} \times 100$).

Effect size has no units, and so allows the combination of results expressed in different units. However, it should be interpreted with caution because it depends not only on differences in the effect itself, but also on differences in standard deviations. The use of effect size is therefore particularly dubious if sample sizes are small.

Heterogeneity

The heterogeneity between studies must always be addressed. Commonly, tests for homogeneity are based on χ^2 or F statistics for categorical (Schlesselman, 1982) and continuous data (Fleiss, 1986), respectively. These are usually interpreted liberally at the 10% level because of the relatively low power of such tests (Breslow and Day, 1980). A sensitivity analysis (see Chapter 19) can also be conducted to determine if exclusion of one or more trials materially affects the heterogeneity. If the heterogeneity is larger than can be inferred from the

results of significance tests, a summary measure is questionable, and the reason for the heterogeneity should be explored.* Note, however, that a high P value does not unequivocally indicate that the results are homogeneous, and the data should be explored by other means, such as graphical representation. Examples include a vertical two-tiered plot of results (e.g., odds ratios, relative risks,† or effect size) with their 95% and 70% confidence intervals, for ease of comparison around the point estimates (Pocock and Hughes, 1990). A 'funnel display' plots results against a measure of precision (e.g., sample size or the reciprocal of the variance); if all studies are estimating a similar value, the spread of results should become narrow as precision increases, producing a funnel shape (Greenland, 1987).

Fixed-effect and random-effect models

Most of the analytical procedures that have been employed in meta-analyses are based on a **fixed-effect** model which assumes that all clinical trials included in the meta-analysis are estimating the **same** treatment effect. They therefore ignore any variability between different studies when producing a summary estimate (e.g., of the odds ratio). An alternative approach, based on a **random-effect** model (e.g., DerSimonian and Laird, 1986), assumes that treatment effect may be **different**, and each study represents a random sample of a (theoretically infinite) number of studies. The variability between studies is then an integral part of the analysis (Bailey, 1987). The net result of such an analysis is that the interval estimate of treatment effect is generally widened relative to the fixed-effect estimate, particularly if there is clear heterogeneity between studies (Dickersin and Berlin, 1992).

Although the random-effect model may be attractive, it needs to be interpreted with caution (Marubini and Valsecchi, 1995). First, the degree of heterogeneity may be such that a random-effect model may greatly modify the inferences made from a fixed-effect model. This will tend to nullify the summary statistic for both models, and there is then a need to investigate the variability further. Secondly, specific statistical distributions of the random-effect model cannot be justified either empirically or by clinical reasoning. Finally, the random-effect model cannot be meaningfully interpreted at the level of the

---

* For example, different dosage levels (analogous to different exposure levels in observational studies: e.g., Frumkin and Berlin, 1988) may induce heterogeneity.
† Odds ratios and relative risks are best plotted on a logarithmic scale.

target population, it is merely the mean of a distribution that generates effects. The random-effect model therefore 'exchanges a questionable homogeneity assumption for a fictitious distribution of effects' (Greenland, 1987).

Debate continues over the relative merits of the fixed-effect and random-effect approaches. Some of the biases can be reduced by excluding poorly designed trials and including all relevant results (e.g., results from germane unpublished studies). With this goal in mind, Meinert (1989) has suggested that meta-analyses should be planned prospectively, with the component trials enlisted into a meta-analysis when they start, rather than being retrospectively identified. This should promote good individual trial design, and therefore consistent quality. Moreover, cumulative meta-analyses may allow both fixed-effect and random-effect models to demonstrate efficacy in the presence of heterogeneity of estimates.*

Meta-analysis is more advanced in human than in veterinary medicine, but is still a contentious issue. Responses to a recent meta-analysis of over 3000 randomized controlled clinical trials of preventive care in human pregnancy and childbirth (Chalmers *et al.*, 1989) ranged from describing it as 'arguably the most important publication in obstetrics since William Smellie wrote his *A Treatise on the Theory and Practice of Midwifery* in 1752' to describing its authors as 'an obstetrical Baader-Meinhof gang' (quoted by Abramson, 1991). However, meta-analysis is a powerful technique which is likely to be applied more in veterinary science, and veterinarians should profit from the experience of their medical counterparts.

References

(References cited in this supplement, but absent from the list below, can be found in the main list of references.)

Abramson, J.H. (1991) Meta-analysis: A review of pros and cons. *Public Health Reviews*, **18**, 1–47

Bailey, K.R. (1987) Inter-study differences: how should they influence the interpretation and analysis of results? *Statistics in Medicine*, **6**, 351–358

Chalmers, I., Enkin, M. and Keirse, M.J.N.V. (1989) *Effective Care in Pregnancy and Childbirth*. Oxford University Press, Oxford

DerSimonian, R. and Laird, N. (1986) Meta-analysis in clinical trials. *Controlled Clinical Trials*, **7**, 177–188

Detsky, A.S., Baker, J.P., O'Rourke, K. and Goel, V. (1987) Perioperative parenteral nutrition: a meta-analysis. *Annals of Internal Medicine*, **107**, 195–203

Dickersin, K. and Berlin, J.A. (1992) Meta-analysis: State-of-the-Science. *Epidemiologic Reviews*, **14**, 154–176

Easterbrook, P.J., Berlin, J.A., Gopolan, R. and Matthews, D.R. (1991) Publication bias in clinical research. *Lancet*, **337**, 867–872

Fleiss, J.L. (1986) Analysis of data from multiclinic trials. *Controlled Clinical Trials*, **7**, 267–275

Frumkin, H. and Berlin, J. (1988) Asbestos exposure and gastrointestinal malignancy: review and meta-analysis. *American Journal of Industrial Medicine*, **14**, 79–95

Glass, G.V. (1976) Primary, secondary, and meta-analysis of research. *Educational Research*, **5**, 3–8

Glass, G.V., McGaw, B. and Smith, M.L. (1981) *Meta-analysis in Social Research*. Sage Publications, Beverly Hills

Green, S.B. and Byar, D.P. (1984) Using observational data from registries to compare treatments: the fallacy of omnimetrics. *Statistics in Medicine*, **3**, 361–370

Greenland, S. (1987) Quantitative methods in the review of epidemiologic literature. *Epidemiologic Reviews*, **9**, 1–30

Greiner, M., Böhning, D. and Dahms, S. (1997) Meta-analytic review of ELISA tests for the diagnosis of human and porcine trichinellosis: which factors are involved in diagnostic accuracy? In: Society for Veterinary Epidemiology and Preventive Medicine, Proceedings, Chester, 9–11 April 1997. Eds Goodall, E.A. and Thrusfield, M.V., pp. 12–21

Horwitz, R.I. (1987) Complexity and contradiction in clinical trial research. *American Journal of Medicine*, **82**, 498–510

Hunter, J.E. and Schmidt, F.L. (1989) *Methods of Meta-Analysis: Correcting Error and Bias in Research Findings*. Sage Publications, Beverly Hills

Marubini, E. and Valsecchi, M.G. (1995) *Analysing Survival Data from Clinical Trials and Observational Studies*. John Wiley, Chichester

Meinert, C.L. (1989) Meta-analysis: Science or Religion? *Controlled Clinical Trials*, **10**, 257S–263S

Naylor, C.D. (1989) Meta-analysis of controlled clinical trials. *Journal of Rheumatology*, **16**, 424–426

Peto, R. (1987) In: Discussion of Light, R.J. (1987) Accumulating evidence from independent studies: what we can win and what we can lose. *Statistics in Medicine*, **6**, 221–231

Pocock, S.J. and Hughes, M.D. (1990) Estimation issues in clinical trials and overviews. *Statistics in Medicine*, **9**, 657–671

Rosenthal, R. (1979) The 'file drawer problem' and tolerance for null results. *Psychological Bulletin*, **85**, 185–193

Sacks, H.S., Berrier, J., Reitman, D., Ancone-Berk, V.A. and Chalmers, T.C. (1987) Meta-analysis of controlled clinical trials. *New England Journal of Medicine*, **316**, 450–455

Wolf, F.M. (1986) *Meta-Analysis: Quantitative Methods for Research Synthesis*. Sage Publications, Beverly Hills

Willeberg, P. (1993) Bovine somatotropin and clinical mastitis: epidemiological analysis of the welfare risk. *Livestock Production Science*, **36**, 55–66

Yusuf, S., Held, P., and Furberg, C. (1991) Update of effects of calcium antagonists in myocardial infarction or angina in light of the second Danish verapamil infarction trials (DAVIT-II) and other recent studies. *American Journal of Cardiology*, **67**, 1295–1297

---

* There is, of course, danger of an increase in Type 1 error such as that which can occur in sequential trials. Yusef *et al.* (1991) suggest methods of significance-level adjustment in this circumstance.

References

Aalund, O., Willeberg, P., Mandrup, M. and Riemann, H. (1976) Lung lesions at slaughter: association to factors in the pig herd. *Nordisk Veterinærmedicin*, **28**, 481−486

Abbey, H. (1952) An examination of the Reed−Frost theory of epidemics. *Human Biology*, **24**, 201−233

Ackoff, R.L. (1971) Towards a system of systems concepts. *Management Science*, **17**, 661−671

ADAS (1989) *Deer Health Scheme*. Ministry of Agriculture, Fisheries and Food, State Veterinary Service, PB 0052. ADAS Publications, London

Agger, J.F. and Willeberg, P. (1986) Epidemiology of teat lesions in a dairy herd. II. Associations with subclinical mastitis. *Nordisk Veterinærmedicin*, **38**, 220−232

Agger, J.F., Willeberg, P., Schmidt Madsen, P. and Klastrup, O. (1986) A case control study of environmental and managerial factors in the Danish national mastitis control program. In: Proceedings of the Fourth International Symposium on Veterinary Epidemiology and Economics, Singapore, 18−22 November 1985, pp. 438−440. Singapore Veterinary Association

Agriculture Canada (1984) Enzyme immunoassay: application to the detection of bovine antibody to *Brucella abortus*. Agriculture Canada, Animal Disease Research Institute, Nepean, PO Box 11 300, Station H, Nepean, Ontario, Canada

Aitken, I.D. (1993) Environmental change and animal disease. In: *The Advancement of Veterinary Science. The Bicentenary Symposium Series, Volume 1: Veterinary Medicine Beyond 2000*. Ed. Michell, A.R., pp. 179−193. CAB International, Wallingford

Akhtar, S., Riemann, H.P., Thurmond, M.C., Farver, T.A. and Franti, C.E. (1990) Multivariate logistic analysis of repeated cross-sectional surveys of *Campylobacter fetus* in dairy cattle. *Preventive Veterinary Medicine*, **10**, 15−24

Akhtar, S., Zahid, S. and Khan, M.I. (1992) Risk factors associated with hydropericardium syndrome in broiler flocks. *Veterinary Record*, **131**, 481−484

Akhtar, S., Riemann, H.P., Thurmond, M.C. and Franti, C.E. (1993a) The association between antibody titres against *Campylobacter fetus* and milk production efficiency in dairy cattle. *Veterinary Research Communications*, **17**, 183−191

Akhtar, S., Riemann, H.P., Thurmond, M.C. and Franti, C.E. (1993b) The association between antibody titres against *Campylobacter fetus* and reproductive efficiency in dairy cattle. *Veterinary Research Communications*, **17**, 95−107

Albert, R.E., Alessandro, D., Lippmann, M. and Berger, J. (1971) Long-term smoking in the donkey. Effect on tracheo-bronchial particle clearance. *Archives of Environmental Health*, **22**, 12−19

Alexander, M. (1971) *Microbial Ecology*. John Wiley, New York

Algers, B. and Hennichs, K. (1985) The effects of exposure to 400 kv transmission lines on the fertility of cows. A retrospective cohort study. *Preventive Veterinary Medicine*, **3**, 351−361

Algers, B. and Hultgren, J. (1987) Effects of long-term exposure to a 400 kv, 50 Hz transmission line on oestrous and fertility in cows. *Preventive Veterinary Medicine*, **5**, 21−36

Algers, B., Ekesbo, I. and Stromberg, S. (1978) The impact of continuous noise on animal health. *Acta Veterinaria Scandinavica*, **19**, Suppl. 67, 1−26

Ambrosio, R.E. and de Waal, D.T. (1990) Diagnosis of parasitic disease. *Revue Scientifique et Technique, Office International des Epizooties*, **9**, 759−788

Anderson, D.E. (1963) Genetic aspects of cancer with special reference to cancer of the eye in the bovine. *Annals of the New York Academy of Sciences*, **108**, 948−962

Anderson, D.E., Lush, J.L. and Chambers, C. (1957) Studies on bovine ocular squamous carcinoma ('cancer eye'). II. Relationships between eyelid pigmentation and occurrence of cancer eye lesions. *Journal of Animal Science*, **16**, 739−746

Anderson, H., Henricson, B., Lundquist, P.-G., Wendenberg, H. and Wesall, J. (1968) Genetic hearing impairment in the Dalmatian dog. *Acta-otolaryngologica*, Suppl., **232**, 1−34

Anderson, J.F. (1988) Mammalian and avian hosts of *Borrelia burgdorferi*. *Annals of the New York Academy of Science*, **539**, 180−191

Anderson, K.L. (Ed.) (1993) Update on bovine mastitis. *Veterinary Clinics of North America: Food Animal Practice*, **9**, 421−630

Anderson, P.L., Morrison, R.B., Molitor, T.W. and Thawley,

D.G. (1990) Factors associated with circulation of pseudorabies virus within swine herds. *Journal of the American Veterinary Medical Association*, **196**, 877–884

Anderson, R.M. (1979) The influence of parasitic infection on the dynamics of host population growth. In: *Population Dynamics*. Eds Anderson, R.M., Turner, B.D. and Taylor, L.R., pp. 245–281. Blackwell Scientific Publications, Oxford

Anderson, R.M. (1981) Population ecology of infectious disease agents. In: *Theoretical Ecology*. Ed. May, R.M., pp. 318–355. Blackwell Scientific Publications, Oxford

Anderson, R.M. and May, R.M. (1986) The invasion, persistence and spread of infectious diseases within animal and plant communities. *Philosophical Transactions of the Royal Society of London, Series B*, **314**, 533–570

Anderson, R.M. and May, R.M. (1988) Epidemiological parameters of HIV infection. *Nature*, **333**, 514–518

Anderson, R.M. and May, R.M. (1991) *Infectious Diseases of Humans: Dynamics and Control*. Oxford University Press, Oxford

Anderson, R.S. (1983) Trends in pet populations. In: Society for Veterinary Epidemiology and Preventive Medicine, Proceedings, Southampton, 12–13 April 1983. Ed. Thrusfield, M.V., pp. 94–97

Anderson, T.W. (1958) *An Introduction to Multivariate Statistical Analysis*. John Wiley, New York

Andersson, M. and Sevelius, E. (1991) Breed, sex and age distribution in dogs with chronic liver disease: a demographic study. *Journal of Small Animal Practice*, **32**, 1–5

Andrewartha, H.G. and Birch, L.C. (1954) *The Distribution and Abundance of Animals*. University of Chicago Press, Chicago

Andrews, J.M. and Langmuir, A.D. (1963) The philosophy of disease eradication. *American Journal of Public Health*, **53**, 1–6

Andrews, L. (1988) Animal health information systems in Australia. *Revue Scientifique et Technique, Office International des Epizooties*, **7**, 569–575

Angelos, J., Oppenheim, Y., Rebhun, W., Mohammed, H. and Antczak, D.F. (1988) Evaluation of breed as a risk factor for sarcoid and uveitis in horses. *Animal Genetics*, **19**, 417–425

Anon. (1984) Tattoos to help keep track of pets. *Veterinary Practice*, **16** (20), 8

Anon. (1985) Turkey rhinotracheitis of unknown aetiology in England and Wales. *Veterinary Record*, **117**, 653–654

Anon. (1989) *Nutrient Requirements of Horses*, 5th edn. National Academy Press, Washington, DC

Anon. (1992) *Completing the Internal Market. Current Status, 1 January 1992. Veterinary and Plant Health Controls*, Vol. 5. Commission of the European Communities, Office for Official Publications of the European Communities, Luxembourg

Ansell, J. (1994) Assessing and understanding risk. In: Dutch Society for Veterinary Epidemiology and Economics, Proceedings (7), Utrecht, December 14 1994. Eds Schukken, Y.H. and Lam, T.J.H.M., pp. 55–66

Ansell, J. and Wharton, F. (Eds) (1992) *Risk: Analysis,*

Assessment and Management. John Wiley, Chichester

Arámbulo, P.V. and Astudillo, V. (1991) Perspectives on the application of remote sensing and geographic information system to disease control and health management. *Preventive Veterinary Medicine*, **11**, 345–352

Archibald, A.L. and Imlah, P. (1985) The halothane sensitivity locus and its linkage relationships. *Animal Blood Groups and Biochemical Genetics*, **16**, 253–263

Arimitsu, Y., Fukumura, K. and Shingaki, Y. (1989) Distribution of leptospirosis among stray dogs in the Okinawa Islands, Japan: comparison of the microcapsule and microscopic agglutination tests. *British Veterinary Journal*, **145**, 473–477

Armenian, H.K. (1987) Incubation periods of cancer: old and new. *Journal of Chronic Diseases*, **40**, Suppl. 2, 9S–15S

Armenian, H.K. and Lilienfeld, A.M. (1974) The distribution of incubation periods of neoplastic disease. *American Journal of Epidemiology*, **99**, 92–100

Armitage, P. (1975) *Sequential Medical Trials*, 2nd edn. John Wiley, New York

Armitage, P. and Berry, G. (1987) *Statistical Methods in Medical Research*, 2nd edn. Blackwell, Oxford

Armitage, P. and Doll, R. (1954) The age distribution of cancer and a multistage theory of carcinogenesis. *British Journal of Cancer*, **8**, 1–12

Armitage, P., McPherson, C.K. and Rowe, B.C. (1969) Repeated significance tests on accumulating data. *Journal of the Royal Statistical Society, Series A*, **132**, 235–244

Asby, C.G., Griffin, T.K., Ellis, P.R. and Kingwill, R.G. (1975) The Benefits and Costs of a System of Mastitis Control in Individual Herds. Study No. 17. University of Reading

Aubert, M. (1994) Control of rabies in foxes: what are the appropriate measures? *Veterinary Record*, **134**, 55–59

Audy, J.R. (1958) The localisation of disease with special reference to the zoonoses. *Transactions of the Royal Society of Tropical Medicine and Hygiene*, **52**, 308–328

Audy, J.R. (1960) *Relation of Foci of Zoonoses to Interspersed or Mosaic Vegetation*. Papers on the First WHO course on natural foci of infections, USSR

Audy, J.R. (1961) The ecology of scrub typhus. In: *Studies in Disease Ecology*. Ed. May, J.M., pp. 389–432. Hafner Publishing, New York

Audy, J.R. (1962) *Behavioral and Sociocultural Aspects of Natural Foci of Infections*. Papers of the Second WHO course on natural foci of infections, Leningrad

Austin, C.C., Weigel, R.M., Hungerford, L.L. and Biehl, L.G. (1993) Factors affecting the risk of infection with pseudorabies virus in Illinois swine herds. *Preventive Veterinary Medicine*, **17**, 161–173

Avgerou, C. and Cornford, T. (1993) *Developing Information Systems: Concepts, Issues and Practice*. The Macmillan Press, London

Babudieri, B. (1958) Animal reservoirs of leptospirosis. *Annals of the New York Academy of Science*, **70**, 393–413

Bäckgren, A.W. (1965) Lymphatic leukosis in dogs. An epizootiological, clinical and haematological study. *Acta Veterinaria Scandinavica*, **6**, Suppl. 1, 1–80

Baggott, D. (1982) Hoof lameness in dairy cattle. *In Practice*, **4**, 133–141

Bailey, N.T.J. (1975) *The Mathematical Theory of Infectious Diseases*, 2nd edn. Charles Griffin, London and High Wycombe

Bailey, N.T.J. (1981) *Statistical Methods in Biology*, 2nd edn. Hodder and Stoughton, London

Baker, M. (1974) *Folklore and Customs of Rural England*. David and Charles, Newton Abbot

Baltussen, W.H.M., Altena, H., Bakker, C.M. and Van Rijnberk, D. (1988) *Results on Dutch swine breeding herds in 1987*. Swine Extension Service and Agricultural Economics Research Institute, Rosmalen

Bang, F.B. (1975) Epidemiological interference. *International Journal of Epidemiology*, **4**, 337–342

Barger, I.A. (1989) Genetic resistance of hosts and its influence on epidemiology. *Veterinary Parasitology*, **32**, 21–35

Barger, I.A., Dash, K.M. and Southcott, W.H. (1978) Epidemiology and control of liver fluke in sheep. In: *The Epidemiology and Control of Gastrointestinal Parasites of Sheep in Australia*. Eds Donald, A.D., Southcott, W.H. and Dineen, J.K., pp. 65–74. Division of Animal Health, Commonwealth Scientific and Industrial Research Organisation, Australia

Barkema, H.W., Schukken, Y.H., Guard, C.L., Brand, A. and van der Weyden, G.C. (1991) Cesarian section in dairy cattle: a study of risk factors. In: Proceedings of the Sixth International Symposium on Veterinary Epidemiology and Economics, Ottawa, 12–16 August 1991. Ed. Martin, S.W., pp. 304–306

Barker, C.G., Herrtage, M.E., Shanahan, F. and Winchester, B.G. (1988) Fucosidosis in English springer spaniels: results of a trial screening programme. *Journal of Small Animal Practice*, **29**, 623–630

Barnard, G.A. (1959) Control charts for stochastic processes. *Journal of the Royal Statistical Society, Series B*, **21**(2), 239–271

Barnouin, J. (1991) Components of the diet in the dry period as risk factors for milk fever in dairy herds in France. *Preventive Veterinary Medicine*, **10**, 185–194

Barnouin, J. and Chacornac, J.P. (1992) A nutritional risk factor for early metritis in dairy farms in France. *Preventive Veterinary Medicine*, **13**, 27–37

Barnouin, J. and Chassagne, M. (1990) Components of the diet in the dry period as risk factors for placental retention in French dairy herds. *Preventive Veterinary Medicine*, **8**, 231–240

Barr, C., Benefield, C., Bunce, B., Ridsdale, H. and Whittaker, M. (1986) *Landscape Changes in Britain*. Institute for Terrestrial Ecology, Huntingdon

Barraclough, G. (Ed.) (1984) *The Times Atlas of World History*, revised edn. Times Books, London

Barron, B.A. (1977) The effects of misclassification on the estimation of relative risk. *Biometrics*, **33**, 414–418

Bartlett, M.S. (1957) Measles periodicity and community size. *Journal of the Royal Statistical Society, Series A*, **120**, 48–60.

(Discussion: 60–70)

Bartlett, P.C. and Miller, G.Y. (1993) Managerial risk factors for intramammary coagulase-positive staphylococci in Ohio dairy herds. *Preventive Veterinary Medicine*, **17**, 33–40

Bartlett, P.C., Kaneene, J., Gibson, C.D., Erickson, R. and Mather, E.C. (1982) Development of a computerised dairy management and disease surveillance system: FAHRMX. In: Proceedings of the first symposium on computer applications in veterinary medicine. College of Veterinary Medicine, Mississippi State University, 13–15 October 1982, pp. 21–29

Bartlett, P.C., Kirk, J.H., Mather, E.C., Gibson, C. and Kaneene, J.B. (1985) FAHRMX: A computerized dairy herd health management network. *The Compendium on Continuing Education for the Practising Veterinarian*, **7**, S124–S133

Bartlett, P.C., Kaneene, J.B., Kirk, J.H., Wilke, M.A. and Martenuik, J.V. (1986) Development of a computerized dairy herd health database for epidemiological research. *Preventive Veterinary Medicine*, **4**, 3–14

Bartlett, P.C., Miller, G.Y., Lance, S.E., Heider, L.E. and Anderson, C.R. (1992) Environmental and managerial risk factors of intramammary infection with coagulase-negative staphylococci in Ohio dairy herds. *Preventive Veterinary Medicine*, **14**, 129–142

Basson, P.A. and Hofmeyr, J.M. (1973) Mortalities associated with wildlife capture operations. In: *The Capture and Care of Wild Animals*. Ed. Young, E., pp. 151–160. Human and Rousseau, Cape Town and Pretoria

Batamuzi, E.K., Kassuku, A.A. and Agger, J.F. (1992) Risk factors associated with canine transmissible venereal tumour in Tanzania. *Preventive Veterinary Medicine*, **13**, 13–17

Baudet, A.E.R.F. (1923) (Mortality in ducks in the Netherlands caused by a filterable virus; fowl plague.) *Tijdschrift Diergeneesk*, **50**, 455–459 (in Dutch)

Beal, V.C. and McCallon, W.R. (1983) The use of mathematical models in animal disease program evaluation. In: Proceedings of the Third International Symposium on Veterinary Epidemiology and Economics. Arlington, Virginia, 6–10 September 1982, pp. 400–407. Veterinary Medical Publishing, Edwardsville

Beard, T.C. (1973) The elimination of echinococcosis from Iceland. *Bulletin of the World Health Organization*, **48**, 653–660

Beard, W.L. and Hayes, H.M. (1993) Risk factors for laryngeal hemiplegia in the horse. *Preventive Veterinary Medicine*, **17**, 57–63

Beck, E. and Strohmaier, K. (1987) Subtyping of European foot-and-mouth disease virus strains by nucleotide sequence determination. *Journal of Virology*, **61**, 1621–1629

Becker, B.A. (1987) The phenomenon of stress: concepts and mechanisms associated with stress-induced response of the neuroendocrine system. *Veterinary Research Communications*, **11**, 443–456

Becker, F.F. (1981) Recent concepts of initiation and promotion in carcinogenesis. *American Journal of Pathology*, **105**, 3–9

Bedard, B.G., Martin, S.W. and Chinombo, D. (1993) A

prevalence study of bovine tuberculosis and brucellosis in Malawi. *Preventive Veterinary Medicine*, **16**, 193−205

Beech, M.W.H. (1911) *The Suk, Their Language and Folklore*. Clarendon Press, Oxford

Beechinor, G. (1993) Regulatory and administrative implications of clinical trials. In: *Field Trial & Error*. Proceedings of the international seminar with workshops on the design, conduct and interpretation of field trials, Berg en Dal, Netherlands, 27−28 April 1993. Eds Noordhuizen, J.P.T.M., Frankena, K., Ploeger, H. and Nell, T., pp. 29−35. Epidecon, Wageningen

Behbehani, K. and Hassounah, O. (1976) The role of native and domestic animals in the dissemination of *Echinococcus* infection among dogs in the State of Kuwait. *Journal of Helminthology*, **50**, 275−280

Beilage, G.B., Salge, H.-J., Krabbe, H. and Blaha, T. (1991) Untersuchungen zur epidemiologie des seuchenhaften spätabortes der zuchtsauen (PRRS). *Collegium Veterinarium*, **22**, 62−64 (in German)

Belák, S. and Ballagi-Pordány, A. (1993) Application of the polymerase chain reaction (PCR) in veterinary diagnostic virology. *Veterinary Research Communications*, **17**, 55−72

Belák, S., Ballagi-Pordány, A., Flensburg, J. and Virtanen, A. (1989) Detection of pseudorabies virus DNA sequences by the polymerase chain reaction. *Archives of Virology*, **108**, 279−286

Bell, K.J. (1980) A study of productivity in sheep flocks. The application and evaluation of health and productivity programmes in south west Australia. In: Proceedings of the 10th Seminar of the Sheep and Beef Cattle Society of the New Zealand Veterinary Association. Lincoln College, Canterbury, 11−12 July 1980, pp. 108−114

Bender, A.P., Bender, G.P., Dorn, C.R. and Schneider, R. (1982) Association between canine benign and malignant neoplasms. *Preventive Veterinary Medicine*, **1**, 77−87

Bendixen, P.H. (1987) Notes about incidence calculations in observational studies (letter). *Preventive Veterinary Medicine*, **5**, 151−156

Bendixen, P.H., Vilson, B., Ekesbo, I. and Astrand, D.B. (1986a) Disease frequencies of tied zero-grazing dairy cows and of dairy cows on pasture during summer and tied during winter. *Preventive Veterinary Medicine*, **4**, 291−306

Bendixen, P.H., Vilson, B., Ekesbo, I. and Astrand, D.B. (1986b) Disease frequencies in Swedish dairy cows. I. Dystokia. *Preventive Veterinary Medicine*, **4**, 291−306

Bendixen, P.H., Vilson, B., Ekesbo, I. and Astrand, D.B. (1987a) Disease frequencies in dairy cows in Sweden. II. Retained placenta. *Preventive Veterinary Medicine*, **4**, 377−387

Bendixen, P.H., Vilson, B., Ekesbo, I. and Astrand, D.B. (1987b) Disease frequencies in dairy cows in Sweden. III. Parturient paresis. *Preventive Veterinary Medicine*, **5**, 87−97

Bendixen, P.H., Vilson, B., Ekesbo, I. and Astrand, D.B. (1987c) Disease frequencies in dairy cows in Sweden. IV. Ketosis. *Preventive Veterinary Medicine*, **5**, 99−109

Bendixen, P.H., Vilson, B., Ekesbo, I. and Astrand, D.B. (1988a) Disease frequencies in dairy cows in Sweden. V. Mastitis. *Preventive Veterinary Medicine*, **5**, 263−274

Bendixen, P.H., Vilson, B., Ekesbo, I. and Astrand, D.B. (1988b) Disease frequencies in dairy cows in Sweden. VI. Tramped teat. *Preventive Veterinary Medicine*, **6**, 17−25

Bendixen, P.H., Emmanuelson, U., Forssberg, P. and Silferberg, L. (1993) Analysis of status of vaccination and development of fever in trotters in Sweden during an outbreak of influenza Type A2 (H3N8). *Preventive Veterinary Medicine*, **16**, 95−102

Benham, P.J.F. and Broom, D.M. (1989) Interactions between cattle and badgers at pasture with reference to bovine tuberculosis transmission. *British Veterinary Journal*, **145**, 226−241

Bergsma, D.R. and Brown, K.S. (1971) White fur, blue eyes and deafness in the domestic cat. *Journal of Heredity*, **62**, 171−185

Bernoulli, M.D. (1766) Essai d'une nouvelle analyse de la mortalité causée par la petite vérole et des avantages de l'inoculation pour la prévenir. In: *Histoire de l'Académie Royale des Sciences, 1760, Avec les Mémoires de Mathématique et de Physique*. L'Imprimerie Royale, Paris. Translated in: Bradley, L. (1971) *Smallpox Inoculation: An Eighteenth Century Mathematical Controversy*. University of Nottingham Adult Education Department, Nottingham

Berry, S.J., Strandberg, J.D., Saunders, W.J. and Coffey, D.S. (1986) Development of canine benign prostatic hyperplasia with age. *The Prostate*, **9**, 363−373

Beyer, W.H. (Ed.) (1968) *CRC Handbook of Probability and Statistics*, 2nd edn. The Chemical Rubber Company, Cleveland

Beyer, W.H. (Ed.) (1981) *CRC Statistical and Mathematical Tables*, 26th edn. CRC Press, Boca Raton

Bibikova, V.A. (1977) Contemporary views on the interrelationships between fleas and the pathogens of human and animal diseases. *Annual Review of Entomology*, **22**, 23−32

Bielflet, S.W., Redman, H.C. and McClellan, R.G. (1971) Sire- and sex-related differences in rates of epileptiform seizures in a purebred beagle dog colony. *American Journal of Veterinary Research*, **32**, 2039−2048

Biggs, P.M. (1982) Vaccination. In: *The Control of Infectious Diseases in Farm Animals*, pp. 21−27. British Veterinary Association Trust Project on the future of animal health control, London

Biggs, P.M. (1993) Developments in vaccines. In: *The Advancement of Veterinary Science. The Bicentenary Symposium Series. Volume 4: Veterinary Medicine — Growth Points and Comparative Medicine*. Ed. Michell, A.R., pp. 13−27. CAB International, Wallingford

Bigras-Poulin, M., Meek, A.H., Martin, S.W. and McMillan, I. (1990) Health problems in selected Ontario Holstein cows: frequency of occurrences, time to first diagnosis and associations. *Preventive Veterinary Medicine*, **10**, 79−89

Biziere, K. and Chambon, J.P. (1987) Modèles animaux d'epilepsie et crises experimentales. *Review Neurologique (Paris)*, **143**, 329−340

Black, A. (1972) Progressive retinal atrophy: a review of the genetics and an appraisal of the eradication scheme. *Journal of Small Animal Practice*, **13**, 295–314

Black, F.L. (1975) Infectious diseases in primitive societies. *Science*, **187**, 515–518

Blackmore, D.K. (1963) The incidence and aetiology of thyroid dysplasia in budgerigars (*Melopsittacus undulatus*). *Veterinary Record*, **75**, 1068–1072

Blackmore, D.K. (1964) A survey of disease in British wild foxes (*Vulpes vulpes*). *Veterinary Record*, **76**, 527–533

Blackmore, D.K. (1983) Practical problems associated with the slaughter of stock. In: *Stunning of Animals for Slaughter*. Ed. Eikelenboom, G., pp. 167–178. Martin Nijhoff Publishers, The Hague

Blackmore, D.K. and Hathaway, S.C. (1980) The nidality of zoonoses. In: *Veterinary Epidemiology and Economics*. Proceedings of the Second International Symposium, Canberra, 7–11 May 1979. Eds Geering, W.A., Roe, R.T. and Chapman, L.A., pp. 207–213. Australian Government Publishing Service, Canberra

Blackmore, D.K. and Schollum, L.M. (1983) The serological investigation of occupational exposure to leptospirosis. In: *Proceedings of the Third International Symposium on Veterinary Epidemiology and Economics*. Arlington, 6–10 September 1982, pp. 544–551. Veterinary Medical Publishing, Edwardsville

Blackmore, D.K., Hill, A. and Jackson, O.F. (1971) The incidence of mycoplasma in pet and colony maintained cats. *Journal of Small Animal Practice*, **12**, 207–216

Blaha, T. (1992) Regional eradication of swine dysentery by gradual elimination of the pathogen from infected herds. In: Society for Veterinary Epidemiology and Preventive Medicine, Proceedings, Edinburgh, 1–3 April 1992. Ed. Thrusfield, M.V., pp. 186–189

Blajan, L. (1979) The systems for veterinary information at the national and worldwide levels. *Bulletin Office International des Epizooties*, **91**, 795–821

Blajan, L. and Chillaud, T. (1991) The OIE world animal disease information system. *Revue Scientifique et Technique, Office International des Epizooties*, **10**, 71–87

Blajan, L. and Welte, V.R. (1988) Information, a prerequisite for veterinary activities. *Revue Scientifique et Technique, Office International des Epizooties*, **7**, 463–478

Blamire, R.V., Crowley, A.J. and Goodhand, R.H. (1970) A review of some animal diseases encountered at meat inspection, 1960–1968. *Veterinary Record*, **87**, 234–238

Blamire, R.V., Goodhand, R.H. and Taylor, K.C. (1980) A review of some animal diseases encountered at meat inspections in England and Wales, 1969–1978. *Veterinary Record*, **106**, 195–199

Bland, J.M. and Altman, D.G. (1986) Statistical methods for measuring agreement between two methods of clinical measurement. *Lancet*, **1**, 307–310

Bloch, D.A. and Kraemer, H.C. (1989) 2 × 2 kappa coefficients: measures of agreement or association. *Biometrics*, **45**, 269–287

Blood, D.C. (1976) The principles of herd health programmes. In: Proceedings No. 28. Refresher course for veterinarians on mastitis, pp. 47–64. The University of Sydney Postgraduate Committee on Veterinary Science in association with the Australian Veterinary Association and the Veterinary Clinic Centre, University of Melbourne

Blood, D.C., Radostits, O.M. and Henderson, J.A. (1983) *Veterinary Medicine*, 6th edn. Baillière Tindall, London

Blot, W.J. and Day, N.E. (1979) Synergism and interaction: are they equivalent? *American Journal of Epidemiology*, **110**, 99–100

Blowey, R.W. and Collis, K. (1992) Effect of premilking teat disinfection on mastitis incidence, total bacterial count and milk yield in three dairy herds. *Veterinary Record*, **130**, 175–178

Bodoh, G.W., Battista, W.J., Schultz, L.H. and Johnston, R.P. (1976) Variation in somatic cell counts in dairy improvement milk samples. *Journal of Dairy Science*, **59**, 1119–1123

Booth, A.J., Stagdale, L. and Gregor, J.A. (1984) Salmon poisoning disease in dogs in Southern Vancouver Island. *Canadian Veterinary Journal*, **25**, 2–6

Booth, J.M. and Warren, M.E. (1984) The use of a computerised herd fertility monitor. In: Society for Veterinary Epidemiology and Preventive Medicine. Proceedings, Edinburgh, 10–11 July 1984. Ed. Thrusfield, M.V., pp. 166–173

Bor, A., Winkler, M. and Gootwine, E. (1989) Non-clinical intramammary infection in lactating ewes and its association with clinical mastitis. *British Veterinary Journal*, **145**, 178–184

Bording, A. (1990) The clinical trial in veterinary practice. In: Proceedings of the International Pig Veterinary Society, 11th Congress, Lausanne, 1–5 Jul 1990, p. 413. Swiss Association of Swine Medicine, Berne

Borg, K. and Hugoson, G. (1980) Wildlife as an indicator of environmental disturbances. In: *Veterinary Epidemiology and Economics*, Proceedings of the Second International Symposium. Eds Geering, W.A., Roe, R.T. and Chapman, L.A., pp. 250–253. Australian Government Publishing Service, Canberra

Borsberry, S. and Dobson, H. (1989) Periparturient diseases and their effect on reproductive performance in five dairy herds. *Veterinary Record*, **124**, 217–219

Bostock, D.E. and Curtis, R. (1984) Comparison of canine oropharyngeal malignancy in various geographical locations. *Veterinary Record*, **114**, 341–342

Bourne, F.J. (1993) Biotechnical and farm animal medicine. In: *The Advancement of Veterinary Science. The Bicentenary Symposium Series, Volume 1: Veterinary Medicine Beyond 2000*. Ed. Michell, A.R., pp. 41–57. CAB International, Wallingford

Bovee, K.C. and McGuire, T. (1984) Qualitative and quantitative analysis of uroliths in dogs: definitive determination of chemical type. *Journal of the American Veterinary Medical Association*, **185**, 983–987

Boycott, J.A. (1971) *Natural History of Infectious Disease*. Studies in Biology No. 26. Edward Arnold, London

Bramley, A.J., Dodd, F.H. and Griffin, T.K. (Eds) (1981) *Mastitis Control and Herd Management*. The proceedings of a course organised by the National Institute for Research in Dairying, 22–24 September 1980. National Institute for Research in Dairying/Hannah Research Institute, Technical Bulletin 4

Braverman, Y., Ungar-Waron, H., Frith, K., Adler, H., Danieli, Y., Baker, K.P. and Quinn, P.J. (1983) Epidemiological and immunological studies of sweet itch in horses in Israel. *Veterinary Record*, **112**, 521–524

Breslow, N.E. and Day, N.E. (1980) *Statistical Methods in Cancer Research, Vol. 1: The Analysis of Case–Control Studies*. IARC Scientific Publications No. 32. International Agency on Cancer Research, Lyon

Breslow, N.E. and Day, N.E. (1987) *Statistical Methods in Cancer Research, Vol. 2: The Design and Analysis of Cohort Studies*. IARC Scientific Publications No. 82. International Agency on Cancer Research, Lyon

Broadbent, D.W. (1979) Field collection of animal disease data in developing countries. *World Animal Review*, **29**, 38–42

Brodey, R.S. (1970) Canine and feline neoplasia. *Advances in Veterinary Science and Comparative Medicine*, **14**, 309–354

Brodey, R.S. (1979) The use of naturally occurring cancer in domestic animals for research into human cancer: general considerations and a review of canine skeletal osteosarcoma. *Yale Journal of Biology and Medicine*, **52**, 345–361

Brodey, R.S., Fidler, I.J. and Howson, B.A. (1966) Relationship of oestrus irregularity, pseudopregnancy and pregnancy to the development of mammary neoplasia. *Journal of the American Veterinary Medical Association*, **149**, 1047–1049

Brodey, R.S., McDonough, S.F., Frye, F.L. and Hardy, W.D. (1970) Epidemiology of feline leukaemia (lymphosarcoma). In: Proceedings of the 4th International Symposium on Comparative Leukaemia Research, Cherry Hill, New Jersey. Ed. Dutcher, R.M. *Bibliotheca Haematologica*, **36**, 333–342

Brooksby, J.B. (1972) Epizootiology of foot-and-mouth disease in developing countries. *World Animal Review*, **1**, 10–13

Brostrom, H. and Larrson, A. (1987) Allergic dermatitis (sweet itch) of Icelandic horses in Sweden: an epidemiological study. *Equine Veterinary Journal*, **19**, 229–236

Brothwell, D. and Sandison, A.T. (Eds) (1967) *Diseases in Antiquity*. Charles C. Thomas, Springfield

Brown, N., Parks, J.L. and Greene, R.W. (1977) Canine urolithiasis: retrospective analysis of 438 cases. *Journal of the American Veterinary Medical Association*, **170**, 414–418

Brownlee, J. (1915) Historical note on Farr's theory of the epidemic. *British Medical Journal*, **ii**, 250–252

Brunsdon, R.V. (1980) Principles of helminth control. *Veterinary Parasitology*, **6**, 185–215

Bryson, R.W. (1982) Kikuyu poisoning and the army worm. *Journal of the South African Veterinary Association*, **53**, 161–165

BSI (1979) *Precision of test methods. I. Guide for the determination of repeatability and reproducibility for a standard test method for inter-laboratory tests*. BS 5497, Part 1. British Standards Institute, London

Buchanan, J.W. (1977) Chronic valvular disease (endocardiosis) in dogs. *Advances in Veterinary Science*, **21**, 75–106

Buck, C. (1975) Popper's philosophy for epidemiologists. *International Journal of Epidemiology*, **4**, 159–168 (comment: 169–172)

Buck, W.B. (1979) Animals as monitors of environmental quality. *Veterinary and Human Toxicology*, **21**, 277–284

Buescher, E.L., Scherer, W.F., McClure, H.E., Moyer, J.T., Rosenberg, M.Z., Yoshii, M. and Okada, Y. (1959) Ecologic studies of Japanese Encephalitis virus in Japan. IV. Avian infection. *American Journal of Tropical Medicine and Hygiene*, **8**, 678–688

Bulpitt, C.J. (1983) *Randomised Controlled Clinical Trials*. Martinus Nijhoff Publishers, The Hague

Burch, P.R.J. (1966) Age and sex distributions for some idiopathic non-malignant conditions in man. Some possible implications for growth-control and natural and radiation-induced ageing. In: *Radiation and Ageing*. Proceedings of a Colloquium held in Semmering, Austria, 23–24 June 1966. Eds Lindop, P.J. and Sacher, G.A., pp. 117–155. Taylor and Francis, London

Burgdorfer, W. (1960) Colorado Tick Fever: II. The behaviour of Colorado Tick Fever virus in rodents. *Journal of Infectious Diseases*, **107**, 384–388

Burger, H.J. (1976) Trichostrongyle infestation in autumn on pastures grazed exclusively by cows or by calves. *Veterinary Parasitology*, **1**, 359–366

Burnet, M. and White, D.O. (1972) *Natural History of Infectious Disease*, 4th edn. Cambridge University Press, London

Burridge, M.J. and McCarthy, S.M. (1979) The Florida veterinary clinical data retrieval system. In: *Proceedings of an International Symposium on Animal Health and Disease Data Banks*, 4–6 December 1978, Washington, DC, pp. 155–161. United States Department of Agriculture, Miscellaneous Publication No. 1381

Calabrese, E.J. (1986) Animal extrapolation and the challenge of human heterogeneity. *Journal of Pharmaceutical Sciences*, **75**, 1041–1046

Caldow, G., Edwards, S., Nixon, P. and Peters, A.R. (1988) Associations between viral infection and respiratory disease in young beef bulls. *Veterinary Record*, **122**, 529–531

Caldow, G.L. (1984) The potential for veterinary involvement in the reproductive management of beef suckler herds. MSc Thesis, University of Edinburgh

Calnek, B.W. (Ed.) (1991) *Diseases of Poultry*, 9th edn. Iowa State University Press, Ames

Cameron, D. and Jones, I.G. (1983) John Snow, the Broad Street pump and modern epidemiology. *International Journal of Epidemiology*, **12**, 393–396

Campbell, C.L. (1989) Geographical information system applications in animal health. In: Proceedings of the 93rd Annual Meeting of the United States Animal Health Association. Las Vegas, Nevada, 28 October–3 November 1989, pp. 47–62

Campbell, J.R., Menzies, P., Waltner-Toews, D., Walton, J.W., Buckrell, B. and Thorsen, J. (1991) An epidemiological study of maedi-visna in Ontario sheep flocks. In: Proceedings of the Sixth International Symposium on Veterinary Epidemiology and Economics, Ottawa, 12−16 August 1991. Ed. Martin, S.W., pp. 373−375

Campos-Filho, N. and Franco, E. (1989) A microcomputer program for multiple logistic regression by unconditional and conditional maximum likelihood methods. *American Journal of Epidemiology*, **129**, 439−444

Canner, P.L., Krol, W.F. and Forman, S.A. (1983) External quality control programs. *Controlled Clinical Trials*, **4**, 441−466

Cannon, R. (1993) ANADIS: Monitoring and eradication of brucellosis and tuberculosis in Australia. *Agricultural Systems and Information Technology*, **5**(1), 11−13

Cannon, R.M. and Roe, R.T. (1982) *Livestock Disease Surveys: A Field Manual for Veterinarians*. Australian Government Publishing Service, Canberra

Cannon, W.B. (1914) The emergency function of the adrenal medulla in pain and major emotions. *American Journal of Physiology*, **33**, 356−372

Caplan, G. and Grunebaum, H. (1967) Perspectives on primary prevention: a review. *Archives of General Psychiatry*, **17**, 331−346

Carles, A.B. (1986) The levels of, and constraints to, productivity of goats and sheep at Ngurunit in Marsabit District. In: *Smallstock and Cattle Productivity, Nutrition and Disease in Northern Kenya*. Integrated Project in Arid Lands, Technical Report No. E-8. Ed. Field, C.R., pp. 33−118. UNESCO, Nairobi

Carles, A.B. (1992) The non-medicinal prevention of livestock disease in African rangeland ecosystems. *Preventive Veterinary Medicine*, **12**, 165−173

Carmichael, L.E. and Binn, L.N. (1981) New enteric viruses in the dog. *Advances in Veterinary Science and Comparative Medicine*, **25**, 1−37

Carpenter, T.E. (1988) Stochastic epidemiologic modeling using a microcomputer spreadsheet package. *Preventive Veterinary Medicine*, **5**, 159−168

Carson, R.L. (1963) *Silent Spring*. Hamish Hamilton, London

Case, J.T. (1994) SNOMED (review). *Preventive Veterinary Medicine*, **21**, 269−273

Case, L.C., Ling, G.V., Ruby, A.L., Johnston, D.L., Franti, C.E. and Stevens, F. (1993) Urolithiasis in Dalmatians: 275 cases (1981−1990). *Journal of the American Veterinary Medical Association*, **203**, 96−100

Cason, R. and Geering, W.A. (1980) An economic evaluation of possible Australian policies to meet the threat of an exotic pest — the screw-worm fly, *Chrysomyia bezziana*. In: *Veterinary Epidemiology and Economics*. Proceedings of the Second International Symposium, Canberra, 7−11 May 1979. Eds Geering, W.A., Roe, R.T. and Chapman, L.A., pp. 463−470. Australian Government Publishing Service, Canberra

Cecchini, G., Bekele, T. and Kasali, O.B. (1992) The effect of repeated freezing and thawing of serum on the activity of antibodies. *Veterinary Research Communications*, **16**, 425−428

Chain, P. (1980) Public participation and communications in Latin American disease control programs. In: *Veterinary Epidemiology and Economics*. Proceedings of the Second International Symposium, Canberra, 4−11 May 1979. Eds Geering, W.A., Roe, R.T. and Chapman, L.A., pp. 335−340. Australian Government Publishing Service, Canberra

Chalmers, A.W. (1968) African horse sickness. *Equine Veterinary Journal*, **1**, 83−86

Chapman, R.N. (1928) The quantitative analysis of environmental factors. *Ecology*, **9**, 111−122

Chapman, R.N. (1931) *Animal Ecology with Special Reference to Insects*. McGraw Hill, New York

Cheeseman, C.L., Wilesmith, J.W. and Stuart, F.A. (1989) Tuberculosis: the disease and its epidemiology in the badger: a review. *Epidemiology and Infection*, **103**, 113−125

Cheeseman, C.L., Jones, G.W., Gallagher, J. and Mallinson, P.J. (1981) The population structure, density and prevalence of tuberculosis (*Mycobacterium bovis*) in badgers (*Meles meles*) from four areas in south-west England. *Journal of Applied Ecology*, **18**, 795−804

Chesterton, R.N., Pfeiffer, D.U., Morris, R.S. and Tanner, C.M. (1989) Environmental and behavioural factors affecting the prevalence of foot lameness in New Zealand dairy herds — a case−control study. *New Zealand Veterinary Journal*, **37**, 135−142

Cheville, N.F. (1975) The gray collie syndrome (cyclic neutropenia). *Journal of the American Animal Hospitals Association*, **11**, 350−352

Christensen, J., Ellegaard, B., Petersen, B.K., Willeberg, P. and Mousing, J. (1994) Pig health and production surveillance in Denmark: sampling design, data recording and measures of disease frequency. *Preventive Veterinary Medicine*, **20**, 47−61

Christensen, L.S., Mousing, J., Mortensen, S., Soerensen, K.J., Strandbygaard, S.B., Henriksen, C.A. and Andersen, J.B. (1990) Evidence of long distance transmission of Aujeszky's disease (pseudorabies) virus. *Veterinary Record*, **127**, 471−474

Christensen, L.S., Mortensen, S., Bøtner, A., Strandbygaard, S.B., Rønsholt, L., Henriksen, C.A. and Andersen, J.B. (1993) Further evidence of long distance airborne transmission of Aujeszky's disease (pseudorabies) virus. *Veterinary Record*, **132**, 317−321

Christiansen, K.H. (1980) Laboratory management and disease surveillance information system. In: *Veterinary Epidemiology and Economics*. Proceedings of the Second International Symposium, Canberra, 7−11 May 1979. Eds Geering, W.A., Roe, R.T. and Chapman, L.A., pp. 59−64. Australian Government Publishing Service, Canberra

Clarke, A. (1987) Air hygiene and equine respiratory disease. *In Practice*, **9**, 196−204

Clarke, K.C., Osleeb, J.P., Sherry, J.M., Meert, J.P. and Larsson, R.W. (1991) The use of remote sensing and geographic information systems in UNICEF's dracunculiasis (Guinea worm) eradication effort. *Preventive Veterinary*

Medicine, **11**, 229–235

Clarkson, M.J. and Faull, W.B. (1990) *Handbook for the Sheep Clinician*. Liverpool University Press, Liverpool

Clemens, J., Sack, D., Rao, M., Chakraborthy, J., Kay, B., Ahmed, F., Khan, M.R., van Loon, F.P.L., Svennerholm, A.-M. and Holmgren, J. (1993) The design and analysis of cholera vaccine trials: recent lessons from Bangladesh. *International Journal of Epidemiology*, **22**, 724–730

Cliff, A.D. and Haggett, P. (1988) *Atlas of Disease Distributions: Analytic Approaches to Epidemiological Data*. Basil Blackwell, Oxford

Cliff, A.D. and Ord, J.K. (1981) *Spatial Processes: Models and Applications*. Pion, London

Clifton-Hadley, R. (1993) The use of a geographical information system (GIS) in the control and epidemiology of bovine tuberculosis in south-west England. In: Society for Veterinary Epidemiology and Preventive Medicine, Proceedings, Exeter, 31 March–2 April 1993. Ed. Thrusfield M.V., pp. 166–179

Cochran, W.G. (1950) The comparison of percentages in matched samples. *Biometrika*, **37**, 256–266

Cockburn, A. (1963) *The Evolution and Eradication of Infectious Diseases*. Johns Hopkins Press, Baltimore

Codd, G.A., Edwards, C., Beattie, K.A., Barr, W.M. and Gunn, G.J. (1992) Fatal attraction to cyanobacteria? (letter). *Nature*, **359**, 110–111

Coffey, D.J. (1988) Stress (letter). *Veterinary Record*, **123**, 476

Cohen, D., Booth, S. and Sussman, O. (1959) An epidemiological study of canine lymphoma and its public health significance. *American Journal of Veterinary Research*, **20**, 1026–1031

Cohen, D., Brodey, R.S. and Chen, S.M. (1964) Epidemiologic aspects of oral and pharyngeal neoplasms of the dog. *American Journal of Veterinary Research*, **25**, 1776–1779

Cohen, D., Reif, J.S., Brodey, R.S. and Keiser, H. (1974) Epidemiologic analysis of the most prevalent sites and types of canine neoplasia observed in a veterinary hospital. *Cancer Research*, **34**, 2859–2868

Cohen, J. (1988) *Statistical Power Analysis for the Behavioral Sciences*, 2nd edn. Lawrence Erlbaum, Hillsdale

Coker-Vann, M., Brown, P. and Gajdusek, D.C. (1984) Serodiagnosis of human cysticercosis using a chromatofocused antigen preparation of *Taenia solium* cysticerci in an enzyme-linked immunosorbent assay (ELISA). *Transactions of the Royal Society of Tropical Medicine and Hygiene*, **78**, 492–496

Cole, P. and MacMahon, B. (1971) Attributable risk percent in case–control studies. *British Journal of Preventive and Social Medicine*, **25**, 242–244

Colinvaux, P.A. (1973) *Introduction to Ecology*. John Wiley, New York

Collett, D. (1991) *Modelling Binary Data*. Chapman and Hall, London

Collick, D.W., Ward, W.R. and Dobson, H. (1989) Associations between types of lameness and fertility. *Veterinary Record*, **125**, 103–106

Collins, M. and Algers, B. (1986) Effects of stable dust on farm

animals — a review. *Veterinary Research Communications*, **10**, 415–428

Congleton, W.R. and Goodwill, R.E. (1980) Simulated comparisons of breeding plans for beef production. Part 1: a dynamic model to evaluate the mating plan on herd age structure and productivity. *Agricultural Systems*, **5**, 207–219

Cook, A.K., Breitschwerdt, E.B., Levine, J.F., Bunch, S.E. and Linn, L.O. (1993) Risk factors associated with acute pancreatitis in dogs: 101 cases (1985–1990). *Journal of the American Veterinary Medical Association*, **203**, 673–679

Coombs, M.M. (1980) Chemical carcinogenesis: a view at the end of the first half-century. *Journal of Pathology*, **130**, 117–146

Copeland, K.T., Checkoway, H., McMichael, A.J. and Holbrook, R.H. (1977) Bias due to misclassification in the estimation of relative risk. *American Journal of Epidemiology*, **105**, 488–495

Coria, M.F. and McClurkin, A.W. (1978) Specific immune tolerance in an apparently healthy bull persistently infected with bovine viral diarrhoea. *Journal of the American Veterinary Medical Association*, **172**, 449–451

Cornfield, J. (1951) A method of estimating comparative rates from clinical data: applications to cancer of the lung, breast and cervix. *Journal of the National Cancer Institute*, **11**, 1269–1275

Cornfield, J. (1956) A statistical problem arising from retrospective studies. In: Proceedings of the Third Berkeley Symposium on Mathematical Statistics and Probability. Ed. Newman, J., pp. 135–148. University of California Press, Berkeley

Corrigan, P.J. and Seneviratna, P. (1989) Pesticide residues in Australian meat. *Veterinary Record*, **125**, 181–182

Cosgrove, A.S. (1962) An apparently new disease of chickens — avian nephrosis. *Avian Diseases*, **6**, 385–389

Cotchin, E. (1984) Veterinary oncology: a survey. *Journal of Pathology*, **142**, 101–127

Cote, R.A., Rothwell, D.J., Beckett, R.S., Palotay, J.L. and Brochu, L. (Eds) (1993) *SNOMED International, The Systematized Nomenclature of Human and Veterinary Medicine*. College of American Pathologists, Northfield/American Veterinary Medical Association, Schaumberg

Cowart, R.P., Boessen, C.R. and Kliebenstein, J.B. (1992) Patterns associated with season and facilities for atrophic rhinitis and pneumonia in swine. *Journal of the American Veterinary Medical Association*, **200**, 190–193

Cowen, P., Pacer, R.A., Van Peteghem, P.N. and Fetrow, J.F. (1990) Management factors affecting trichinosis seropositivity among 91 North Carolina swine farms. *Preventive Veterinary Medicine*, **9**, 165–172

Cowen, P., McGinn, T.J., Pyle, G.F., Routh, P.A. and Burstein, J.T. (1991) The influence of farm location, management characteristics and medical geographic factors on Aujeszky's disease status of swine farms in Sampson County, North Carolina. In: Proceedings of the Sixth International Symposium on Veterinary Epidemiology and Economics, Ottawa, 12–16 August 1991. Ed. Martin, S.W., pp. 409–411

Cramer, D.W., Welch, W.R., Scully, R.E. and Wojciechowski, C.A. (1982) Ovarian cancer and talc. A case-control study. *Cancer*, **50**, 372-376

Cregier, S.E. (1990) Shocking docking: mutilation before education? *Journal of Equine Veterinary Science*, **10**, 252-255

Creighton, C. (1965) *A History of Epidemics in Britain*, 2nd edn. Frank Cass, London

Croll, N.A., Anderson, R.M., Gyorkos, T.W. and Ghadirian, E. (1982) The population biology and control of *Ascaris lumbricoides* in a rural community in Iran. *Transactions of the Royal Society of Tropical Medicine and Hygiene*, **76**, 187-197

Crossman, P.J. (1978) Gastric torsion in cows. *The Pig Veterinary Society Proceedings*, **2**, 47-49

Csiza, C.K., Scott, F.W., Lahunta, A. de and Gillespie, J.H. (1971) Feline viruses. XIV: Transplacental infections in spontaneous panleukopenia of cats. *Cornell Veterinarian*, **61**, 423-439

Cummings, S.R. and Richard, R.J. (1988) Optimum cutoff points for biochemical validation of smoking status. *American Journal of Public Health*, **78**, 575-585

Cunningham, M.P., McIntyre, W.I.M. and Ives, J.C.J. (1957) The incidence of canine leptospirosis in Glasgow. *Veterinary Record*, **69**, 903-906

Curtis, C.R. and Farrar, J.A. (Eds) (1990) The National Animal Health Monitoring System in the United States. *Preventive Veterinary Medicine*, **8**, 87-225

Curtis, C.R., Erb, H.N., Sniffen, C.J. and Smith, R.D. (1984) Epidemiology of parturient paresis: predisposing factors with emphasis on dry cow feeding and management. *Journal of Dairy Science*, **67**, 817-825

Curtis, C.R., White, M.E. and Erb, H.N. (1989) Effects of calfhood morbidity on long-term survival in New York Holstein herds. *Preventive Veterinary Medicine*, **7**, 173-186

Curtis, R. and Barnett, K.C. (1989) A survey of cataracts in golden and labrador retrievers. *Journal of Small Animal Practice*, **30**, 277-286

Cuthbertson, J.C. (1983) Sheep disease surveillance based on condemnations at three Scottish abattoirs. *Veterinary Record*, **112**, 219-221

CVMP (1993) Demonstration of efficacy of ectoparasiticides. CVMP Working Party on the Efficacy of Veterinary Medicines. Notes for Guidance, Document No. III/3682/92-EN, Commission of the European Communities, Brussels

D'Allaire, S., Morris, R.S., Martin, F.B., Robinson, R.A. and Leman, A.D. (1989) Management and environmental factors associated with annual sow culling rate: a path analysis. *Preventive Veterinary Medicine*, **7**, 255-265

Daniel, M. and Kolár, K. (1990) Using satellite data to forecast the occurrence of the common tick *Ixodes ricinus* (L.). *Journal of Hygiene, Epidemiology, Microbiology and Immunology*, **34**, 243-252

Dargent-Molina, P., Scarlett, J., Pollock, R.V.H., Erb, H.N. and Sears, P. (1988) Herd-level risk factors for *Staphylococcus aureus* and *Streptococcus agalactiae* intramammary infections. *Preventive Veterinary Medicine*, **6**, 127-142

Darke, P.G.G. (1982) The value of clinical case records in small animal cases. In: *Epidemiology in Animal Health*. Proceedings of a symposium held at the British Veterinary Association's Centenary Congress, Reading, 22-25 September 1982, pp. 103-106. Society for Veterinary Epidemiology and Preventive Medicine

Darke, P.G.G., Thrusfield, M.V. and Aitken, C.G.G. (1985) Association between tail injuries and docking in dogs. *Veterinary Record*, **116**, 409

Das, K.M. and Tashjian, R.J. (1965) Chronic mitral valve disease in the dog. *Veterinary Medicine/Small Animal Clinician*, **60**, 1209-1216

Daubney, R., Hudson, J.R. and Garnham, P.C. (1931) Enzootic hepatitis or Rift Valley fever. An undescribed virus disease of sheep, cattle and man from East Africa. *Journal of Pathology and Bacteriology*, **34**, 545-579

David, F.N. and Barton, D.E. (1966) Two space-time interaction tests for epidemicity. *British Journal of Preventive and Social Medicine*, **20**, 44-48

David-West, K.B. (1980) Planning and implementation of contagious bovine pleuropneumonia control programs in Nigeria. In: *Veterinary Epidemiology and Economics*. Proceedings of the Second International Symposium, Canberra, 7-14 May 1979. Eds Geering, W.A., Roe, R.T. and Chapman, L.A., pp. 575-580. Australian Government Publishing Service, Canberra

Davidson, M.K., Lindsey, J.R. and Davis, J.K. (1987) Requirements and selection of an animal model. *Israel Journal of Medical Sciences*, **23**, 551-555

Davies, E.B. and Watkinson, J.H. (1966) Uptake of native and applied selenium by pasture species. I. Uptake of Se by browntop, ryegrass, cocksfoot and white clover from Atiamuri sand. *New Zealand Journal of Agricultural Research*, **9**, 317-327

Davies, F.G. (1975) Observations on the epidemiology of Rift Valley Fever in Kenya. *Journal of Hygiene, Cambridge*, **75**, 219-230

Davies, F.G., Shaw, T. and Ochieng, P. (1975) Observations on the epidemiology of ephemeral fever in Kenya. *Journal of Hygiene, Cambridge*, **75**, 231-235

Davies, G. (1980) Animal disease surveillance. In: *Veterinary Epidemiology and Economics*. Proceedings of the Second International Symposium. Eds Geering, W.A., Roe, R.T. and Chapman, L.A., pp. 3-10. Australian Government Publishing Service, Canberra

Davies, G. (1983) The development of veterinary epidemiology. In: Society for Veterinary Epidemiology and Preventive Medicine, Proceedings, Southampton, 12-13 April 1983. Ed. Thrusfield, M.V., pp. ix-xvi

Davies, G. (1993) Do we need a European surveillance system? In: Society for Veterinary Epidemiology and Preventive Medicine, Proceedings, Exeter, 31 March-2 April 1993. Ed. Thrusfield, M.V., pp. 153-163

Davies, O.L. and Goldsmith, P.L. (1972) *Statistical Methods in Research and Production*, 4th edn. Longman, New York and

London

De Boer, C.J. (1967) Studies to determine neutralizing antibody in sera from animals recovered from African Swine Fever and laboratory animals inoculated with African virus adjuvants. *Archiv für die Gesamte Virusforschung*, **20**, 164–179

De Candolle, A.P.A. (1874) Constitution dans le regne vegetal de groupes physiologiques applicables a la geographie ancienne et moderne. *Archives des Sciences Physiques et Naturelles*, **50**, 5–42

Degner, R.L., Rodan, L.W., Mathis, W.K. and Gibbs, E.P.J. (1983) The recreational and commercial importance of feral swine in Florida: relevance to the possible introduction of African Swine Fever into the USA. *Preventive Veterinary Medicine*, **1**, 371–381

De Kruif, A. (1978) Factors influencing the fertility of a cattle population. *Journal of Reproduction and Fertility*, **54**, 507–518

De Kruif, A. (1980) Efficiency of a fertility control programme in dairy herds. In: Proceedings of the Ninth International Congress on Animal Reproduction and Artificial Insemination, Madrid, 16–20 June 1980, Volume II, pp. 381–388

Demets, D.L. and Ware, J.H. (1980) Group sequential methods in clinical trials with a one-sided hypothesis. *Biometrika*, **67**, 651–660

Denny, G.O., Wilesmith, J.W., Clements, R.A. and Hueston, W.D. (1992) Bovine spongiform encephalopathy in Northern Ireland: epidemiological observations, 1988–1990. *Veterinary Record*, **130**, 113–116

Descour, L. (1922) *Pasteur and His Work*. Wedd, A.F. and Wedd, B.H. (translators). T. Fisher Unwin, London

De Troyer, V. and D. Schepper, J. (1989) Pyometra in bitches: more frequently observed and a more serious illness in the Chow Chow? *Vlaams Diergeneeskundig Tijdschrift*, **58**, 73–76

Dickerman, R.W. and Scherer, W.F. (1983) Equine herds as sentinels for Venezuelan equine encephalitis virus activity, Nicaragua, 1977. *Bulletin of the Pan American Health Organization*, **17**, 14–18

Diekmann, O., Heesterbeek, J.A.P. and Metz, J.A.J. (1990) On the definition and the computation of the basic reproduction ratio R_0 in models for infectious diseases in heterogeneous populations. *Journal of Mathematical Biology*, **28**, 365–382

Diesch, S.L. (1979) Disease recording at the farm level. In: Proceedings of an International Symposium on Animal Health and Disease Data Banks, 4–6 December 1978, Washington, DC, pp. 97–100. United States Department of Agriculture, Miscellaneous Publications No. 1381

Diesch, S.L. and Ellinghausen, H.C. (1975) Leptospiroses. In: *Diseases Transmitted from Animals to Man*, 6th edn. Eds Hubbert, W.T., McCulloch, W.F. and Schnurrenberger, P.R., pp. 436–462. Charles C. Thomas, Springfield

Dietrich, R.A., Amosson, S.H. and Hopkin, J.A. (1980) Epidemiologic and economic analysis of the USA bovine brucellosis program and selected program alternatives via an open-ended simulation model. In: *Veterinary Epidemiology and Economics*. Proceedings of the Second International

Symposium, Canberra, 7–11 May 1979. Eds Geering, W.A., Roe, R.T. and Chapman, L.A., pp. 623–632. Australian Government Publishing Service, Canberra

Dijkhuizen, A.A., Morris, R.S. and Morrow, M. (1986) Economic optimization of culling strategies in swine breeding herds using the PorkCHOP computer program. *Preventive Veterinary Medicine*, **4**, 431–453

Dillon, J.L. and Anderson, J.R. (1990) *The Analysis of Response in Crop and Livestock Production*, 3rd edn. Pergamon Press, Oxford

Di Salvo, A.F. and Johnson, W.M. (1979) Histoplasmosis in South Carolina: support for the microfocus concept. *American Journal of Epidemiology*, **109**, 408–492

Dixon, J.S. and Bird, H.A. (1981) Reproducibility along a 10 cm vertical visual analogue scale. *Annals of Rheumatic Diseases*, **40**, 87–89

Dobben, W.H. van (1952) The food of the cormorants in the Netherlands. *Ardea*, **40**, 1–63

Dobson, A.P. (1988) Restoring island ecosystems: the potential of parasites to control introduced mammals. *Conservation Biology*, **2**, 31–39

Dobson, A.P., Hudson, P.J. and Lyles, A.M. (1992) Macroparasites: worms and others. In: *Natural Enemies: The Population Biology of Predators, Parasites and Diseases*. Ed. Crawley, M.J., pp. 329–348. Blackwell Scientific Publications, Oxford

Dodd, F.H. and Neave, F.K. (1970) *Mastitis Control*. Biennial Review, Paper No. 3559. National Institute for Research in Dairying, Reading

Dohms, J.E. and Metz, A. (1991) Stress mechanisms of immunosuppression. *Veterinary Immunology and immunopathology*, **30**, 89–109

Dohoo, I.R. (1988) Animal Productivity and Health Information Network. *Canadian Veterinary Journal*, **29**, 281–287

Dohoo, I.R. (1992) Dairy APHIN — an information service for the dairy industry in Prince Edward Island, Canada. *Preventive Veterinary Medicine*, **12**, 259–268

Dohoo, I.R. (1993) Monitoring livestock health and production: service — epidemiology's last frontier? *Preventive Veterinary Medicine*, **18**, 43–52

Dohoo, I.R. and Martin, S.W. (1984) Disease, production and culling in Holstein–Friesian cows. III. Disease and production as determinants of disease. *Preventive Veterinary Medicine*, **2**, 671–690

Dohoo, I.R., Martin, S.W., McMillan, I. and Kennedy, B.W. (1984) Disease, production and culling in Holstein–Friesian cows. II. Age, season and sire effects. *Preventive Veterinary Medicine*, **2**, 655–670

Dohoo, I.R., Morris, R.S., Martin, S.W., Perry, B.D., Bernado, T., Thrusfield, M., Smith, R. and Welte, V.R. (1994) Epidemiology (letter). *Nature*, **368**, 284

Dolan, R.B. (1987) Genetics and trypanotolerance. *Parasitology Today*, **3**, 137–143

Doll, R. (1959) Smoking and cancer. Report to the subcommittee for the study of the risks of cancer from air pollution and the consumption of tobacco. *Acta Uniaris*

Internationalis Contra Cancrum, **15**, 1283–1296

Doll, R. (1977) Strategy for detection of cancer hazards to man. *Nature*, **265**, 589–596

Doll, R. (1992) Sir Austin Bradford Hill and the progress of medical science. *British Medical Journal*, **305**, 1521–1528

Doll, R. and Hill, A.B. (1964a) Mortality in relation to smoking. Ten years' observations of British doctors. *British Medical Journal*, **i**, 1399–1410

Doll, R. and Hill, A.B. (1964b) Mortality in relation to smoking. Ten years' observations of British doctors. *British Medical Journal*, **i**, 1460–1467

Donald, W.A., Gardner, I.A. and Wiggins, A.D. (1994) Cut-off points for aggregate herd testing in the presence of disease clustering and correlation of test errors. *Preventive Veterinary Medicine*, **19**, 167–187

Donaldson, A.I. and Doel, T.R. (1992) Foot-and-mouth disease: the risk for Great Britain after 1992. *Veterinary Record*, **131**, 114–120

Donaldson, A.I., Gloster, J., Harvey, L.D.J. and Deans, D.H. (1982) Use of prediction models to forecast and analyse airborne spread during the foot-and-mouth disease outbreaks in Brittany, Jersey and the Isle of Wight in 1981. *Veterinary Record*, **110**, 53–57

Done, J.T. (1985) Eradication, elimination or control? *Veterinary Record*, **117**, 253

Donham, K.J., Berg, J.W. and Sawin, R.S. (1980) Epidemiologic relationships of the bovine population and human leukaemia in Iowa. *American Journal of Epidemiology*, **112**, 80–92

Donner, A. (1993) The comparison of proportions in the presence of litter effects. *Preventive Veterinary Medicine*, **18**, 17–26

Dorn, C.R. (1966) An animal tumour registry as a source of morbidity information. In: Proceedings of the United States Livestock Sanitation Association, pp. 443–454

Dorn, C.R. and Priester, W.A. (1976) Epidemiologic analysis of oral and pharyngeal cancer in dogs, cats, horses and cattle. *Journal of the American Veterinary Association*, **169**, 1202–1206

Dorn, C.R. and Priester, W.A. (1987) Epidemiology. In: *Veterinary Cancer Medicine*, 2nd edn. Eds Theilen, G.H. and Madewell, B.R., pp. 27–52. Lea and Febiger, Philadelphia

Dorn, C.R. and Schneider, R. (1976) Inbreeding and canine mammary cancer: a retrospective study. *Journal of the National Cancer Institute*, **57**, 545–548

Dorn, C.R., Taylor, D.O.N. and Hibbard, H.H. (1967) Epizootiologic characteristics of canine and feline leukaemia and lymphoma. *American Journal of Veterinary Research*, **28**, 993–1001

Dorn, C.R., Terbrusch, F.G. and Hibbard, H.H. (1967) Zoographic and Demographic Analysis of Dog and Cat Ownership in Alameda County, California, 1965. State of California Department of Public Health, Berkeley

Dorn, C.R., Taylor, D.O.N., Schneider, R., Hibbard, H.H. and Klauber, M.R. (1968) Survey of animal neoplasms in Alameda and Contra Costa Counties, California. II. Cancer morbidity in dogs and cats from Alameda County. *Journal of*

the National Cancer Institute, **40**, 307–318

Dorn, C.R., Taylor, D.O.N. and Schneider, R. (1971) Sunlight exposure and risk of developing cutaneous and oral squamous cell carcinomas in white cats. *Journal of the National Cancer Institute*, **46**, 1073–1081

Dorn, C.R., Garner, H.E., Coffman, J.R., Hahn, A.W. and Tritschler, L.G. (1975) Castration and other factors affecting the risk of equine laminitis. *Cornell Veterinarian*, **65**, 57–64

Douglas, A. (1984) Disease prevention in pig herds. *In Practice*, **6**, 108–115

Doyle, T.M. (1927) A hitherto unrecorded disease of fowls due to a filter-passing virus. *Journal of Comparative Pathology and Therapeutics*, **40**, 144–169

Draper, N. and Smith, H. (1966) *Applied Regression Analysis*, 2nd edn. John Wiley, New York

Drolia, H., Luescher, U.A. and Meek, A.H. (1990) Tail-tip necrosis in Ontario feedlot cattle: two case–control studies. *Preventive Veterinary Medicine*, **9**, 195–205

Dubos, R. (1965) *Man Adapting*. Yale University Press, New Haven

Ducrot, C. and Cimarotsi, I. (1991) Complementary aspects of the logistic model and of the correspondence analysis to investigate risk factors in animal pathology: application to the study of orf risk factors in sheep breeders. In: Proceedings of the Sixth International Symposium on Veterinary Epidemiology and Economics, Ottawa, 12–16 August 1991. Ed. Martin, S.W., pp. 97–100

Dunbar, I. (1979) *Dog Behaviour: Why Dogs Do What They Do*. T.F.H. Publications, Neptune, New Jersey

Duppong, B.L. and Ettinger, S.J. (1983) The medical record. In: *Textbook of Veterinary Internal Medicine: Diseases of the Dog and Cat*, Vol. 2, 2nd edn. Ed. Ettinger, S.J., pp. 3–29. W.B. Saunders, Philadelphia

Dyer, J. (1990) *Ancient Britain*. Batsford, London

Dykhuizen, A.A. (1993) Modelling animal health economics. In: Society for Veterinary Epidemiology and Preventive Medicine, Proceedings, Exeter, 31 March–2 April 1993. Ed. Thrusfield, M.V., pp. ix–xx

Eddy, R.G. (1992) Private health schemes. In: *Livestock Health and Welfare*. Ed. Moss, R., pp. 183–291. Longman Scientific & Technical, Harlow

Edney, A.T.B. and Smith, P.M. (1986) Study of obesity in dogs visiting veterinary practices in the United Kingdom. *Veterinary Record*, **118**, 391–396

Edney, A.T.B., Gaskell, C.J. and Sharp, N.J.H. (Eds) (1987) Feline dysautonomia — an emerging disease. *Journal of Small Animal Practice*, **28**, 333–416

Edwards, B. (1980) Foot lameness in cattle. *In Practice*, **2**(4), 25–31

Edwards, J.R. (1990) Surveys and questionnaires: design, conduct and analysis. In: *Epidemiological Skills in Animal Health*. Refresher Course for Veterinarians, Proceedings 143, Sydney, 1–5 October 1990, pp. 151–158. Postgraduate Committee in Veterinary Science, University of Sydney

Edwards, J.T. (1928) Rinderpest: active immunization by means of the serum simultaneous method; goat virus. *Agricultural*

Journal of India, **23**, 185–189

Edwards, P. (Ed.) (1967) *The Encyclopedia of Philosophy*, Vol. 8. The Macmillan Company and the Free Press, New York

Edwards, S.A. and Lightfoot, A.L. (1986) The effect of floor type in farrowing pens on pig injury. II. Leg and teat damage of sows. *British Veterinary Journal*, **142**, 441–445

Egeberg, R.O. (1954) Coccidioidomycosis: its clinical and climatological aspects with remarks on treatment. *American Journal of Medical Science*, **227**, 268–271

Egerton, J.R. (1981) Foot-rot. In: Refresher course on sheep, 10–14 August. Postgraduate Committee in Veterinary Science, University of Sydney, Proceedings No. 58, pp. 647–651

Egwu, G.O., Faull, W.B., Bradbury, J.M. and Clarkson, M.J. (1989) Ovine infectious keratoconjunctivitis: a microbiological study of clinically unaffected and affected sheep's eyes with special reference to *Mycoplasma conjunctiviae*. *Veterinary Record*, **125**, 253–256

Ekesbo, I. (1966) Disease incidence in tied and loose housed dairy cattle and causes of incidence variation with particular reference to cowshed type. *Acta Agriculturae Scandinavica*, Suppl. 15, 1–74

Ekesbo, I. (1992) Monitoring systems using clinical, subclinical and behavioural records for improving health and welfare. In: *Livestock Health and Welfare*. Ed. Moss, R., pp. 20–50. Longman Scientific & Technical, Harlow

Elbers, A.R.W., Tielen, M.J.M., Cromwijk, W.A.J. and Hunneman, W.A. (1992) Variation in seropositivity for some respiratory disease agents in finishing pigs: epidemiological studies on some health parameters and farm management conditions in the herds. *The Veterinary Quarterly*, **14**, 8–13

Elder, J.K. (1976) A functional computer recording system for a veterinary diagnostic laboratory. *Australian Veterinary Journal*, **52**, 24–35

Elliott, A.C. (1988) KWIKSTAT: a low-cost interactive statistical analysis package for IBM-PC-compatible computers. *The American Statistician*, **42**, 228–229

Ellis, P.R. (1980) International aspects of animal disease surveillance. In: *Veterinary Epidemiology and Economics*, Proceedings of the Second International Symposium. Eds Geering, W.A., Roe, R.T. and Chapman, L.A., pp. 11–15. Australian Government Publishing Service, Canberra

Ellis, P.R., James, A.D. and Shaw, A.P. (1977) Studies on the Epidemiology and Economics of Swine Fever Eradication in the EEC, EUR 5738e. Commission of the European Communities, Luxembourg

Elton, C.S. (1927) *Animal Ecology*. Macmillan, New York

Elwood, J.M. (1988) *Causal Relationships in Medicine. A Practical System for Critical Appraisal*. Oxford University Press, Oxford

Emanuelson, U. and Bendixen, P.H. (1991) Occurrence of cystic ovaries in dairy cows in Sweden. *Preventive Veterinary Medicine*, **10**, 261–271

Emanuelson, U., Scherling, K. and Pettersson, H. (1992) Relationship between herd bovine leukaemia infection status and reproduction, disease incidence and productivity in

Swedish dairy herds. *Preventive Veterinary Medicine*, **12**, 121–131

Emery, R.S., Hafs, H.D., Armstrong, D. and Snyder, W.W. (1969) Prepartum grain feeding effects on milk production, mammary edema and incidence of diseases. *Journal of Dairy Science*, **52**, 345–351

Enevoldsen, C., Grohn, Y.T. and Thysen, I. (1990) Physical injuries in dairy cows: associations with season, cow characteristics, disease and production. In: Society for Veterinary Epidemiology and Preventive Medicine, Proceedings, Belfast, 4–6 April 1990. Ed. Thrusfield, M.V., pp. 133–144

Erb, H. (1984) Economics for veterinary farm practice. *In Practice*, **6**, 33–37

Erickson, B.H. and Nosanchuk, T.A. (1979) *Understanding Data*. Open University Press, Milton Keynes

Ernst, S.N. and Fabrega, F. (1989) A time series analysis of the rabies control programme in Chile. *Epidemiology and Infection*, **103**, 651–657

Erskine, R.J., Eberhart, R.J., Hutchinson, L.J. and Spencer, S.B. (1987) Herd management and prevalence of mastitis in dairy herds with high and low somatic cell counts. *Journal of the American Veterinary Medical Association*, **190**, 1411–1416

Esslemont, R.J. (1993) Measuring fertility in dairy herds. In: Society for Veterinary Epidemiology and Preventive Medicine, Proceedings, Exeter, 31 March–2 April 1993. Ed. Thrusfield, M.V., pp. 96–109

Esslemont, R.J., Wassell, B.R., Wassell, T.R., Grimbleby, L., Lamb, J.M. and Horne, S. (1991) The application of planned animal health and production to dairy farms: DAISY — The Dairy Information System. *The Bovine Practitioner*, **26**, 38–41

Estola, T. and Neuvonen, E. (1976) Experience of efficacy of equine influenza vaccinations. *Nordisk Veterinærmedicin*, **28**, 353–356

Eugster, A.K., Bendele, R.A. and Hones, C.P. (1978) Parvovirus infection in dogs. *Journal of the American Veterinary Medical Association*, **173**, 1340–1341

Evans, A.S. (1976) Causation and disease. The Henle–Koch postulates revisited. *Yale Journal of Biology and Medicine*, **49**, 175–195

Evans, A.S. (1987) Subclinical epidemiology. *American Journal of Epidemiology*, **125**, 545–555

Evans, A.S. (1993) *Causation and Disease: A Chronological Journey*. Plenum Publishing, New York

Evans-Pritchard, E.E. (1956) *Nuer Religion*. Oxford University Press, London

Everitt, R.S. (1989) *Statistical Methods for Medical Investigations*. Oxford University Press, New York/Edward Arnold, London

Everitt, R.S. and Dunn, G. (1991) *Applied Multivariate Data Analysis*. Edward Arnold, London

Ewbank, D. and Wray, J.D. (1980) Population and public health. In: *Maxcy-Rosenau: Public Health and Preventive Medicine*, 11th edn. Ed. Last, J.M., pp. 1504–1548

Ewbank, R. (1986) Animal welfare — is an epidemiological

approach possible? In: Society for Veterinary Epidemiology and Preventive Medicine, Proceedings, Edinburgh, 2–4 April 1986. Ed. Thrusfield, M.V., pp. 92–96

Ewbank, R. (1988) Animal welfare. In: *Management and Welfare of Farm Animals*. The UFAW Handbook, 3rd edn, pp. 1–14. Baillière Tindall, London

Ewbank, R. and Cullinan, A. (1984) The effect of simulated sonic booms on horses. In: Proceedings of the International Congress on Applied Ethology in Farm Animals, Kiel. Eds Unschelm, J., van Putten, G. and Zeeb, K., pp. 325–328. Kuratorium für Technik und Bauwesen in der Landwirtschaft, Darmstadt

Eyster, G.E., Eyster, J.T., Cords, G.B. and Johnston, J. (1976) Patent ductus arteriosus in the dog: characteristics of occurrence and results of surgery in one hundred consecutive cases. *Journal of the American Veterinary Medical Association*, **168**, 435–438

Fabia, J., Boivin, J.-F., Bernard, P.-M., Ducic, S. and Thuriaux, M. (1988) English–French and French–English dictionary of terms used in epidemiology. *International Journal of Epidemiology*, **17**(1), Suppl., 1–49

FAHRMX (1984) FAHRMX dairy herd health management computer network. In: Proceedings of the Second Symposium on Computer Applications in Veterinary Medicine. College of Veterinary Medicine, Mississippi State University, 23–25 May 1984, pp. 45–50

Falconer, D.S. (1989) *Introduction to Quantitative Genetics*, 3rd edn. Longman, London

Fang, D.Y. and Wang, Y.K. (1981) Studies on the aetiology and specific control of goose parvovirus infection. *Scienta Agricultura Sinica*, **4**, 1–8 (in Chinese).

FAO (1991) *FAO Production Yearbook 1990*, Vol. 44. Food and Agriculture Organization of the United Nations, Rome

FAO/WHO (1967) *Report of a Joint Food and Agriculture Organization/World Health Organization Expert Committee on Zoonoses*. Technical Report Series No. 3. World Health Organization, Geneva

FAO-WHO-OIE (1992) *Animal Health Yearbook 1991*. Food and Agriculture Organization of the United Nations, World Health Organization, Office International des Epizooties. Food and Agriculture Organization of the United Nations, Rome

Farr, W. (1840) Appendix to the Second Annual Report of the Registrar-General of Births, Deaths and Marriages in England, pp. 3–22. William Clowes and Sons, London. In: *House of Commons Parliamentary Papers, Vol. XVII. Reports from Commissioners, 2, Births; Deaths; Marriages; Poor Laws, Session 16 January–11 August 1840*, pp. 39–58

Faye, B. and Lescourret, F. (1989) Environmental factors associated with lameness in dairy cattle. *Preventive Veterinary Medicine*, **7**, 267–287

Fekadu, M. and Baer, G.M. (1980) Recovery from clinical rabies of 2 dogs inoculated with a rabies virus strain from Ethiopia. *American Journal of Veterinary Research*, **41**, 1632–1634

Felton, M.R. and Ellis, P.R. (1978) *Studies in the Control of*

Rinderpest in Nigeria. Study No. 23. University of Reading

Fennell, C. (1975) Some demographic characteristics of the domestic cat population in Great Britain with particular reference to feeding habits and the incidence of the feline urological syndrome. *Journal of Small Animal Practice*, **16**, 775–783

Fenner, F. and Ratcliffe, F.N. (1965) *Myxomatosis*. Cambridge University Press, Cambridge

Fenner, F., Henderson, D.A., Arita, I., Jezek, Z. and Ladnyi, I.D. (1988) *Smallpox and its Eradication*. World Health Organization, Geneva

Ferns, L., Dohoo, I. and Donald, A. (1991) A case–control study of *Nocardia* mastitis in Nova Scotia dairy herds. *Canadian Veterinary Journal*, **32**, 673–677

Ferris, D.H. (1967) Epizootiology. *Advances in Veterinary Science*, **11**, 261–320

Ferris, D.H. (1971) Epizootiologic features of transmissible swine gastroenteritis. *Journal of the American Veterinary Medical Association*, **159**, 184–194

Fidler, I.J., Brodey, R.S., Howson, A.E. and Cohen, D. (1966) Relationship of estrus irregularity, pseudopregnancy and pregnancy to canine pyometra. *Journal of the American Veterinary Medical Association*, **149**, 1043–1046

Finnegan, D.J. (1976) *Bacterial Conjugation*. Meadowfield Press, Shildon

Finney, D.J. (1971) *Probit Analysis*, 3rd edn. Cambridge University Press, Cambridge

Finney, D.J. (1978) *Statistical Method in Biological Assay*, 3rd edn. Charles Griffin, London and High Wycombe

Fisk, D. (1959) *Dr Jenner of Baltimore*. William Heinemann, London

Fleiss, J.L. (1981) *Statistical Methods for Rates and Proportions*, 2nd edn. John Wiley, New York

Flesja, K.I. and Solberg, I. (1981) Pathological lesions in swine at slaughter. IV. Pathological lesions in relation to rearing system and herd size. *Acta Veterinaria Scandinavica*, **22**, 272–282

Flesja, K.I., Forus, I.B. and Solberg, I. (1982) Pathological lesions in swine at slaughter. V. Pathological lesions in relation to some environmental factors in the herds. *Acta Veterinaria Scandinavica*, **23**, 169–183

Fletcher, R.H., Fletcher, S.W. and Wagener, E.H. (1988) *Clinical Epidemiology: the Essentials*, 2nd edn. Williams and Wilkins, Baltimore

Foley, C.W., Lasley, J.F. and Osweiler, G.D. (1979) *Abnormalities of Companion Animals: Analysis of Heritability*. Iowa State University Press, Ames

Forbes, R.N., Sanson, R.L. and Morris, R.S. (1994) Application of subjective methods to the determination of the likelihood and consequences of the entry of foot-and-mouth disease into New Zealand. *New Zealand Veterinary Journal*, **42**, 81–88

Ford, J. (1971) *The Role of the Trypanosomiases in African Ecology: A Study of the Tsetse Fly Problem*. Clarendon Press, Oxford

Forster, F. (1966) Use of a demographic base map for the

presentation of aerial data in epidemiology. *British Journal of Preventive and Social Medicine*, **20**, 156−171

Foster, D.A. and Sullivan, K.M. (1989a) A discrete-time, stochastic system for the simulation of infectious disease epidemics (abstract). *American Journal of Epidemiology*, **130**, 847

Foster, D.A. and Sullivan, K.M. (1989b) Microcomputer programs for exact calculation or maximum likelihood estimation of selected epidemiologic parameters. *The American Statistician*, **43**, 126

Fourichon, C., Madec, F., Pansart, J.F. and Paboeuf, F. (1990) The application of some multivariate statistical methods in epidemiology — an example: a cohort study of respiratory disease in pigs. In: Society for Veterinary Epidemiology and Preventive Medicine, Proceedings, Belfast, 4−6 April 1990. Ed. Thrusfield, M.V., pp. 153−166

Fox, J.P. (1958) Prophylaxis against rabies in humans. *Annals of the New York Academy of Sciences*, **70**, 480−494

Fox, M.T. and Sykes, T.J. (1985) Establishment of the tropical dog tick, *Rhipicephalus sanquineus*, in a house in London. *Veterinary Record*, **116**, 661−662

Francis, P.G., Sumner, J. and Joyce, D.A. (1979) *The Environment in Relation to Mastitis: A Field Study*. Agricultural Development Advisory Services, South-Western Region, UK

Francis, P.G., Wilesmith, J.W. and Wilson, C.D. (1986) Observations on the incidence of clinical bovine mastitis in non-lactating cows in England and Wales. *Veterinary Record*, **118**, 549−552

Frankena, K., Noordhuizen, J.P., Willeberg, P., van Voorthuysen, P.F. and Goelema, J.O. (1990) EPISCOPE: Computer programs for veterinary epidemiology. *Veterinary Record*, **126**, 573−576

Frankena, K., Stassen, E.N., Noordhuizen, J.P. and Goelema, J.O. (1991a) Lameness in dairy cattle during housing: general descriptive results and risk analysis for dermatitis digitalis. In: Proceedings of the Sixth International Symposium on Veterinary Epidemiology and Economics, Ottawa, 12−16 August 1991. Ed. Martin, S.W., pp. 276−279

Frankena, K., van Keulen, K.A.S., Noordhuizen, J.P., Noordhuizen-Stassen, E.N., Gundelach, J., de Jong, D.-J. and Saedt, I. (1991b) Prevalence and risk indicators of digital laminitis in dairy breeding calves. Studievereniging voor Veterinaire Epidemiologie en Economie, Proceedings, Utrecht, 11 December 1991. Eds. Hogeveen, H. and Nielen, M., pp. 41−52

Frankena, K., van Keulen, K.A.S., Noordhuizen, J.P., Noordhuizen-Stassen, E.N., Gundelach, J., de Jong, D.-J. and Saedt, I. (1992) A cross-sectional study into prevalence and risk indicators of digital haemorrhages in female dairy calves. *Preventive Veterinary Medicine*, **14**, 1−12

Frankena, K., van Keulen, K.A.S., Noordhuizen, J.P., Noordhuizen-Stassen, E.N., Gundelach, J., de Jong, D.-J. and Saedt, I. (1993) A cross-sectional study into prevalence and risk factors of dermatitis interdigitalis in female dairy calves in the Netherlands. *Preventive Veterinary Medicine*, **17**, 137−144

Franti, C.E. and Kraus, J.F. (1974) Aspects of pet ownership in Yolo County, California. *Journal of the American Veterinary Medical Association*, **164**, 166−171

Franti, C.E., Kraus, J.F. and Borhani, N.O. (1974) Pet ownership in a suburban−rural area of California, 1970. *Public Health Reports*, **89**, 473−484

Franti, C.E., Kraus, J.F., Borhani, N.O., Johnson, S.L. and Tucker, S.D. (1980) Pet ownership in rural northern California (El Dorado County). *Journal of the American Veterinary Medical Association*, **176**, 143−149

Fraser, A.C. (1969) Advisory and preventive medicine in equine practice. *Veterinary Record*, **85**, 249−250

Fraser, A.F. (1976) *Topics in Theriogenology*. A supplementary handbook on special practical and clinical features of veterinary reproduction. Western College of Veterinary Medicine, Saskatoon

Fraumeni, J.F. (1967) Stature and malignant tumours of bone in childhood and adolescence. *Cancer*, **20**, 967−973

Frazer, J.G. (1890) *The Golden Bough: A Study in Comparative Religion*, Vol. 2. Macmillan, London

French, N.P., Wall, R., Cripps, P.J. and Morgan, K.L. (1992) Prevalence, regional distribution and control of blowfly strike in England and Wales. *Veterinary Record*, **131**, 337−342

Frenkel, J.K. (1969) Choice of animal models for the study of disease processes in man. *Federation Proceedings*, **28**, 160−161

Freshman, J.L., Reif, J.S., Allen, T.A. and Jones, R.L. (1989) Risk factors associated with urinary tract infection in female dogs. *Preventive Veterinary Medicine*, **7**, 59−67

Fritschen, R.D. (1979) Housing and its effect on feet and leg problems. *The Pig Veterinary Society Proceedings*, **5**, 95−98

Frost, W.H. (1976) Some conceptions of epidemics in general. *American Journal of Epidemiology*, **103**, 141−151

Frye, F.L., Dorn, C.R., Taylor, D.O.N., Hibbard, H.H. and Klauber, M.R. (1967) Characteristics of canine mammary gland tumour cases. *Animal Hospital*, **3**, 1−12

Furniss, S.J., Edwards, S.A., Lightfoot, A.L. and Spechter, H.H. (1986) The effect of floor type in farrowing pens on pig injury. I. Leg and teat damage of suckling piglets. *British Veterinary Journal*, **142**, 434−440

Gaddum, J.H. (1933) *Reports of Biological Standards. III. Methods of Biological Assay Depending on a Quantal Response*. Special Report Series No. 183. Medical Research Council, London

Galen, R.S. and Gambino, S.R. (1975) *Beyond Normality — The Predictive Value and Efficiency of Medical Diagnoses*. John Wiley, New York

Galuzo, I.G. (1975) Landscape epidemiology (epizootiology). *Advances in Veterinary Science and Comparative Medicine*, **19**, 73−96

Ganchi, C., Di Sacco, B., Formaggini, L., Venco, L., Vezzoni, A. and Guerro, J. (1992) Spreading of *Dirofilaria immitis* infections in dogs and cats in Italy. In: Proceedings of the 17th World Small Animal Veterinary Association Congress, Vol. 1, Rome, 24−27 September 1992. Ed. Delfino, A., pp. 203−209

Gardiner, W.P. and Gettinby, G. (1983) A weather-based prediction model for the life-cycle of the sheep tick *Ixodes ricinus* (L). *Veterinary Parasitology*, **13**, 77−84

Gardner, M.J. and Altman, D.G. (1989) *Statistics with Confidence*. British Medical Journal, London

Gaskell, C.J. (1983) Dilated pupil (Key−Gaskell) syndrome in cats. In: Society for Veterinary Epidemiology and Preventive Medicine, Proceedings, Southampton, 12−13 April 1983. Ed. Thrusfield, M.V., pp. 99−100

Gause, G.F. (1934) *The Struggle for Existence*. Williams and Wilkins, Baltimore

Gerstman, B. (1987) Epidemiologic calculations, graphs and 'what if' analysis on a microcomputer spreadsheet (abstract). *American Journal of Epidemiology*, **126**, 778

Gettinby, B., Bairden, K., Armour, J. and Benitez-Usher, C. (1979) A prediction model for bovine ostertagiasis. *Veterinary Record*, **105**, 57−59

Gettinby, G. (1989) Computational veterinary parasitology with an application to chemical resistance. *Veterinary Parasitology*, **32**, 57−72

Gettinby, G. and Byrom, W. (1989) ECFXPERT: A computer model for the study of East Coast fever. Eighth Biennial Conference and Bushfire Dynamics Workshop Proceedings, 25−27 September 1989, Australian National University, Canberra. Simulation Society of Australia Inc. affiliated with the International Association for Mathematics and Computers in Simulation, pp. 123−127

Gettinby, G. and Gardiner, W.P. (1980) Disease incidence forecasts by means of climatic data. *Biometeorology*, **7**, 87−103

Gettinby, G. and McClean, S. (1979) A matrix formulation of the life-cycle of liver fluke. *Proceedings of the Royal Irish Academy*, **79B**, 155−167

Ghirotti, M. (1992) Rapid appraisal techniques: a tool for planning and managing animal health and production programmes. In: Society for Veterinary Epidemiology and Preventive Medicine, Proceedings, Edinburgh, 1−3 April 1992. Ed. Thrusfield, M.V., pp. 190−206

Gibson, M. and Warren, K.S. (1970) Capture of *Schistosoma mansoni* miracidia and cercariae by carnivorous aquatic vascular plants of the genus *Utricularia*. *Bulletin of the World Health Organization*, **42**, 833−835

Gibson, T.E. (1978) The 'Mt' system for forecasting the prevalence of fascioliasis. In: *Weather and Parasitic Animal Disease*. Ed. Gibson, T.E., pp. 3−5, World Meteorological Organization Technical Note No. 159

Gibson, T.E. and Smith, L.P. (1978a) Forecasting the prevalence of nematodiriasis in England and Wales. In: *Weather and Parasitic Animal Disease*. Ed. Gibson, T.E., pp. 74−75. World Meteorological Organization Technical Note No. 159

Gibson, T.E. and Smith, L.P. (1978b) Forecasting outbreaks of parasitic gastroenteritis in ruminants in England and Wales. In: *Weather and Parasitic Animal Disease*. Ed. Gibson, T.E., pp. 76−77. World Meteorological Organization Technical Note No. 159

Gill, J.L. (1987) Biased statistical analysis when the animal is not the experimental unit (letter). *Journal of the American Veterinary Medical Association*, **190**, 5−6

Gilmour, J.S. (1989) Grass sickness in horses. *Animal Diseases Research Association News Sheet No. 17*. Moredun Research Institute, Edinburgh

Gittinger, J.P. (1972) *Economic Analysis of Agricultural Projects*. The Johns Hopkins University Press, Baltimore and London

Glickman, L.T. (1980) Preventive medicine in kennel management. In: *Current Veterinary Therapy VII. Small Animal Practice*. Ed. Kirk, R.W., pp. 67−76. W.B. Saunders, Philadelphia

Glickman, L.T., Domanski, L.M., Maguire, T.G., Dubielzig, R.R. and Churg, A. (1983) Mesothelioma in pet dogs associated with exposure of their owners to asbestos. *Environmental Research*, **32**, 305−313

Glickman, L.T., Domanski, L.M., Patronek, G.J. and Visintainer, F. (1985) Breed-related risk factors for canine parvovirus enteritis. *American Journal of Veterinary Research*, **187**, 589−594

Glickman, L.T., Schofer, F.S., McKee, L.J., Reif, J.S. and Goldschmidt, M.H. (1989) Epidemiologic study of insecticide exposures, obesity and risk of bladder cancer in household dogs. *Journal of Toxicology and Environmental Health*, **28**, 407−414

Glosser, J.W. (1988) Back to the future: the Animal Health Monitoring System — a political necessity being addressed in the United States. *Acta Veterinaria Scandinavica*, Suppl. 84, 42−48

Gloster, J., Blackall, R.M., Sellers, R.F. and Donaldson, A.I. (1981) Forecasting the airborne spread of foot-and-mouth disease. *Veterinary Record*, **108**, 370−374

Goggin, J.E., Li, A. and Franti, C.E. (1970) Canine intervertebral disc disease: characterization by age, sex, breed and anatomic site of involvement. *American Journal of Veterinary Research*, **31**, 1687−1692

Gogolin-Ewens, K.J., Meeusen, E.N.T., Scott, P.C., Adams, T.E. and Brandon, M.R. (1990) Genetic selection for disease resistance and traits of economic importance in animal production. *Revue Scientifique et Technique, Office International des Epizooties*, **9**, 865−896

Goldberger, J., Waring, C.H. and Tanner, W.F. (1923) Pellagra prevention by diet among institutional inmates. *Public Health Reports*, **38**, 2361−2368

Goldspink, G. and Gerlach, G.-F. (1990) Prospective use of recombinant DNA methods in animal disease control. In: Proceedings of the Society for Veterinary Epidemiology and Preventive Medicine, Belfast, 4−6 April 1990. Ed. Thrusfield, M.V., pp. 1−14

Goldspink, G.E. (1993) The impact of recombinant DNA techniques on veterinary diagnosis and genetic screening. In: *The Advancement of Veterinary Science. The Bicentenary Symposium Series. Volume 1: Veterinary Medicine Beyond 2000*. Ed. Michell, A.R., pp. 59−71. CAB International, Wallingford

Goldstein, R. (1988) Epistat (Version 3.3) and True Epistat (Version 2.0). *The American Statistician*, **42**, 217–219

Goodall, E.A., McCaughey, W.J., McMurray, C.H. and Rice, D. (1984) SIRO — a computer system for dairy herd recording. In: Society for Veterinary Epidemiology and Preventive Medicine, Proceedings, Edinburgh, 10–11 July 1984. Ed. Thrusfield, M.V., pp. 174–183

Goodger, W.J. and Ruppanner, R. (1982) Why the dairy industry does not make greater use of veterinarians. *Journal of the American Veterinary Medical Association*, **181**, 706–710

Goodwin, R.F.W. (1971) A procedure for investigating the influence of disease status on productivity efficiency in a pig herd. *Veterinary Record*, **88**, 387–392

Gopal, T. (1977) Carcinogenesis. In: *Current Veterinary Therapy VI. Small Animal Practice*. Ed. Kirk, R.W., pp. 164–166. W.B. Saunders, Philadelphia

Gordon, J.C. and Angrick, E.J. (1985) Stray dogs as sentinels for canine parvovirus. *Preventive Veterinary Medicine*, **3**, 311–316

Gordon Smith, C.E. (1976) *Epidemiology and Infections*. Meadowfield Press, Shildon

Gordon Smith, C.E. (1982) Major factors in the spread of infections. In: *Animal Disease in Relation to Animal Conservation*. Symposium of the Zoological Society of London No. 50. Eds Edwards, M.A. and McDonald, U., pp. 207–235. Academic Press, London and New York

Gorman, B.M., Taylor, J. and Walker, P.J. (1979) Variation in arboviruses. In: *Arbovirus Research in Australia*. Proceedings of the Second Symposium, 17–19 July 1979. Eds St George, T.D. and French, E.L., pp. 71–76. The Commonwealth Scientific and Industrial Research Organization/Queensland Institute of Medical Research, Brisbane

Gottstein, B. (1984) An immunoassay for the detection of circulating antigens in human echinococcosis. *American Journal of Tropical Medicine and Hygiene*, **33**, 1185–1191

Goulden, C.H. (1952) *Methods of Statistical Analysis*, 2nd edn. Chapman and Hall, London

Graat, L, Noordhuizen, J., Frankena, K., Henken, A. and Goelema, J. (1990) Epidemiological aspects of salmonellosis in poultry. In: Studievereniging voor Veterinaire Epidemiologie en Economie, Proceedings, Wageningen, 12 December 1990. Ed. Frankena, K., pp. 61–72

Gracey, J.F. (1960) *Survey of Livestock Diseases in Northern Ireland*. Her Majesty's Stationery Office, Belfast

Gracey, J.F. (1986) *Meat Hygiene*, 8th edn. Baillière Tindall, London

Grachev, M.A., Kumarev, V.P., Mamaev, L.V., Zorin, V.L., Baranova, L.V., Denikina, N.N., Belikov, S.I., Petrov, E.A., Kolesnik, V.S., Kolesnik, R.S., Dorofeev, V.M., Beim, A.M., Kudelin, V.N., Nagieva, F.G. and Sidorov, V.N. (1989) Distemper virus in Baikal seals. *Nature*, **338**, 209

Graunt, J. (1662) *Natural and Political Observations in a Following Index, and Made Upon the Bills of Mortality*. London. Reprinted 1939: The Johns Hopkins Press, Baltimore

Greenland, S. and Kleinbaum, D.G. (1983) Correcting for misclassification in two-way tables and matched-pair studies. *International Journal of Epidemiology*, **12**, 93–97

Greenland, S., Morgenstern, H. and Thomas, D.C. (1981) Considerations in determining matching criteria and stratum sizes for case–control studies. *International Journal of Epidemiology*, **10**, 389–392

Greenwood, Major (1943) Medical statistics from Graunt to Farr. VI. Some English medical statisticians in the eighteenth century. *Biometrika*, **33**, 1–24

Griffin, J.M., Hahesy, T., Lynch, K., Salman, M.D., McCarthy, J. and Hurley, T. (1993) The association of cattle husbandry practices, environmental factors and farmer characteristics with the occurrence of chronic bovine tuberculosis in dairy herds in the Republic of Ireland. *Preventive Veterinary Medicine*, **17**, 145–160

Griffiths, A.O. and Brenner, A. (1977) Survey of cat and dog ownership in Champagne County, Illinois, 1976. *Journal of the American Veterinary Medical Association*, **170**, 1333–1340

Griffiths, I.B. and Done, S.H. (1991) Citrinin as a possible cause of the pruritis, pyrexia, haemorrhagic syndrome in cattle. *Veterinary Record*, **129**, 113–117

Grindle, R.J. (1980) Appropriate methodology in economic analysis of disease control projects. In: *Veterinary Epidemiology and Economics*. Proceedings of the Second International Symposium, Canberra, 7–11 May 1979. Eds Geering, W.A., Roe, R.T. and Chapman, L.A., pp. 506–510. Australian Government Publishing Service, Canberra

Grindle, R.J. (1986) The use and abuse of economic methods as applied to veterinary problems. In: Proceedings of the Fourth International Symposium on Veterinary Epidemiology and Economics, Singapore, 18–22 November 1985, pp. 60–70. Singapore Veterinary Association, Singapore

Griner, L.A. (1980) Storage and retrieval of necropsy records at San Diego zoo. In: *The Comparative Pathology of Zoo Animals*. Eds Montali, R.J. and Miguki, G., pp. 663–667. Smithsonian Institution Press, Washington, DC

Groehn, J.A., Kaneene, J.B. and Foster, D. (1992) Risk factors associated with lameness in lactating dairy cattle in Michigan. *Preventive Veterinary Medicine*, **14**, 77–85

Grohn, Y.T., Erb, H.N. and Saloniemi, H.S. (1988) Risk factors for the disorders of the mammary gland in dairy cattle. *Acta Veterinaria Scandinavica*, Suppl. 84, 170–172

Grohn, Y.T., Erb, H.M., McCulloch, C.E. and Saloniemi, H.S. (1990) Epidemiology of reproductive disorders in dairy cattle: associations among host characteristics, disease and production. *Preventive Veterinary Medicine*, **8**, 25–39

Grondalen, J. and Lingaas, F. (1991) Arthrosis in the elbow joint of young rapidly growing dogs: a genetic investigation. *Journal of Small Animal Practice*, **32**, 460–464

Grønvold, J., Henriksen, S.A., Nansen, P., Wolstrup, J. and Thylin, J. (1989) Attempts to control infection with *Ostertagia ostertagi* (Trichostrongylidae) in grazing calves by adding mycelium of the nematode-trapping fungus *Arthrobotrys oligospora* (Hyphomycetales) to cow pats. *Journal of Helminthology*, **63**, 115–126

Grønvold, J., Wolstrup, J., Nansen, P., Henriksen, S.A.,

Larsen, M. and Bresciani, J. (1993) Biological control of nematode parasites in cattle with nematode-trapping fungi: a survey of Danish studies. *Veterinary Parasitology*, **48**, 311–325

Gross, L. (1955) Mouse leukaemia: an egg-borne virus disease (with a note on mouse salivary gland carcinoma). *Acta Haematologica*, **13**, 13–29

Groves, R.M., Biemer, P.P., Lyberg, L.E., Massey, J.T., Nicholls, W.L. and Waksberg, J. (Eds) (1988) *Telephone Survey Methodology*. John Wiley, New York

Grufferman, S. and Kimm, S.Y.S. (1984) Clinical epidemiology defined. *The New England Journal of Medicine*, **311**, 541–542

Grunsell, C.S., Penny, R.H.C., Wragg, S.R. and Allcock, J. (1969) The practicability and economics of veterinary preventive medicine. *Veterinary Record*, **84**, 26–41

Guerrero, J., Newcomb, K.M. and Fukase, T. (1992) Prevalence of *Dirofilaria immitis* in dogs and cats in the USA and Japan. In: Proceedings of the 17th World Small Animal Veterinary Association Congress, Rome, 24–27 September 1992, Vol. 1. Ed. Dolfino, A., pp. 211–217

Guess, H.A. and Thomas, J.E. (1990) A rapidly converging algorithm for exact binomial confidence intervals about the relative risk in follow-up studies with stratified incidence-density data. *Epidemiology*, **1**, 75–77

Guess, H.A., Lydick, E.G., Small, R.D. and Miller, L.P. (1987) Exact binomial confidence intervals for the relative risk in follow-up studies with sparsely stratified incidence density data. *American Journal of Epidemiology*, **125**, 340–347

Gustavsson, I. (1969) Cytogenetics, distribution and phenotypic effects of a translocation in Swedish cattle. *Hereditas*, **63**, 68–169

Habtemariam, T., Ruppanner, R., Farver, T.B. and Riemann, H.P. (1986) Determination of risk groups to African trypanosomiasis using discriminant analysis. *Preventive Veterinary Medicine*, **4**, 45–56

Habtemariam, T., Gharty-Tagoe, A., Robnett, V. and Trammel, G. (1988) Computational epidemiology: new research avenues. *Acta Veterinaria Scandinavica*, Suppl. 84, 439–441

Haelterman, E.O. (1963) Epidemiological studies of transmissible gastroenteritis of swine. Proceedings of the 66th Annual Meeting of the United States Livestock Sanitary Association, 29 October–2 November 1962, Washington, DC, pp. 305–315

Haenszel, W., Loveland, D.B. and Sirken, M.G. (1962) Lung cancer mortality as related to residence and smoking histories. 1. White males. *Journal of the National Cancer Institute*, **200**, 947–1001

Häggström, J., Hansson, K., Kvart, C. and Swenson, L. (1992) Chronic valvular disease in the cavalier King Charles spaniel in Sweden. *Veterinary Record*, **131**, 549–553

Haig, D.A. (1977) Rabies in animals. In: *Rabies: The Facts*. Ed. Kaplan, C., pp. 53–69. Oxford University Press, Oxford

Haladej, S. and Hurcik, V. (1988) Computerised management system of the Veterinary Service in the Slovak Socialist Republic. *Revue Scientifique et Technique, Office Internatio-nal des Epizooties*, **7**, 517–541

Hall, S.A. (1978) Farm animal disease data banks. *Advances in Veterinary Science and Comparative Medicine*, **22**, 265–286

Hall, S.A., Dawson, P.S. and Davies, G. (1980) VIDA II: A computerised diagnostic recording system for veterinary investigation centres in Great Britain. *Veterinary Record*, **106**, 260–264

Halliwell, R.E.W. (1978) Autoimmune disease in the dog. *Advances in Veterinary Science*, **22**, 221–263

Hallstrom, A.P. and Trobaugh, G.B. (1985) Specificity, sensitivity, and prevalence in the design of randomized trials: a univariate analysis. *Controlled Clinical Trials*, **6**, 128–135

Hammond, R.F. and Lynch, K. (1992) The use and application of geographical information system technology in the Tuberculosis Investigation Unit. Tuberculosis Investigation Unit, University College Dublin, selected papers, pp. 28–30

Hanna, S.R., Briggs, G.A. and Hosker, R.P. (1982) *Handbook on Atmospheric Diffusion*. Technical Information Center, US Department of Energy. Document DE82002045 (DOE/TIC-11223). National Technical Information Service, US Department of Commerce, Springfield, Virginia

Hanssen, I. (1991) Hip dysplasia in dogs in relation to their month of birth. *Veterinary Record*, **128**, 425–426

Haresnape, J.M. and Wilkinson, P.J. (1989) A study of African swine fever virus infected ticks (*Ornithodoros moubata*) collected from villages in the ASF enzootic area of Malawi following an outbreak of the disease in domestic pigs. *Epidemiology and Infection*, **102**, 507–522

Harkness, J.W. (1987) Technical aspects of bovine virus diarrhoea. In: Society for Veterinary Epidemiology and Preventive Medicine, Proceedings, Solihull, 1–3 April 1987. Ed. Thrusfield, M.V., pp. 1–6

Harris, D.J. (1981) Factors predisposing to parturient paresis. *Australian Veterinary Journal*, **57**, 357–361

Harris, D.J., Lambell, R.G. and Oliver, C.J. (1983) Factors predisposing dairy and beef cows to grass tetany. *Australian Veterinary Journal*, **60**, 230–234

Hartsough, G.R. and Burger, D. (1965) Encephalopathy of milk. I. Epizootiologic and clinical observations. *Journal of Infectious Diseases*, **115**, 387–392

Hartsough, G.R. and Gorham, J.R. (1956) Aleutian disease in mink. *National Fur News*, **28**, 10–11

Hashmi, H.A. and Connan, R.M. (1989) Biological control of ruminant trichostrongylids by *Arthrobotrys oligospora*, a predacious fungus. *Parasitology Today*, **5**, 28–30

Hathaway, S.C. (1981) Leptospirosis in New Zealand: an ecological view. *New Zealand Veterinary Journal*, **29**, 109–112

Hayes, H.M. (1974a) Congenital umbilical and inguinal hernias in cattle, horses, swine, dogs and cats: risk by breed and sex among hospital patients. *American Journal of Veterinary Research*, **35**, 839–842

Hayes, H.M. (1974b) Ectopic ureter in dogs: epidemiologic features. *Teratology*, **10**, 129–132

Hayes, H.M. (1975) An hypothesis for the aetiology of canine chemoreceptor system neoplasms, based upon an epidemiological study of 73 cases among hospital patients. *Journal of Small Animal Practice*, **16**, 337–343

Hayes, H.M. (1976) Canine bladder cancer: epidemiologic features. *American Journal of Epidemiology*, **104**, 673–677

Hayes, H.M. (1984) Breed association of canine ectopic ureter: a study of 217 female cases. *Journal of Small Animal Practice*, **25**, 501–504

Hayes, H.M. (1986) Epidemiological features of 5009 cases of equine cryptorchism. *Equine Veterinary Journal*, **18**, 467–471

Hayes, H.M. and Fraumeni, J.F. (1974) Chemodectomas in dogs: epidemiologic comparisons with man. *Journal of the National Cancer Institute*, **52**, 1455–1458

Hayes, H.M. and Fraumeni, J.F. (1975) Canine thyroid neoplasms: epidemiologic features. *Journal of the National Cancer Institute*, **55**, 931–934

Hayes, H.M. and Fraumeni, J.F. (1977) Epidemiological features of canine renal neoplasms. *Cancer Research*, **37**, 2553–2556

Hayes, H.M. and Pendergrass, T.W. (1976) Canine testicular tumours: epidemiologic features of 410 dogs. *International Journal of Cancer*, **18**, 482–487

Hayes, H.M. and Priester, W.A. (1973) Feline infectious anaemia: risk by age, sex and breed; prior disease; seasonal occurrence; mortality. *Journal of Small Animal Practice*, **14**, 797–804

Hayes, H.M. and Wilson, G.P. (1986) Hospital incidence of hypospadias in dogs in North America. *Veterinary Record*, **118**, 605–606

Hayes, H.M., Priester, W.A. and Pendergrass, T.W. (1975) Occurrence of nervous-tissue tumours in cattle, horses, cats and dogs. *International Journal of Cancer*, **15**, 39–47

Hayes, H.M., Selby, L.A., Wilson, G.P. and Hohn, R.B. (1979) Epidemiologic observations on canine elbow disease (emphasis on dysplasia). *Journal of the American Animal Hospitals Association*, **15**, 449–453

Hayes, H.M., Hoover, R. and Tarone, R.E. (1981) Bladder cancer in pet dogs: a sentinel for environmental cancer? *American Journal of Epidemiology*, **114**, 229–233

Hayes, H.M., Wilson, G.P. and Fraumeni, J.F. (1982) Carcinoma of the nasal cavity and paranasal sinuses in dogs: descriptive epidemiology. *Cornell Veterinarian*, **72**, 168–179

Hayes, H.M., Wilson, G.P., Pendergrass, T.W. and Cox, V.S. (1985) Canine cryptorchism and subsequent testicular neoplasia: case–control study with epidemiologic update. *Teratology*, **32**, 51–56

Haygarth, J. (1800) *Of the Imagination, as a Cause and as a Cure of Disorders of the Body; Exemplified by Fictious Tractors, and Epidemical Convulsions.* R. Cruttwell, Bath

Heady, E.O. and Dillon, J.L. (1961) *Agricultural Production Functions.* Iowa State University Press, Ames

Helle, O. (1971) The effect on sheep parasites of grazing in alternate years by sheep and cattle. A comparison with set-stocking, and the use of anthelmintics with these grazing arrangements. *Acta Veterinaria Scandinavica*, Suppl. 33, 1–59

Henderson, W.M. (1982) Priorities for research. In: *The Control of Infectious Diseases in Farm Animals.* British Veterinary Association Trust Project on the future of animal health control, London, pp. 50–55

Herbert, W.J. (1970) *Veterinary Immunology.* Blackwell Scientific, Oxford

Herd, R., Strong, L. and Wardhaugh, K. (Eds) (1993) Environmental impact of avermectin usage in livestock. *Veterinary Parasitology*, **48**, 1–340

Herløv, L. and Vedel, T. (1992) An information system for pig producers and advisory service. Proceedings of EAAP Satellite Symposium on pig management information systems, 12 September 1992, pp. 17–23; 43rd Annual Meeting of the European Association of Animal Production. Madrid, 13–17 September 1992

Heuer, C., Nothelle, N. and Bode, E. (1991) Clinical disease and fertility associated with low phosphorus supply in water buffaloes. In: Proceedings of the Sixth International Symposium on Veterinary Epidemiology and Economics, Ottawa, 12–16 August 1991. Ed. Martin, S.W., pp. 491–493

Higgs, A.R.B., Norris, R.T. and Richards, R.B. (1991) Season, age and adiposity influence death rates in sheep exported by sea. *Australian Journal of Agricultural Research*, **42**, 205–214

Hill, T., Carmichael, D., Maylin, G. and Krook, L. (1986) Track condition and racing injuries in thoroughbred horses. *Cornell Veterinarian*, **76**, 361–379

Hills, M. and Armitage, P. (1979) The two-period cross-over clinical trial. *British Journal of Clinical Pharmacology*, **8**, 7–20

Himsworth, H. (1970) *The Development and Organisation of Scientific Knowledge.* William Heinemann, Medical Books, London

Hindmarsh, F., Fraser, J. and Scott, K. (1989) Efficacy of a multivalent *Bacteroides nodosus* vaccine against foot rot in sheep in Britain. *Veterinary Record*, **125**, 128–130

Hindson, J. (1982) Sheep health schemes. *In Practice*, **4**, 53–58

Hird, D.W. and Christiansen, K.H. (1991) California national animal health monitoring system for meat turkey flocks. In: Proceedings of the 6th International Symposium on Veterinary Epidemiology and Economics, Ottawa, 12–16 August 1991. Ed. Martin, S.W., pp. 504–506

Hird, D.W., Pappaioanou, M. and Smith, B.P. (1984) Case–control study of risk factors associated with isolation of *Salmonella saintpaul* in hospitalized horses. *American Journal of Epidemiology*, **120**, 852–864

Hird, D.W., Casebolt, D.B., Carter, J.D., Pappaionou, M. and Hjerpe, C.A. (1986) Risk factors for salmonellosis in hospitalized horses. *Journal of the American Veterinary Medical Association*, **188**, 173–177

Hird, D.W., Carpenter, T.E., Snipes, K.P., Hirsh, D.C. and McCapes (1991) Case–control study of fowl cholera outbreaks in meat turkeys in California from August 1985 through July 1986. *American Journal of Veterinary Research*, **52**, 212–216

HMSO (1954) *Mortality and Morbidity during the London Fog of*

December 1952. Reports on Public Health and Medical Subjects, No. 95. Her Majesty's Stationery Office, London

HMSO (1958) *1951 Occupational Mortality, Part II, Vol. 2.* Registrar General's Decennial Supplement, 1958. Her Majesty's Stationery Office, London

HMSO (1968) *A Century of Agricultural Statistics, Great Britain, 1866–1966.* Ministry of Agriculture, Fisheries and Food; Department of Agriculture and Fisheries for Scotland. Her Majesty's Stationery Office, London

HMSO (1969) *Report of the Committee of Enquiry on Foot-and-Mouth Disease 1968. Part 1.* Her Majesty's Stationery Office, London

HMSO (1982) *Agricultural Statistics, United Kingdom 1980 and 1981.* Ministry of Agriculture, Fisheries and Food; Department of Agriculture and Fisheries for Scotland; Department of Agriculture for Northern Ireland; Welsh Agricultural Department. Her Majesty's Stationery Office, London

HMSO (1991) *Agricultural Statistics, United Kingdom 1989.* Ministry of Agriculture, Fisheries and Food; Department of Agriculture and Fisheries for Scotland; Department of Agriculture for Northern Ireland; Welsh Agricultural Department. Her Majesty's Stationery Office, London

Hogeveen, H., Noordhuizen-Stassen, E.N., Nielen, M. and Brand, A. (1993) Use of knowledge representation methodologies to diagnose mastitis. In: Society for Veterinary Epidemiology and Preventive Medicine, Proceedings, Exeter, 31 March–2 April 1993. Ed. Thrusfield, M.V., pp. 225–235

Holland, W. (1984) A standard advisory system for lowland sheep flocks. In: Society for Veterinary Epidemiology and Preventive Medicine, Proceedings, Edinburgh, 10–11 July 1984. Ed. Thrusfield, M.V., pp. 39–52

Holman, C.D.J. (1984) Analysis of inter-observer variation on a programmable calculator. *American Journal of Epidemiology*, **120**, 154–160

Holst, P.A., Kromhout, D. and Brand, R. (1988) For debate: pet birds as an independent risk factor for lung cancer. *British Medical Journal*, **297**, 1319–1321

Holt, P.E. (1976) *Toxocara canis*: an estimation of the incidence of infection in puppies in an industrial town. *Veterinary Record*, **98**, 383

Holt, P.E. and Thrusfield, M.V. (1993) Association in bitches between breed, size, neutering and docking, and acquired urinary incontinence due to incompetence of the urethral sphincter mechanism. *Veterinary Record*, **133**, 177–180

Hoogstraal, H. (1966) Ticks in relation to human diseases caused by viruses. *Annual Review of Entomology*, **11**, 261–308

Hoogstraal, H. (1979) The epidemiology of tick-borne Crimean–Congo haemorrhagic fever in Asia, Europe and Africa. *Journal of Medical Entomology*, **15**, 307–417

Hoover, R. and Cole, P. (1973) Temporal aspects of occupational bladder carcinogenesis. *New England Journal of Medicine*, **288**, 1040–1043

Hope-Cawdery, M.J., Gettinby, G. and Grainger, J.N. (1978) Mathematical models for predicting the prevalence of liver-fluke disease and its control from biological and meteorological data. In: *Weather and Parasitic Animal Disease*. Ed.

Gibson, T.E., pp. 21–38. World Meteorological Organization Technical Note No. 159

Horrobin, D.F. (Ed.) (1990) *Omega-6 Essential Fatty Acids: Pathophysiology and Roles in Clinical Medicine.* Alan R. Liss, New York

Horse and Hound (1992) *The Horse and Hound Equestrian Survey, October 1992.* IPC Magazines, London

Hosie, M.J., Robertson, C. and Jarrett, O. (1989) Prevalence of feline leukaemia virus and antibodies to feline immunodeficiency virus in cats in the United Kingdom. *Veterinary Record*, **128**, 293–297

Hoskins, J.D. (1988a) Preventive health program for dogs. *Veterinary Technician*, **9**, 187–192

Hoskins, J.D. (1988b) Preventive health program for cats. *Veterinary Technician*, **9**, 273–278

Hoskins, J.D., Seahorn, T.L. and Claxton-Gill, M.S. (1994) Preventive health programs. In: *Clinical Textbook for Veterinary Technicians*, 3rd edn. Ed. McCurnin, D.M., pp. 600–632. W.B. Saunders, Philadelphia

Houe, H., Pedersen, K.M. and Meyling, A. (1993) The effect of bovine virus diarrhoea virus infection on conception rate. *Preventive Veterinary Medicine*, **15**, 117–123

Hourrigan, J.L. and Klingsporn, A.L. (1975) Epizootiology of bluetongue: the situation in the United States of America. *Australian Veterinary Journal*, **51**, 203–208

Houwers, D.J. (1989) Importance of ewe/lamb relationship and breed in the epidemiology of maedi-visna virus infections. *Research in Veterinary Science*, **46**, 5–8

Howard, E.B. and Nielsen, S.W. (1965) Neoplasia of the Boxer dog. *American Journal of Veterinary Research*, **26**, 1121–1131

Howe, K.S. (1985) An economist's view of animal disease. In: Society for Veterinary Epidemiology and Preventive Medicine, Proceedings, Reading, 27–29 March 1985. Ed. Thrusfield, M.V., pp. 122–129

Howe, K.S. (1989) An economist's view of veterinary epidemiology. In: Society for Veterinary Epidemiology and Preventive Medicine, Proceedings, Exeter, 12–14 April 1989. Ed. Thrusfield, M.V., pp. 60–71

Howe, K.S. (1992) Epidemiologists' views of economics — an economist's reply. In: Society for Veterinary Epidemiology and Preventive Medicine, Denary Proceedings, Edinburgh, 1–3 April 1992. Ed. Thrusfield, M.V., pp. 157–167

Hubbert, W.T. and Hermann, G.J. (1970) A winter epizootic of infectious bovine keratoconjunctivitis. *Journal of the American Veterinary Medical Association*, **157**, 452–454

Hudson, L. and Hay, F.C. (1989) *Practical Immunology*, 3rd edn. Blackwell Scientific Publications, Oxford

Hudson, P.J. (1986) *Red Grouse: the Biology and Management of a Wild Gamebird.* The Game Conservancy Trust, Fordingbridge

Hueston, W.D. and Walker, K.D. (1993) Macroepidemiological contributions to quantitative risk assessment. *Revue Scientifique et Technique, Office International des Epizooties*, **12**, 1197–1201

Hueston, W.D., Heider, L.E., Harvey, W.R. and Smith, K.L.

(1987) The use of high somatic cell count prevalence in epidemiologic investigations of mastitis control practices. *Preventive Veterinary Medicine*, **4**, 447−461

Hueston, W.D., Heider, L.E., Harvey, W.R. and Smith, K.L. (1990) Determinants of high somatic cell count prevalence in dairy herds practising teat dipping and dry cow therapy and with no evidence of *Streptococcus agalactiae* on repeated bulk tank milk examination. *Preventive Veterinary Medicine*, **9**, 131−142

Hugh-Jones, M.E. (1972) Epidemiological studies on the 1967/68 foot-and-mouth disease epidemic: attack rates and cattle density. *Research in Veterinary Science*, **13**, 411−417

Hugh-Jones, M.E. (1975) Some pragmatic aspects of animal disease monitoring. In: *Animal Disease Monitoring*. Eds Ingram, D.G., Mitchell, W.F. and Martin, S.W., pp. 220−236. Charles C. Thomas, Springfield

Hugh-Jones, M.E. (1983) Conclusions for the symposium and lessons for the future. In: Proceedings of the Third International Symposium on Veterinary Epidemiology and Economics, Arlington, Virginia, 6−10 September 1982, pp. 650−654. Veterinary Medical Publishing Company, Edwardsville

Hugh-Jones, M.E. (1986a) Utilization of a working serum bank. In: Proceedings of the Fourth International Symposium on Veterinary Epidemiology and Economics, Singapore, 18−22 November 1985, pp. 179−182. Singapore Veterinary Association, Singapore

Hugh-Jones, M.E. (1986b) A mathematical model of antigenic drift. *Mathematical Modelling*, **7**, 765−775

Hugh-Jones, M.E. (1989) Applications of remote sensing to the identification of the habitats of parasites and disease vectors. *Parasitology Today*, **5**, 244−251

Hugh-Jones, M.E. (1991a) Remote sensing and geographic information systems, epidemiology and Igor Piskun's rule. In: Proceedings of the 6th International Symposium on Veterinary Epidemiology and Economics, Ottawa, 12−16 August 1991. Ed. Martin, S.W., pp. 541−543

Hugh-Jones, M.E. (1991b) Satellite imaging as a technique for obtaining disease-related data. *Revue Scientifique et Technique, Office International des Epizooties*, **10**, 197−204

Hugh-Jones, M.E. (1991c) The remote recognition of tick habitats. *Journal of Agricultural Entomology*, **8**, 309−315

Hugh-Jones, M.E. and Hubbert, W. (1988) Seroconversion rates to bovine leucosis virus, bluetonge virus, *Leptospira hardjo* and *Anaplasma marginale* infections in a random series of Louisiana beef cattle. *Acta Veterinaria Scandinavica*, Suppl. 84, 107−109

Hugh-Jones, M.E. and O'Neil, P. (1986) The epidemiological uses of remote sensing and satellites. In: Proceedings of the 4th International Conference on Veterinary Epidemiology and Economics, 18−22 November 1985, Singapore, pp. 113−118. Singapore Veterinary Association, Singapore

Hugh-Jones, M.E. and Wright, P.B. (1970) Studies on the 1967−68 foot-and-mouth disease epidemic. The relation of weather to spread of disease. *Journal of Hygiene, Cambridge*, **68**, 253−271

Hugh-Jones, M.E., Pugh, G.W. and McDonald, T.J. (1965)

Ultraviolet radiation and *Moraxella bovis* in the etiology of bovine infectious keratoconjunctivitis. *American Journal of Veterinary Research*, **26**, 1331−1338

Hugh-Jones, M.E., Ivory, D.W., Loosmore, R.M. and Gibbins, J. (1969) Veterinary Investigation Diagnosis Analysis: an information recording and retrieval system for veterinary diagnostic laboratories in the Ministry of Agriculture, Fisheries and Food. *Veterinary Record*, **84**, 304−307

Hugh-Jones, M.E.,, Parkin, R.S. and Whitney, J.C. (1975) The cost of premature death in young rabbits. *Veterinary Record*, **96**, 353−356

Hugh-Jones, M.E., Ellis, P.R. and Felton, M.R. (1976) The use of a computer model of brucellosis in the dairy herd. In: *New Techniques in Veterinary Epidemiology and Economics*, Proceedings of a symposium, University of Reading, 12−15 July 1976. Eds Ellis, P.R., Shaw, A.P.M. and Stephens, A.J., pp. 96−112

Hugh-Jones, M.E., Barre, N., Nelson, G., Wehnes, K., Warner, J., Garvin, J. and Garris, G. (1992) Landstat-TM identification of *Amblyomma variegatum* (Acari: Ixodidae) habitats in Guadeloupe. *Remote Sensing of Environment*, **40**, 43−55

Huirne, R.B.M. and Dijkhuizen, A.A. (1994) CHESS: a decision support system to analyse individual sow-herd performance. In: Society for Veterinary Epidemiology and Preventive Medicine, Proceedings, Belfast, 13−15 April 1994. Ed. Thrusfield, M.V., pp. 136−145

Huirne, R.B.M., Dijkhuizen, A.A., Pijpers, A., Verheijden, J.H.M. and van Gulick, P. (1991) An economic expert system on the personal computer to support sow replacement decisions. *Preventive Veterinary Medicine*, **11**, 79−93

Huirne, R.B.M., Dijkhuizen, A.A., Renkema, J.A. and Van Beek, P. (1992) Computerized analysis of individual sow-herd performance. *American Journal of Agricultural Economics*, **74**, 388−399

Hulka, B.S., Wilcosky, T.C. and Griffith, J.D. (Eds) (1990) *Biological Markers in Epidemiology*. Oxford University Press, New York

Hurd, H.S. and Kaneene, J.B. (1993) The application of simulation models and systems analysis in epidemiology: a review. *Preventive Veterinary Medicine*, **15**, 81−99

Hurnik, D. and Dohoo, I.R. (1991) Evaluation of management risk factors in swine respiratory disease. In: Proceedings of the Sixth International Symposium on Veterinary Epidemiology and Economics, Ottawa, 12−16 August 1991. Ed. Martin, S.W., pp. 412−415

Hutchison, J.M., Salman, M.D., Fowler, M.E., Zinkl, J.G. and Garry, F.B. (1991) Guidelines for the establishment of reference ranges in veterinary medicine. In: Proceedings of the 6th International Symposium on Veterinary Epidemiology and Economics, Ottawa, 12−16 August 1991. Ed. Martin, S.W., pp. 465−467

Hutton, C.T., Fox, L.K. and Hancock, D.D. (1991) Risk factors associated with herd-group milk somatic cell count and prevalence of coagulase-positive staphylococcal intramammary infections. *Preventive Veterinary Medicine*, **11**, 25−35

Hutton, N.E. and Halvorson, L.C. (1974) *A Nationwide System for Animal Health Surveillance*. National Academy of Sciences, Washington, DC

IAEE (1991) *The Sero-monitoring of Rinderpest Throughout Africa. Phase One*. Proceedings of a Final Research Co-ordination Meeting of the FAO/IAEA/SIDA/OAU/BAR/PARC Co-ordinated Research Programme, Bingerville, Cote d'Ivoire, 19–23 November 1990. IAEA-TECDOC-623. International Atomic Energy Agency, Vienna

Ianovich, T.D., Bliznichenko, A.G., Zaburina, L.V., Mstibovskii, S.A., Berkovich, A.I. and Dushevin, I.P. (1957) Leptospirosis of the *canicola* type in one of the districts of Rostov-on-the-Don. *Journal of Microbiology, Epidemiology and Immunology*, **28**, 259–264

Isaacson, R.E., Moon, H.W. and Schneider, R.A. (1978) Distribution and virulence of *Escherichia coli* in the small intestines of calves with and without diarrhoea. *American Journal of Veterinary Research*, **39**, 1750–1755

Ismaiel, M.O., Greenman, J., Morgan, K., Glover, M.G., Rees, A.S. and Scully, C. (1989) Periodontitis in sheep: a model for human periodontal disease. *Journal of Periodontology*, **60**, 279–284

Jackson, G.H. and Baker, J.R. (1981) The occurrence of unthriftiness in piglets post-weaning. *The Pig Veterinary Society Proceedings*, **7**, 63–67

Jacobs, R.M. Heeney, J.L., Godkin, M.A., Leslie, K.E., Taylor, J.A., Davies, C. and Valli, V.E.O. (1991) Production and related variables in bovine leukaemia virus-infected cows. *Veterinary Research Communications*, **15**, 463–474

Jactel, B., Espinasse, J., Viso, M. and Valiergue, H. (1990) An epidemiological study of winter dysentery in fifteen herds in France. *Veterinary Research Communications*, **14**, 367–379

Jakab, G.J. (1977) Pulmonary defense mechanisms and the interaction between viruses and bacteria in acute respiratory infections. *Bulletin Européen de Physiopathologie Respiratoire*, **13**, 119–135

Janzen, D.H. (1971) Seed predation by animals. *Annual Review of Ecology and Systematics*, **2**, 465–492

Jarrett, J.A. (Ed.) (1984) Symposium on bovine mastitis. *The Veterinary Clinics of North America*, **6**, 231–431

Jarrett, O. (1985) Update: feline leukaemia virus. *In Practice*, **7**, 125–126

Jarrett, W.F.H. (1980) Bracken fern and papilloma virus in bovine alimentary cancer. *British Medical Bulletin*, **36**, 79–81

Jasper, D.E., Dellinger, J.D., Rollins, H. and Hakanson, H.D. (1979) Prevalence of mycoplasmal bovine mastitis in California. *American Journal of Veterinary Research*, **40**, 1043–1047

Jepson, P.G.H. and Hinton, M.H. (1986) An inquiry into the causes of liver damage in lambs. *Veterinary Record*, **118**, 584–587

Jericho, K.W.F. (1979) Update on pasteurellosis in young cattle. *Canadian Veterinary Journal*, **20**, 333–335

Johnston, G.M. (1994) Epidemiological aspects of the confidential enquiry of perioperative equine fatalities (CEPEF) and some preliminary results. In: Society for Veterinary Epidemiology and Preventive Medicine, Proceedings, Belfast, 13–15 April 1994. Ed. Thrusfield, M.V., pp. 174–184

Johnston, P.I., Henry, N., de Boer, R. and Braidwood, J.C. (1992) Phenoxymethyl penicillin potassium as an in-feed medication for pigs with streptococcal meningitis. *Veterinary Record*, **130**, 138–139

Jolley, J.L. (1968) *Data Study*. World University Library, Weidenfeld and Nicolson, London

Jolly, R.D. and Townsley, R.J. (1980) Genetic screening programmes: an analysis of benefits and costs using the bovine mannosidosis scheme as a model. *New Zealand Veterinary Journal*, **28**, 3–6

Jolly, R.D., Tse, C.A. and Greenway, R.M. (1973) Plasma α-mannosidase activity as a means of detecting mannosidosis heterozygotes. *New Zealand Veterinary Journal*, **21**, 64–69

Jolly, R.D., Dodds, W.J., Ruth, G.R. and Trauner, D.B. (1981) Screening for genetic diseases: principles and practice. *Advances in Veterinary Science and Comparative Medicine*, **25**, 245–275

Jones, G.E. and Gilmour, J.S. (1983) Atypical pneumonia. In: *Diseases of Sheep*. Ed. Martin, W.B., pp. 17–23. Blackwell, Oxford

Jones, W.H.S. (Translator) (1923) *Hippocrates*, Vol. 1. The Loeb Classical Library, William Heinemann, London

Jorm, L.R. (1990) Strangles in horse studs: incidence, risk factors and effect of vaccination. *Australian Veterinary Journal*, **67**, 436–439

Jubb, K.V.F. and Kennedy, P.C. (1971) *Pathology of Domestic Animals*, 2nd edn. Academic Press, London and New York

Julian, A.F. (1981) Tuberculosis in the possum (*Trichosurus vulpecula*). In: Proceedings of the First Symposium on Marsupials in New Zealand. Ed. Bell, B.D., pp. 163–174. Zoology Publications from Victoria University of Wellington No. 74. Victoria University, Wellington

Kahn, H.A. and Sempos, C.T. (1989) *Statistical Methods in Epidemiology*. Oxford University Press, New York

Kaleta, E.F., Alexander, D.J. and Russell, P.H. (1985) The first isolation of the avian PMV1 virus responsible for the current panzootic in pigeons. *Avian Pathology*, **14**, 553–557

Kaneene, J.B. and Willeberg, P. (1988) Influence of management factors on the occurrence of antibiotic residues in milk: a case–control study in Michigan dairy herds, with examples of suspected information bias. *Acta Veterinaria Scandinavica*, Suppl. 84, 473–476

Kaneene, J.B., Miller, R., Herdt, T. and Gardenier, J. (1991) Haematological indices of feed utilization as predictors of postpartum diseases: metritis, retained placenta and mastitis. In: Proceedings of the Sixth International Symposium on Veterinary Epidemiology and Economics, Ottawa, 12–16 August 1991. Ed. Martin, S.W., pp. 301–303

Kaneko, J.J. (Ed.) (1989) *Clinical Biochemistry of Domestic Animals*, 4th edn. Academic Press, London and New York

Kapetsky, J.M., Wijkstrom, U.N., Macpherson, N.J., Vincke, M.M.J., Ataman, E. and Caponera, F. (1991) Where are the best opportunities for fish farming in Ghana? The Ghana aquaculture geographical information system as a decision-making tool. In: *Geographical Information Systems and Remote Sensing in Inland Fisheries*. FAO Fisheries Technical Paper No. 318, pp. 228–233

Kaplan, M.M. (1982) Influenza in nature. In: *Animal Diseases in Relation to Animal Conservation*. Symposium of the Zoological Society of London No. 50. Eds Edwards, M.A. and McDonald, U., pp. 121–135. Academic Press, London and New York

Karber, G. (1931) Beitrag zur kollektiven behandlung pharmakologischer reihenversuche. *Archiv für experimentelle Pathologie und Pharmakologie*, **162**, 480–487

Karstad, L. (1962) Epizootiology in disease investigations. *Canadian Veterinary Journal*, **3**, 145–149

Kass, P.H. and Greenland, S. (1991) Conflicting definitions of confounding and their ramifications for veterinary epidemiologic research: collapsibility vs comparability. *Journal of the American Veterinary Medical Association*, **199**, 1569–1573

Kass, P.H., Barnes, W.G., Spangler, W.L., Chomel, B.B. and Cuthbertson, M.R. (1993) Epidemiologic evidence for a causal relation between vaccination and fibrosarcoma tumorigenesis in cats. *Journal of the American Veterinary Medical Association*, **203**, 396–405 (Correction: p. 1046)

Katz, D., Baptista, J., Azen, S.P. and Pike, M.C. (1978) Obtaining confidence intervals for the risk ratio in cohort studies. *Biometrics*, **34**, 469–474

Kay, R.D. (1986) *Farm Management, Planning, Control and Implementation*. McGraw-Hill, New York

Keffaber, K.K. (1989) Reproductive failure of unknown aetiology. *American Association of Swine Practitioners Newsletter*, **1**(2), 1, 4–9

Kellar, J., Marra, R. and Martin, W. (1976) Brucellosis in Ontario: a case–control study. *Canadian Journal of Comparative Medicine*, **40**, 119–128

Kellar, J.A. (1983) Canada's bovine serum bank — a practical approach. In: Proceedings of the Third International Symposium on Veterinary Epidemiology and Economics, Arlington, Virginia, 6–10 September 1982, pp. 138–143. Veterinary Medical Publishing Company, Edwardsville

Keller, G.G. and Corley, E.A. (1989) Canine hip dysplasia: investigating the sex predilection and the frequency of unilateral CHD. *Veterinary Medicine*, **84**, 1162–1166

Keller, G.H. and Manak, M.M. (Eds) (1989) *DNA Probes*. Macmillan, London

Kelly, J.M., Whitaker, D.A. and Smith, E.J. (1988) A dairy herd health and productivity service. *British Veterinary Journal*, **144**, 470–480

Kelton, D.F., Martin, S.W. and Hansen, D.S. (1992) Development and implementation of the Ontario dairy monitoring and analysis program. In: Proceedings of the 17th World Buiatrics Congress and the 25th American Association of Bovine Practitioners Conference, St Paul, Minnesota, 31 August–4 September 1992. Ed. Williams, I.E., Vol. 1, pp. 285–289

Kendall, D.G. (1957) La propogation d'une épidémie ou d'un bruit dans une population limitée. *Publications of the Institute of Statistics, University of Paris*, **6**, 307–331

Kendall, M.G. and Buckland, W.R. (1982) *A Dictionary of Statistical Terms*, 4th edn. Longman Group, London and New York

Khmaladze, E.V. (1975) Estimation of the necessary number of observations for discriminating simple close hypotheses. *Theory of Probability and its Applications*, **20**, 116–126

King, L.J. (1985) Unique characteristics of the National Animal Disease Surveillance System in the United States. *Journal of the American Veterinary Medical Association*, **186**, 35–39

Kingwill, R.G., Neave, F.K., Dodd, F.H., Griffin, T.K. and Westgarth, D.R. (1970) The effect of a mastitis control system on levels of subclinical and clinical mastitis in two years. *Veterinary Record*, **87**, 94–100

Kiper, M.L., Traub-Dargatz, J.L., Salman, M.D. and Rikihisa, Y. (1992) Risk factors for equine monocytic ehrlichiosis seropositivity in horses in Colorado. *Preventive Veterinary Medicine*, **13**, 251–259

Kirkwood, T.B.L. (1985) Comparative and evolutionary aspects of longevity. In: *Handbook of the Biology of Aging*, 2nd edn. Eds Finch, C.E. and Schneider, E.L., pp. 27–44. Van Nostrand Reinhold Company, New York

Kitchin, P.A., Almond, N., Szotyori, Z., Fromhole, C.E., McAlpine, L., Silvera, P., Stott, E.J., Cranage, M., Baskerville, A. and Schild, G. (1990) The use of the polymerase chain reaction for the detection of Simian immunodeficiency virus in experimentally infected macaques. *Journal of Virological Methods*, **28**, 85–100

Kitron, U., Bouseman, J.K. and Jones, C.J. (1991) Use of the ARC/INFO GIS to study the distribution of Lyme disease ticks in an Illinois county. *Preventive Veterinary Medicine*, **11**, 243–248

Kleinbaum, D.G., Kupper, L.L. and Morgenstern, H. (1982) *Epidemiologic Research. Principles and Quantitative Measures*. Lifetime Learning Publications, Belmont

Klimczak, J.C. (1994) SNOMED (review). *Preventive Veterinary Medicine*, **21**, 266–269

Knecht, C.D. and Phares, J. (1971) Characterization of dogs with salivary cyst. *Journal of the American Veterinary Medical Association*, **158**, 612–613

Knowles, D.P. and Gorham, J.R. (1990) Diagnosis of viral and bacterial diseases. *Revue Scientifique et Technique, Office International des Epizooties*, **9**, 733–757

Knox, G.A. (1964) The detection of space–time interactions. *Applied Statistics*, **13**, 25–29

Konig, C.D.W. (1985) Bedrijfsdiergeneeskundige aspecten van de schapenhouderij (Planned animal health and production service on sheep farms. An inventory and evaluation). PhD Thesis. University of Utrecht

Konner, M. (1993) *The Trouble with Medicine*. BBC Books, London

Kovacs, A.B. and Beer, G.Y. (1979) The mechanical properties and qualities of floors for pigs in relation to limb disorders. *The Pig Veterinary Society Proceedings*, **5**, 99–104

Krabbe, H. (1864) Observations for Icelanders on hydatids and precautions against them. J. Schultz (Copenhagen). Translated by Maxwell, I.R. (1973). *Australian Veterinary Journal*, **49**,

395–401

Kral, F. (1966) Canine pruritus (desire for scratching). *Animal Hospital*, **2**, 40–43

Krehbiel, J.D. and Langham, R.F. (1975) Eyelid neoplasms of dogs. *American Journal of Veterinary Research*, **36**, 115–119

Kricka, L.J. (Ed.) (1992) *Nonisotopic DNA Probe Techniques*. Academic Press, San Diego

Kroneman, A., Vellenga, L., van der Wilt, F.J. and Vermeer, H.M. (1993) Review of health problems in group-housed sows, with special emphasis on lameness. *The Veterinary Quarterly*, **15**, 26–29

Krook, L., Larsson, S. and Rooney, J.R. (1960) The interrelationship of diabetes mellitus, obesity and pyometra in the dog. *American Journal of Veterinary Research*, **21**, 120–124

Kubes, V. and Rios, F.A. (1939) The causative agent of infectious equine encephalomyelitis in Venezuela. *Science*, **90**, 20–21

Kuhn, T.S. (1970) *The Structure of Scientific Revolutions*. International Encyclopaedia of Unified Science, Vol. 2, No. 2, 2nd edn. University of Chicago Press, Chicago and London

Kupper, L.L. and Hogan, M.D. (1978) Interaction in epidemiologic studies. *American Journal of Epidemiology*, **108**, 447–453

Kwok, S. and Higuchi, R. (1989) Avoiding false positives with PCR. *Nature*, **339**, 237–238

Lafi, S.Q. and Kaneene, J.B. (1992) Epidemiological and economic study of the repeat breeder syndrome in Michigan dairy cattle. I. Epidemiological modeling. *Preventive Veterinary Medicine*, **14**, 87–98

Lance, S.E., Miller, G.Y., Hancock, D.D., Bartlett, P.C., Heider, L.E. and Moeschberger, M.L. (1992) Effects of environment and management on mortality in preweaned dairy calves. *Journal of the American Veterinary Medical Association*, **201**, 1197–1202

Lane-Claypon, J.E. (1926) A further report on cancer of the breast. *Reports on Public Health and Medical Subjects*, **32**. His Majesty's Stationery Office, London

Langmuir, A.D. (1965) Developing concepts in surveillance. *The Millbank Memorial Fund Quarterly*, **43**(2), 369–372

Larsen, C.T., Domermuth, C.H., Sponenberg, D.P. and Gross, W.B. (1985) Colibacillosis of turkeys exacerbated by haemorrhagic enteritis virus. Laboratory studies. *Avian Diseases*, **29**, 729–732

Last, J.M. (1988) *A Dictionary of Epidemiology*, 2nd edn. Oxford University Press, New York

Laut, P. (1986) Land evaluation for bovine tuberculosis eradication in Northern Australia. *Australian Geographical Studies*, **24**, 259–271

Lebeau, A. (1953) L'age du chien et celui de l'homme. Essai de statistique sur la mortalité canine. *Bulletin de l'Academie Veterinaire de France*, **26**, 229–232

Lee, E.T. (1992) *Statistical Methods for Survival Data Analysis*, 2nd edn. John Wiley, New York

Leech, A., Howarth, R.J., Thornton, I. and Lewis, G. (1982) Incidence of bovine copper deficiency in England and the Welsh borders. *Veterinary Record*, **111**, 203–204

Leech, F.B. (1980) Relations between objectives and observations in epidemiological studies. In: *Veterinary Epidemiology and Economics*. Proceedings of the Second International Symposium, Canberra, 7–11 May 1979. Eds Geering, W.A., Roe, R.T. and Chapman, L.A., pp. 254–257. Australian Government Publishing Services, Canberra

Lehenbauer, T. and Harman, B. (1982) Statistical modelling of real world health problems with an electronic spreadsheet program. In: Symposium on Computer Applications in Veterinary Science. Mississippi State University, Starkville, 13–15 October 1982, pp. 519–530

Leimbacher, F. (1978) Experience with the 'Mt' system of forecasting fascioliasis in France. In: *Weather and Parasitic Animal Disease*. Ed. Gibson, T.E., pp. 6–13. World Meteorological Organization Technical Note No. 159

Lemire, G.E., Lemire, M.R., Tiemann, M. and Verdon, L. (1991) Analytical study of small dairy herds with high pregnancy loss rates. In: Proceedings of the Sixth International Symposium on Veterinary Epidemiology and Economics, Ottawa, 12–16 August 1991. Ed. Martin, S.W., pp. 320–322

Lengerich, E.J., Teclaw, R.F., Mendlein, J.M., Mariolis, P. and Garbe, P.L. (1992) Pet populations in the catchment area of the Purdue Comparative Oncology Program. *Journal of the American Veterinary Medical Association*, **200**, 51–56

Lentner, C. (Ed.) (1982) *Geigy Scientific Tables*, 8th edn, Vol. 2. Ciba-Geigy, Basle

Lepissier, H.E. and MacFarlane, I.M. (1966) Organisation for African Unity. Scientific, Technical and Research Commission. Joint campaign against rinderpest. Phase I Final Report, November 1965. *Bulletin of Epizootic Diseases of Africa*, **14**, 193–224

Lesch, T.E. (Ed.) (1981) Symposium on herd health management — dairy cow. *Veterinary Clinics of North America: Large Animal Practice*, **3**, 251–490

Leslie, B.E., Meek, A.H., Kawash, G.F. and McKeown, D.B. (1994) An epidemiological investigation of pet ownership in Ontario. *Canadian Veterinary Journal*, **35**, 218–222

Leslie, P.. (1945) On the use of matrices in certain population mathematics. *Biometrika*, **35**, 183–212

Lessard, P., L'Eplattenier, R., Norval, R.A.I., Perry, B.D., Dolan, T.T., Burrill, A., Croze, H., Sorensen, M., Grootenhuis, J.G. and Irvin, A.D. (1988) The use of geographical information systems in estimating East Coast fever risk to African livestock. *Acta Veterinaria Scandinavica*, Suppl. 84, 234–236

Lessard, P., L'Eplattenier, R., Norval, R.A.I., Kundert, K., Dolan, T.T., Croze, H., Walker, J.B., Irvin, A.D. and Perry, B.D. (1990) Geographical information systems for studying the epidemiology of cattle disease caused by *Theileria parva*. *Veterinary Record*, **126**, 225–262

Levine, J.M. and Hohenboken, W. (1982) Modelling of beef production systems. *World Animal Review*, **43**, 33–39

Levine, P.P. and Fabricant, J. (1950) A hitherto-undescribed virus disease of ducks in North America. *Cornell Veterinarian*, **40**, 71–86

Leviton, A. (1973) Definitions of attributable risk (letter). *American Journal of Epidemiology*, **98**, 231

Levy, P.S. and Lemeshow, S. (1991) *Sampling of Populations: Methods and Applications*. John Wiley, New York

Lewis, E.R. (1977) *Network Models in Population Biology*. Springer-Verlag, Berlin

Lienhardt, G. (1961) *Divinity and Experience, the Religion of the Dinka*. Oxford University Press, Oxford

Liess, B. and Plowright, W. (1964) Studies on the pathogenesis of rinderpest in experimental cattle. I. Correlations of clinical signs, viraemia and virus excretion by various routes. *Journal of Hygiene, Cambridge*, **62**, 81–100

Lilienfeld, A.M. and Lilienfeld, D.E. (1980) *Foundations of Epidemiology*, 2nd edn. Oxford University Press, New York

Lilienfeld, D.E. (1978) Definitions of epidemiology. *American Journal of Epidemiology*, **107**, 87–90

Lincoln, F.C. (1930) Calculating waterfowl abundance on the basis of banding returns. *USDA Circular No. 118, May 1930*, pp. 1–4. United States Department of Agriculture, Washington, DC

Lind, J. (1753) *A Treatise of the Scurvy in Three Parts: Containing an Inquiry into the Nature, Causes and Cure of That Disease, Together with a Critical Chronological View of What has been Published on the Subject*. Murray and Cochran, Edinburgh

Lindemann, R.L. (1942) The trophic dynamic aspects of ecology. *Ecology*, **36**, 587–600

Lindley, D.V. and Scott, W.F. (1984) *New Cambridge Elementary Statistical Tables*. Cambridge University Press, Cambridge

Lindstrom, U.B. (1983) Effects of some herd factors and traits of the cow on bacterial scores and cell counts in quarter milk samples. *Acta Agriculturae Scandinavica*, **33**, 389–394

Lingaas, F. (1991a) Epidemiological and genetic studies in Norwegian pig herds. IV. Breed effects, recurrence of disease, and relationship between disease and some performance traits. *Acta Veterinaria Scandinavica*, **32**, 107–114

Lingaas, F. (1991b) Epidemiological and genetical studies in Norwegian pig herds. III. Herd effects. *Acta Veterinaria Scandinavica*, **32**, 97–105

Lingaas, F. and Ronningen, K. (1991) Epidemiological and genetical studies in Norwegian pig herds. II. Overall disease incidence and seasonal variation. *Acta Veterinaria Scandinavica*, **32**, 89–96

Linklater, K.A. and Speedy, A.W. (1980) Health and management programmes for lowland sheep flocks. Paper presented at the British Veterinary Association's Annual Congress, 14 September 1980, York, unpublished

Lipsey, M.W. (1990) *Design Sensitivity. Statistical Power for Experimental Design*. Sage Publications, Newbury Park

Lister, D. and Gregory, N.G. (Eds) (1978) *The Use of Blood Metabolites in Animal Production*. Proceedings of a symposium organised by the British Society of Animal Production, Harrogate, March 1976. BSAP occasional publication No. 1, British Society of Animal Production, Milton Keynes

Lister, J. (1870) On the effects of the antiseptic system of treatment upon the salubrity of a surgical hospital. *Lancet*, **1**, 4–6, 40–42

Little, I.M.D. and Mirrlees, J.A. (1974) *Project Appraisal and Planning for Developing Countries*. Heinemann, London

Little, T.W.A., Swan, C., Thompson, H.V. and Wilesmith, J.W. (1982) Bovine tuberculosis in domestic and wild mammals in an area of Dorset. II. The badger population, its ecology and tuberculosis status. *Journal of Hygiene, Cambridge*, **89**, 211–224

Liu, S.J., Xue, H.P., Pu, B.Q. and Qian, N.H. (1984) A new viral disease in rabbits. *Animal Husbandry and Veterinary Medicine (Xumu yu Shouyi)*, **16**, 253–255 (in Chinese)

Lobb, T. (1745) *Letters Relating to the Plague and other Contagious Distempers*. Buckland, London

Logan, E.F., McBeath, D.G. and Lowman, B.G. (1974) Quantitative studies on serum immunoglobulin levels in suckled calves from birth to five weeks. *Veterinary Record*, **94**, 367–370

Lomas, M.J. (1993) State Veterinary Service — Pig Health Scheme. *Pig Veterinary Journal*, **30**, 69–71

Lord, R.D. (1983) Ecological strategies for the prevention and control of health problems. *Bulletin of the Pan American Health Organization*, **17**, 19–34

Lord, R.D., Calisher, C.H., Metzger, W.R. and Fischer, G.W. (1974) Urban St Louis encephalitis surveillance through wild birds. *American Journal of Epidemiology*, **99**, 360–363

Lorenz, K. (1977) *Behind the Mirror: A Search for the Natural History of Human Knowledge*. Methuen, London

Lotka, A.J. (1925) *Elements of Physical Biology*. Williams and Wilkins, Baltimore

Lowe, J.E. (1974) Sex, breed and age incidence of navicular disease. In: Proceedings of the Twentieth Annual Convention of the American Association of Equine Practitioners, 3–5 December 1974, Las Vegas, Nevada, pp. 37–46

Luckins, A.G. and Gray, A.R. (1983) Interference with anti-trypanosome immune responses in rabbits infected with cyclically-transmitted *Trypanosoma congolense*. *Parasite Immunology*, **5**, 547–556

Lutnaes, B. and Simensen, E. (1983) An epidemiological study of abomasal bloat in young lambs. *Preventive Veterinary Medicine*, **1**, 335–345

MacDiarmid, S.C. (1987) A theoretical basis for the use of a skin test for brucellosis surveillance in extensively-managed cattle herds. *Revue Scientifique et Technique, Office International des Epizooties*, **6**, 1029–1035

MacDiarmid, S.C. (1991) Risk analysis and the importation of animals. *Surveillance*, **18**(5), 8–11

MacDiarmid, S.C. (1993) Risk analysis and the importation of animals and animal products. *Revue Scientifique et Technique, Office International des Epizooties*, **12**, 1093–1107

Macdonald, D.W. and Bacon, P.J. (1980) To control rabies: vaccinate foxes. *New Scientist*, **87**, 640–645

Mackintosh, C.G., Schollum, L.M., Harris, R.E., Blackmore, D.K., Willis, A.F., Cook, N.R. and Stoke, J.C.J. (1980) Epidemiology of leptospirosis in dairy farm workers in the Manawatu. Part I: A cross-sectional serological survey and associated occupational factors. *New Zealand Veterinary Journal*, **28**, 245–250

Maclure, M. (1985) Popperian refutation in epidemiology. *American Journal of Epidemiology*, **121**, 343–350

Maclure, M. and Willett, W.C. (1987) Misinterpretation and misuse of the kappa statistic. *American Journal of Epidemiology*, **126**, 161–169

MacMahon, B. (1972) Concepts of multiple factors. In: *Multiple Factors in the Causation of Environmentally Induced Disease*. Fogarty International Center Proceedings No. 12. Eds Lee, D.H.K. and Kotin, P., pp. 1–12. Academic Press, New York and London

MacMahon, B. and Pugh, T.F. (1970) *Epidemiology, Principles and Methods*. Little Brown, Boston

Macquarrie, J. (1978) *The Humility of God*. SCM Press, London

MacVean, D.W., Monlux, A.W., Anderson, P.S., Silberg, S.L. and Roszel, J.F. (1978) Frequency of canine and feline tumours in a defined population. *Veterinary Pathology*, **15**, 700–715

Maddy, K.T. (1958) Disseminated coccidioidomycosis of the dog. *Journal of the American Veterinary Medical Association*, **132**, 483–489

Madec, F. (1988) Multifactorial analysis of return to oestrus and low litter size in the sow. *Acta Veterinaria Scandinavica*, Suppl. 84, 167–169

Madewell, B.R., Priester, W.A., Gillette, E.L. and Snyder, S.P. (1976) Neoplasms of the nasal passages and paranasal sinuses in domesticated animals as reported by 13 veterinary colleges. *American Journal of Veterinary Research*, **37**, 851–856

MAF (1977) *Brucellosis: A Veterinarian's Guide to the Literature*. Ministry of Agriculture and Fisheries, Government Printer, Wellington, New Zealand

MAFF (1976) *Animal Disease Surveillance in Great Britain*. The Report of a Ministry of Agriculture, Fisheries and Food Working Party, May 1976

MAFF (1977) Animal Disease Report, **1**(2), July 1977. Ministry of Agriculture, Fisheries and Food

MAFF (1983) *Brucellosis — A History of the Disease and its Eradication from Cattle in Great Britain*. Her Majesty's Stationery Office, London

MAFF/ADAS (1976a) Distribution of cattle in England and Wales (map). Ministry of Agriculture, Fisheries and Food; Agricultural Development and Advisory Service

MAFF/ADAS (1976b) Distribution of sheep in England and Wales (map). Ministry of Agriculture, Fisheries and Food; Agricultural Advisory and Development Service

MAFF/ADAS (1976c) Distribution of pigs in England and Wales (map). Ministry of Agriculture, Fisheries and Food; Agricultural Development Advisory Service

MAFF/DAFS (1984) *Blood Characteristics and the Nutrition of Ruminants*. Ministry of Agriculture, Fisheries and Food; Department of Agriculture and Fisheries for Scotland. Reference Book No. 260. Her Majesty's Stationery Office, London

Maguire, D.J. (1991) An overview and definition of GIS. In: *Geographical Information Systems, Vol. 1, Principles*. Eds Maguire, D.J., Goodchild, M.F. and Rhind, D.W.,

pp. 9–20. Longman Scientific and Technical, Harlow

Malik, R., Hunt, G.B. and Allan, G.S. (1992) Prevalence of mitral valve insufficiency in cavalier King Charles spaniels. *Veterinary Record*, **130**, 302–303

Mantel, N. (1963) Chi-square tests with one degree of freedom: extension of the Mantel–Haenszel procedure. *Journal of the American Statistical Association*, **58**, 690–700

Mantel, N. (1967) The detection of disease clustering and a generalized regression approach. *Cancer Research*, **27**, 209–220

Mantel, N. and Haenszel, W. (1959) Statistical aspects of the analysis of data from retrospective studies of disease. *Journal of the National Cancer Institute*, **22**, 719–748

Marchevsky, N., Held, J.R. and Garcia-Carrillio, C. (1989) Probability of introducing diseases because of false negative test results. *American Journal of Epidemiology*, **130**, 611–614

Markusfeld, O. (1985) Relationship between overfeeding, metritis and ketosis in high yielding dairy cows. *Veterinary Record*, **116**, 489–491

Markusfeld, O. (1986) The association of displaced abomasum with various preparturient factors in dairy cows. *Preventive Veterinary Medicine*, **4**, 173–183

Markusfeld, O. (1987) Inactive ovaries in high-yielding dairy cows before service: aetiology and effect on conception. *Veterinary Record*, **121**, 149–153

Markusfeld, O. (1990) Risk recurrence of eight periparturient and reproductive traits in dairy cows. *Preventive Veterinary Medicine*, **9**, 279–286

Marmor, M., Willeberg, P., Glickman, L.T., Priester, W.A., Cypess, R.H. and Hurvitz, A.L. (1982) Epizootiologic patterns of diabetes mellitus in dogs. *American Journal of Veterinary Research*, **43**, 465–471

Marsh, W.E., Dijkhuizen, A.A. and Morris, R.S. (1987) An economic comparison of four culling decision rules for reproductive failure in United States dairy herds using DairyORACLE. *Journal of Dairy Science*, **70**, 1274–1280

Marsh, W.E., Damrongwatanapokin, T., Lartz, K. and Morrison, R.B. (1991) The use of a geographical information system in an epidemiological study of pseudorabies (Aujeszky's disease) in Minnesota swine herds. *Preventive Veterinary Medicine*, **11**, 249–254

Martin, B., Mainland, D.D. and Green, M.A. (1982a) VIRUS: A computer program for herd health and productivity. *Veterinary Record*, **110**, 446–448

Martin, C.M. (1964) Interactions of hydrocarbon carcinogens with viruses and nucleic acids in vivo and in vitro. *Progress in Experimental Tumor Research*, **5**, 134–156

Martin, D. and Austin, H. (1991) An efficient program for computing conditional likelihood estimates and exact confidence limits for a common odds ratio. *Epidemiology*, **2**, 359–362

Martin, P.M., Cotard, M., Mialott, J.-P., Andre, F. and Raynaud, J.-P. (1984) Animal models for hormone-dependent human breast cancer. Relationship between steroid receptor profiles in canine and feline mammary tumours and survival rate. *Cancer Chemotherapy and Pharmacology*, **12**, 13−17

Martin, S.W. (1977) The evaluation of tests. *Canadian Journal of Comparative Medicine*, **41**, 19−25

Martin, S.W. (1988) The interpretation of laboratory results. In: Investigation of disease outbreaks and impaired productivity. Eds Lessard, P.R. and Perry, B.D. *The Veterinary Clinics of North America: Food Animal Practice*, **4**(1), 61−78

Martin, S.W. and Bonnett, B. (1987) Clinical epidemiology. *Canadian Veterinary Journal*, **28**, 318−325

Martin, S.W., Aziz, S.A., Sandals, W.C.D. and Curtis, R.A. (1982b) The association between clinical disease, production and culling in Holstein−Friesian cows. *Canadian Journal of Animal Science*, **62**, 622−640

Martin, S.W., Meek, A.H., Davis, D.G., Johnson, J.A. and Curtis, R.A. (1982c) Factors associated with mortality and treatment costs in feedlot calves: the Bruce County beef project, years 1978, 1979, 1980. *Canadian Journal of Comparative Medicine*, **46**, 341−349

Martin, S.W., Meek, A.H. and Willeberg, P. (1987) *Veterinary Epidemiology: Principles and Methods*. Iowa State University Press, Ames

Martin, S.W., Shoukri, M. and Thorburn, M. (1992) Evaluating the test status of herds based on tests applied to individuals. *Preventive Veterinary Medicine*, **14**, 33−43

Martin, W., Lissemore, K. and Kelton, D. (1990) Animal health monitoring systems in Canada. In: Society for Veterinary Epidemiology and Preventive Medicine, Proceedings, Belfast, 4−6 April 1990. Ed. Thrusfield, M.V., pp. 62−69

Maslakov, V.I. (1968) On the problem of the elimination of communicable diseases. *Zeichift für Mikrobiologie, Epidemiologie und Immunologie*, **45**, 118−122

Mason, J.W. (1971) A re-evaluation of the concept of 'non-specificity' in stress theory. *Journal of Psychiatric Research*, **8**, 323−333

Mason, J.W., Wool, M.S., Mougey, E.H., Wherry, F.E., Collins, D.R. and Taylor, E.D. (1968) Psychological vs nutritional factors in the effects of 'fasting' on hormonal balance. *Psychosomatic Medicine*, **30**, 554−555

Mateu-de-Antonio, E.M., Martin, M. and Soler, M. (1993) Use of indirect enzyme-linked immunosorbent assay with hot saline solution extracts of a variant (M-) strain of *Brucella canis* for diagnosis of brucellosis in dogs. *American Journal of Veterinary Research*, **54**, 1043−1046

Matthews, S.A. (1989) GIS methodology and spatial statistics. In: First National Conference and Exhibition, GIS — A Corporate Resource. National Motorcycle Museum Conference Centre, Birmingham, 11−12 October 1989. Conference papers, pp. 6.4.1−6.4.6. Association for Geographic Information

May, R.M. and Anderson, R.M. (1979) Population biology of infectious diseases. *Nature*, **280**, 455−461

Mayer, S.J. (1992) Stratospheric ozone depletion and animal health. *Veterinary Record*, **131**, 120−122

McAllum, H.J.F. (1985) Stress and postcapture myopathy in red deer. In: *Biology of Deer Production*. Proceedings of an International Conference, Dunedin, New Zealand, 13−18

February 1983. Eds Fennessy, P.F. and Drew, K.R., pp. 65−72. Bulletin 22. The Royal Society of New Zealand, Wellington

McArthur, A.J. (1991) Thermal interaction between animal and microclimate: specification of a 'standard environmental temperature' for animals outdoors. *Journal of Theoretical Biology*, **148**, 331−343

McCaughey, W.J. (1992) Residues: sample selection. In: Society for Veterinary Epidemiology and Preventive Medicine, Proceedings, Edinburgh, 1−3 April 1992. Ed. Thrusfield, M.V., pp. 13−23

McCauley, E.H. (1985) Hog cholera in Honduras. Evaluation of the economic and technical aspects of the impact on production and consequences of vaccination programs; and report of 1985 owner survey results, February−April 1985. College of Veterinary Medicine, Department of Large Animal Clinical Sciences, University of Minnesota

McCauley, E.H., Majid, A.A., Tayeb, A. and Bushara, H.O. (1983a) Clinical diagnosis of schistosomiasis in Sudanese cattle. *Tropical Animal Health and Production*, **15**, 129−136

McCauley, E.H., Tayeb, A. and Majid, A.A. (1983b) Owner survey of schistosomiasis mortality in Sudanese cattle. *Tropical Animal Health and Production*, **15**, 227−233

McClintock, P.M. (1988) *The Economic Contribution of the British Equine Industry*. British Horse Society, Stoneleigh

McClure, J.J. (1988) Equine disease association studies: a clinician's perspective. *Animal Genetics*, **19**, 409−415

McCracken, J.A., Pretty, J.N. and Conway, G.R. (1988) *An Introduction to Rapid Rural Appraisal for Agricultural Development*. International Institute for Environment and Development, London

McCrea, C.T. and Head, K.W. (1978) Sheep tumours in north-east Yorkshire. I. Prevalence on seven moorland farms. *British Veterinary Journal*, **134**, 454−461

McCrea, C.T. and Head, K.W. (1981) Sheep tumours in north-east Yorkshire. II. Experimental production of tumours. *British Veterinary Journal*, **137**, 21−30

McDermott, J.J., Deng, K.A., Jayatileka, T.N. and El Jack, M.A. (1987) A cross-sectional cattle disease study in Kongor Rural Council, Southern Sudan. I. Prevalence estimates and age, sex and breed associations for brucellosis and contagious bovine pleuropneumonia. *Preventive Veterinary Medicine*, **5**, 111−123

McGee, D.L. (1986) A program for logistic regression on the IBM PC. *American Journal of Epidemiology*, **124**, 702−705

McIlroy, S.G., Goodall, E.A., Rainey, J. and McMurray, C.H. (1988) A computerised management and disease information retrieval system for profitable broiler production. *Agricultural Systems*, **27**, 11−22

McInerney, J.P. (1988) The economic analysis of livestock disease: the developing framework. *Acta Veterinaria Scandinavica*, Suppl. 84, 66−74

McInerney, J.P. (1991) Economic aspects of the animal welfare issue. In: Society for Veterinary Epidemiology and Preventive Medicine, Proceedings, London, 17−19 April 1991. Ed. Thrusfield, M.V., pp. 83−91

McInerney, J.P., Howe, K.S. and Schepers, J.A. (1992) A framework for the economic analysis of disease in farm livestock. *Preventive Veterinary Medicine*, **13**, 137−154

McKay, B., McCallum, S. and Morris, R.S. (1988) An expert system program for diagnosing reproductive problems in seasonal dairy herds. *Acta Veterinaria Scandinavica*, Suppl. 84, 480−482

McKinnell, R.G. and Ellis, V.L. (1972) Epidemiology of the frog renal tumour and the significance of tumour nuclear transplantation studies to a viral aetiology of the tumour — a review. In: *Oncogenesis and Herpesviruses*. Proceedings of a symposium held at Christ's College, Cambridge, 20−25 June 1971. Eds Biggs, P.M., de-The, G. and Payne, L.N., pp. 183−197. IARC Scientific Publications No. 2, International Agency for Research on Cancer, Lyon

McLauchlan, J.D. and Henderson, W.M. (1947) The occurrence of foot-and-mouth disease in the hedgehog under natural conditions. *Journal of Hygiene, Cambridge*, **45**, 474−479

McNeil, P.H., Rhodes, A.P. and Willis, B.H. (1984) *A Flock Health and Productivity Service for New Zealand*. Report of a trial involving ten farms in the Dannevirke area, November 1979−June 1983. Veterinary Services Council, New Zealand

McTaggart, H.S., Laing, A.H., Imlah, P., Head, K.W. and Brownlie, S.E. (1979) The genetics of hereditary lymphosarcoma in pigs. *Veterinary Record*, **105**, 36

Mehta, C.R. and Patel, N.R. (1983) A network algorithm for performing Fisher's exact test in $r \times c$ contingency tables. *Journal of the American Statistical Association*, **78**, 427−434

Mehta, C.R., Patel, N.R. and Gray, R. (1985) Computing an exact confidence interval for the common odds ratio in several 2×2 contingency tables. *Journal of the American Statistical Association*, **80**, 969−973

Meinert, C.L. and Tonascia, S. (1986) *Clinical Trials: Design, Conduct and Analysis*. Oxford University Press, New York

Meischke, H.R.C., Ramsey, W.R. and Shaw, F.D. (1974) The effect of horns on bruising in cattle. *Australian Veterinary Journal*, **50**, 432−434

Mellaart, J.C. (1967) *Catal Huyuk*. McGraw-Hill, New York

Mellor, P.S., Jennings, D.M., Wilkinson, P.J. and Boorman, J.P.T. (1985) *Culicoides imicola*: a bluetongue virus vector in Spain and Portugal. *Veterinary Record*, **116**, 589−590

Menzies, F.D., Goodall, E.A., McLoughlin, M.F. and Wheatley, S. (1992) Computerised monitoring of disease and production in farmed Atlantic salmon (Salmo salar). In: Society for Veterinary Epidemiology and Preventive Medicine, Denary Proceedings, Edinburgh, 1−3 April 1992. Ed. Thrusfield, M.V., pp. 138−147

Merriam, C.H. (1893) *The Geographic Distribution of Life in North America*. Smithsonian Institute Annual Report, pp. 365−415

Merry, D.L. and Kolar, J.R. (1984) A comparative study of four rabies vaccines. *Veterinary Medicine and Small Animal Clinician*, **79**, 661−664

Meyers, P.J., Bonnett, B.N., Hearn, P. and McKee, S.L. (1991) Epidemiological approach to studying reproductive performance on equine breeding farms. In: Proceedings of the Sixth International Symposium on Veterinary Epidemiology and Economics, Ottawa, 12−16 August 1991. Ed. Martin, S.W., pp. 488−490

Michell, A.R. (Ed.) (1993) *The Advancement of Veterinary Science. The Bicentenary Symposium Series. Volume 1: Veterinary Medicine Beyond 2000*. CAB International, Wallingford

Miettinen, O.S. (1970) Matching and design efficiency in retrospective studies. *American Journal of Epidemiology*, **91**, 111−118

Miettinen, O.S. (1974) Confounding and effect modification. *American Journal of Epidemiology*, **100**, 350−353

Miettinen, O.S. (1976) Estimability and estimation in case-referent studies. *American Journal of Epidemiology*, **103**, 226−235

Miettinen, P.V.A. and Setälä, J.J. (1993) Relationships between subclinical ketosis, milk production and fertility in Finnish dairy cattle. *Preventive Veterinary Medicine*, **17**, 1−8

Milian-Suazo, F., Erb, H.N. and Smith, R.D. (1988) Descriptive epidemiology of culling in dairy cows from 34 herds in New York State. *Preventive Veterinary Medicine*, **6**, 243−251

Milian-Suazo, F., Erb, H.N. and Smith, R.D. (1989) Risk factors for reason-specific culling of dairy cows. *Preventive Veterinary Medicine*, **7**, 19−29

Millar, R. and Francis, J. (1974) The relation of clinical and bacteriological findings to fertility in thoroughbred mares. *Australian Veterinary Journal*, **50**, 351−355

Miller, L., McElvaine, M.D., McDowell, R.M. and Ahl, A.S. (1993) Developing a quantitative risk assessment process. *Revue Scientifique et Technique, Office International des Epizooties*, **12**, 1153−1164

Milne, A. (1950) The ecology of the sheep tick, *Ixodes ricinus* (L.). Spatial distribution. *Parasitology*, **41**, 189−207

Mims, C.A. (1987) *The Pathogenesis of Infectious Disease*, 3rd edn. Academic Press, London and New York

Misdorp, W. (1987) The impact of pathology on the study and treatment of cancer. In: *Veterinary Cancer Medicine*, 2nd edn. Eds Theilen, G.H. and Madewell, B.R., pp. 53−70. Lea and Febiger, Philadelphia

Mishan, E.J. (1976) *Elements of Cost−Benefit Analysis*. George Allen and Unwin, London

Miura, Y., Hayashi, S., Ishihara, T., Inaba, Y., Omori, T. and Matumoto, M. (1974) Neutralizing antibody against Akabane virus in precolostral sera from calves with congenital arthrogryposis — hydranencephaly syndrome. Brief report. *Archiv für die Gesamte Virusforschung*, **46**, 377−380

Moberg, G.P. (Ed.) (1985) *Animal stress*. American Physiological Society, Bethesda

Mohammed, H.O. (1990a) Factors associated with the risk of developing osteochondrosis in horses: a case−control study. *Preventive Veterinary Medicine*, **10**, 63−71

Mohammed, H.O. (1990b) A multivariate indexing system for hygiene in relation to the risk of *Mycoplasma gallisepticum* infection in chickens. *Preventive Veterinary Medicine*, **9**, 75−83

Mohammed, H.O., Hill, T. and Lowe, J. (1991a) Risk factors

associated with injuries in thoroughbred horses. *Equine Veterinary Journal*, **23**, 445–448

Mohammed, H.O., Oltenacu, P.A. and Erb, H.N. (1991b) A simple multivariate index for scaling breeding management variables in relation to diseases in dairy herds. In: Proceedings of the Sixth International Symposium on Veterinary Epidemiology and Economics, Ottawa, 12–16 August 1991. Ed. Martin, S.W., pp. 292–294.

Mohammed, H.O., Rebhun, W.C. and Antczak, D.F. (1992) Factors associated with the risk of developing sarcoid tumours in horses. *Equine Veterinary Journal*, **24**, 165–168 (Correspondence: (1993) **25**, 169)

Monaghan, M.L.M. and Hannan, J. (1983) Abattoir survey of bovine kidney disease. *Veterinary Record*, **113**, 55–57

Monath, T.P., Newhouse, V.F., Kemp, G.E., Setzer, H.W. and Cacciapuoti, A. (1974) Lassa virus isolation from *Mastomys natalensis* rodents during an epidemic in Sierra Leone. *Science*, **185**, 263–265

Montgomery, R.D., Stein, G., Stotts, V.D. and Settle, F.H. (1979) The 1978 epornitic of avian cholera on the Chesapeake Bay. *Avian Diseases*, **23**, 966–978

Montgomery, R.E. (1917) On a tick-borne gastroenteritis of sheep and goats occurring in British East Africa. *Journal of Comparative Pathology and Therapeutics*, **30**, 28–57

Montgomery, R.E. (1921) On a form of swine fever occurring in British East Africa (Kenya Colony). *Journal of Comparative Pathology and Therapeutics*, **34**, 159–191, 247–262

Moore, B. (1957) Observations pointing to the conjunctiva as a portal of entry in salmonella infections of guinea-pigs. *Journal of Hygiene, Cambridge*, **55**, 414–433

Moorhouse, P.D. and Hugh-Jones, M.E. (1981) Serum banks. *The Veterinary Bulletin*, **51**, 277–290

Moorhouse, P.D. and Hugh-Jones, M.E. (1983) The results of retesting bovine sera stored at −18 °C for twenty years, with lessons for future serum banks. In: Proceedings of the Third International Symposium on Veterinary Epidemiology and Economics, Arlington, Virginia, 6–10 September 1982, pp. 44–51. Veterinary Medicine Publishing Company, Edwardsville

Morant, S.V. (1984) Factors affecting reproductive performance including the importance and effect of problem cows. In: *Dairy Cow Fertility*. Proceedings of a joint British Veterinary Association and British Society of Animal Production Conference, Bristol University, 28–29 June 1984. Eds Eddy, R.G. and Ducker, M.J., pp. 15–23. British Veterinary Association, London

Morgan, J.P., Bahr, A., Franti, C.E. and Barley, C.S. (1993) Lumbosacral transitional vertebrae as a predisposing cause of cauda equine syndrome in German Shepherd dogs: 161 cases (1987–1990). *Journal of the American Veterinary Medical Association*, **202**, 1877–1882

Morgan, K.L. and Tuppen, A.T.A. (1988) Sheep health, productivity and the IBM PC. In: *The Research and Academic Users' Guide to the IBM Personal Computer*. Ed. Barnetson, P., pp. 147–153. Oxford University Press, Oxford

Morley, F.H.W., Watt, B.R., Grant, I.McL. and Galloway,

D.B. (1983) A flock health and production program for sheep. In: Proceedings of the Third International Symposium on Veterinary Epidemiology and Economics, Arlington, Virginia, 6–10 September 1982, pp. 186–194. Veterinary Medical Publishing Company, Edwardsville

Morley, R.S. (1988) National Animal Health Information System, Agriculture Canada. *Revue Scientifique et Technique, Office International des Epizooties*, **7**, 577–581

Morley, R.S. (Coordinator) (1993) Risk analysis, animal health and trade. *Revue Scientifique et Technique, Office International des Epizooties*, **12**, 1001–1362

Morley, R.S. and Hugh-Jones, M.E. (1989) The effect of management and ecological factors on the epidemiology of anaplasmosis in the Red River Plains and south-east areas of Louisiana. *Veterinary Research Communications*, **13**, 359–369

Morris, D.D., Moore, J.N. and Ward, S. (1989) Comparison of age, sex, breed, history and management in 229 horses with colic. In: Proceedings of the Third Equine Colic Research Symposium, University of Georgia, 1–3 November 1988. Eds Gerring, E.L., Morris, D.D., Moore, J.N. and White, N.A. *Equine Veterinary Journal*, Suppl. 7, 129–132

Morris, R.S. (1969) Assessing the economic value of veterinary services to primary industries. *Australian Veterinary Journal*, **45**, 295–300

Morris, R.S. (1982) New techniques in veterinary epidemiology — providing workable answers to complex problems. In: *Epidemiology in Animal Health*. Proceedings of a symposium held at the British Veterinary Association's Centenary Congress, Reading, 22–25 September 1982, pp. 1–16. Society for Veterinary Epidemiology and Preventive Medicine

Morris, R.S., Sanson, R.L. and Stern, M.W. (1992) EpiMAN — a decision support system for managing a foot-and-mouth disease epidemic. In: Dutch Society for Veterinary Epidemiology and Economy, Proceedings, **5**, Wageningen, 9 December 1992. Eds Frankena, K. and van der Hoofd, C.M., pp. 1–35

Morris, R.S., Sanson, R.L., McKenzie, J.S. and Marsh, W.E. (1993) Decision support systems in animal health. In: Society for Veterinary Epidemiology and Preventive Medicine, Proceedings, Exeter, 31 March–2 April 1993. Ed. Thrusfield, M.V., pp. 188–199

Morrow, D.A. (1980) Examination schedule for a dairy reproductive health programme. In: *Current Therapy in Theriogenology*. Ed. Morrow, D.A., pp. 549–562. W.B. Saunders, Philadelphia, London, Toronto

Mortensen, S. and Madsen, K. (1992) The occurrence of PRRS in Denmark. *American Association of Swine Practitioners Newsletter*, **4**(4), 48

Morton, D. (1992) Docking of dogs: practical and ethical aspects. *Veterinary Record*, **131**, 301–306

Morton, N.E. (1982) *Outline of Genetic Epidemiology*. Karger, New York

Moss, R. (Coordinator) (1994) Animal welfare and veterinary services. *Revue Scientifique et Technique, Office International des Epizooties*, **13**, 1–302

Moulder, J.W. (1974) Intracellular parasitism: life in an extreme environment. *Journal of Infectious Diseases*, **130**, 300−306

Moulton, J.E., Taylor, D.O.N., Dorn, C.R. and Andersen, A.C. (1970) Canine mammary tumors. *Pathologia Veterinaria*, **7**, 289−320

Mousing, J. (1988) The Danish Pig Health Scheme: a questionnaire survey and analysis of swine producers' attitudes and willingness to pay. *Preventive Veterinary Medicine*, **6**, 157−170

Mousing, J., Lybye, H., Barfod, K., Meyling, A., Ronsholt, L. and Willeberg, P. (1990) Chronic pleuritis in pigs for slaughter: an epidemiological study of infections and rearing system-related risk factors. *Preventive Veterinary Medicine*, **9**, 107−119

Mousing, J., Mortensen, S., Ewald, C. and Christensen, L.S. (1991) Epidemiological and meteorological aspects of Aujeszky's disease in Denmark and Northern Germany. In: Society for Veterinary Epidemiology and Preventive Medicine, Proceedings, London, 17−19 April 1991. Ed. Thrusfield, M.V., pp. 18−26

Moxley, J.E., Kennedy, B.W., Downey, B.R. and Bowman, J.S.T. (1978) Survey of milking hygiene practices and their relationships to somatic cell counts and milk production. *Journal of Dairy Science*, **61**, 1637−1644

MRC (1938) *Epidemics in Schools. An Analysis of the Data collected during the First Five Years of a Statistical Inquiry by the Schools Epidemic Committee*. Medical Research Council Special Report Series No. 227. His Majesty's Stationery Office, London

Mtambo, M.M.A., Nash, A.S., Blewett, D.A., Smith, H.V. and Wright, S. (1991) Cryptosporidium infection in cats: prevalence of infection in domestic and feral cats in the Glasgow area. *Veterinary Record*, **129**, 502−504

Muench, H. (1959) *Catalytic Models in Epidemiology*. Harvard University Press, Cambridge, MA

Muirhead, M.R. (1976) Veterinary problems of intensive pig husbandry. *Veterinary Record*, **99**, 288−292

Muirhead, M.R. (1978) Intensive pig production: studies in preventive medicine. Fellowship thesis, Royal College of Veterinary Surgeons.

Muirhead, M.R. (1980) The pig advisory visit in preventive medicine. *Veterinary Record*, **106**, 170−173

Mulder, C.A.T., Bonnett, B.N., Martin, S.W., Lissemore, K. and Page, P.D. (1994) The usefulness of the computerized medical records of one practice for research into pregnancy loss in dairy cows. *Preventive Veterinary Medicine*, **21**, 43−63

Müller, W.W. (1991) New areas of oral fox vaccination in Europe, 1991. *Rabies Bulletin Europe*, **15**(3), 11−12. WHO Collaborating Centre for Rabies Surveillance and Research, Tübingen

Mulvihill, J.J. and Priester, W.A. (1973) Congenital heart disease in dogs: epidemiologic similarities to man. *Teratology*, **7**, 73−78

Murphy, B.R. and Webster, R.G. (1990) Orthomyxoviruses. In: *Virology*. Eds Fields, B.N. and Knipe, D.M., Vol. 1, pp. 1091−1152. Raven Press, New York

Murray, A., Moriarty, K.M. and Scott, D.B. (1989) A cloned DNA probe for the detection of *Mycobacterium paratuberculosis*. *New Zealand Veterinary Journal*, **37**, 47−50

Murray, J. (1968) Some aspects of ovicaprid and pig breeding in neolithic Europe. In: *Studies in Ancient Europe. Essays Presented to Stuart Piggott*. Eds Coles, J.M. and Simpson, D.D.A., pp. 71−81. Leicester University Press, Leicester

Mussman, H.C., McCallon, W.R. and Otte, E. (1980) Planning and implementation of animal disease control programs in developing countries. In: *Veterinary Epidemiology and Economics*. Proceedings of the Second International Symposium, Canberra, 4−11 May 1979. Eds Geering, W.A., Roe, R.T. and Chapman, L.A., pp. 551−557. Australian Government Publishing Service, Canberra

Myers, J.H. (1988) Can a general hypothesis explain population cycles of forest Lepidoptera? *Advances in Ecological Research*, Vol. 18. Eds Begon, M., Fitter, A.H., Ford, E.D. and Macfadyen, A., pp. 179−242. Academic Press, London

Nasser, R. and Mosier, J.E. (1980) Canine population dynamics: a study of the Manhattan, Kansas, canine population. *American Journal of Veterinary Research*, **41**, 1798−1803

Nasser, R. and Mosier, J.E. (1982) Feline population dynamics: a study of the Manhattan, Kansas, feline population. *American Journal of Veterinary Research*, **43**, 167−170

Nasser, R., Mosier, J.E. and Williams, L.W. (1984) Study of the canine and feline populations in the Greater Las Vegas area. *American Journal of Veterinary Research*, **45**, 282−287

Neaton, J.D., Duchene, A.G., Svendsen, K.H. and Wentworth, D. (1990) Examination of the efficiency of some quality assurance methods commonly employed in clinical trials. *Statistics in Medicine*, **9**, 115−124

Neitz, W.O. (1948) Immunological studies on bluetongue in sheep. *Onderstepoort Journal of Veterinary Science*, **23**, 93−135

Nelson, A.W. and White, L.K. (1990) Medical Records. In: *Clinical Textbook for Veterinary Technicians*, 2nd edn. Ed. McCurnin, D.M., pp. 43−55. W.B. Saunders, Philadelphia

Newcombe, H.B. (1964) Session VII discussion. In: *Second International Conference on Congenital Malformations*. Papers and Discussions presented at the Second International Conference on Congenital Malformations, New York City, 14−19 July 1963, pp. 345−349. International Medical Congress, New York

Newell, K.W., Ross, A.D. and Renner, R.M. (1984) Phenoxy and picolinic acid herbicides and small intestinal adenocarcinoma in sheep. *Lancet*, **ii**, 1301−1305

Nicholas, F.W. (1987) *Veterinary Genetics*. Oxford University Press, Oxford

Nicholls, T.J., Barton, M.G. and Anderson, B.P. (1981) An outbreak of mastitis in dairy cows due to *Pseudomonas aeruginosa* contamination of dry cow therapy at manufacture. *Veterinary Record*, **108**, 93−96

Nicod, F., Coche, B., Desjouis, G. and Benet, J.J. (1991) Foot-and-mouth disease vaccine-related accidents in France in 1985: retrospective study by practitioners. In: Proceedings of the Sixth International Symposium on Veterinary Epidemiology and Economics, Ottawa, 12–16 August 1991. Ed. Martin, S.W., pp. 323–326

Nilsson, S.A. (1978) Bovine laminitis and sequelae of it. In: Report on the Second Symposium on Bovine Digital Disease, 25–28 September 1978, Skara, Sweden

Noack, H. (1987) Concepts of health and health promotion. In: *Measurement in Health Promotion and Protection*. Eds Abelin, T., Brzeziński, Z.J. and Carstairs, V.D.L., pp. 5–28. World Health Organization Regional Office for Europe, Copenhagen

Nokes, J.D. (1992) Microparasites: viruses and bacteria. In: *Natural Enemies: The Population Biology of Predators, Parasites and Diseases*. Ed. Crawley, M.J., pp. 349–374. Blackwell Scientific Publications, Oxford

Noordhuizen, J.P.T.M. and Buurman, J. (1984) Veterinary automated management and production control programme for dairy herds (VAMPP). The application of MUMPS for data processing. *The Veterinary Quarterly*, **6**, 62–77

Noordhuizen, J.P.T.M., Frankena, K., Ploeger, H. and Nell, T. (Eds) (1993) *Field Trial and Error*. Proceedings of the International Seminar with Workshops on the Design, Conduct and Interpretation of Field Trials, Berg en Dal, Netherlands, 27–28 April 1993. Epidecon, Wageningen

Nordenstam, T. and Tornebohm, H. (1979) Research, ethics and development. *Zeitschrift für Allgemeine Wissenschaftstheorie*, **10**, 54–66

Norton-Griffiths, M. (1978) *Counting Animals*, 2nd edn. African Wildlife Leadership Foundation, Nairobi

Nurmi, E. (1988) Modern methods of public health practice: exclusion of food-borne pathogens. *Acta Veterinaria Scandinavica*, Suppl. 84, 49–56

Nyaga, P.N.N. (1975) Epidemiology of equine influenza: risk by age, breed and sex. MPVM thesis, University of California, Davis

Odend'hal, S. (1983) *The Geographical Distribution of Animal Viral Diseases*. Academic Press, New York and London

OIE (1987) *Procedures for Immediate and Monthly Reporting of Significant Disease Outbreaks to the Office International des Epizooties. Guidelines*. Office International des Epizooties, Paris

OIE (1992) *International Animal Health Code: Mammals, Birds and Bees*, 6th edn. Office International des Epizooties, Paris

OIE (1993) Biotechnology applied to the diagnosis of animal diseases. *Revue Scientifique et Technique, Office International des Epizooties*, **12**, 1–672

Ollerenshaw, C.B. (1966) The approach to forecasting the incidence of fascioliasis over England and Wales, 1958–1962. *Agricultural Meteorology*, **3**(1/2), 35–54

Ollerenshaw, C.B. and Rowlands, W.T. (1959) A method of forecasting the incidence of fascioliasis in Anglesey. *Veterinary Record*, **71**, 591–598

Oltenacu, P.A., Bendixen, P.H., Vilson, B. and Ekesbo, I. (1988) Evaluation of the tramped teats-clinical mastitis disease complex. Risk factors and interrelationships with other diseases. In: *Environment and Animal Health*. Proceedings of the 6th International Congress on Animal Hygiene, 14–17

June 1988, Skara, Sweden, Vol. 1. Ed. Ekesbo, I., pp. 46–50. Swedish University of Agricultural Sciences, Skara

Oltenacu, P.A., Frick, P. and Lindhe, B. (1990) Epidemiological study of several clinical diseases, reproductive performance and culling in primiparous Swedish cattle. *Preventive Veterinary Medicine*, **9**, 59–74

Opit, L.J. (1987) How should information on health care be generated and used? *World Health Forum*, **8**, 409–417. (Discussion: 417–438)

Orr, M.B. and Chalmers, M. (1988) A field study of the association between periodontal disease and body condition in sheep. *New Zealand Veterinary Journal*, **36**, 171–172

Osteras, O. and Lund, A. (1988a) Epidemiological analyses of the associations between bovine udder health and housing. *Preventive Veterinary Medicine*, **6**, 79–90

Osteras, O. and Lund, A. (1988b) Epidemiological analyses of the associations between bovine udder health and milking machine and milking management. *Preventive Veterinary Medicine*, **6**, 91–108

Osterhaus, A.D.M.E. and Vedder, E.J. (1988) Identification of virus causing recent seal deaths. *Nature*, **335**, 20

Ouelett, B.L., Romeder, J.M. and Lance, J.M. (1979) Premature mortality attributable to smoking and hazardous drinking in Canada. *American Journal of Epidemiology*, **109**, 451–463

Owen, J.M. (1985) Preventive medicine in stud and stable. In: Society for Veterinary Epidemiology and Preventive Medicine, Proceedings, Reading, 27–29 March 1985. Ed. Thrusfield, M.V., pp. 56–60

Owen, M. (1989) *SPC and Continuous Improvement*. IFS Publications/Springer-Verlag, Berlin

Oxford English Dictionary (1972) *A Supplement to the Oxford English Dictionary*. Ed. Burchfield, R.W. Oxford University Press

Oxford, J.S. (1985) Biochemical techniques for the genetic and phenotypic analysis of viruses: 'Molecular Epidemiology'. *Journal of Hygiene, Cambridge*, **94**, 1–7

Page, E.S. (1961) Cumulative sum charts. *Technometrics*, **3**, 1–9

Page, S., Davenport, M. and Hewitt, A. (1991) *The GATT Uruguay Round: Effects on Developing Countries*. Overseas Development Institute, London

Panciera, D.L., Thomas, C.B., Eicker, S.W. and Atkins, C.E. (1990) Epizootiologic patterns of diabetes mellitus in cats: 333 cases (1980–1986). *Journal of the American Veterinary Medical Association*, **197**, 1504–1508

Pappaioanou, M., Schwabe, C.W. and Polydorou, K. (1984) Epidemiological analysis of the Cyprus anti-echinococcosis campaign. I. The prevalence of *Echinococcus granulosus* in Cypriot village dogs, the first dog-test period of the campaign, June–December 1972. *Preventive Veterinary Medicine*, **3**, 159–180

Paraf, A. and Peltre, G. (1991) *Immunoassays in Food and Agriculture*. Kluwer Academic Publishers, Dordrecht

Parente, E.J., Richardson, D.W. and Spencer, P. (1993) Basal sesamoidean fractures in horses: 57 cases (1980–91). *Journal* of the American Veterinary Medical Association, **202**, 1293–1297

Park, Y.G., Gordon, J.G., Bech-Nielsen, S. and Slemonds, R.D. (1992) Factors for seropositivity to leptospirosis in horses. *Preventive Veterinary Medicine*, **13**, 121–127

Parsons, J.H. (1982) Funding of control measures. In: *The Control of Infectious Diseases in Farm Animals*. British Veterinary Association Trust Project on the future of animal health control, London, pp. 58–62

Pascoe, P.J., McDonnell, W.N., Trim, C.M. and van Gorder, J. (1983) Mortality rates and associated factors in equine colic operations — a retrospective study of 341 operations. *Canadian Veterinary Journal*, **24**, 76–85

Paton, G. and Gettinby, G. (1983) The control of a parasitic nematode population in sheep represented by a discrete time network with stochastic inputs. *Proceedings of the Royal Irish Academy*, **83B**, 267–280

Paton, G. and Gettinby, G. (1985) Comparing control strategies for parasitic gastroenteritis in lambs grazed on previously contaminated pasture: a network modelling approach. *Preventive Veterinary Medicine*, **3**, 301–310

Paton, G., Thomas, R.J. and Waller, P.J. (1984) A prediction model for parasitic gastroenteritis in lambs. *International Journal of Parasitology*, **14**, 439–445

Patterson, D.F. (1968) Epidemiologic and genetic studies of congenital heart disease in the dog. *Circulation Research*, **23**, 171–202

Patterson, D.F. (1980) A catalog of genetic disorders of the dog. In: *Current Veterinary Therapy VII. Small Animal Practice*. Ed. Kirk, R.W., pp. 82–103. W.B. Saunders, Philadelphia

Patterson, D.F. and Medway, W. (1966) Hereditary diseases of the dog. *Journal of the American Veterinary Medical Association*, **149**, 1741–1754

Patterson, D.F., Pyle, R.L., Buchanan, J.W., Trautveter, E. and Abt, D.A. (1971) Hereditary patent ductus arteriosus and its sequelae in the dog. *Circulation Research*, **29**, 1–13

Patterson, D.F., Haskins, M.E. and Jezyk, P.F. (1982) Models of human genetic disease in domestic animals. In: *Advances in Human Genetics*, Vol. 12. Eds Harris, H. and Hirschhorn, K., pp. 263–339. Plenum Press, New York and London

Paul, J.R. and White, C. (Eds) (1973) *Serological Epidemiology*. Academic Press, New York and London

Pavlovsky, E.N. (1964) *Prirodnaya Ochagovost' Transmissivnykh Bolezney v Svyazi s Landshaftnoy Epidemiologiey Zooantroponozo*. Translated as *Natural Nidality of Transmissible Disease with Special Reference to the Landscape Epidemiology of Zooanthroponoses*. Plous, F.K. (Translator), Levine, N.D. (Ed.), 1966. University of Illinois Press, Urbana

Payne, A.M. (1963) Basic concepts of eradication. *American Review of Respiratory Diseases*, **88**, 449–455

Payne, C.D. (Ed.) (1986) *The GLIM System Release 3.77 Generalised Linear Interactive Modelling*. The Royal Statistical Society, London

Payne, J.M., Dew, S.M., Manston, R. and Faulks, M. (1970) The use of a metabolic profile test in dairy herds. *Veterinary Record*, **87**, 150–158

Payne, L.N. (1982) Breeding resistant shock. In: *The Control of Infectious Diseases in Farm Animals*. British Veterinary Association Trust Project on the future of animal health control, London, pp. 37–42

Pearce, D.W. (1971) *Cost–Benefit Analysis*. The Macmillan Press, London

Pearce, D.W. and Sturmey, S.G. (1966) Private and social costs and benefits: a note on terminology. *Economic Journal*, March 1966, 152–158

Pearson, J.K.L., Greer, D.O., Spence, B.K., McParland, P.J., McKinley, D.L., Dunlop, W.L. and Acheson, A.W. (1972) Factors involved in mastitis control: a comparative study between high and low incidence herds. *Veterinary Record*, **91**, 615–624

Pearson, R.A. (1983) Prevention of foot lesions in broiler breeder hens kept in individual cages. *British Poultry Science*, **24**, 183–190

Pendergrass, T.W. and Hayes, H.M. (1975) Cryptorchism and related defects in dogs: epidemiologic comparisons with man. *Teratology*, **12**, 51–56

Penny, R.H.C., Cameron, R.D.A., Johnson, S., Kenyon, P.J., Smith, H.A., Bell, A.W.P., Cole, J.P.L. and Taylor, J. (1980) Foot rot of pigs: the influence of biotin supplementation on foot lesions in cows. *Veterinary Record*, **107**, 350–351

Peraino, C., Fry, R.J.M. and Staffeldt, E. (1977) Effects of varying the onset and duration of exposure to phenobarbital on its enhancement of 2-acetylaminofluorene-induced hepatic tumorigenesis. *Cancer Research*, **37**, 3623–3627

Peralta, E.A., Carpenter, T.E. and Farver, T.B. (1982) The application of time series analysis to determine the pattern of foot-and-mouth disease in cattle in Paraguay. *Preventive Veterinary Medicine*, **1**, 27–36

Perera, F.P. and Weinstein, I.B. (1982) Molecular epidemiology and carcinogen-DNA adduct detection: new approaches to studies of human cancer causation. *Journal of Chronic Diseases*, **35**, 581–600

Perry, B.D. and McCauley, E.H. (1984) Owner interview surveys as a basis for estimating animal productivity and disease impact in developing countries. In: Society for Veterinary Epidemiology and Preventive Medicine, Proceedings, Edinburgh, 10–11 July 1984. Ed. Thrusfield, M.V., pp. 54–62

Perry, B.D., Matthewman, R.W., Eicher, E. and Snacken, M. (1983) An evaluation of the efficacy of a questionnaire survey by comparison with data from sentinel herds. In: Proceedings of the Third International Symposium on Veterinary Epidemiology and Economics. Arlington, Virginia, 6–10 September 1982, p. 667. Veterinary Medical Publishing, Edwardsville

Perry, B.D., Mwanauma, B., Schels, H.F., Eicher, E. and Zaman, M.R. (1984a) A study of health and productivity in traditionally managed cattle in Zambia. *Preventive Veterinary Medicine*, **2**, 633–653

Perry, B.D., Palmer, J.E., Birch, J.B., Magnusson, R.A., Morris, D. and Troutt, H.F. (1984b) Epidemiological characterization of an acute equine diarrhoea syndrome: the case−control approach. In: Society for Veterinary Epidemiology and Preventive Medicine, Proceedings, Edinburgh, 10−11 July 1984. Ed. Thrusfield, M.V., pp. 148−153

Perry, B.D., Palmer, J.E., Troutt, H.F., Birch, J.B., Morris, D., Ehrich, M. and Rikihisa, Y. (1986) A case−control study of Potomac horse fever. *Preventive Veterinary Medicine*, **4**, 69−82

Perry, B.D., Lessard, P., Norval, R.A.I., Kundert, K. and Kruska, R. (1990) Climate, vegetation and the distribution of *Rhipicephalus appendiculatus* in Africa. *Parasitology Today*, **6**, 100−104

Persing, D.H., Smith, T.F., Tenover, F.C. and White, T.J. (Eds) (1993) *Diagnostic Molecular Microbiology: Principles and Applications*. American Society for Microbiology, Washington, DC

Peters, J.A. (1969) Canine mastocytoma: excess risk as related to ancestry. *Journal of the National Cancer Institute*, **42**, 435−443

Peterse, D.J. and Antonisse, W. (1981) Genetic aspects of feet soundness in cattle. *Livestock Production Science*, **8**, 253−261

Petersen, G.V. (1983) The effect of swimming lambs and subsequent resting periods on the ultimate pH of meat. *Meat Science*, **9**, 237−246

Peto, R. (1977) Epidemiology, multistage models and short-term mutagenicity tests. In: *Origins of Human Cancer*. Eds Hiatt, H.H., Watson, J.D. and Winsten, J.A., pp. 1403−1429. Cold Spring Harbor Laboratory, New York

Peto, R. (1978) Clinical trial methodology. *Biomedicine Special*, 24−36

Pfeiffer, D., Cortes, C.E., Otte, E. and Morris, R.S. (1988) Management factors affecting the prevalence of brucellosis in traditionally managed cattle herds in Northern Colombia. *Acta Veterinaria Scandinavica*, Suppl. 84, 133−135

Pfeiffer, D.U., Morris, R.S., Harris, A., Jockson, R. and Paterson, B. (1991) The epidemiology of bovine tuberculosis in the common brushtail possum. In: Proceedings of the Sixth International Symposium on Veterinary Epidemiology and Economics, Ottawa, 12−16 August 1991. Ed. Martin, S.W., pp. 430−433

Pharo, H.J. (1983) DAISY — Health and fertility monitoring for dairy herds. In: Society for Veterinary Epidemiology and Preventive Medicine, Proceedings, Southampton, 12−13 April 1983. Ed. Thrusfield, M.V., pp. 37−44

Pharo, H.J., Esslemont, R.J. and Putt, S.N.H. (1984) Assessing the benefits and costs of a computerised information system in dairy herd management. In: Society for Veterinary Epidemiology and Preventive Medicine, Proceedings, Edinburgh, 10−11 July 1984. Ed. Thrusfield, M.V., pp. 80−89

Physick-Sheard, P.W. (1986a) Career profile of the Canadian Standardbred I. Influence of age, gait and sex upon chances of racing. *Canadian Journal of Veterinary Research*, **50**, 449−456

Physick-Sheard, P.W. (1986b) Career profile of the Canadian Standardbred II. Influence of age, gait and sex upon number of races, money won and race times. *Canadian Journal of Veterinary Research*, **50**, 457−470

Physick-Sheard, P.W. and Russell, M. (1986) Career profile of the Canadian Standardbred III. Influence of temporary absence from racing and season. *Canadian Journal of Veterinary Research*, **50**, 471−478

Piantadosi, S., Byar, D.P. and Green, S.B. (1988) The ecological fallacy. *American Journal of Epidemiology*, **127**, 893−904

Pierrepoint, C.G. (1985) Possible benefits to veterinary medicine of considering dogs as a model for human cancer. *Journal of Small Animal Practice*, **26**, 43−47

Pierrepoint, C.G., Thomas, S. and Eaton, C.L. (1984) Hormones and cancer. In: *Progress in Cancer Research and Therapy*, Vol. 31. Eds Bresciani, F., King, R.J.B., Lippman, M.E., Namer, M. and Raynaud, J.-P., pp. 357−365. Raven Press, New York

Pike, M.C. and Casagrande, J.T. (1979) Re: cost considerations and sample size requirements in cohort and case−control studies (letter). *American Journal of Epidemiology*, **110**, 100−102

Pike, M.C. and Smith, P.G. (1968) Disease clustering: a generalization of Knox's approach to the detection of space −time interactions. *Biometrics*, **24**, 541−556

Pilchard, E.I. (1979) The world situation for animal health and disease information. *Journal of the American Veterinary Medical Association*, **175**, 1297−1300

Pilchard, E.I. (1985) Standardized nomenclature of veterinary medicine: taking the first step. *Journal of the American Veterinary Medical Association*, **187**, 798−799

Pilliner, S. (1992) *Horse Nutrition and Feeding*. Blackwell Scientific Publications, Oxford

Pinney, M.E. (1981) How I learned live with the computer. *Veterinary Record*, **109**, 431−432

Pinsent, P.J.N. (1989) Grass sickness of horses (grass disease: equine dysautonomia). In: Grunsell, C.S.G., Raw, M.-E. and Hill, F.W.G. (Eds). *The Veterinary Annual*, **29**, 1−12. Wright, London

Pisano, R.G. and Storer, T.I. (1948) Burrows and feeding of the Norway rat. *Journal of Mammalogy*, **29**, 374−383

Pivnick, H. and Nurmi, E. (1982) The Nurmi concept and its role in the control of *Salmonellae* in poultry. In: *Developments in Food Microbiology − 1*. Ed. Davies, R., pp. 41−70. Applied Science Publishers, Barking

Plackett, P. and Alton, G.G. (1975) A mechanism for prozone formation in the complement fixation test for bovine brucellosis. *Australian Veterinary Journal*, **52**, 136−140

Plowright, R.C. and Paloheimo, J.E. (1977) A theoretical study of population dynamics in the sheep tick. *Theoretical Population Biology*, **12**, 286−297

Plowright, W., Ferris, R.D. and Scott, G.R. (1960) Blue wildebeest and the aetiological agent of bovine malignant catarrhal fever. *Nature, London*, **188**, 1167−1169

Plowright, W., Perry, C.T. and Greig, A. (1974) Sexual transmission of African swine fever virus in the tick, *Ornithodoros moubata porcinus*, Walton. *Research in Veterin-*

ary Science, **17**, 106–113

Pocock, S.J. (1977) Group sequential methods in the design and analysis of clinical trials. *Biometrika*, **64**, 191–199

Pocock, S.J. (1983) *Clinical Trials: A Practical Approach*. John Wiley, Chichester and New York

Pointon, A. and Hueston, W.D. (1990) The National Animal Health Monitoring System (NAHMS): evolution of an animal health information database system in the USA. In: Society for Veterinary Epidemiology and Preventive Medicine, Proceedings, Belfast, 4–6 April 1990. Ed. Thrusfield, M.V., pp. 70–82

Pointon, A.M. (1989) *Campylobacter* associated intestinal pathology in pigs. *Australian Veterinary Journal*, **66**, 90–91

Pointon, A.M., Heap, P. and McCloud, P. (1985) Enzootic pneumonia of pigs in South Australia — factors relating to incidence of disease. *Australian Veterinary Journal*, **62**, 98–101

Pollard, J.C., Littlejohn, R.P., Johnstone, P., Laas, F.J., Corson, I.D. and Suttie, J.M. (1992) Behavioural and heart rate responses to velvet antler removal in red deer. *New Zealand Veterinary Journal*, **40**, 65–71

Pollitzer, R. and Meyer, K.F. (1961) The ecology of plague. In: *Studies in Disease Ecology*. Ed. May, J.M., pp. 433–510. Hafner Publishing, New York

Poppensiek, G.C., Budd, D.E. and Scholtens, R.G. (1966) *A Historical Survey of Animal Disease Morbidity and Mortality Reporting*. National Academy of Sciences, Washington, DC, Publication No. 1346

Porter, P. (1979) Hazards of recycling enteropathogens (letter). *Veterinary Record*, **105**, 515–516

Powell, D.G. (1985) International movement of horses and its influence on the spread of infection. In: Society for Veterinary Epidemiology and Preventive Medicine, Proceedings, Reading, 27–29 March 1985. Ed. Thrusfield, M.V., pp. 90–94

Prabhakaran, P., Soman, M., Iyer, R.P. and Abraham, J. (1980) Common disease conditions among cattle slaughtered in Trichur municipal slaughterhouse: a preliminary study. *Kerala Journal of Veterinary Science*, **11**, 159–163

Pratt, D.J., Greenway, P.J. and Gwynne, M.D. (1966) A classification of East African rangeland, with an appendix on terminology. *Journal of Applied Ecology*, **3**, 369–382

Priester, W.A. (1964) *Standard Nomenclature of Veterinary Diseases and Operations*. USHEW/PHS National Cancer Institute, Bethesda, MD. 1st edition revised 1966. 2nd (abridged) edition 1975

Priester, W.A. (1967) Canine lymphoma: relative risk in the boxer breed. *Journal of the National Cancer Institute*, **39**, 833–845

Priester, W.A. (1971) *Coding Supplement to Standard Nomenclature of Veterinary Diseases and Operations*. USHEW/PHS National Cancer Institute, Bethesda, MD. Revised 1977

Priester, W.A. (1972a) Congenital ocular defects in cattle, horses, cats and dogs. *Journal of the American Veterinary Medical Association*, **160**, 1504–1511

Priester, W.A. (1972b) Sex, size and breed as risk factors in canine patellar dislocation. *Journal of the American Veterinary Medical Association*, **160**, 740–742

Priester, W.A. (1973) Skin tumors in domestic animals. Data from 12 United States and Canadian colleges of veterinary medicine. *Journal of the National Cancer Institute*, **50**, 457–466

Priester, W.A. (1974a) Canine progressive retinal atrophy: occurrence by age, breed and sex. *American Journal of Veterinary Research*, **35**, 571–574

Priester, W.A. (1974b) Data from eleven United States and Canadian colleges of veterinary medicine on pancreatic carcinoma in domestic animals. *Cancer Research*, **34**, 1372–1375

Priester, W.A. (1974c) Pancreatic islet cell tumors in domestic animals. Data from 11 colleges of veterinary medicine in the United States and Canada. *Journal of the National Cancer Institute*, **53**, 227–229

Priester, W.A. (1975) Collecting and using veterinary clinical data. In: *Animal Disease Monitoring*. Eds Ingram, D.G., Mitchell, W.F. and Martin, S.W., pp. 119–128. Charles C. Thomas, Springfield

Priester, W.A. (1976a) Canine intervertebral disc disease: occurrence by age, breed and sex among 8,117 cases. *Theriogenology*, **6**, 293–303

Priester, W.A. (1976b) Hepatic angiosarcomas in dogs: an excessive frequency as compared with man. *Journal of the National Cancer Institute*, **57**, 451–453

Priester, W.A. and Hayes, H.M. (1973) Feline leukaemia after feline infectious anaemia. *Journal of the National Cancer Institute*, **51**, 289–291

Priester, W.A. and Mantel, N. (1971) Occurrence of tumours in domestic animals. Data from twelve United States and Canadian colleges of veterinary medicine. *Journal of the National Cancer Institute*, **47**, 1333–1344

Priester, W.A. and McKay, F.W. (1980) *The Occurrence of Tumours in Domestic Animals*. National Cancer Institute Monograph No. 54. United States Department of Health and Human Services. National Cancer Institute, Bethesda

Priester, W.A. and Mulvihill, J.J. (1972) Canine hip dysplasia: relative risk by sex, size and breed, and comparative aspects. *Journal of the American Veterinary Medical Association*, **160**, 735–739

Priester, W.A., Glass, A.G. and Waggoner, N.S. (1970) Congenital defects in domesticated animals: general considerations. *American Journal of Veterinary Research*, **31**, 1871–1879

Primrose, S.B. (1976) *Bacterial Transduction*. Meadowfield Press, Shildon

Pritchard, D.G., Carpenter, G.A., Morzaria, S.P., Harkness, J.W., Richards, M.S. and Brewer, J.I. (1981) Effect of air filtration on respiratory disease in intensively housed veal calves. *Veterinary Record*, **109**, 5–9

Pritchard, D.G., Edwards, S., Morzaria, S.P., Andrews, A.H., Peters, A.R. and Gilmour, N.J.L. (1983) Case–control studies in the evaluation of serological data from respiratory disease outbreaks in cattle. In: Society for Veterinary

Epidemiology and Preventive Medicine, Proceedings, South-ampton, 12−13 April 1983. Ed. Thrusfield, M.V., pp. 131−138

Pritchard, D.G., Little, T.W.A., Wrathall, A.E. and Jones, P. (1985) Epidemiology of leptospirosis in relation to repro-ductive disease in pigs. *The Pig Veterinary Society Proceed-ings*, **12**, 65−82

Pritchard, D.G., Allsup, T.N., Pennycott, T.W., Palmer, N.M.A., Woolley, J.C. and Richards, M.S. (1989) Analysis of risk factors for infection of cattle herds with *Leptospira interrogans* serovar *hardjo*. In: Society for Veterinary Epide-miology and Preventive Medicine, Proceedings, Exeter, 12−14 April 1989. Ed. Rowlands, G.J., pp. 130−138

Pritchard, W.R. (1986) Veterinary education for the 21st century. *Journal of the American Veterinary Medical Associa-tion*, **189**, 172−177

Pritchard, W.R. (Ed.) (1989) *Current Status and Future Directions for Veterinary Medicine*. Pew National Veterinary Education Program Report. Duke University, Durham, North Carolina

Prothro, R.M. (1977) Disease and mobility: a neglected factor in epidemiology. *International Journal of Epidemiology*, **6**, 259−267

Proudman, C.J. (1992) A two-year prospective survey of equine colic in general practice. *Equine Veterinary Journal*, **24**, 90−93

Proudman, C.J. and Edwards, G.B. (1992) Validation of a centrifugation/flotation technique for the diagnosis of equine cestodiasis. *Veterinary Record*, **131**, 71−72

Prymak, C., McKee, L.J., Goldschmidt, M.H. and Glickman, L.T. (1988) Epidemiologic, clinical, pathologic and prognos-tic characteristics of splenic haemangiosarcoma and splenic haematoma in dogs: 217 cases (1985). *Journal of the American Veterinary Medical Association*, **193**, 706−712

Pugsley, S.L. (1981) The veterinary computer system at London zoo. In: *A Computerised Veterinary Clinical Data Base*. Proceedings of a symposium, Edinburgh, 30 September 1981. Ed. Thrusfield, M.V., p. 55. Department of Animal Health, Royal (Dick) School of Veterinary Studies, Edinburgh

Radostits, O.M. (Ed.) (1983) Symposium on herd health management — cow-calf and feedlot. *Veterinary Clinics of North America: Large Animal Practice*, **5**, 1−209

Radostits, O.M., Leslie, K.E. and Fetrow, J. (1994) *Herd Health: Food Animal Production Medicine*, 2nd edn. W.B. Saunders, Philadelphia

Ragland, W.L., Keown, G.H. and Spencer, G.R. (1970) Equine sarcoid. *Equine Veterinary Journal*, **2**, 2−11

Rahko, T. (1968) A statistical study of tumours in dogs. *Acta Veterinaria Scandinavica*, **9**, 328−349

Ramsey, F.K. and Chivers, W.H. (1953) Mucosal disease of cattle. *North American Veterinarian*, **34**, 629−633

Ratcliffe, H. (1850) *Observations on the mortality and sickness existing among Friendly Societies: particularised for various trades, occupations and localities, with a series of tables, showing the value of annuities, sick gift, assurance for death, and contributions to be paid equivalent thereto: calculated*

from the experience of the members composing the Manchester Unity of the Independent Order of Odd Fellows. George Falkener, Manchester. Reprinted in *Mortality in Mid-19th Century Britain*. Introduced by Wall, R. (1974) Gregg International, Amersham

Rattenborg, E.E. and Agger, J.F. (1991) Disease and mortality in the European hare (*Lepus europaeus* Pallas) population in Denmark, 1932−1985. In: Proceedings of the Sixth Interna-tional Symposium on Veterinary Epidemiology and Econ-omics, Ottawa, 12−16 August 1991. Ed. Martin, S.W., pp. 437−439

Reece, R.L. and Beddome, V.D. (1983) Causes of culling and mortality in three flocks of broiler chickens in Victoria during 1979. *Veterinary Record*, **112**, 450−452

Rees, W.G.H. and Davies, G. (1992) Legislation for health. In: *Livestock Health and Welfare*. Ed. Moss R., pp. 118−159. Longman Scientific & Technical, Harlow

Reeves, M.J., Gay, J.M., Hilbert, B.J. and Morris, R.S. (1989) Association of age, sex and breed factors in acute equine colic: a retrospective study of 320 cases admitted to a veterinary teaching hospital in the USA. *Preventive Veterinary Medicine*, **7**, 149−160

Reid, J. and Nolan, A.M. (1991) A comparison of the post-operative analgesic and sedative effects of flunixin and papaveretum in the dog. *Journal of Small Animal Practice*, **32**, 603−608

Reid, S.W.J. and Gettinby, G. (1994) Modelling the equine sarcoid. In: Society for Veterinary Epidemiology and Preven-tive Medicine, Proceedings, Belfast, 13−15 April 1994. Ed. Thrusfield, M.V., pp. 167−173

Reif, J.S. (1976) Seasonality, natality and herd immunity in feline panleukopenia. *American Journal of Epidemiology*, **103**, 81−87

Reif, J.S. (1983) Ecologic factors and disease. In: *Textbook of Veterinary Internal Medicine. Volume 1. Diseases of the Dog and Cat*, 2nd edn. Ed. Ettinger, S.J., pp. 147−173. W.B. Saunders, Philadelphia

Reif, J.S. and Brodey, R.S. (1969) The relationship between cryptorchidism and canine testicular neoplasia. *Journal of the American Veterinary Medical Association*, **155**, 2005−2010

Reif, J.S. and Cohen, D. (1970) Canine pulmonary disease. II. Retrospective radiographic analysis of pulmonary disease in rural and urban dogs. *Archives of Environmental Health*, **20**, 684−689

Reif, J.S. and Cohen, D. (1971) The environmental distribution of canine respiratory tract neoplasms. *Archives of Environ-mental Health*, **22**, 136−140

Reif, J.S. and Cohen, D. (1979) Canine pulmonary disease: a spontaneous model for environmental epidemiology. In: *Animals as Monitors of Environmental Pollutants*, pp. 241−250. National Academy of Sciences, Washington, DC

Reif, J.S., Maguire, T.G., Kenney, R.M. and Brodey, R.S. (1979) A cohort study of canine testicular neoplasia. *Journal of the American Veterinary Medical Association*, **175**, 719−723

Reif, J.S., Schweitzer, D.J., Ferguson, S.W. and Benjamin, S.A. (1983) Canine neoplasia and exposure to uranium mill tailings in Mesa County, Colorado. In: *Epidemiology Applied to Health Physics*. Proceedings of the 16th Midyear Topical Meeting of the Health Physics Society, Albuquerque, New Mexico, 9 – 13 January 1983, pp. 461 – 469. Rio Grande Chapter of the Health Physics Society

Reif, J.S., Dunn, K., Ogilvie, G.K. and Harris, C.K. (1992) Passive smoking and canine lung cancer. *American Journal of Epidemiology*, **135**, 234 – 239

Report (1983) *Risk Assessment: A Study Group Report*. The Royal Society, London

Report (1990) Potential use of live viral and bacterial vectors for vaccines. *Vaccine*, **8**, 425 – 437

Report (1992) *Risk Analysis, Perception and Management. Report of a Royal Society Study Group*. The Royal Society, London

Reutlinger, S. (1970) *Techniques for Project Appraisal Under Uncertainty*. World Bank Staff Occasional Paper No. 10, Washington, DC

Reynolds, D.J., Morgan, J.H., Chanter, N., Jones, P.W., Bridger, J.C., Debney, T.G. and Bunch, K.J. (1986) Microbiology of calf diarrhoea in southern Britain. *Veterinary Record*, **119**, 34 – 39

Ribble, C.S. (1989) Principles of implementing and marketing bovine health management programs. *Proceedings of the American Association of Bovine Practitioners*, **21**, 27 – 33

Ribelin, W.E. and Bailey, W.S. (1958) Oesophageal sarcomas associated with *Spirocirca lupi* infection in the dog. *Cancer*, **11**, 1242 – 1246

Rice, L. (1980a) Reproductive health management in beef cows. In: *Current Therapy in Theriogenology: Diagnosis, Treatment and Prevention of Reproductive Diseases in Animals*. Ed. Morrow, D., pp. 534 – 545. W.B. Saunders, Philadelphia

Rice, L. (1980b) Reproductive health program for beef cattle. In: *Current Therapy in Theriogenology: Diagnosis, Treatment and Prevention of Reproductive Diseases in Animals*. Ed. Morrow, D., pp. 545 – 548. W.B. Saunders, Philadelphia

Richards, M. (1954) *The Laws of Hywel Dda (The Book of Blegywryd)*. The University of Liverpool Press, Liverpool

Ricketts, S.W. and Alonso, S. (1991) The effect of age and parity on the development of equine chronic endometrial disease. *Equine Veterinary Journal*, **23**, 189 – 192

Riggenbach, C. (1988) National animal health information system in Switzerland. *Revue Scientifique et Technique, Office International des Epizooties*, **7**, 503 – 507

Riser, W.H. (1974) Canine hip dysplasia: cause and control. *Journal of the American Veterinary Medical Association*, **165**, 360 – 362

Roberts, D.F. (1985) A definition of genetic epidemiology. In: *Diseases of Complex Aetiology in Small Populations: Ethnic Differences and Research Approaches*. Proceedings of a symposium on Genetic Epidemiology in an Anthropological Context, Victoria, British Columbia, 18 – 19 August 1983. Eds Chakraborty, R. and Szathmary, E.J.E., pp. 9 – 20. Alan R. Liss, New York

Roberts, D.S. (1969) Synergic mechanisms in certain mixed infections. *Journal of Infectious Diseases*, **120**, 720 – 724

Roberts, L., Lawson, G.H.K., Rowland, A.C. and Laing, A.H. (1979) Porcine intestinal adenomatosis and its detection in a closed pig herd. *Veterinary Record*, **104**, 366 – 368

Roberts, L.S. and Cohen, J. (1985) Good with stats: Systat and Epistat. *PC Magazine*, **5**, 179 – 186

Robertson, F.J. (1971) Brucellosis: a possible symptomless carrier. *Veterinary Record*, **88**, 313 – 314

Robinson, R.A., Kobluk, C., Clanton, C., Martin, F., Gordon, B., Ames, T., Trent, M. and Ruth, G. (1988) Epidemiological studies of musculoskeletal racing and training injuries in thoroughbred horses, Minnesota, USA. *Acta Veterinaria Scandinavica*, Suppl. 84, 340 – 341

Robinson, W.S. (1950) Ecological correlations and the behavior of individuals. *American Sociological Review*, **15**, 351 – 357

Rodrigues, L. and Kirkwood, B.R. (1990) Case – control designs in the study of common diseases: updates on the demise of the rare disease assumption and the choice of sampling scheme for controls. *International Journal of Epidemiology*, **19**, 205 – 213

Roe, R.T. (1980) Features of the Australian National Animal Disease Information System. In: *Veterinary Epidemiology and Economics*. Proceedings of the Second International Symposium, Canberra, 7 – 11 May 1979. Eds Geering, W.A., Roe, R.T. and Chapman, L.A., pp. 26 – 34. Australian Government Publishing Service, Canberra

Rogan, W.J. and Gladen, B. (1978) Estimating prevalence from the results of a screening test. *American Journal of Epidemiology*, **107**, 71 – 76

Rogers, D.J. (1991) Satellite imagery: tsetse and trypanosomiasis in Africa. *Preventive Veterinary Medicine*, **11**, 201 – 220

Roitt, I.M. (1988) *Essential Immunology*, 6th edn. Blackwell Scientific Publications, Oxford

Rolfe, D.C. (1986) The development of an animal disease information system. In: Proceedings of the 4th International Symposium on Veterinary Epidemiology and Economics, Singapore, 18 – 22 November 1985, pp. 362 – 364

Rooney, J.R. (1982) The relationship of season of the year to lameness and breakdown in thoroughbred racehorses. *Journal of Equine Veterinary Science*, **2**, 174 – 176

Roos, L.L., Sharp, S.M. and Wajda, A. (1989) Assessing data quality: a computerized approach. *Social Science Medicine*, **28**, 175 – 182

Rosenberg, F.J., Astudillo, V.M. and Goic, R. (1980) Regional strategies for the control of foot-and-mouth disease — an ecological outlook. In: *Veterinary Epidemiology and Economics*. Proceedings of the Second International Symposium, Canberra, 7 – 11 May 1979. Eds Geering, W.A., Roe, R.T. and Chapman, L.A., pp. 587 – 596

Roslow, S. and Roslow, L. (1972) Unlisted phone subscribers are different. *Journal of Advertising Research*, **12**, 35 – 38

Ross, J.G. (1978) Stormont 'wet-day' fluke forecasting. In: *Weather and Parasitic Animal Disease*. Ed. Gibson, T.E., pp. 4 – 20. World Meteorological Organization Technical Note No. 159

Roth, H.H., Keymer, I.F. and Appleby, E.C. (1973) Computerised data recording from captive and free-living wild animals. *International Zoo Yearbook*, **13**, 252−257

Rothman, K.J. (1975) A pictorial representation of confounding in epidemiologic studies. *Journal of Chronic Diseases*, **28**, 101−108

Rothman, K.J. (1976) Causes. *American Journal of Epidemiology*, **104**, 587−592

Rothman, K.J. (1986) *Modern Epidemiology*. Little, Brown and Co., Boston and Toronto

Rothman, K.J. (1987) Clustering of disease. *American Journal of Public Health*, **77**, 13−15

Rothman, K.J. and Boice, J.D. (1982) *Epidemiologic Analysis with a Programmable Calculator*. Epidemiology Resources, Boston

Roudebush, P. (1984) Canine cough knowledge coupler. In: Proceedings of the Second Symposium on Computer Applications in Veterinary Medicine, College of Veterinary Medicine, Mississippi State University, 23−25 May 1984, pp. 127−129

Roueché, B. (1991) *The Medical Detectives*. Truman Talley Books/Plume, New York

Rowlands, G.J. and Booth, J.M. (1989) Methods of analysis of disease incidence data in a survey of bovine clinical mastitis. In: Society for Veterinary Epidemiology and Preventive Medicine, Proceedings, Exeter, 12−14 April 1989. Ed. Rowlands, G.J., pp. 25−36

Rowlands, G.J., Russell, A.M. and Williams, L.A. (1983) Effects of season, herd size, management system and veterinary practice on the lameness incidence in dairy cattle. *Veterinary Record*, **113**, 441−445

Rowlands, G.J., Lucey, S. and Russell, A.M. (1986) Susceptibility to disease in the dairy cow and its relationship with occurrences of other diseases in the current or preceding lactation. *Preventive Veterinary Medicine*, **4**, 223−234

Roy, J.H.B. (1980) *The Calf. Studies in the Agricultural and Food Sciences*, 4th edn. Butterworths, London and Boston

Ruble, R.P. and Hird, D.W. (1993) Congenital abnormalities in immature dogs from a pet store: 253 cases (1987−1988). *Journal of the American Veterinary Medical Association*, **202**, 633−636

Rudman, R. and Keiper, R.R. (1991) The body condition score of feral ponies on Assateague Island. *Equine Veterinary Journal*, **23**, 453−456

Ruppanner, R. (1972) Measurement of disease in animal populations based on interviews. *Journal of the American Veterinary Medical Association*, **161**, 1033−1038

Rushen, J. (1986) Some problems with the physiological concept of 'stress'. *Australian Veterinary Journal*, **63**, 359−361

Russel, A. (1985) Nutrition of the pregnant ewe. *In Practice*, **7**, 23−28

Russell, A.M. and Rowlands, G.J. (1983) COSREEL: Computerised recording system for herd health information management. *Veterinary Record*, **112**, 189−193

Russell, A.M., Rowlands, G.J., Shaw, S.R. and Weaver, A.D. (1982) Survey of lameness in British dairy cattle. *Veterinary Record*, **111**, 155−160

Russell, M. and Gruber, A. (1987) Risk assessment in environmental policy-making. *Science*, **236**, 286−290

Rutter, J.M. (1982) Diseases caused by mixed agents and factors. In: *The Control of Infectious Diseases in Farm Animals*, pp. 5−10. British Veterinary Association Trust Project on the future of animal health control, London

Saatkamp, H.W., Huirne, R.B.M., Dijkhuizen, A.A., Geers, R., Noordhuizen, J.P.T.M. and Goedseels, V. (1994) The potential value of identification and recording systems in contagious disease control. In: Proceedings of the 7th International Symposium on Veterinary Epidemiology and Economics, Nairobi, 15−19 August 1994. Eds Rowlands, G.J., Kyule, M.N. and Perry, B.D. *The Kenya Veterinarian*, **18**(2), 391−393

Sackett, D.I. (1979) Bias in analytic research. *Journal of Chronic Diseases*, **32**, 51−68

Salman, M.D., Reif, J.S., Rupp, L. and Aaronson, M.J. (1990) Chlorinated hydrocarbon insecticides in Colorado beef cattle − a pilot environmental monitoring system. *Journal of Toxicology and Environmental Health*, **31**, 125−132

Saloniemi, H. and Roine, K. (1981) Incidence of some metabolic diseases in dairy cows. *Nordisk Veterinærmedicin*, **33**, 289−296

Saloniemi, H., Grohn, Y.T. and Erb, H.N. (1988) Epidemiology of reproductive disorders in Finnish Ayrshire dairy cattle. In: *Environment and Animal Health*. Proceedings of the 6th International Congress on Animal Hygiene, 14−17 June 1988, Skara, Sweden, Vol. 1. Ed. Ekesbo, I., pp. 56−59

Salt, J. (1994) The epidemiological significance of foot-and-mouth disease virus carriers: a review. In: Society for Veterinary Epidemiology and Preventive Medicine, Proceedings, Belfast, 13−15 April 1994. Ed. Thrusfield, M.V., pp. 71−84

Samuels, M.L. (1989) *Statistics for the Life Sciences*. Deller Publishing, San Francisco

Sandals, W.C.D., Curtis, R.A., Cote, J.F. and Martin, S.W. (1979) The effect of retained placenta and metritis complex on reproductive performance in dairy cattle: a case−control study. *Canadian Veterinary Journal*, **20**, 131−135

Sanson, R.L., Pfeiffer, D.U. and Morris, R.S. (1991a) Geographic information systems: their applications in animal disease control. *Revue Scientifique et Technique, Office International des Epizooties*, **10**, 179−195

Sanson, R.L., Liberona, H. and Morris, R.S. (1991b) The use of a geographical information system in the management of a foot-and-mouth disease epidemic. *Preventive Veterinary Medicine*, **11**, 309−313

Sard, D.M. (1979) *Dealing with Data: The Practical Use of Numerical Information*. British Veterinary Association Publications, London

Sartwell, P.E. (1950) The distribution of incubation periods of infectious disease. *American Journal of Hygiene*, **51**, 310−318

Sartwell, P.E. (1966) The incubation period and the dynamics of infectious disease. *American Journal of Epidemiology*, **83**,

204–216

Sartwell, P.E. (1973) *Preventive Medicine and Public Health*. Appleton, Century Crofts, New York

Sasaki, M. (1991) Eradication of rinderpest — a review. In: South Asia Rinderpest Eradication Campaign. Proceedings of the Regional Expert Consultation on Rinderpest Eradication in South Asia, Bangkok, Thailand, 5–8 June 1990. RAPA Publication 1991/8, pp. 67–77. Food and Agriculture Organization, Bangkok

Scarff, D.H. and Lloyd, D.H. (1992) Double blind, placebo-controlled, crossover study of evening primrose oil in the treatment of canine atopy. *Veterinary Record*, **131**, 97–99

Scarlett, J.M., Moise, N.S. and Rayl, J. (1988) Feline hyperthyroidism: a descriptive and case–control study. *Preventive Veterinary Medicine*, **6**, 295–309

Schachter, J., Sugg, N. and Sung, M. (1978) Psittacosis: the reservoir persists. *Journal of Infectious Diseases*, **137**, 44–49

Scheaffer, R.L., Mendenhall, W. and Ott, L. (1979) *Elementary Survey Sampling*, 2nd edn. Duxbury Press, Belmont

Schepers, J.A. (1990) Data requirements and objectives for economic analyses of disease in farm livestock. In: Society for Veterinary Epidemiology and Preventive Medicine, Proceedings, Belfast, 4–6 April 1990. Ed. Thrusfield, M.V., pp. 120–132

Scherer, W.F., Moyer, J.T., Izumi, T., Gresser, I. and McCown, J. (1959) Ecologic studies of Japanese Encephalitis virus in Japan. VI. Swine infection. *American Journal of Tropical Medicine and Hygiene*, **8**, 698–706

Schlesselman, J.J. (1982) *Case–Control Studies: Design, Conduct, Analysis*. Oxford University Press, New York

Schmelzer, L.L. and Tabershaw, I.R. (1968) Exposure factors in occupational coccidioidomycosis. *American Journal of Public Health*, **58**, 107–113

Schneider, R. (1970) Comparison of age, sex and incidence rates in human and canine breast cancer. *Cancer*, **26**, 419–426

Schneider, R. (1976) Epidemiologic studies of cancer in man and animals sharing the same environment. In: *Prevention and Detection of Cancer. Vol. 2. Part I: Etiology: Prevention Methods*. Proceedings of the 3rd International Symposium on the Detection and Prevention of Cancer, New York, 26 April–1 May 1976. Ed. Nieburgs, H.E., pp. 1377–1387. Marcel Dekker, New York

Schneider, R. (1983) Comparison of age- and sex-specific incidence rate patterns of the leukaemia complex in the cat and dog. *Journal of the National Cancer Institute*, **70**, 971–977

Schneider, R. and Vaida, M.L. (1975) Survey of canine and feline populations: Alameda and Contra Costa Counties, California, 1970. *Journal of the American Veterinary Medical Association*, **166**, 481–486

Schneider, R., Dorn, C.R. and Taylor, D.O.N. (1969) Factors influencing canine mammary cancer development and postsurgical survival. *Journal of the National Cancer Institute*, **43**, 1249–1261

Schnurrenberger, P.R., Kangilaski, E., Berg, L.E. and Bashe, W.J. (1961) Characteristics of a rural Ohio dog population. *Veterinary Medicine*, **56**, 519–523

Schofield, F.W. (1949) Virus enteritis in mink. *North American Veterinarian*, **30**, 651–654

Schukken, Y.H., Erb, H.N. and Smith, R.D. (1988) The relationship between mastitis and retained placenta in a commercial population of Holstein dairy cows. *Preventive Veterinary Medicine*, **5**, 181–190

Schukken, Y.H., Erb, H.N., White, M.E., Schwager, S.J. and Scholl, D.T. (1990) A review of statistical techniques to evaluate space–time clustering in disease occurrence. In: Society for Veterinary Epidemiology and Preventive Medicine, Proceedings, Belfast, 4–6 April 1990. Ed. Thrusfield, M.V., pp. 167–178

Schwabe, A.E. and Hall, S.J.G. (1989) Dystocia in nine British breeds of cattle and its relationship to the dimensions of the dam and calf. *Veterinary Record*, **125**, 636–639

Schwabe, C. (1982) The current epidemiological revolution in veterinary medicine. Part 1. *Preventive Veterinary Medicine*, **1**, 5–15

Schwabe, C.W. (1980a) Animal disease control. Part I. Developments prior to 1960. *Sudan Journal of Veterinary Science and Animal Husbandry*, **21**, 43–54

Schwabe, C.W. (1980b) Animal disease control. Part II. Newer methods, with possibility for their application in the Sudan. *Sudan Journal of Veterinary Science and Animal Husbandry*, **21**, 55–65

Schwabe, C.W. (1984) *Veterinary Medicine and Human Health*, 3rd edn. Williams and Wilkins, Baltimore and London

Schwabe, C.W., Riemann, H. and Franti, C. (1977) *Epidemiology in Veterinary Practice*. Lea and Feibiger, Philadelphia

Scott, R.J. (1981) Zoonoses in the abattoir. In: *Advances in Veterinary Public Health*, Vol. 2. Ed. Senevirata, P., pp. 68–82. Australian College of Veterinary Scientists, Brisbane

Seamer, J.H. and Quimby, F.W. (Eds) (1992) Animal Welfare. Proceedings of the Animal Welfare Sessions, XXIV World Veterinary Congress, Rio de Janeiro, 1991. Animal Welfare Committee of the World Veterinary Association, London

Selby, L.A., Edmonds, L.D., Parke, D.W., Stewart, R.W., Marienfeld, C.J. and Heidlage, W.F. (1973) Use of mailed questionnaire data in a study of swine congenital malformations. *Canadian Journal of Comparative Medicine*, **37**, 413–417

Selby, L.A., Edmonds, L.D. and Hyde, L.D. (1976) Epidemiological field studies of animal populations. *Canadian Journal of Comparative Medicine*, **40**, 135–141

Selby, L.A., Corwin, R.M. and Hayes, H.M. (1980) Risk factors associated with canine heartworm infection. *Journal of the American Veterinary Medical Association*, **176**, 33–35

Selikoff, I.J., Hammond, E.C. and Seidman, H. (1979) Mortality experience of insulation workers in the United States and Canada, 1943–1976. *Annals of the New York Academy of Sciences*, **330**, 91–116

Sellers, R.F. (1982) Eradication — local and national. In: *The Control of Infectious Diseases in Farm Animals*, pp. 18–21. British Veterinary Association Trust Project on the future of animal health control, London

Sellers, R.F. and Gloster, J. (1980) The Northumberland epidemic of foot-and-mouth disease, 1966. *Journal of Hygiene, Cambridge*, **85**, 129−140

Sellers, R.F. and Maarouf, A.R. (1990) Trajectory analysis of winds and vesicular stomatitis virus in North America, 1982−85. *Epidemiology and Infection*, **104**, 313−328

Sellers, R.F., Pedgley, D.E. and Tucker, M.R. (1978) Possible windborne spread of bluetongue to Portugal, June−July 1956. *Journal of Hygiene, Cambridge*, **81**, 189−196

Selye, H. (1946) The general adaptation syndrome and the diseases of adaptation. *Journal of Clinical Endocrinology*, **6**, 117−230

Sembrat, R.F. (1975) The acute abdomen in the horse. Epidemiologic considerations. *Archives of the American College of Veterinary Surgeons*, **4**(2), 34−39

Senn, S. (1993) *Cross-over Trials in Clinical Research*. John Wiley, Chichester and New York

Shane, S.M., Gyimah, J.E., Harrington, K.S. and Snider, T.G. (1985) Etiology and pathogenesis of necrotic enteritis. *Veterinary Research Communications*, **9**, 269−287

Shewhart, W.A. (1931) *The Economic Control of the Quality of the Manufactured Product*. Macmillan, New York

Shope, R.E. (1931) Swine influenza. III. Filtration experiment and etiology. *Journal of Experimental Medicine*, **54**, 373−385

Short, C.E. (Ed.) (1987) *Principles and Practice of Veterinary Anesthesia*. Williams and Wilkins, Baltimore

Shott, S. (1985) Statistics in veterinary research. *Journal of the American Veterinary Medical Association*, **187**, 138−141

Shuster, J. (1992) *Practical Handbook of Sample Size Guidelines for Clinical Trials*. CRC Press, Boca Raton

Siegel, S. and Castellan, N.J. (1988) *Nonparametric Statistics for the Behavioral Sciences*, 2nd edn. McGraw-Hill, New York

Simmons, A. and Cuthbertson, J.C. (1985) Time series analysis of ovine pneumonia using Scottish slaughterhouse data. In: Society for Veterinary Epidemiology and Preventive Medicine, Proceedings, Reading, 27−29 March 1985. Ed. Thrusfield, M.V., pp. 130−141

Simpson, B.H. and Wright, D.F. (1980) The use of questionnaires to assess the importance of clinical disease in sheep. In: *Veterinary Epidemiology and Economics*. Proceedings of the Second International Symposium, Canberra, 7−11 May 1979. Eds Geering, W.A., Roe, R.T. and Chapman, L.A., pp. 97−105. Australian Government Publishing Service, Canberra

Sinclair, I.J., Tarry, D.W. and Wassall, D.A. (1989) Serological survey of the incidence of *Hypoderma bovis* in cattle in 1988. *Veterinary Record*, **124**, 243−244

Singh, K.P.R., Khorshed, M.P. and Anderson, C.R. (1964) Transmission of Kyasanur Forest Disease virus by *Haemaphysalis turturis*, *Haemaphysalis papuana kinneari* and *Haemaphysalis minuta*. *Indian Journal of Medical Research*, **52**, 566−573

Singleton, W.B. (1993) Companion animal medicine: future outlook. In: *The Advancement of Veterinary Science. The Bicentenary Symposium Series. Volume 1: Veterinary Medicine Beyond 2000*. Ed. Michell, A.R., pp. 249−263. CAB International, Wallingford

Sinnecker, H. (1976) *General Epidemiology* (translated by Walker, N.). John Wiley, London

Slater, M.R., Scarlett, J.M. and Erb, H.N. (1991) A comparison of five strategies for selecting control groups: a canine osteochondritis dissecans example. *Preventive Veterinary Medicine*, **10**, 319−326

Slater, M.R., Scarlett, J.M., Donoghue, S. and Erb, H.N. (1992) The repeatability and validity of a telephone questionnaire on diet and exercise in dogs. *Preventive Veterinary Medicine*, **13**, 77−91

Slettbakk, T., Jorstad, A., Farver, T.B. and Hird, D.W. (1990) Impact of milking characteristics and teat morphology on somatic cell counts in first-lactation Norwegian cattle. *Preventive Veterinary Medicine*, **8**, 253−267

Slocombe, J.O.D. (1975) Surveillance for parasitism in domestic animals. In: *Animal Disease Monitoring*. Eds Ingram, D.G., Mitchell, W.F. and Martin, S.W., pp. 129−135. Charles C. Thomas, Springfield

Smith, E.J., Kelly, J.M. and Whitaker, D.A. (1983) Health and fertility data recorded by members of the Dairy Herd Health and Productivity Service. In: Society for Veterinary Epidemiology and Preventive Medicine, Proceedings, Southampton, 12−13 April 1983. Ed. Thrusfield, M.V., pp. 8−12

Smith, G. (1984) Density-dependent mechanisms in the regulation of *Fasciola hepatica* populations in sheep. *Parasitology*, **88**, 449−461

Smith, K.G.V. (Ed.) (1973) *Insects and Other Arthropods of Medical Importance*. The Trustees of the British Museum (Natural History), London

Smith, L.P. and Hugh-Jones, M.E. (1969) The weather factor in foot-and-mouth disease epidemics. *Nature*, **223**, 712−715

Smith, R.D. (1988) Veterinary clinical research: a survey of study designs and clinical issues appearing in a practice journal. *Journal of Veterinary Medical Education*, **15**(1), 2−7

Smith, R.D. (1991) *Veterinary Clinical Epidemiology: A Problem-Oriented Approach*. Butterworth-Heinemann, Stoneham

Smith, W.J. (1981) Rectal prolapse in swine. *The Pig Veterinary Society Proceedings*, **7**, 68−72

Smithcors, J.F. (1957) *Evolution of the Veterinary Art*. Veterinary Medicine Publishing Company, Kansas

Snedecor, G.W. and Cochran, W.G. (1980) *Statistical Methods*, 7th edn. Iowa State University Press, Ames

Snodgrass, D.R. (1974) Studies on bovine petechial fever and tick-borne fever. PhD Thesis, University of Edinburgh

Snodgrass, D.R., Terzolo, H.R., Sherwood, D., Campbell, I., Menzies, J.D. and Synge, B.A. (1986) Aetiology of diarrhoea in young calves. *Veterinary Record*, **119**, 31−34

Snow, J. (1855) *On the Mode of Communication of Cholera*, 2nd edn. Churchill, London. Reproduced in *Snow on Cholera*. Commonwealth Fund, New York, 1936. Reprinted by Hafner, New York, 1965

Somvanshi, R. (1991) Horn cancer in Indian cattle. *Veterinary Bulletin*, **61**, 901−911

Sonnenschein, E., Glickman, L.T., McKee, L. and Goldschmidt, M. (1987) Nutritional risk factors for spontaneous breast cancer in pet dogs: a case–control study. *American Journal of Epidemiology*, **126**, 736

Sonnenschein, E.G., Glickman, L.T., Goldschmidt, M.H. and McKee, L.J. (1991) Body conformation, diet and risk of breast cancer in pet dogs: a case–control study. *American Journal of Epidemiology*, **133**, 694–703

Sørensen, J.T. and Enevoldsen, C. (1992) Modelling the dynamics of the health-production complex in livestock herds: a review. *Preventive Veterinary Medicine*, **13**, 287–297

Soulsby, E.J.L. (1982) *Helminths, Arthropods and Protozoa of Domestic Animals*, 7th edn. Baillière Tindall, London

Southwood, T.R.E. (1978) *Ecological Methods with Particular Reference to the Study of Insect Populations*, 2nd edn. Chapman and Hall, London

Spangler, E., Dohoo, I.R., Kendall, O. and Hurnik, D. (1991) Influence of pre-slaughter processing factors in the development of pale, soft and exudative pork. In: Proceedings of the Sixth International Symposium on Veterinary Epidemiology and Economics, Ottawa, 12–16 August 1991. Ed. Martin, S.W., pp. 422–424

Sparkes, A.H., Gruffydd-Jones, T.J., Shaw, S.W., Wright, A.I. and Stokes, C.R. (1993) Epidemiological and diagnostic features of canine and feline dermatophytosis in the United Kingdom from 1956 to 1991. *Veterinary Record*, **133**, 57–61

Spearman, C. (1908) The method of 'right and wrong' cases ('constant stimuli') without Gauss's formulae. *British Journal of Psychology*, **2**, 227–242

Spinu, I. and Biberi-Moroianu, S. (1969) Theoretical and practical problems concerning the eradication of communicable diseases. *Archives Roumaines de Pathologie Experimentale et de Microbiologie*, **28**, 725–742 (in English)

Sprague, R.H. and Carlson, E.D. (1982) *Building Effective Decision Support Systems*. Prentice Hall, Englewood Cliffs

Srebernik, N. and Appleby, E.C. (1991) Breed prevalence and sites of haemangioma and haemangiosarcoma in dogs. *Veterinary Record*, **129**, 408–409

Stallbaumer, M. and Skrzynecki, E. (1987) The use of discriminant analysis in a case–control study of coccidiosis in European broiler flocks. In: Society for Veterinary Epidemiology and Preventive Medicine, Proceedings, Solihull, 1–3 April 1987. Ed. Thrusfield, M.V., pp. 108–117

Stallbaumer, M.F. (1983) The prevalence of *Cysticercus tenuicollis* in slaughtered sheep in Britain. In: Society for Veterinary Epidemiology and Preventive Medicine, Proceedings, Southampton, 12–13 April 1983. Ed. Thrusfield, M.V., pp. 124–130

Stark, D.A. and Anderson, N.G. (1990) A case–control study of *Nocardia* mastitis in Ontario dairy herds. *Canadian Veterinary Journal*, **31**, 197–201

Stärk, K.D.C., Vicari, A. and Nicolet, J. (1994) Contagious bovine pleuropneumonia (CBPP) surveillance in Switzerland: a pilot study. In: Society for Veterinary Epidemiology and Preventive Medicine, Proceedings, Belfast, 13–15 April 1994. Ed. Thrusfield, M.V., pp. 96–103

Stedman (1982) *Stedman's Medical Dictionary*, 24th edn. Williams and Wilkins, Baltimore

Steele, J.H., Hendricks, S.L., Barr, R. and Parker, R.L. (1972) Brucellosis in the United States, 1970. *Archives of Environmental Health*, **25**, 66–72

Steere, A.C., Malawista, S.E., Snydman, D.R., Shope, R.E., Andiman, W.A., Ross, M.R. and Steele, F.M. (1977) Lyme arthritis. An epidemic of oligoarticular arthritis in children and adults in three Connecticut communities. *Arthritis and Rheumatism*, **20**, 7–17

Stein, T., Molitor, T., Joo, H.S. and Leman, A.D. (1982) Porcine parvovirus infection and its control. *The Pig Veterinary Society Proceedings*, **9**, 158–167

Stein, T.E. (1986) Marketing health management to food animal enterprises. Part II. The structure of herd health management services. *Compendium on Continuing Education for the Practising Veterinarian*, **8**, S330–S336

Stein, T.E. (1988) Problem-oriented population medicine in swine breeding herds. *Compendium on Continuing Education for the Practising Veterinarian*, **10**, 871–879

Stein, T.E., Dijkhuizen, A., D'Allaire, S. and Morris, R.S. (1990) Sow culling and mortality in commercial swine breeding herds. *Preventive Veterinary Medicine*, **9**, 85–94

Stephen, L.E. (1980) An index for coding and recording veterinary diseases and pathological states, according to body system(s) involved and aetiology or indicated cause. In: *Veterinary Epidemiology and Economics*. Proceedings of the Second International Symposium, Canberra, 7–11 May 1979. Eds Geering, W.A., Roe, R.T. and Chapman, L.A., pp. 247–249. Australian Government Publishing Service, Canberra

Stewart, G.T. (1968) Limitations of the germ theory. *The Lancet*, **1**, 1077–1081

Stewart, I. (1992) Risky business. In: *The New Scientist: Inside Science*. Ed. Fifield, R., pp. 329–342. Penguin Books, Harmondsworth

Steyn, P.F. and Wittum, T.B. (1993) Radiographic, epidemiologic and clinical aspects of simultaneous pleural and peritoneal effusions in dogs and cats: 48 cases (1982–1991). *Journal of the American Veterinary Medical Association*, **202**, 307–312

Stites, D.P., Stobo, J.D., Fundenberg, H.H. and Wells, J.V. (1982) *Basic and Clinical Immunology*, 4th edn. Lange Medical Publications, Los Altos

Stites, D.P. and Rodgers, R.P.C. (1991) Clinical laboratory methods for detection of antigen and antibodies. In: *Basic and Clinical Immunology*, 7th edn. Eds Stites, D.P. and Terr, A.I., pp. 217–262. Appleton and Lange, East Norwalk

Stone, D.J.W. and Thrusfield, M.V. (1989) A small animal clinical and epidemiological relational database. *Preventive Veterinary Medicine*, **7**, 289–302

Stuart, R.D. (1946) Canine leptospirosis in Glasgow. *Veterinary Record*, **58**, 131–132

Stuart-Harris, C.H. and Schild, G.C. (1976) *Influenza, the Viruses and the Disease*. Edward Arnold, London

Sugden, R. and Williams, A. (1978) *The Principles of Practical Cost–Benefit Analysis*. Oxford University Press, London

Sukura, A., Gröhn, Y.T., Junttila, J. and Palolahti, T. (1992) Association between feline immunodeficiency virus antibodies and host characteristics in Finnish cats. *Acta Veterinaria Scandinavica*, **33**, 325–334

Summers, M. (1961) *The Vampire in Europe*. University Books, New York

Sung, H.-T. (1992) Disease reporting systems in Taiwan, R.O.C. *Office International des Epizooties Quarterly Epidemiology Report (Asian and Pacific Region)*, **1**, 40–44

Sunguya, F.P.A. (1981) Disease surveillance, economic losses and trace back of pigs in the abattoir. MSc Thesis, University of Edinburgh

Tanaka, J. (1992) Outline of animal health information processing in Japan. *Office International des Epizooties Quarterly Epidemiology Report (Asian and Pacific Region)*, **1**, 36–39

Tannahill, R. (1968) *The Fine Art of Food*. The Folio Society, London

Tansley, A.G. (1935) The use and abuse of vegetational concepts and terms. *Ecology*, **16**, 284–307

Taylor, R. (1967) Causation. In: *The Encyclopedia of Philosophy*, Vol. 2. Ed. Edwards, P. The Macmillan Company and The Free Press, New York

Taylor, W.P. and Marshall, I.E. (1975) Adaptation studies with Ross River virus: retention of field level virulence. *Journal of General Virology*, **28**, 73–83

Teclaw, R., Mendlein, J., Garbe, P. and Mariolis, P. (1992) Characteristics of pet populations and households in the Purdue Comparative Oncology Program catchment area, 1988. *Journal of the American Veterinary Medical Association*, **201**, 1725–1729

Tedor, J. and Reif, J.S. (1978) Natal patterns among registered dogs in the United States. *Journal of the American Veterinary Medical Association*, **172**, 1179–1185

Terris, M. (1962) Scope and methods of epidemiology. *American Journal of Public Health*, **52**, 1371–1376

The Times (1983) Running dogs banned. *The Times*, 13 October 1983, p. 6

Thoday, K.L. (1980) Canine pruritus: an approach to diagnosis. Stage I. Preliminary investigation. *Journal of Small Animal Practice*, **21**, 399–408

Thomas, A.D. and Maré, C.v.E. (1945) Knopvelsiekte. *Journal of the South African Veterinary Medical Association*, **16**, 36–43

Thomas, C.B., Willeberg, P. and Jasper, D.E. (1981) Case–control study of bovine mycoplasmal mastitis in California. *American Journal of Veterinary Research*, **42**, 511–515

Thomas, C.B., Jasper, D.E. and Willeberg, P. (1982) Clinical bovine mycoplasmal mastitis. An epidemiologic study of factors associated with problem herds. *Acta Veterinaria Scandinavica*, **23**, 53–64

Thomas, D.G. (1975) Exact and asymptotic methods for the combination of 2 × 2 tables. *Computers and Biomedical Research*, **8**, 423–466

Thomas, D.G. and Gart, J.J. (1992) Improved and extended exact and asymptotic methods for the combination of 2 × 2 tables. *Computers and Biomedical Research*, **25**, 75–84

Thomas, D.R. (1989) Simultaneous confidence intervals for proportions under cluster sampling. *Survey Methodology*, **18**, 187–201

Thomas, R.J. (1978) Forecasting the onset of nematodiriasis in sheep. In: *Weather and Parasitic Animal Disease*. Ed. Gibson, T.E., pp. 68–73. World Meteorological Organization Technical Note No. 159

Thomas, R.J. and Starr, J.R. (1978) Forecasting the peak of gastrointestinal nematode infection in lambs. *Veterinary Record*, **103**, 465–468

Thompson, E.T. and Hayden, A.C. (1961) *Standard Nomenclature of Diseases and Operations*, 5th edn. McGraw-Hill, New York

Thorburn, M.A., Carpenter, T.E., Jasper, D.E. and Thomas, C.B. (1983) The use of the log-linear model to evaluate the effects of three herd factors on *Streptococcus agalactiae* mastitis occurrence in California, 1977. *Preventive Veterinary Medicine*, **1**, 243–256

Thorns, C.J. and Morris, J.A. (1983) The immune spectrum of *Mycobacterium bovis* infection in some mammalian species: a review. *Veterinary Bulletin*, **53**, 543–550

Thrusfield, M.V. (Ed.) (1981) *A Computerised Veterinary Clinical Data Base*. Proceedings of a Symposium, Edinburgh, 30 September 1981. Department of Animal Health, Royal (Dick) School of Veterinary Studies, Edinburgh

Thrusfield, M.V. (1983a) Recording and manipulating clinical data. *Journal of Small Animal Practice*, **24**, 703–717

Thrusfield, M.V. (1983b) Application of computer technology to the collection, analysis and use of veterinary data. *Veterinary Record*, **112**, 538–543

Thrusfield, M.V. (1985a) How to use a knowledge of epidemiology in practice. *The Pig Veterinary Society Proceedings*, **12**, 25–37

Thrusfield, M.V. (1985b) Data recording in general practice. *In Practice*, **7**, 128–138

Thrusfield, M.V. (1985c) Association between urinary incontinence and spaying in bitches. *Veterinary Record*, **116**, 695

Thrusfield, M.V. (1989) Demographic characteristics of the canine and feline populations of the UK in 1986. *Journal of Small Animal Practice*, **30**, 76–80

Thrusfield, M.V. (1991) A computerised small animal practice health management system with a centralised data-analysis facility. In: Proceedings of the 6th International Symposium on Veterinary Epidemiology and Economics, Ottawa, 12–16 August 1991. Ed. Martin, S.W., pp. 459–461

Thrusfield, M.V. (1992) Canine kennel cough: a review. In: Raw, M.-E. and Parkinson, T.J. (Eds) *The Veterinary Annual*, **32**, 1–12. Blackwell Scientific Publications, Oxford

Thrusfield, M.V. (1993) Quantitative approaches to veterinary epidemiology. In: *The Advancement of Veterinary Science. The Bicentenary Symposium Series. Volume 1: Veterinary Medicine Beyond 2000*. Ed. Michell, A.R., pp. 121–142. CAB International, Wallingford

Thrusfield, M.V., Aitken, C.G.G. and Darke, P.G.G. (1985) Observations on breed and sex in relation to canine heart valve incompetence. *Journal of Small Animal Practice*, **26**,

709−717

Thrusfield, M.V., Aitken, C.G.G. and Muirhead, R.H. (1989a) A field investigation of kennel cough. Efficacy of vaccination. *Journal of Small Animal Practice*, **30**, 550−560

Thrusfield, M.V., Mullineaux, E., MacTaggart, D.C. and Trinder, N.J. (1989b) Some epidemiological observations on canine testicular tumours. In: Society for Veterinary Epidemiology and Preventive Medicine, Proceedings, Exeter, 12−14 April 1989. Ed. Rowlands, G.J., pp. 98−109

Thurber, E.T., Bass, E.P. and Beckenhauer, W.H. (1977) Field trial evaluation of a reo-coronavirus calf diarrhoea vaccine. *Canadian Journal of Comparative Medicine*, **41**, 131−146

Timbs, D.V. (1980) The New Zealand national bovine serum bank. In: *Veterinary Epidemiology and Economics*, Proceedings of the Second International Symposium, Canberra, 7−11 May 1979. Eds Geering, W.A., Roe, R.T. and Chapman, L.A., pp. 76−80. Australian Government Publishing Service, Canberra

Timoney, J.F., Gillespie, J.H., Scott, F.W. and Balough, J.E. (1988) *Hagan and Bruner's Microbiology and Infectious Diseases of Domesticated Animals*, 8th edn. Comstock Publishing Associates, Ithaca

Tinline, R. (1970) Lee wave hypothesis for the initial pattern of spread during the 1967−68 foot-and-mouth disease epizootic. *Nature*, **227**, 860−862

Tinline, R. (1972) A simulation study of the 1967−68 foot-and-mouth epizootic in Great Britain. PhD Thesis, University of Bristol

Tizard, I.R. (1982) *An Introduction to Veterinary Immunology*, 2nd edn. J.B. Saunders, Philadelphia

Tjalma, R.A. (1966) Canine bone sarcoma: estimation of relative risk as a function of body size. *Journal of the National Cancer Institute*, **36**, 1137−1150

Tjalma, R.A. (1968) Implications of animal cancers to human neoplasia: epidemiologic considerations. *International Journal of Cancer*, **3**, 1−6

Toma, B., Bénet, J.-J., Dufour, B., Eloit, M., Moutou, F. and Sanaa, M. (1991) *Glossaire d'epidemiologie animale*. Editions du Point Vétérinaire, Maisons-Alfort

Topley, W.W.C. (1942) The biology of epidemics. *Proceedings of the Royal Society of London*, **130**, 337−359

Torres-Anjel, M.J. and Tshikuka, J.G. (1988) The microepidemiology of the animal acquired immunodeficiency syndrome (AIDS) in the context of human AIDS (HAIDS). In: *Environment and Animal Health*, Proceedings of the 6th International Congress on Animal Hygiene, Skara, Sweden, Vol. 2. Ed. Ekesbo, I., pp. 745−749. Swedish University of Agricultural Sciences, Report No. 21

Townsend, H.G.G., Morley, P.S. and Haines, D.M. (1991) Risk factors associated with upper respiratory tract disease during an outbreak of influenza. In: Proceedings of the Sixth International Symposium on Veterinary Epidemiology and Economics, Ottawa, 12−16 August 1991. Ed. Martin, S.W., pp. 479−481

Tranter, W.P., Morris, R.S., Dohoo, I.R. and Williamson, N.B. (1993) A case−control study of lameness in dairy cows.

Preventive Veterinary Medicine, **15**, 191−203

Travis, C.C. (1987) Interspecies extrapolations in risk analysis. *Toxicology*, **47**, 3−13

Trewhella, W.R. and Anderson, R.M. (1983) Modelling bovine tuberculosis in badgers. In: Society for Veterinary Epidemiology and Preventive Medicine, Proceedings, Southampton, 12−13 April 1983. Ed. Thrusfield, M.V., pp. 78−84

Tribe, H.T. (1980) Prospects for the biological control of plant-parasitic nematodes. *Parasitology*, **81**, 619−639

Trotter, W. (1930) Observation and experiment and their use in the medical sciences. *British Medical Journal*, **ii**, 129−134

Trotter, W. (1932) *Art and Science in Medicine*. (Quoted by Himsworth, 1970)

Tukey, J.W. (1977) *Exploratory Data Analysis*. Addison-Wesley, Philippines

Tuovinen, V.K., Grohn, Y.T., Straw, B.E. and Boyd, D. (1992) Feeder unit environmental factors associated with partial carcass condemnations in market swine. *Preventive Veterinary Medicine*, **12**, 175−195

Turner, T. and Pegg, E. (1977) A survey of patent nematode infestations in dogs. *Veterinary Record*, **100**, 284−285

Turner, T.A., Kneller, S.K., Badertscher, R.R. and Stowater, J.L. (1987) Radiographic changes in the navicular bones of normal horses. In: Proceedings of the 32nd Annual Convention of the American Association of Equine Practitioners, Nashville, 29 November−3 December 1986, pp. 309−314

Tyler, L. (1991) PARC sero-monitoring: survey design, implementation and the analysis, presentation and use of results. In: *The Sero-monitoring of Rinderpest Throughout Africa. Phase One*. Proceedings of a Final Research Co-ordination Meeting of the FAO/IAEA/SIDA/OAU/BAR/PARC Co-ordinated Research Programme, Bingerville, Cote d'Ivoire, 19−23 November 1990. IAEA-TECDOC-623, pp. 67−79. International Atomic Energy Agency, Vienna

Udomprasert, P. and Williamson, N.B. (1990) The Dairy-CHAMP program: a computerised recording system for dairy herds. *Veterinary Record*, **127**, 256−262

Uhaa, I.J., Riemann, H.P., Thurmond, M.C. and Franti, C.E. (1990a) A cross-sectional study of bluetongue virus and *Mycoplasma bovis* infections in dairy cattle: I. The association between a positive antibody response and production efficiency. *Veterinary Research Communications*, **14**, 461−470

Uhaa, I.J., Riemann, H.P., Thurmond, M.C. and Franti, C.E. (1990b) A cross-sectional study of bluetongue virus and *Mycoplasma bovs* infections in dairy cattle: II. The association between a positive antibody response and reproduction performance. *Veterinary Research Communications*, **14**, 471−480

Uhaa, I.J., Mandel, E.J., Whiteway, R. and Fishbein, D.B. (1992) Rabies surveillance in the United States during 1990. *Journal of the American Veterinary Medical Association*, **200**, 920−929

Urquhart, G.M. (1980) Application of immunity in the control of parasitic disease. *Veterinary Parasitology*, **6**, 217−239

USDA (1982) *International Directory of Animal Health and*

Disease Data Banks. National Agricultural Library. United States Department of Agriculture. Miscellaneous Publication No. 1423

Vail, D.M., Withrow, S.J., Schwarz, P.D. and Powers, B.E. (1990) Perianal adenocarcinoma in the canine male: a retrospective study of 41 cases. *Journal of the American Animal Hospital Association*, **26**, 329 – 334

Vaillancourt, J.-P., Martineau, G., Morrow, M., Marsh, W. and Robinson, A. (1991) Construction of questionnaires and their use in veterinary medicine. In: Society for Veterinary Epidemiology and Preventive Medicine, Proceedings, London, 17 – 19 April 1991. Ed. Thrusfield, M.V., pp. 94 – 106

Valensin, A. (1972) Satan in the Old Testament. In: *Soundings in Satanism*. Ed. Sheed, F.J., pp. 105 – 120. Mowbrays, Oxford

Van de Braak, A.E., van't Klooster, A. Th. and Malestein, A. (1987) Influence of a deficient supply of magnesium during the dry period on the rate of calcium mobilisation by dairy cows at parturition. *Research in Veterinary Science*, **42**, 101 – 108

Van den Broek, A.H.M., Thrusfield, M.V., Dobbie, G.R. and Ellis, W.A. (1991) A serological and bacteriological survey of leptospiral infection in dogs in Edinburgh and Glasgow. *Journal of Small Animal Practice*, **32**, 118 – 124

Van den Geer, D., Schukken, Y.H., Grommers, F.J. and Brand, A. (1988) A matched case – control study of clinical mastitis in Holstein – Friesian dairy cows. In: *Environment and Animal Health*. Proceedings of the 6th International Congress on Animal Hygiene, 14 – 17 June 1988, Skara, Sweden, Vol. 1. Ed. Ekesbo, I., pp. 60 – 64

Vandegraaff, R. (1980) The use of discriminant analysis in a case – control study of salmonellosis in East Gippsland dairy herds. In: *Veterinary Epidemiology and Economics*. Proceedings of the Second International Symposium, Canberra, 7 – 11 May 1979. Eds Geering, W.A., Roe, R.T. and Chapman, L.A., pp. 258 – 263. Australian Government Publishing Service, Canberra

Vecchio, T.J. (1966) Predictive value of a single diagnostic test in unselected populations. *New England Journal of Medicine*, **274**, 1171 – 1173

Verberne, L.R.M. and Mirck, M.H. (1976) A practical health programme for prevention of parasitic and infectious diseases in horses and ponies. *Equine Veterinary Journal*, **8**, 123 – 125

Visser, I.J.R., Ingh, T.S.G.A.M. van den, Kruijf, J.M., Tielen, M.J.M., Urlings, H.A.P. and Gruys, E. (1988) Atrofische rhinitis: beoordeling van de lengtedoorsnede van varkenskoppen aan de slachtlijn ter bepaling van voorkomen en mate van concha-atrofie. (Atrophic rhinitis: the use of longitudinal sections of pigs' heads in the diagnosis of atrophy of the turbinate bones at the slaughter line.) *Tijdschrift voor Diergeneeskunde*, **113**, 1345 – 1355 (in Dutch)

Vizard, A.L., Anderson, G.A. and Gasser, R.B. (1990) Determination of the optimum cut-off value of a diagnostic test. *Preventive Veterinary Medicine*, **10**, 137 – 143

Vögeli, P., Kuhn, B., Kühne, R., Obrist, R., Stranzinger, G., Huang, S.C., Hu, Z.L., Hasler-Rapacz, J. and Rapacz, J. (1992) Evidence for linkage between the swine L blood group and the loci specifying the receptors mediating adhesion of

K88 *Escherichia coli* pilus antigens. *Animal Genetics*, **23**, 19 – 29

Voisin, C., Tonnel, A.B., Lahoute, C., Robin, H., Lebas, J. and Aerts, C. (1983) Bird fanciers lung: studies of bronchiolar lavage and correlations with inhalation provocation tests. *Lung*, **159**, 17 – 22

Vollset, S.E. and Hirji, K.F. (1991) A computer program for exact and symptotic analysis of several 2 × 2 tables. *Epidemiology*, **2**, 217 – 219

Vollset, S.E., Hirji, K.F. and Elashoff, R.M. (1991) Fast computation of exact confidence limits for the common odds ratio in a series of 2 × 2 tables. *Journal of the American Statistical Association*, **86**, 404 – 409

Vraa-Andersen, L. (1991) Analysis of risk factors related to infection with *Actinobacillus pleuropneumonia* and *Mycoplasma hyopneumonia* in swine. In: Proceedings of the Sixth International Symposium on Veterinary Epidemiology and Economics, Ottawa, 12 – 16 August 1991. Ed. Martin, S.W., pp. 419 – 422

Wachendörfer, G. and Frost, J.W. (1992) Epidemiology of red fox rabies: a review. In: *Wildlife Rabies Control*. Eds Bögel, K., Meslin, F.X. and Kaplan, M., pp. 19 – 31. Wells Medical, Tunbridge Wells

Wagener, J.S., Sobonya, R., Minnich, L. and Taussig, L.M. (1984) Role of canine parainfluenza virus and *Bordetella bronchiseptica* in kennel cough. *American Journal of Veterinary Research*, **45**, 1862 – 1866

Waksberg, J. (1978) Sampling methods for random digit dialing. *Journal of the American Statistical Association*, **73**, 40 – 46

Waller, P.J. (1992) Prospects for biological control of nematode parasites of ruminants. *New Zealand Veterinary Journal*, **40**, 1 – 3

Walter, S.D. (1977) Determination of significant relative risks and optimal sampling procedures in prospective and retrospective comparative studies of various sizes. *American Journal of Epidemiology*, **105**, 387 – 397

Walters, J.R. (1978) Problems associated with the movement and marketing of weaners. *The Pig Veterinary Society Proceedings*, **3**, 37 – 44

Waltner-Toews, D. (1983) Questionnaire design and administration. In: Proceedings of the Third International Symposium on Veterinary Epidemiology and Economics, Arlington, Virginia, 6 – 10 September 1982, pp. 31 – 37. Veterinary Medical Publishing Company, Edwardsville

Waltner-Toews, D. and McEwen, S.A. (1994) Human health risks from chemical contaminants in foods of animal origin. *Preventive Veterinary Medicine*, **20**, 159 – 247

Waltner-Toews, D., Martin, S.W. and Meek, A.H. (1986a) Dairy calf management, morbidity and mortality in Ontario Holstein herds. II. Age and seasonal patterns. *Preventive Veterinary Medicine*, **4**, 125 – 135

Waltner-Toews, D., Martin, S.W. and Meek, A.H. (1986b) Dairy calf management, morbidity and mortality in Ontario Holstein herds. III. Association of management with morbidity. *Preventive Veterinary Medicine*, **4**, 137 – 158

Waltner-Toews, D., Martin, S.W. and Meek, A.H. (1986c)

Estimating disease prevalence using a test with no false positives. In: Proceedings of the 4th International Symposium on Veterinary Epidemiology and Economics, Singapore, 18–22 November 1985, pp. 414–415

Waltner-Toews, D., Mondesire, R. and Menzies, P. (1991) The seroprevalence of *Toxoplasma gondii* in Ontario sheep flocks. *Canadian Veterinary Journal*, **32**, 734–737

Wang, C.Y., Chiu, C.W., Pamukcu, A.M. and Bryan, G.T. (1976) Identification of carcinogenic tannin isolated from bracken fern (*Pteridium aquilinum*). *Journal of the National Cancer Institute*, **56**, 33–36

Warble, A. (1994) Veterinary Medical Data Base (VMDB) update. *American Veterinary Computer Society Newsletter*, September–October 1994, pp. 8–10

Ward, K.A. Nancarrow, C.D., Byrne, C.R., Shanahan, C.M., Murray, J.D., Leish, Z., Townrow, C., Rigby, N.W., Wilson, B.W. and Hunt, C.L.H. (1990) The potential of transgenic animals for improved agricultural productivity. *Revue Scientifique et Technique, Office International des Epizooties*, **9**, 847–864

Ward, M.P. (1991) Bluetongue virus infection in cattle in Queensland: a retrospective study of climatic factors. In: Proceedings of the Sixth International Symposium on Veterinary Epidemiology and Economics, Ottawa, 12–16 August 1991. Ed. Martin, S.W., pp. 230–234

Wathes, C.M. (1987) Airborne microorganisms in pig and poultry houses. In: *Environmental Aspects of Respiratory Disease in Intensive Pig and Poultry Houses, including Implications for Human Health*. Proceedings of a meeting, Aberdeen, 29–30 October 1986. Eds Bruce, J.M. and Sommer, M., pp. 57–71. Commission of the European Communities, Luxembourg, Report EUR 10820 EN

Wathes, C.M. (1989) Ventilation of stables. *Farm Buildings and Engineering*, **6**, 21–25

Wathes, C.M., Jones, C.D.R. and Webster, A.J.F. (1983) Ventilation, air hygiene and animal health. *Veterinary Record*, **113**, 554–559

Wathes, C.M., Zaidan, W.A.R., Pearson, G.R., Hinton, M. and Todd, J.N. (1988) Aerosol infection of calves and mice with *Salmonella typhimurium*. *Veterinary Record*, **123**, 590–594

Watson, J.C. (1982) Food hygiene. Methods of linking meat inspection findings with disease on the farm and in human populations. In: *Epidemiology in Animal Health*. Proceedings of a Symposium held at the British Veterinary Association's Centenary Congress, Reading, 22–25 September 1982, pp. 131–140. Society for Veterinary Epidemiology and Preventive Medicine

Watt, G.E.L. (1980) An approach to determining the prevalence of liver fluke in a large region. In: *Veterinary Epidemiology and Economics*. Proceedings of the Second International Symposium, Canberra, 7–11 May 1979. Eds Geering, W.A., Roe, R.T. and Chapman, L.A., pp. 152–155. Australian Government Publishing Service, Canberra

Way, M.J. (1977) Pest and disease status in mixed stands vs. monocultures; the relevance of ecosystem stability. In: *Origins of Pest, Parasite, Disease and Weed Problems*. 18th Symposium of the British Ecological Society, Bangor, 12–14 April 1976. Eds Cherrett, J.M. and Sagar, G.R., pp. 127–138. Blackwell Scientific Publications, Oxford

Weaver, A.D. (1983) Survey with follow-up of 67 dogs with testicular sertoli cell tumours. *Veterinary Record*, **113**, 105–107

Webb, J.S., Thornton, I., Thompson, M., Howarth, R.J. and Lowenstein, P.L. (1978) *The Wolfston Geochemical Atlas of England and Wales*. Oxford University Press, London

Webster, A.J.F. (1981) Weather and infectious disease in cattle. *Veterinary Record*, **108**, 183–187

Webster, A.J.F. (1982) Improvements of environment, husbandry and feeding. In: *The Control of Infectious Diseases in Farm Animals*. British Veterinary Association Trust Project on the future of animal health control, London, pp. 28–35

Webster, R.G., Bean, W.J., Gorman, O.T., Chambers, T.M. and Kawaoka, Y. (1992) Evolution and ecology of influenza A viruses. *Microbiological Reviews*, **56**(1), 152–179

Weed, D.L. (1986) On the logic of causal inference. *American Journal of Epidemiology*, **123**, 965–979

Weigel, R.M., Austin, C.C., Siegel, A.M., Biehl, L.G. and Taft, A.C. (1992) Risk factors associated with the seroprevalence of pseudorabies virus in Illinois swine herds. *Preventive Veterinary Medicine*, **12**, 1–13

Weijer, K. and Hart, A.A.M. (1983) Prognostic factors in feline mammary carcinoma. *Journal of the National Cancer Institute*, **70**, 709–716

Weinberg, R.A. (1983) A molecular basis of cancer. *Scientific American*, **249**(5), 102–116

Weinstein, M.C. and Fineberg, H.V. (1980) *Clinical Decision Analysis*. W.B. Saunders, Philadelphia

Wells, G.A.H., Scott, A.C., Johnson, C.T., Cunning, R.F., Hancock, R.D., Jeffrey, M., Dawson, M. and Bradley, R. (1987) A novel progressive spongiform encephalopathy in cattle. *Veterinary Record*, **121**, 419–420

Wells, S.J., Trent, A.M., Marsh, W.E., McGovern, P.G. and Robinson, R.A. (1993a) Individual cow risk factors for clinical lameness in lactating dairy cows. *Preventive Veterinary Medicine*, **17**, 95–109

Wells, S.J., Trent, A.M., Marsh, W.E. and Robinson, R.A. (1993b) Prevalence and severity of lameness in lactating dairy cows in a sample of Minnesota and Wisconsin herds. *Journal of the American Veterinary Medical Association*, **202**, 78–82

Welsh, E.M., Gettinby, G. and Nolan, A.M. (1993) Comparison of a visual analogue scale and a numerical rating scale for assessment of lameness, using sheep as a model. *American Journal of Veterinary Research*, **54**, 976–983

West, G.P. (1972) *Rabies in Animals and Man*. David and Charles, Newton Abbot

Wetherill, G.B. (1969) *Sampling Inspection and Quality Control*. Methuen, London

Wheelwright, S.C. and Makridakis, S. (1973) *Forecasting Methods for Management*. Wiley-Interscience, New York

Whitaker, D.A. and Kelly, J.M. (1982) Incidence of clinical and subclinical hypomagnesaemia in dairy cows in England and Wales. *Veterinary Record*, **110**, 450–451

Whitaker, D.A., Kelly, J.M. and Smith, E.J. (1983a) Incidence of lameness in dairy cows. *Veterinary Record*, **113**, 60–62

Whitaker, D.A., Kelly, J.M. and Smith, E.J. (1983b) Subclinical ketosis and serum Beta hydroxybutyrate levels in dairy cattle. *British Veterinary Journal*, **139**, 462–463

White, M.E. and Vellake, E. (1980) A coding system for veterinary clinical signs. *Cornell Veterinarian*, **70**, 160–182

White, N.A. and Lessard, P. (1986) Risk factors and clinical signs associated with cases of equine colic. In: Proceedings of the Thirty-second Annual Convention of the American Association of Equine Practitioners, Nashville, Tennessee, 29 November–3 December 1986, pp. 637–644

Whitehair, J.G., Vasseur, P.B. and Willits, N.H. (1993) Epidemiology of cranial cruciate ligament rupture in dogs. *Journal of the American Veterinary Medical Association*, **203**, 1016–1019

Whittaker, M. (1960) The supernatural in the Roman Empire. *Church Quarterly Review*, **161**, 185–199

WHO (1959) *Immunological and Haematological Surveys*. Report of a study group. World Health Organization Technical Report Series No. 181

WHO (1970) *Multipurpose Serological Surveys and WHO Serum Reference Banks*. Report of a World Health Organization scientific group. World Health Organization Technical Report Series No. 454

WHO (1978) Proposals for the nomenclature of salivarian trypanosomes and for the nomenclature of reference collections. *Bulletin of the World Health Organization*, **56**, 467–480

WHO (1983) *Basic Documents*, 35th edn. World Health Organization, Geneva

WHO (1993) *Evaluation of Certain Veterinary Drug Residues in Food*. Fortieth Report of the Joint FAO/WHO Expert Committee on Food Additives. World Health Organization Technical Report Series No. 832. World Health Organization, Geneva

Wierup, M. (1983) The Swedish canine parvovirus epidemic — an epidemiological study in a dog population of defined size. *Preventive Veterinary Medicine*, **1**, 273–288

Wierup, M., Wold-Troell, M., Nurmi, E. and Hakkinen, M. (1988) Epidemiological evaluation of the Salmonella-controlling effect of a nationwide use of a competitive exclusion culture in poultry. *Poultry Science*, **67**, 1026–1033

Wilesmith, J.W. (1993) BSE: epidemiological approaches, trials and tribulations. *Preventive Veterinary Medicine*, **18**, 33–42

Wilesmith, J.W. and Clifton-Hadley, R.S. (1991) Observations from an epidemiological study of tuberculosis in a naturally-infected badger population. In: Society for Veterinary Epidemiology and Preventive Medicine, Proceedings, London, 17–19 April 1991. Ed. Thrusfield, M.V., pp. 133–144

Wilesmith, J.W. and Gitter, M. (1986) Epidemiology of ovine listeriosis in Great Britain. *Veterinary Record*, **119**, 467–470

Wilesmith, J.W. and Ryan, J.B.M. (1992) Bovine spongiform encephalopathy: recent observations on the age-specific incidences. *Veterinary Record*, **130**, 491–492

Wilesmith, J.W., Little, T.W.A., Thompson, H.V. and Swan, C. (1982) Bovine tuberculosis in domestic and wild mammals in an area of Dorset. I. Tuberculosis in cattle. *Journal of Hygiene, Cambridge*, **89**, 195–210

Wilesmith, J.W., Francis, P.G. and Wilson, C.D. (1986) Incidence of clinical mastitis in a cohort of British dairy herds. *Veterinary Record*, **118**, 199–204

Wilesmith, J.W., Wells, G.A.H., Cranwell, M.P. and Ryan, J.B.M. (1988) Bovine spongiform encephalopathy: epidemiological studies. *Veterinary Record*, **123**, 638–644

Wilkinson, P.J. (1984) The persistence of African swine fever in Africa and the Mediterranean. *Preventive Veterinary Medicine*, **2**, 71–82

Willeberg, P. (1975a) A case–control study of some fundamental determinants in the epidemiology of the feline urological syndrome. *Nordisk Vetereinærmedicin*, **27**, 1–14

Willeberg, P. (1975b) Diets and the feline urological syndrome: a retrospective case–control study. *Nordisk Veterinærmedicin*, **27**, 15–19

Willeberg, P. (1975c) Outdoor activity level as a factor in the feline urological syndrome. *Nordisk Veterinærmedicin*, **27**, 523–524

Willeberg, P. (1976) Interaction effects of epidemiologic factors in the feline urological syndrome. *Nordisk Veterinærmedicin*, **28**, 193–200

Willeberg, P. (1977) Animal disease information processing: epidemiologic analyses of the feline urological syndrome. *Acta Veterinaria Scandinavica*, **18**, Suppl. 64, 1–48

Willeberg, P. (1979) The Danish swine slaughter inspection data bank and some epidemiological applications. In: Proceedings of an International Symposium on Animal Health and Disease Data Banks, 4–6 December 1978, pp. 133–145. United States Department of Agriculture, Washington, DC. Miscellaneous Publication No. 1381

Willeberg, P. (1980a) Abattoir surveillance in Denmark. *The Pig Veterinary Society Proceedings*, **6**, 43–54

Willeberg, P. (1980b) The analysis and interpretation of epidemiological data. In: *Veterinary Epidemiology and Economics*. Proceedings of the Second International Symposium, Canberra, 7–11 May 1979. Eds Geering, W.A., Roe, R.T. and Chapman, L.A., pp. 185–198. Australian Government Publishing Service, Canberra

Willeberg, P. (1981) Epidemiology of the feline urological syndrome. *Advances in Veterinary Science*, **25**, 311–344

Willeberg, P. (1986) Epidemiologic use of routinely collected veterinary data: risks and benefits. In: Proceedings of the 4th International Symposium on Veterinary Epidemiology and Economics, Singapore, 18–22 November 1985, pp. 40–45

Willeberg, P. (1991) Animal welfare studies: epidemiological considerations. In: Society for Veterinary Epidemiology and Preventive Medicine, Proceedings, London, 17–19 April 1991. Ed. Thrusfield, M.V., pp. 76–82

Willeberg, P. (1992) Disease monitoring in Denmark. In: Minnesota Swine Conference for Veterinarians. High-Health Strategies, College of Veterinary Medicine, University of Minnesota. *Veterinary Continuing Education and Extension, USA*, **19**, 95–101

Willeberg, P. and Priester, W.A. (1976) Feline urological syndrome: association with some time, space and individual patient factors. *American Journal of Veterinary Research*, **37**, 975–978

Willeberg, P., Gerbola, M.-A., Madsen, A., Mandrup, M., Nielsen, E.K., Riemann, H.P. and Aalund, O. (1978) A retrospective study of respiratory disease in a cohort of bacon pigs: I. Clinico-epidemiological analyses. *Nordisk Veterinærmedicin*, **30**, 513–525

Willeberg, P., Grymer, J. and Hesselholt, M. (1982) Left displacement at the abomasum: relationship to age and medical history. *Nordisk Veterinærmedicin*, **34**, 404–411

Willeberg, P., Gerbola, M.-A., Kirkegaard Petersen, B. and Andersen, J.B. (1984) The Danish pig health scheme; nationwide computer-based abattoir surveillance and follow-up at the herd level. *Preventive Veterinary Medicine*, **3**, 79–91

Willemse, T. (1986) Atopic skin disease: a review and a reconsideration of diagnostic criteria. *Journal of Small Animal Practice*, **27**, 771–778.

Willett, W. (1990) *Nutritional Epidemiology*. Oxford University Press, New York

Willetts, N. and Cobon, G. (1993) Antiparasite vaccines. In: *Vaccines for Veterinary Applications*. Ed. Peters, A.R., pp. 259–294. Butterworth-Heinemann, Oxford

Williams, G.W. (1984) Time–space clustering of disease. In: *Statistical Methods for Cancer Studies*. Ed. Cornell, R.G., pp. 167–227. Marcel Dekker, New York and Basel

Williams, M.E. and Esslemont, R.J. (1993) A decision support system using milk progesterone tests to improve fertility in commercial dairy herds. *Veterinary Record*, **132**, 503–506

Williams, P.C.W. and Ward, W.R. (1989a) Development of a coding system for recording clinical findings in farm animal practice. *Veterinary Record*, **124**, 118–122

Williams, P.C.W. and Ward, W.R. (1989b) Development of a microcomputer system for recording veterinary visits, preparing accounts and as an aid to herd fertility and health schemes. *Veterinary Record*, **124**, 265–268

Williamson, M.H. and Wilson, R.A. (1978) The use of mathematical models for predicting the incidence of fascioliasis. In: *Weather and Parasitic Animal Disease*. Ed. Gibson, T.E., pp. 39–48. World Meteorological Organization Technical Note No. 159

Williamson, N.B. (1980) The economic efficiency of a veterinary preventive medicine and management program in Victorian dairy herds. *Australian Veterinary Journal*, **56**, 1–9

Williamson, N.B. (1987) Evaluating herd reproductive status. *Proceedings of the American Association of Bovine Practitioners*, **19**, 117–121

Williamson, N.B. (1993) The economics of preventive veterinary medicine schemes in sheep and cattle. In: *The William Dick Bicentenary Proceedings*. The University of Edinburgh, 7–10 July 1993, pp. 13–16. Royal (Dick) School of Veterinary Studies, University of Edinburgh

Wilson, C.D. and Richards, M.S. (1980) A survey of mastitis in the British dairy herd. *Veterinary Record*, **106**, 431–435

Wilson, C.D., Richards, M.S., Stevenson, F.J. and Davies, G. (1983) *The National Mastitis Survey: A Survey of Udder Infection and Related Factors in the British Dairy Herd, 1977*. Ministry of Agriculture, Fisheries and Food Booklet 2433

Wilson, G.P., Hayes, H.M. and Casey, H.W. (1979) Canine urethral cancer. *Journal of the American Animal Hospital Association*, **15**, 741–744

Wilson, J.B., McEwen, S.A., Clarke, R.C., Leslie, K.E., Waltner-Toews, D. and Gyles, C.L. (1993) Risk factors for bovine infection with verocytotoxigenic *Escherichia coli* in Ontario, Canada. *Preventive Veterinary Medicine*, **16**, 159–170

Wilson, S.M. (1993) Application of nucleic acid-based technologies to the diagnosis and detection of disease. *Transactions of the Royal Society of Tropical Medicine and Hygiene*, **87**, 609–611

Wilson, T.M. and Howes, B. (1980) An epizootic of bovine tuberculosis in Barbados, West Indies. Proceedings of the Second International Symposium of Veterinary Laboratory Diagnosticians, 24–26 June 1980, Lucerne, Switzerland, Vol. 1, pp. 136–144

Wilton, J.W., Van Vleck, L.D., Everett, R.W., Guthrie, R.S. and Roberts, S.J. (1972) Genetic and environmental aspects of udder infections. *Journal of Dairy Science*, **55**, 183–193

Winkler, W.G. (1975) Fox rabies. In: *The Natural History of Rabies*, Vol. 2. Ed. Baer, G.M., pp. 3–22. Academic Press, New York

Wise, J.K. and Yang, J.-J. (1992) Demographic and employment shifts of US veterinarians, 1980 to 1990. *Journal of the American Veterinary Medical Association*, **201**, 684–687

Wittum, T.E., King, M.E. and Salman, M.D. (1991) Determinants of health and performance of calves in Colorado beef herds. In: Proceedings of the Sixth International Symposium on Veterinary Epidemiology and Economics, Ottawa, 12–16 August 1991. Ed. Martin, S.W., pp. 336–338

Wojciechowski, K.J. (1991) Global strategies for rinderpest eradication. In: South Asia Rinderpest Eradication Campaign. Proceedings of the Regional Expert Consultation on Rinderpest Eradication in South Asia, Bangkok, Thailand, 5–8 June 1990. RAPA Publication 1991/8, pp. 78–90. Food and Agriculture Organization, Bangkok

Wong, W.T. and Lee, M.K.C. (1985) Some observations on the population and natal patterns among purebred dogs in Malaysia. *Journal of Small Animal Practice*, **26**, 111–119

Wood, B., Washino, R., Beck, L., Hibbard, K., Pitcairn, M., Roberts, D., Rejmankova, E., Paris, J., Hacker, C., Salute, J., Sebesta, P. and Legters, L. (1991) Distinguishing high and low anopheline-producing rice fields using remote sensing and GIS technologies. *Preventive Veterinary Medicine*, **11**, 277–288

Wood, E.N. (1978) The incidence of stillborn piglets associated with high atmospheric carbon monoxide levels. *The Pig Veterinary Society Proceedings*, **3**, 117–118

Woodruff, A.W. (1976) Toxocariasis as a public health problem. *Environmental Health*, **84**, 29–31

Woods, J.M. and Howard, T.H. (1980) Reproductive management in large dairy herds. In: *Current Therapy in Theriogenology: Diagnosis, Treatment and Prevention of Reproductive Diseases in Animals*. Ed. Morrow, D.A., pp. 524–528. W.B. Saunders, Philadelphia, London and Toronto

Woodward, R.H. and Goldsmith, P.L. (1964) *Cumulative Sum Techniques*. Imperial Chemical Industries Mathematical and Statistical Techniques for Industry Monograph No. 3. Oliver and Boyd, Edinburgh

Woolcock, J.B. (1991) Microbial interactions in health and disease. In: *Microbiology of Animals and Animal Products*. World Animal Science, Vol. A6. Ed. Woolcock, J.B., pp. 61–76. Elsevier, Amsterdam

Wooldridge, M.J.A., Hoinville, L.J. and Wilesmith, J.W. (1992) A scrapie survey by postal questionnaire: aims, problems and results. In: Society for Veterinary Epidemiology and Preventive Medicine, Denary Proceedings, Edinburgh, 1–3 April 1992. Ed. Thrusfield, M.V., pp. 78–89

Woolf, B. (1955) On estimating the relation between blood group and disease. *Annals of Human Genetics*, **19**, 251–253

Worthington, R.W. (1982) Serology as an aid to diagnosis: uses and abuses. *New Zealand Veterinary Journal*, **30**, 93–97

Wrathall, A.E. (1975) *Reproductive Disorders in Pigs*. Review Series No. 11 of the Commonwealth Bureau of Animal Health. Commonwealth Agricultural Bureaux, Farnham Royal

Wrathall, A.E. and Hebert, C.N. (1982) Monitoring reproductive performance in the pig herd. *The Pig Veterinary Society Proceedings*, **9**, 136–148

Wratten, S.D., Mead-Briggs, M., Gettinby, G., Ericsson, G. and Baggott, D.G. (1993) An evaluation of the potential effects of ivermectin on the decomposition of cattle dung pats. *Veterinary Record*, **133**, 365–371

Wray, C. and Woodward, M.J. (1990) Biotechnology and veterinary science. *Revue Scientifique et Technique, Office International des Epizooties*, **9**, 779–794

Wright, S. (1959) Genetics and hierarchy of biological sciences. *Science, New York*, **130**, 959–965

Wynder, E.L. (1985) Applied epidemiology. *American Journal of Epidemiology*, **121**, 781–782

Wynne-Edwards, V.C. (1962) *Animal Dispersion in Relation to Social Behaviour*. Oliver and Boyd, Edinburgh

Yapi, C.V., Boylan, W.J. and Robinson, R.A. (1990) Factors associated with causes of preweaning lamb mortality. *Preventive Veterinary Medicine*, **10**, 145–152

Yates, F. (1981) *Sampling Methods for Censuses and Surveys*, 4th edn. Charles Griffin, London and High Wycombe

Yekutiel, P. (1980) *Eradication of Infectious Disease — A Critical Study*. Contributions to Epidemiology and Biostatistics, Vol. 2. S. Karger, Basel

Yoon, J.W., Kim, C.M., Pak, C.Y. and McArthur, R.G. (1987) Effects of environmental factors on the development of insulin-dependent diabetes mellitus. *Clinical and Investigative Medicine*, **10**, 457–469

Yorke, J.A. and London, W.P. (1973) Recurrent outbreaks of measles, chickenpox and mumps. II. Systematic differences in contact rates and stochastic effects. *American Journal of Epidemiology*, **98**, 469–482

Yoshida, N., Miyamoto, T., Fukusho, N.S. and Tajima, M. (1977) Properties of paramyxovirus isolated from budgerigars with an acute fatal disease. *Journal of the Japanese Veterinary Medical Association*, **30**, 599–603

Young, G.B., Lee, G.J., Waddington, D., Sales, D.I., Bradley, J.S. and Spooner, R.L. (1983) Culling and wastage in dairy cows in East Anglia. *Veterinary Record*, **113**, 107–111

Yuasa, N., Taniguchi, T. and Yashida, I. (1979) Isolation and some characteristics of an agent inducing anaemia in chicks. *Avian Diseases*, **23**, 366–385

Zeiger, R. (1990) True Epistat review. *Journal of the American Medical Association*, **264**, 97

Zelen, M. (1969) Play the winner rule and the controlled clinical trial. *Journal of the American Statistical Association*, **64**, 131–146

Zelen, M. (1974) The randomization and stratification of patients to clinical trials. *Journal of Chronic Diseases*, **27**, 365–375

Zetterquist, P. (1972) *A Clinical and Genetic Study of Congenital Heart Defects*. Institute for Medical Genetics, University of Uppsala, Sweden

Zuckerman, Lord (1980) *Badgers, Cattle and Tuberculosis*. Report to the Right Honourable Peter Walker. Her Majesty's Stationery Office, London

Zukowski, S.H., Hill, J.M., Jones, F.W. and Malone, J.B. (1991) Development and validation of a soil-based geographic information system model of habitat of *Fossario bulimoides*, a snail intermediate host of *Fasciola hepatica*. *Preventive Veterinary Medicine*, **11**, 221–227

Index

USBORNE ACTIVITIES

Magic Tricks to make and do

Ben Denne

Designed by Russell Punter
Illustrated by Andi Good

Photographs by Howard Allman
Edited by Gillian Doherty
Cover design by Michelle Lawrence

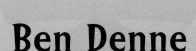

Cards © by Piatnik, Vienna

Contents

Q. How do you make your audience leave after the show?
A. Tell them the terrible jokes in this book.

Making a wand

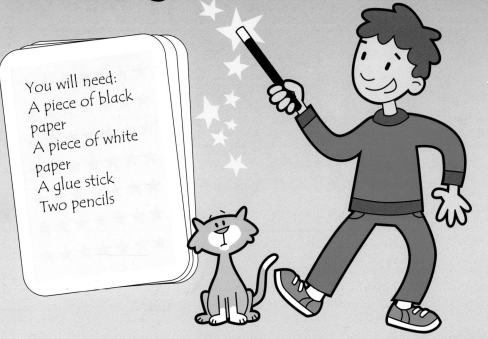

You will need:
A piece of black paper
A piece of white paper
A glue stick
Two pencils

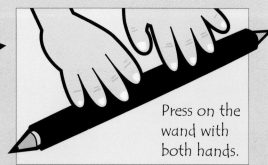

You could use purple or gold paper to make your wand.

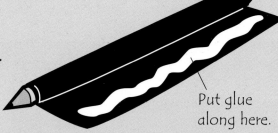

Put glue along here.

Press on the wand with both hands.

1. Cut out a piece of black paper, about the same size as this page. Roll it up tightly around two pencils.

2. When you have rolled up all the paper, unroll it a little and put some glue along the edge. Then roll it up again.

3. Hold the wand down firmly for about a minute, until the glue dries. Make sure you hold it with the glued edge underneath.

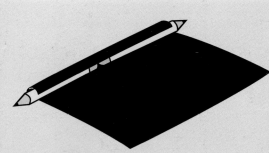

Use some of the stickers in this book to brighten up your wand.

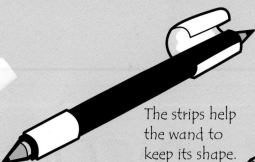

The strips help the wand to keep its shape.

4. Cut out two thin strips of white paper. Cover one side of them with glue. Wrap them around the ends of the wand.

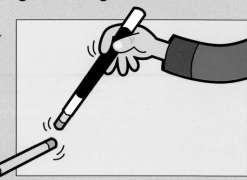

5. Hold your wand with one end facing the floor. Shake it until the pencils fall out. Now you're ready to do some magic.

2

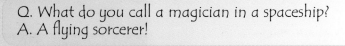

Q. What do you call a magician in a spaceship?
A. A flying sorcerer!

The incredible shrinking wand

Getting ready

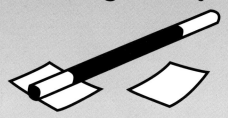

1. Cut out two strips of white paper. They should be wide enough to cover the strips on the ends of your wand.

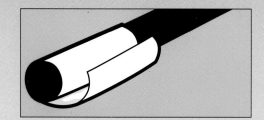

2. Roll a strip around one end of your wand. Unroll it a little, put some glue along the edge and roll it up again quite loosely.

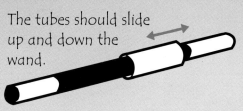

The tubes should slide up and down the wand.

3. Do the same with the other end of your wand. The tubes should fit well, but be loose enough to slide along the wand.

Doing the trick

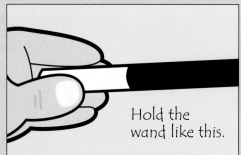

Hold the wand like this.

1. Hold the tubes between your middle finger and thumb. Cover the front with your fingers.

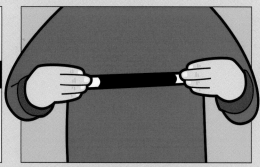

2. Close your fingers, so people can't see between them. Then say that you can make your wand change size.

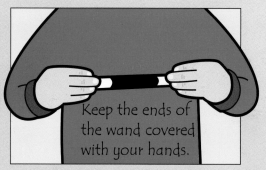

Keep the ends of the wand covered with your hands.

3. Look like you are really concentrating. Then slowly bring your hands together, so the tubes slide along the wand.

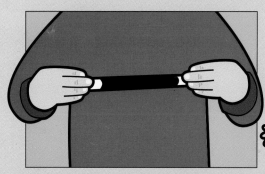

4. Say you can make the wand grow again. Slowly pull your hands apart, so the tubes slide back out along the wand.

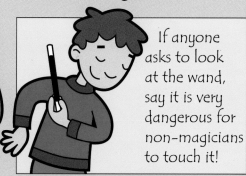

If anyone asks to look at the wand, say it is very dangerous for non-magicians to touch it!

5. Take a bow. Then, put your wand away before anyone can see it. Continue your show with a normal wand.

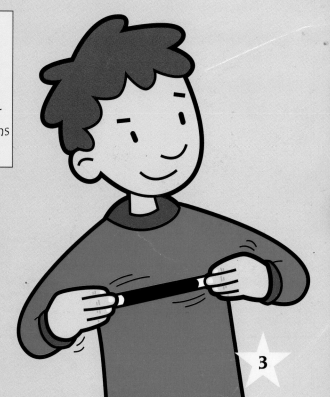

Q. Which book do magicians like best?
A. Alice in Wand-erland.

3

Finger in a matchbox

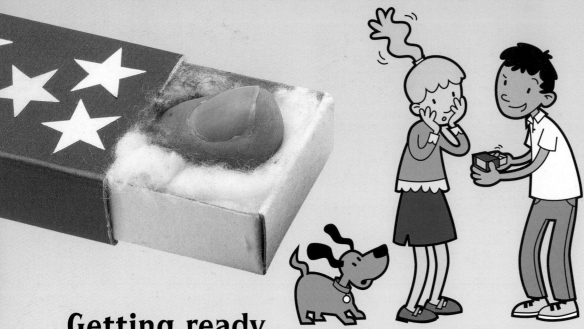

Getting ready

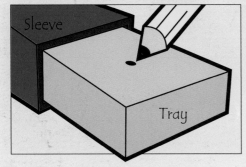

Sleeve

Tray

1. Slide the sleeve off the matchbox. Poke a small hole in the bottom of the matchbox tray with a pencil.

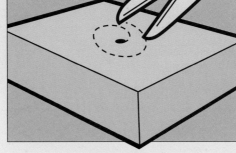

2. Cut around the hole, making it a little bigger. Keep making it bigger, until your middle finger just fits through it.

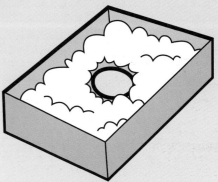

3. Put glue around the hole. Pull a cotton ball apart and press the cotton onto the glue. Be careful not to cover the hole.

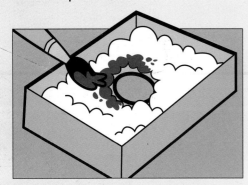

4. Dip a paintbrush into some red food dye or poster paint. Dab a small amount onto the cotton around the hole.

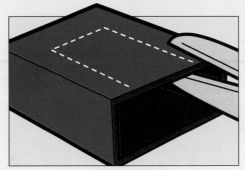

5. Cut a rectangle out of the bottom of one end of the matchbox sleeve. Make it wide enough for your finger to fit through.

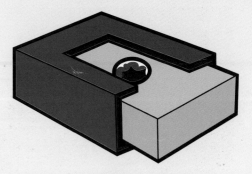

6. Slide the sleeve onto the matchbox tray, so that the cutout part of the sleeve is over the hole in the tray.

4

Q. Why are fingers reliable?
A. Because you can count on them.

Doing the trick

Q. What did one match say to the other?
A. Let's go on strike.

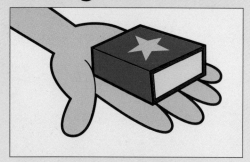

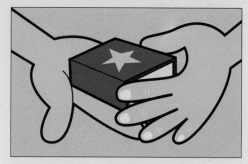

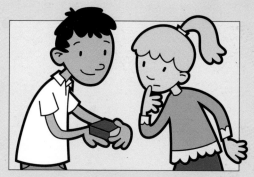

1. Hold your hand out, with your palm facing up. Put the matchbox on it, with the cutout part underneath, like this.

2. Curl your other hand around the front of the matchbox, holding the sides of it with your finger and thumb.

3. Show your audience the closed matchbox. Tell them you have something special inside it that you want to show them.

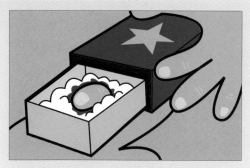

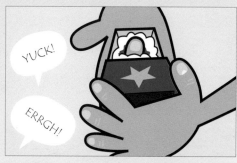

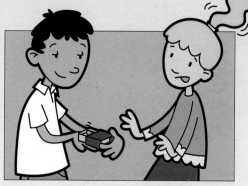

4. Put your middle finger through the hole in the tray, then open the sleeve. Try this beforehand, until you can do it smoothly.

5. Show your audience the matchbox with your finger inside. Make sure you keep the front covered with your other hand.

6. Pause for a few seconds, then wiggle your finger around in the matchbox. This should really make your audience scream!

Here are some ideas for how to decorate your matchbox.

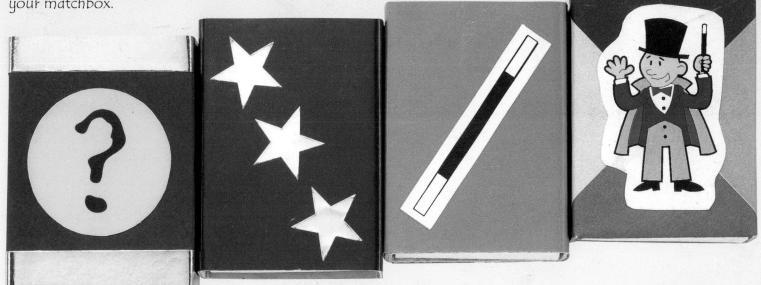

A ready-sliced banana

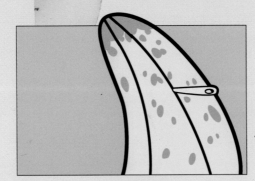

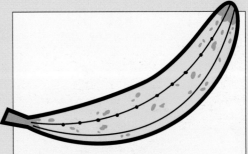

You will need:
A banana
A clean sewing
needle
A magic wand

Getting ready

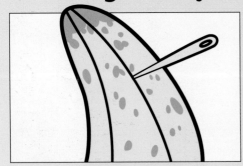

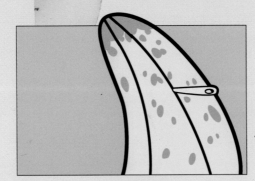

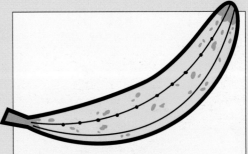

1. Take a banana. A slightly brown or freckled one works best. Poke a needle into it along an edge near one end.

2. Push the needle through the banana but not through the skin on the other side. Wiggle it from side to side and pull it out.

3. Repeat step 2 until you have made ten tiny holes along the banana. Make the holes an equal distance apart.

Doing the trick

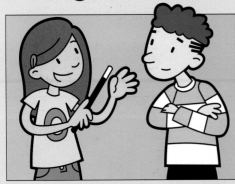

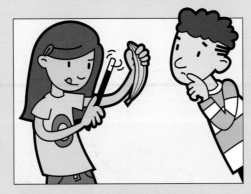

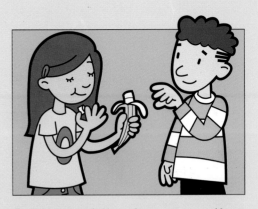

1. Tell your audience you can control the banana with your wand. Say you will command the banana to cut itself into slices.

2. Hold the banana up and point your wand at it. Say some magic words and stare very hard at the banana.

3. Unpeel the banana. It will be in slices. To end the trick, eat a slice of banana and offer the rest to your audience.

Q. Why are bananas never lonely?
A. Because they hang around in bunches.

The unburstable balloon

You will need:
Two balloons
Clear sticky tape
A knitting needle

Getting ready

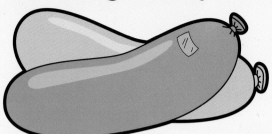

Blow up two balloons and tie the ends. Press a small piece of tape onto one of the balloons.

Doing the trick

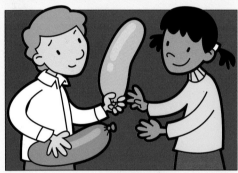

1. Tell your audience that you can make a balloon unburstable. Then give somebody the balloon without any tape on it.

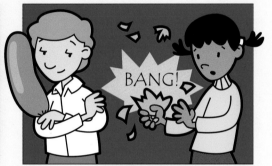

2. Challenge the volunteer to stick a knitting needle into the balloon without bursting it. Then get ready for a loud bang.

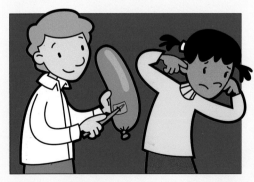

3. Hold the other balloon with the tape facing you. Carefully poke the knitting needle through the tape. The balloon won't burst.

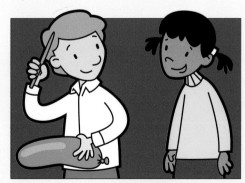

4. Take out the needle. Then hide the balloon. It won't burst even when you take out the needle, but it will start to go down.

Q. What sort of music do balloons listen to?
A. Pop.

7

Counting cards

Getting ready

1. A pack of cards is called a deck. Look through a deck of cards and take out a joker, an ace (with an A on it) and one of each number from 2 to 10.

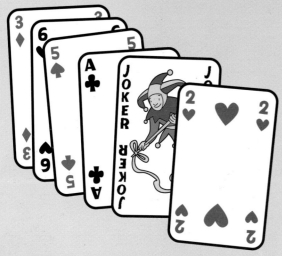

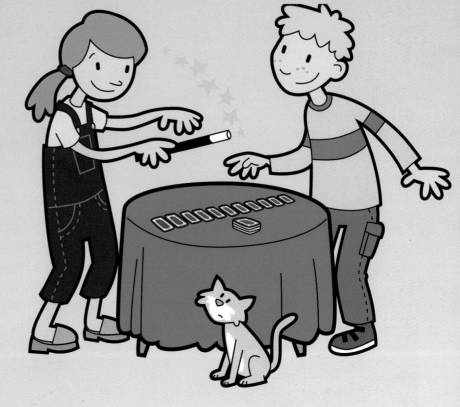

2. Put the cards on a table, face up in a line. They should be in this order from left to right: 6, 5, 4, 3, 2, ace, joker, 10, 9, 8, 7.

3. Keeping the cards in order, gather them up and place them face down. Keep the 6 on top and the 7 on the bottom.

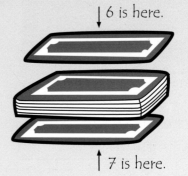

↓ 6 is here.

↑ 7 is here.

There is no card with the number 1 on it. An ace is the same as number 1.

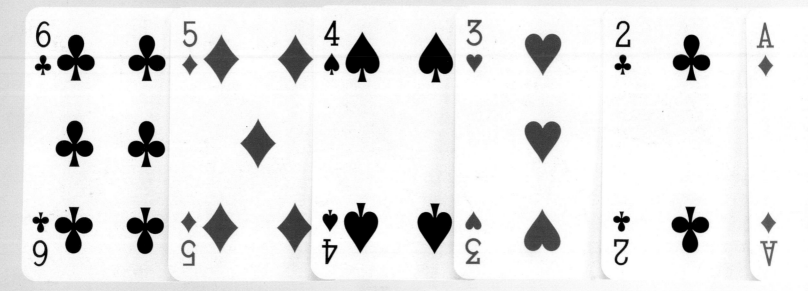

Q. How do playing cards walk?
A. They shuffle.

Doing the trick

6 is here.   7 is here.

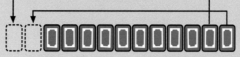

You are here.

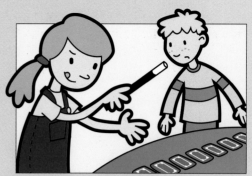

The person moving the cards can move up to 10 cards.

1. Deal the cards out. Place them face down in front of you, with the 6 on the left and the 7 on the right.

2. Turn away. Then ask someone to move cards one by one from the right end to the left, but not to tell you how many.

3. Turn back. Say you will ask the cards how many were moved. Wave your wand around over the cards.

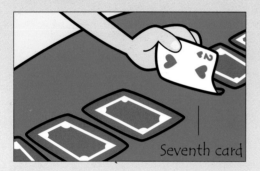

Seventh card

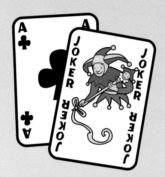

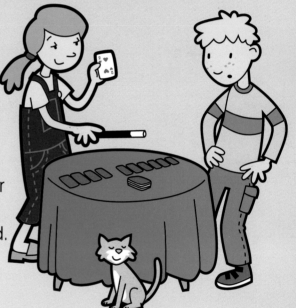

4. Turn over the seventh card from the left. The number on it will be the same as the number of cards the person moved.

5. If the card you turn over is the ace, it means that only one card was moved. If it's the joker, then no cards were moved.

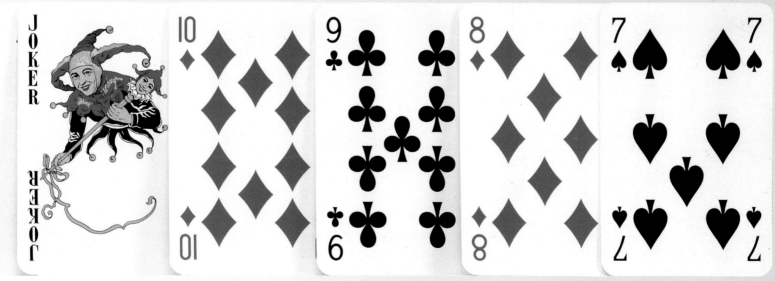

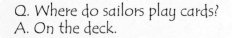

Q. Where do sailors play cards?
A. On the deck.

Cards © by Piatnik, Vienna

Self-joining paperclips

It is difficult to see why this trick works, but it always does.

You will need:
Two paperclips
A strip of paper

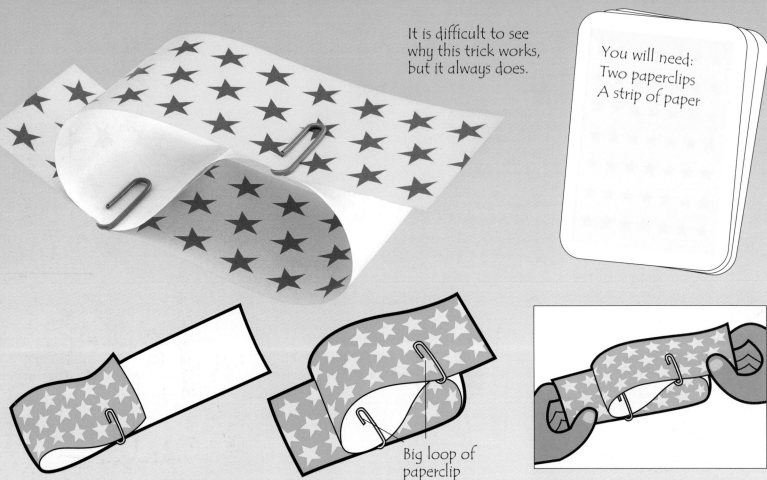

Big loop of paperclip

1. Take a strip of paper. Bend a third of it over on itself (but don't fold it). Clip a paperclip on, with the big loop facing you.

2. Now bend the other third of paper back on itself, to make an S-shape. Clip it, with the big loop of the paperclip facing you.

3. Hold the ends of the strip of paper and slowly pull them apart. The paperclips will move closer to each other.

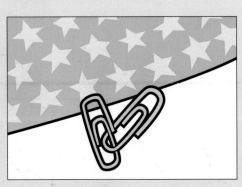

4. When the paperclips are touching each other, pull sharply. They will jump off the strip of paper and join together.

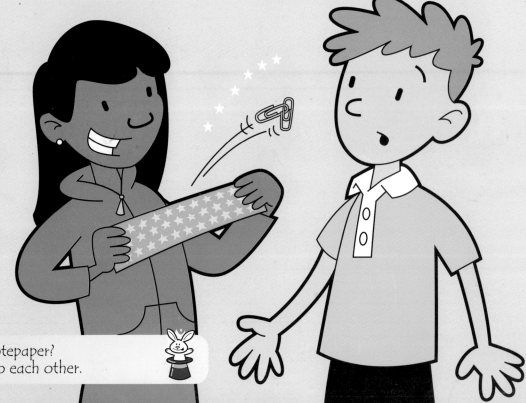

Q. Why do paperclips date notepaper?
A. Because they're attached to each other.

10

Changing cards

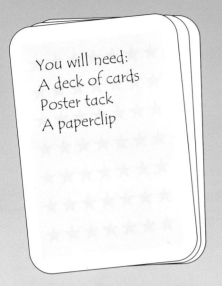

Cards © by Piatnik, Vienna

You will need:
A deck of cards
Poster tack
A paperclip

This is more of a puzzle than a trick, but it fools everybody.

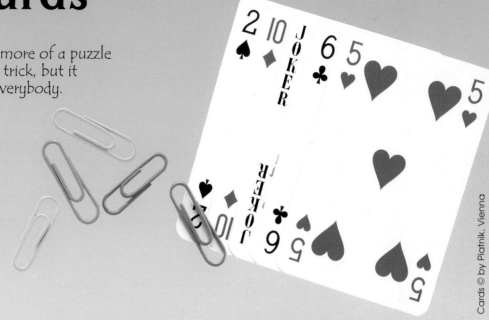

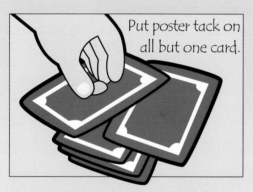

Put poster tack on all but one card.

1. Take a joker and four other cards from a deck. Put a ball of poster tack on the backs of four of them, including the joker.

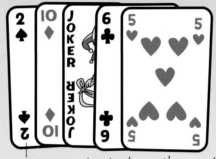

There is no poster tack on this card.

2. Stick the cards together, like this. Put the card without poster tack on at the back and the joker in the middle.

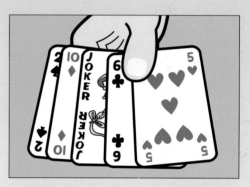

3. Now show the cards to your audience. Tell them to look carefully at where the joker is. Then turn the cards over.

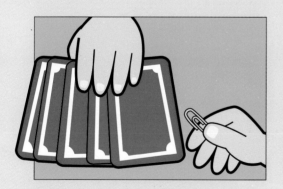

4. Challenge a volunteer from the audience to clip a paper clip over the joker, without turning the cards over.

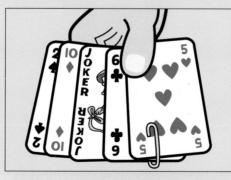

5. Your volunteer will probably clip the middle card. Turn the cards over and see where the clip really is.

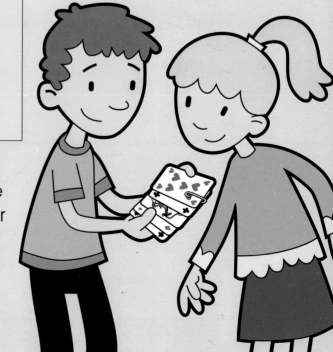

Q. What happens at a card school?
A. People learn a great deal.

Moving matchbox

You will need:
An empty
matchbox
A pencil
A used match
A pair of scissors
String

Getting ready

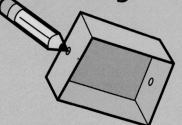

Make holes
in the short
sides of the
tray, at the
bottom.

1. Take the tray out of an
empty matchbox. Use a
sharp pencil to make a
small hole at each end
of the tray.

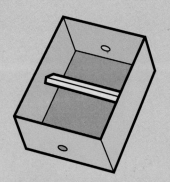

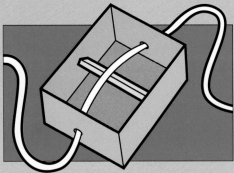

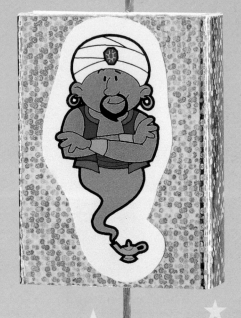

2. Trim a used match with
scissors to make it just
bigger than the width of
the tray. Wedge it across
the inside of the tray.

3. Thread a long piece of
string through the holes in
the tray and over the
match. Then put the
sleeve back on the box.

Doing the trick

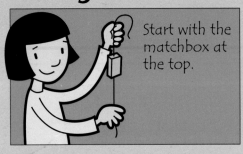

Start with the
matchbox at
the top.

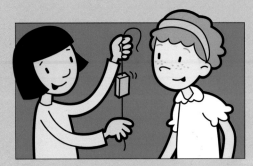

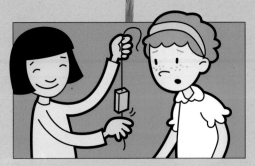

1. Push the matchbox to
one end of the string. Pull
the string to stretch it
tight. Hold it up vertically
with the box at the top.

2. Tell the audience that
you can control the
matchbox. Ask a volunteer
to say the commands "go"
and "stop".

3. Relax the string to make
the matchbox move. To
stop it, stretch the string
tight. Make it move at the
volunteer's command.

Q. Why are matchboxes like soccer teams?
A. Because they're full of strikers.

Escaped prisoner

You could draw your own prisoner, or use the sticker in this book.

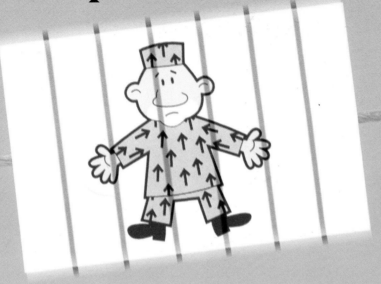

You will need:
A piece of paper
A pair of scissors
A pencil
A glue stick
String

Getting ready

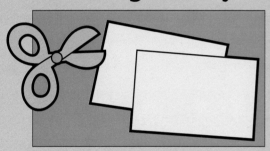

1. Cut out two rectangles of paper, about the size of a playing card. Make them exactly the same size.

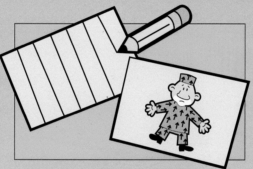

2. Draw straight lines down one piece of paper. Draw a picture of a man on the other (or use the prisoner sticker in this book).

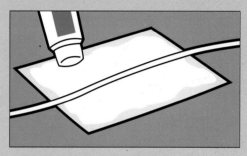

3. Cover the back of one piece of paper in glue. Put a piece of string about the width of this page across the middle of it.

Doing the trick

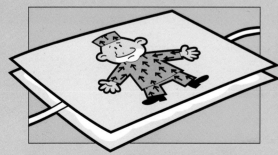

4. Press the back of the other piece of paper on top, so it completely covers the first piece. Leave it to dry.

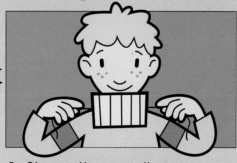

1. Show the audience both sides of the sign. Say the man is an escaped prisoner and you are going to recapture him.

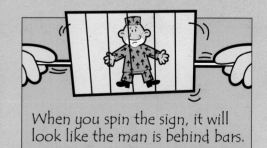

When you spin the sign, it will look like the man is behind bars.

2. Hold the ends of the string, so the man is upside down, facing you. Then spin it quickly between your fingers and thumbs.

Q. How did the female prisoner escape from jail?
A. She used the ladder in her stockings.

Coin drop

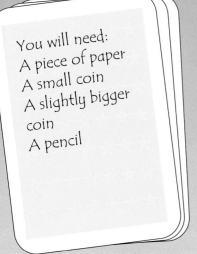

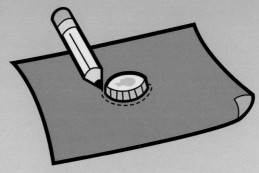

1. You can prepare this trick while the audience is watching. Put a small coin on a piece of paper and draw around it.

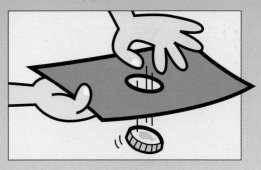

2. Cut out the circle you have drawn. Then hold up the piece of paper and drop the small coin through the hole.

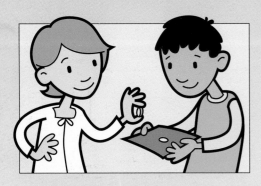

3. Now challenge a volunteer from the audience to fit the bigger coin through the hole. It seems impossible.

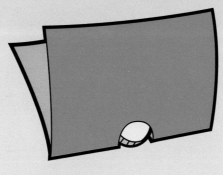

4. Take the paper and the coin back. Fold the paper in half, so the fold is across the middle of the hole. Put the big coin in it, like this.

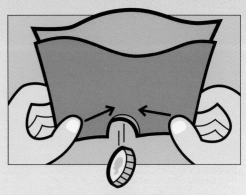

5. Hold the folded piece of paper at the bottom. push the sides up and into the middle. The coin will fall through.

Any two round coins will work for this trick, as long as one is slightly bigger than the other.

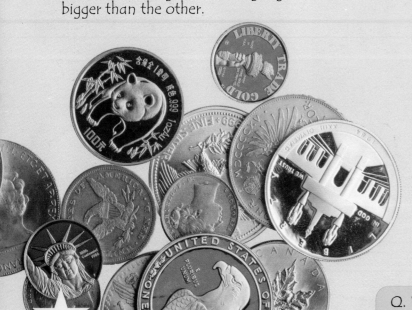

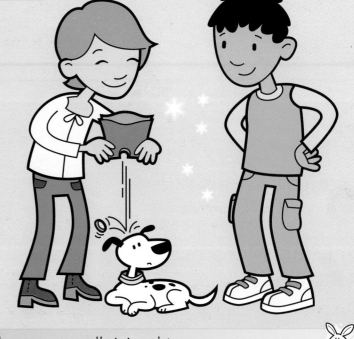

Q. Why is money called dough?
A. Because we knead it.

14

Magic paper

Getting ready

Make two rips in a small piece of paper, from the top to a third of the way down. Fold down the part between the rips.

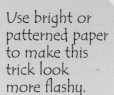

The two rips should be exactly the same length.

Use bright or patterned paper to make this trick look more flashy.

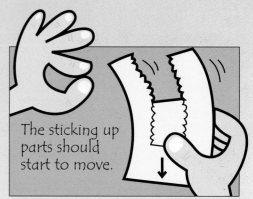

Doing the trick

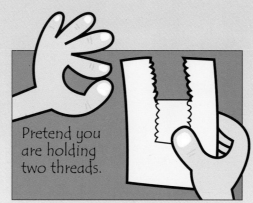

Hold the paper between your fingers and thumb.

Pretend you are holding two threads.

The sticking up parts should start to move.

1. Face your audience. Hold the paper up in your right hand, with the folded part facing you, and your thumb over it.

2. Hold up your left hand behind the paper. Say you are holding invisible threads attached to the sticking-up parts.

3. Slowly pull your left hand away from the paper, as if holding the strings. At the same time, slide your right thumb down.

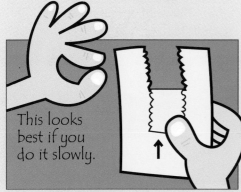

This looks best if you do it slowly.

4. Look like you are really concentrating. Move your left hand forward again and push your right thumb back up.

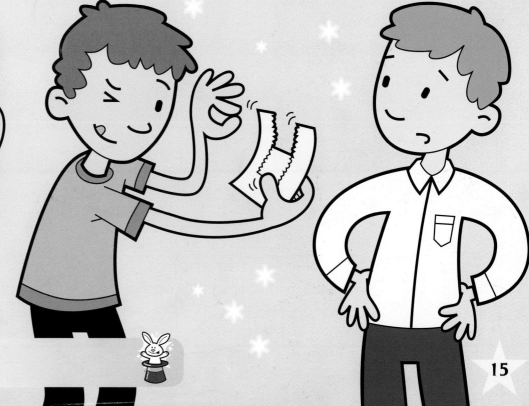

Q. Why is paper like a piano?
A. You can make notes on it.

Wobbly wand

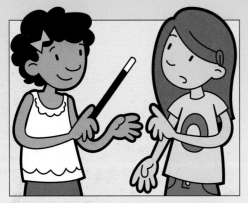

1. Hold out your wand for your audience to examine. Tell them that you can turn it into a bendy wand by saying some magic words.

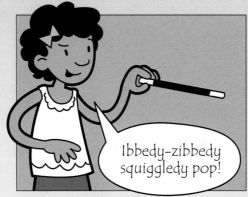

Ibbedy-zibbedy squiggledy pop!

2. Hold your wand loosely at one end, between your first finger and thumb. Look at your wand and say some magic words.

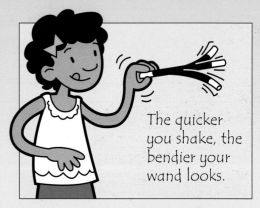

The quicker you shake, the bendier your wand looks.

3. Now move your hand quickly up and down. Make quite small movements. Your wand will look as if it's bending.

Knotty problem

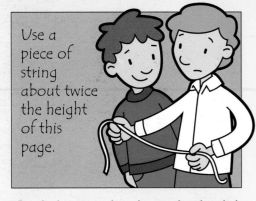

Use a piece of string about twice the height of this page.

1. Ask a volunteer to hold the ends of a piece of string and tie a knot in it without letting go of the ends. It seems impossible.

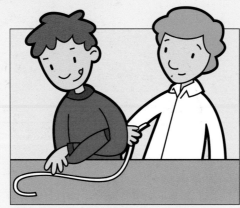

2. When he gives up, lay the string on the table. Cross your arms. Pick up the ends of the string, one end at a time.

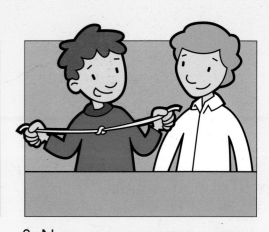

3. Now uncross your arms without letting go of the ends of the string. A knot will magically appear in the middle of it.

Q. Why can't magicians stay in one place?
A. Because they're always wand-ering around.

Magic matchbox

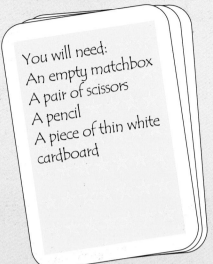

You will need:
An empty matchbox
A pair of scissors
A pencil
A piece of thin white cardboard

In this trick, a picture magically appears in an empty matchbox.

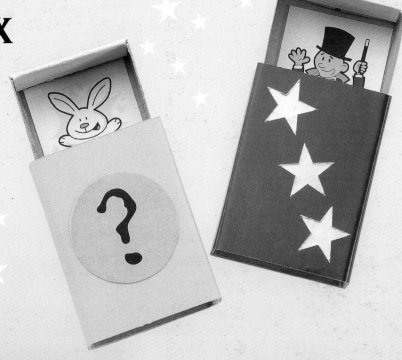

Getting ready

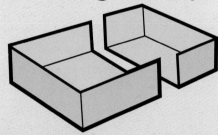

1. Take the tray out of an empty matchbox. Cut a piece off the end of the tray, about a third of the way along it.

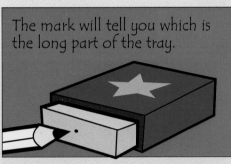

The mark will tell you which is the long part of the tray.

2. Put both parts of the tray back in the sleeve, with the long part sticking out slightly. Make a mark on the end of the long part.

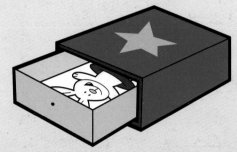

3. Cut out a piece of cardboard small enough to fit into the tray. Draw a picture on it, or put a sticker on it. Put it in the tray.

Doing the trick

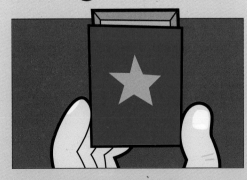

1. Hold the matchbox vertically, with the long part of the tray at the top. Tell the audience that it is a magic matchbox.

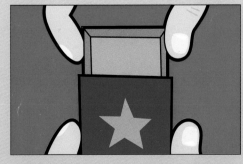

2. Pull up the long part of the tray. The picture will stay hidden inside the matchbox, so it will look as if the tray is empty.

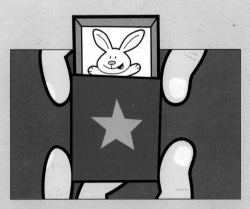

3. Close the box. Tap it with your wand. Then push the short part of the tray up from underneath, like this. The picture will appear.

Q. What did the matchbox say to the used match?
A. You're fired!

17

Disappearing coin

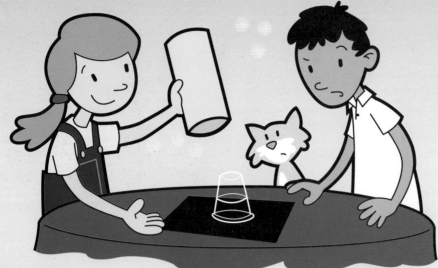

Getting ready

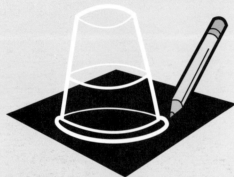

1. Turn the plastic cup upside down on a piece of cardboard. Hold it steady and carefully draw around it with a pencil.

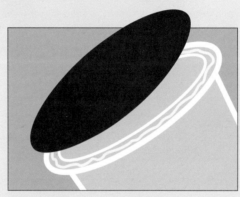

2. Cut out the circle of cardboard. Put a thin layer of glue around the rim of the cup. Press the cardboard onto it.

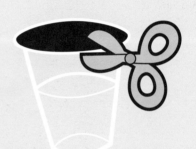

3. Let the glue dry. Then carefully cut off any cardboard sticking out around the rim of the cup. Wipe off any extra glue too.

Never let your audience see underneath the cup.

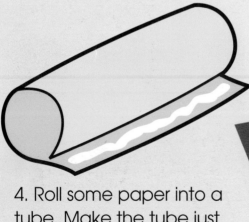

4. Roll some paper into a tube. Make the tube just wide enough to fit over the cup. Glue the edges together. Leave it to dry.

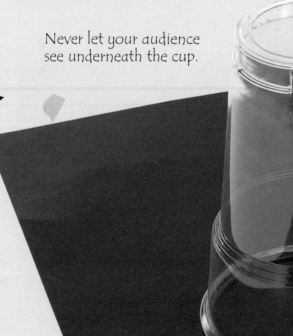

Q. Where do frogs keep their money?
A. At the riverbank.

Doing the trick

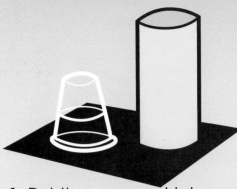

1. Put the cup and tube next to each other on the cardboard, like this. Ask your audience for a coin. A thin one works best.

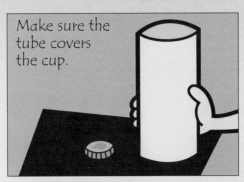

Make sure the tube covers the cup.

2. Put the coin on the cardboard and say that you are going to make it disappear. Then slide the paper tube over the cup.

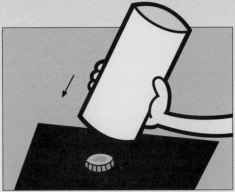

3. Squeeze the tube between your fingers and thumb, so it grips the cup. Lift them both up and put them on top of the coin.

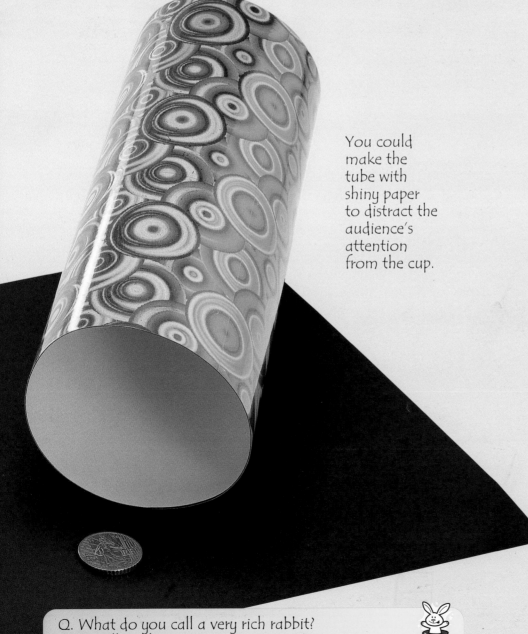

You could make the tube with shiny paper to distract the audience's attention from the cup.

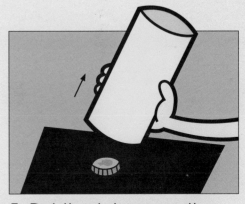

4. Now lift the tube all the way off, leaving the cup where it is. It will look as if the coin has disappeared.

5. Put the tube over the cup and tap it with your wand. Lift them both off to make the coin reappear.

Q. What do you call a very rich rabbit?
A. A million-hare.

Magic handkerchief

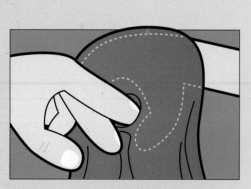

In this trick, you push a wand straight through a handkerchief.

This trick works best if you use a big handkerchief.

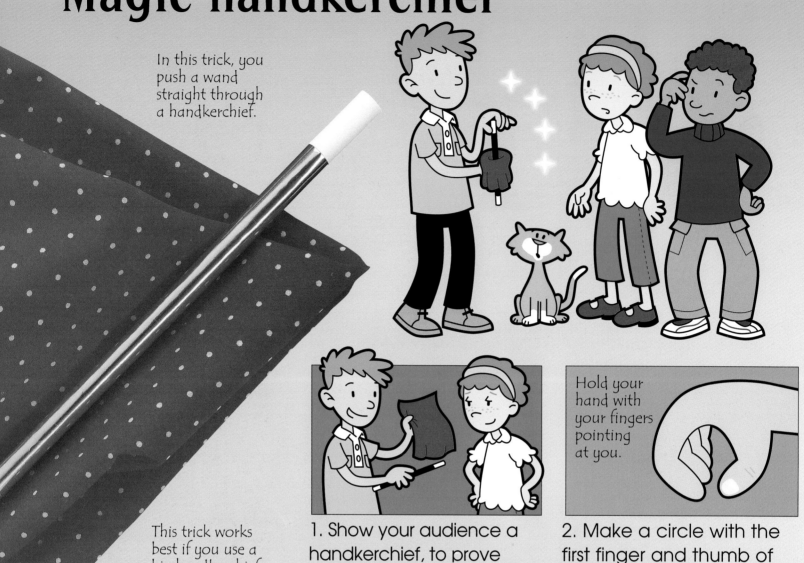

1. Show your audience a handkerchief, to prove that there are no holes in it. Tell them you can push your wand through it.

Hold your hand with your fingers pointing at you.

2. Make a circle with the first finger and thumb of your right hand, but leave a gap between them. Put the handkerchief over it.

3. Push the first finger of your left hand into the circle. Bring your middle finger in through the gap, to make a tunnel.

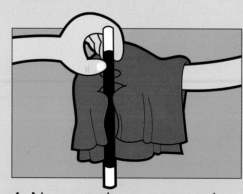

4. Now push your wand through the tunnel. It will look as if your wand is going straight through the handkerchief.

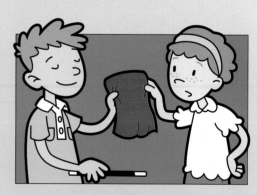

5. Shake the handkerchief out and show it to the audience, so they can see that there are still no holes in it.

Q. Why couldn't the viper viper nose?
A. Because the adder adder handkerchief!

Jumping rubber band

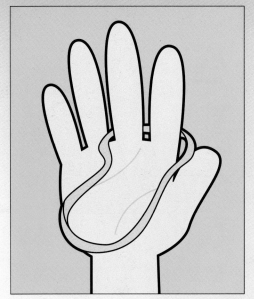

1. Put a rubber band over your first and middle fingers. Hold it up like this, so the back of your hand faces the audience.

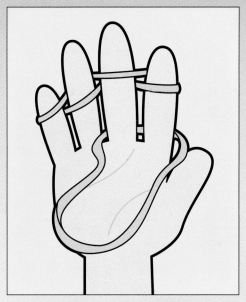

2. On the same hand, twist another rubber band around the tops of your fingers. Do this while the audience watches.

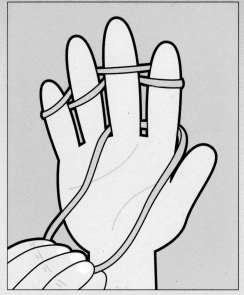

3. Now take the first rubber band between your fingers and thumb. Stretch it back quite far, like this.

The back of your hand should always face the audience, so they can't see what your fingers are doing.

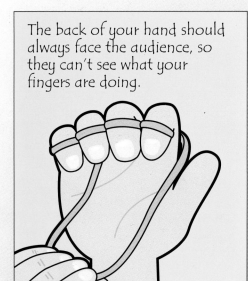

4. With the rubber band stretched back, curl your fingers over to make a fist. Let the rubber band go and straighten your fingers.

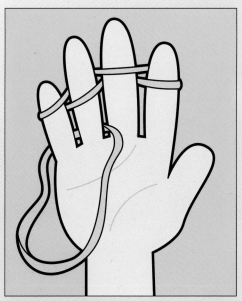

5. The band will magically jump across the barrier made by the second rubber band, onto your other two fingers.

If you do this trick quickly, it looks really impressive.

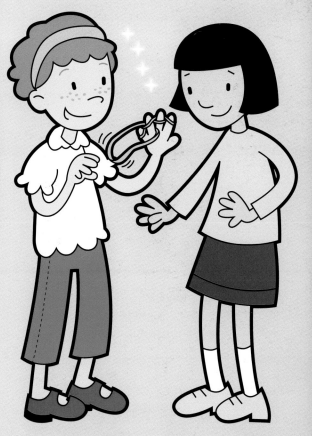

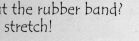
Q. Have you heard the one about the rubber band?
A. They could play anything at a stretch!

21

Find the card

Getting ready

1. Look through a deck of cards. Some of the numbers and letters have rounded tops and some of them don't.

Not rounded tops

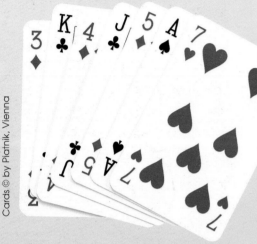

Rounded tops

Count the tens as cards with rounded tops, even though the one isn't rounded.

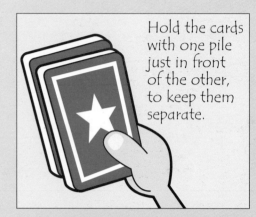

Hold the cards with one pile just in front of the other, to keep them separate.

2. Place all the cards with rounded tops in a pile and all the other cards in another pile. Place the piles together, like this.

Cards © by Piatnik, Vienna

Doing the trick

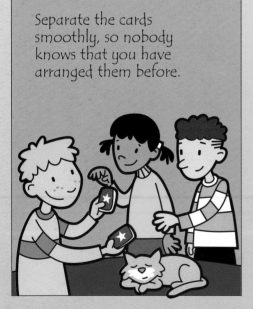

Separate the cards smoothly, so nobody knows that you have arranged them before.

1. Ask for two volunteers. Give the cards with rounded numbers to one of them and the other cards to the other.

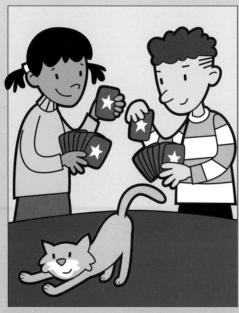

2. Ask your volunteers to pick a card each and memorize it. They mustn't show you the cards they pick.

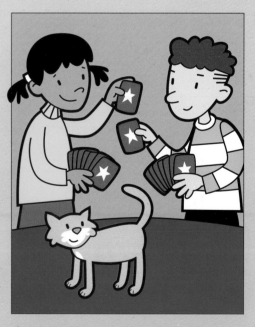

3. Ask them to swap the two cards they picked. Then ask them to put the new card anywhere in their part of the deck.

Q. Why did the thief steal the deck of cards?
A. Because it was full of diamonds.

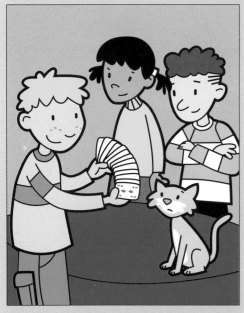

4. Take both piles of cards back. Put them together, without mixing them up, and fan them out in front of you.

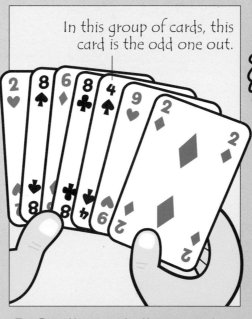

In this group of cards, this card is the odd one out.

5. Go through the cards with rounded tops looking for one without a rounded top. Do the opposite with the other pile of cards.

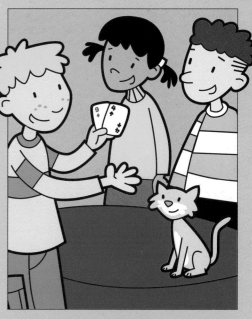

6. The two cards that you pick out will be the cards that your volunteers chose. Show them and take a bow.

Magic knot

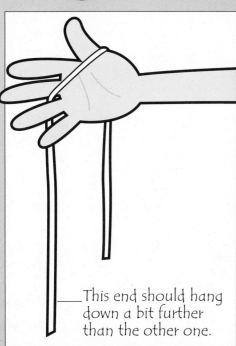

This end should hang down a bit further than the other one.

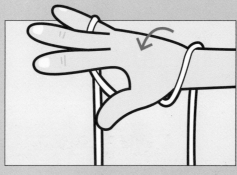

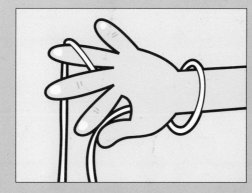

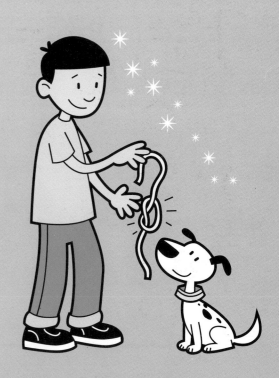

1. Cut a piece of string, about twice the length of this page. Lay it over your right hand, like this.

2. Angle your hand forward. Take the shorter end of the string between your finger and thumb.

3. Still holding the string, shake your hand, so the string falls off. A knot will appear.

Q. Why are cards like businessmen?
A. They come in suits.

23

Abracadabra magic cards

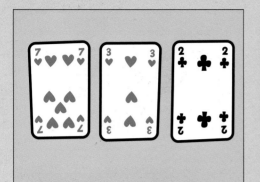

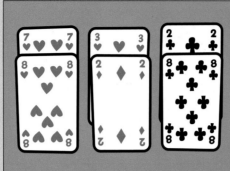

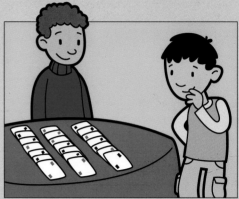

1. Deal a row of three cards onto a table. Deal them out from left to right, facing up so your audience can see them.

2. Deal three more cards from left to right, just under the first three. Keep doing this until you have three columns of seven cards.

3. Ask a volunteer from the audience to memorize one of the cards on the table, but not to tell you which one.

Lay out the three columns of cards like this.

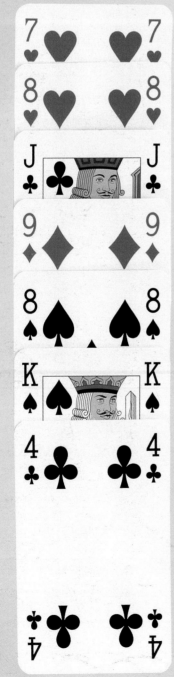

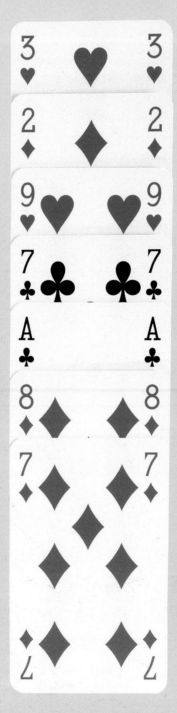

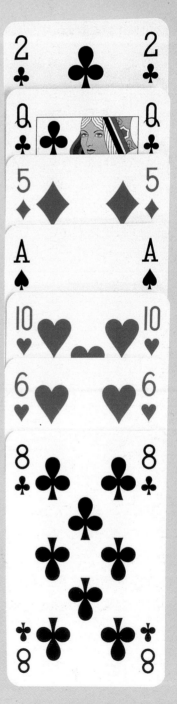

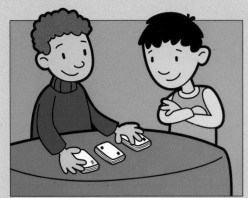

4. Ask your volunteer to say which column the card is in. Then gather each column up, so you have three piles.

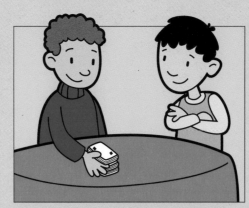

5. Put the three piles of cards together, with the pile that contains your volunteer's card in the middle.

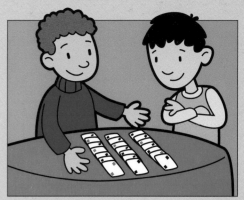

6. Deal out three columns of cards in exactly the same way, and repeat steps 4 and 5. Then do this step again.

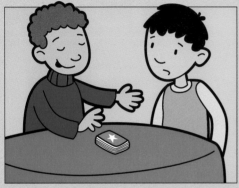

7. Now tell the audience that "abracadabra" is a very magic word. Say that you are about to prove it.

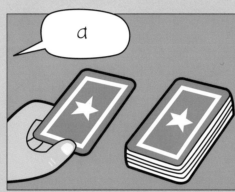

8. Take a card from the top of the pile. Put it face down on the table. As you do this, say "a": the first letter of "abracadabra".

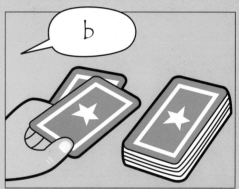

9. Now do the same thing with the next card in the pile, and say "b". Lay it face down, on top of the first card.

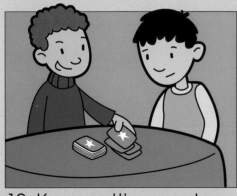

10. Keep putting cards down one by one on the table. Each time you put one down, say the next letter of "abracadabra".

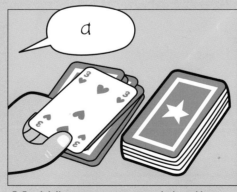

11. When you get to the last "a", put the card face up on the table. It will be the card your volunteer chose.

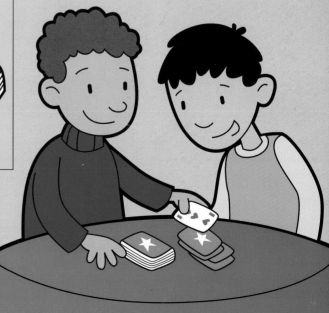

Q. What card game do alligators like best?
A. Snap, of course!

25

Card control

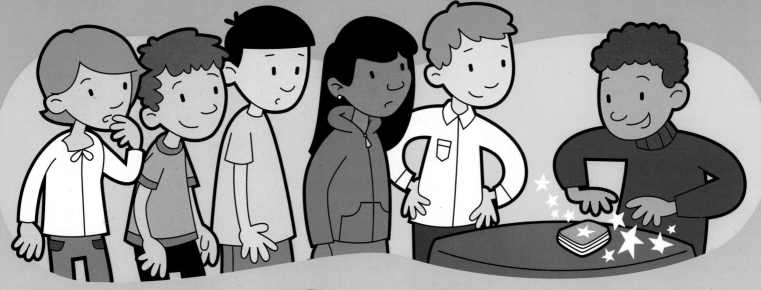

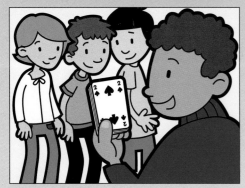

1. Hold a deck of cards up with the backs facing the audience. Tell them you need a volunteer for a mind control trick.

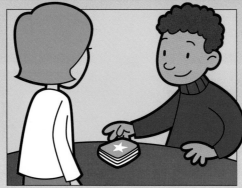

2. As you do step 1, secretly memorize the card that is facing you. Then put the deck of cards face down on the table.

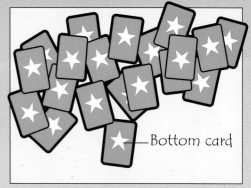

Bottom card

3. Mess up all the cards on the table, like this. Do it so the bottom card ends up slightly separate and remember where it is.

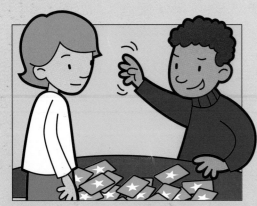

4. Say you will ask the volunteer to pick a certain card and that you will control her mind to guide her to the right one.

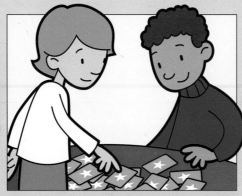

5. Ask the volunteer to pick the card you memorized. For example, if it was the two of spades, say, "Point to the two of spades."

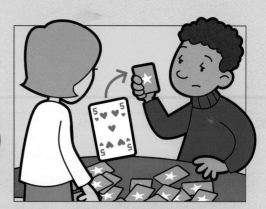

6. Ask the volunteer to give you the card without looking at it. Look at the new card, memorize it and put it to one side.

Q. What do magicians wear to keep warm?
A. Card-igans.

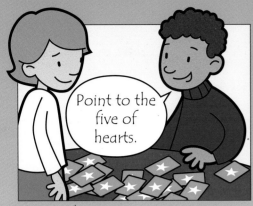

7. Now ask for the card that your volunteer just gave you. She won't know she has already picked it.

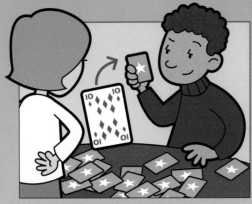

8. Once again, look at the card and memorize it, then put it with the other card your volunteer chose.

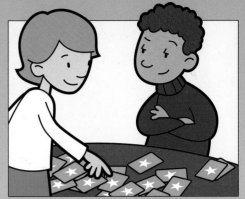

9. Ask for the card your volunteer just gave you, but when she chooses one, shake your head and tell her to try again.

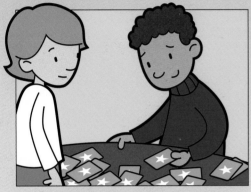

10. When she chooses another one, tell her she is wrong again. Say you will pick it. Pick up the card you memorized in step 3.

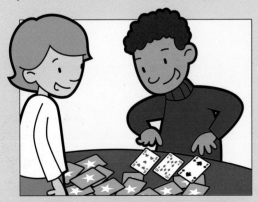

11. Pick up the three cards. Lay them in a line face down on the table, then turn them over. The audience will be amazed.

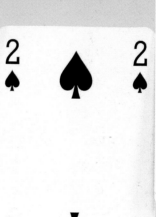
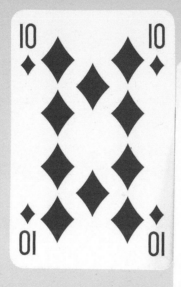
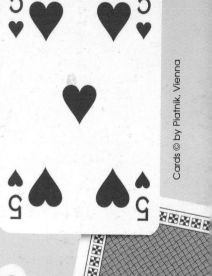

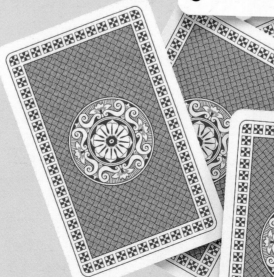
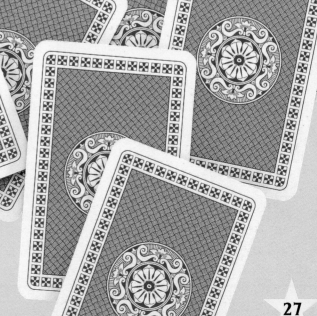

Cards © by Piatnik, Vienna

Q. Which animal always wins at cards?
A. A cheetah!

Jumping coin

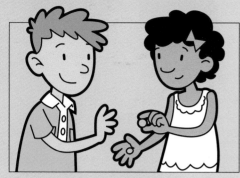

1. Ask your audience for two coins. The coins don't need to be the same.

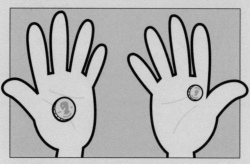

2. Put one coin in the middle of your left palm and the other on the right side of your right palm.

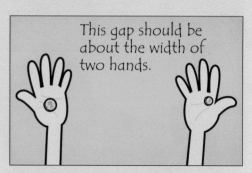

This gap should be about the width of two hands.

3. Lay your hands on the table with a gap between them and your palms facing up.

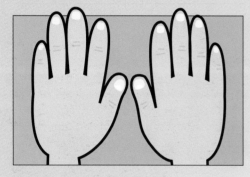

4. Turn your hands over quickly with the coins on them, like this. The coin on your right hand will jump across to your left hand.

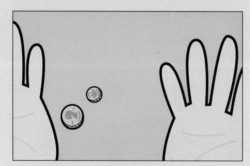

5. Ask the audience where the coins are. When they tell you there is one under each hand, lift your hands up and show them.

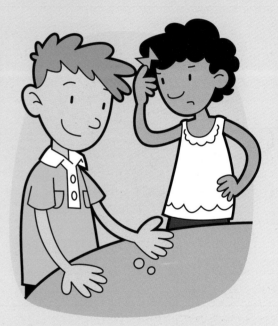

Changing coins

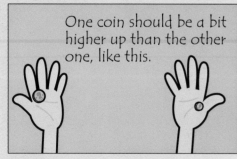

One coin should be a bit higher up than the other one, like this.

1. For another version of the jumping coin trick, put two different coins on the sides of your palms.

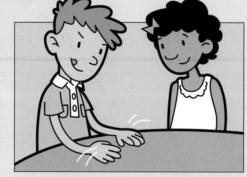

2. Tell the audience to look closely at which coin is in which hand. Then do steps 3 and 4 of "Jumping coin".

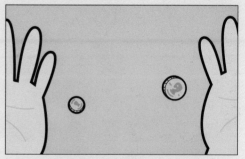

3. Ask the audience which coin is under which hand, then lift your hands. They will have swapped places.

Q. What happened when the cat swallowed a coin?
A. There was money in the kitty!

One-sided paper

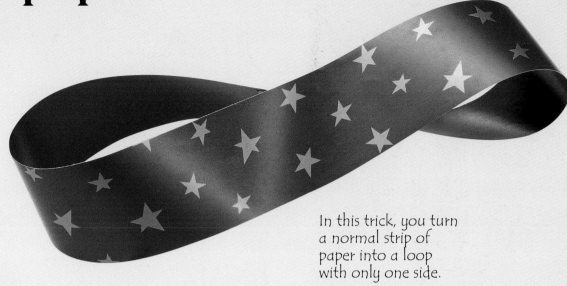

In this trick, you turn a normal strip of paper into a loop with only one side.

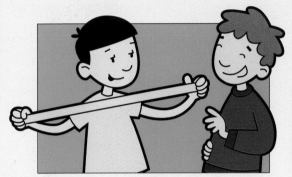

1. Hold up the strip of paper and tell your audience that it only has one side. If they laugh, say you will prove it.

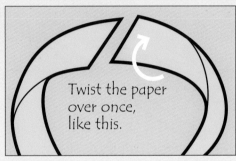

Twist the paper over once, like this.

2. Hold the strip up like this, to make a loop. Twist one of the ends over once, to make a single twist in the loop.

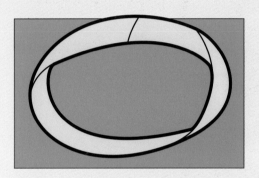

3. Hold the ends of the loop together and stick them with tape. Then ask for a volunteer from the audience.

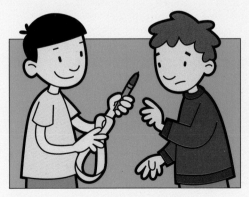

4. Ask the volunteer to draw a line along the middle of the strip, without taking the pen off the paper.

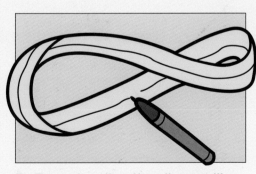

5. Eventually, the line will join up with itself. Point out that the pen has never left the paper, so the paper must be one-sided.

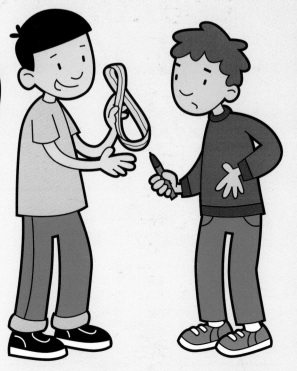

Q. What's the angriest part of a newspaper?
A. The crossword!

29

Loopy loops

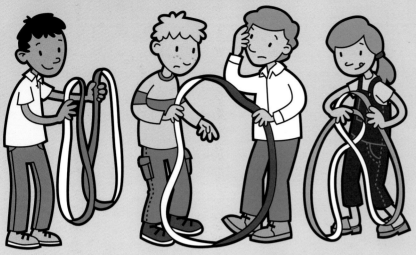

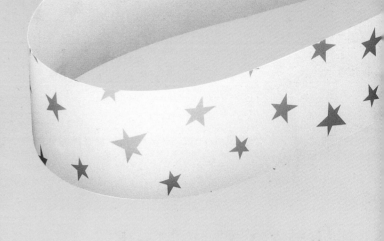

Getting ready

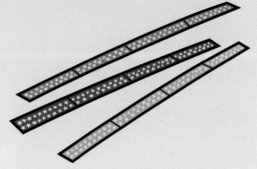

You will need:
Lots of long strips of paper, about the width of a matchbox (Giftwrap or newspaper works well.)
Scissors
Clear sticky tape

1. Stick strips of paper together with tape until you have a strip about 1.5m (5ft) long. Make three of these long strips.

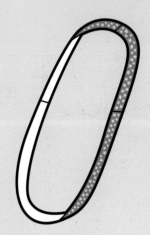

2. Use the first strip to make a big loop without any twists in it. Hold the ends together and stick them with tape.

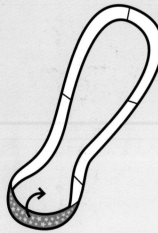

3. Take the bottom of the loop and carefully turn it over once, like this, so that part of it is twisted.

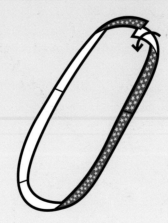

4. Pick up another strip. Make it into a loop. Turn one of the ends over, like this, and stick the ends together with tape.

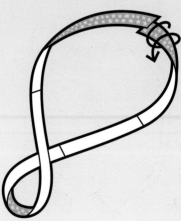

5. Pick up the third strip and make a loop. Turn one end over twice, like this. Then stick the ends together with tape.

30

Q. What's black and white and read all over?
A. A newspaper.

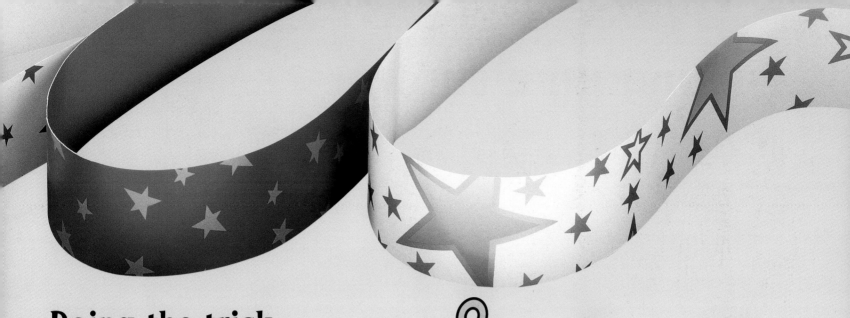

Doing the trick

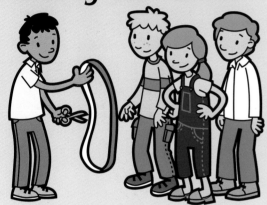

1. Show the three loops of paper to the audience. Put the last two loops you made on one side and hold up the first one.

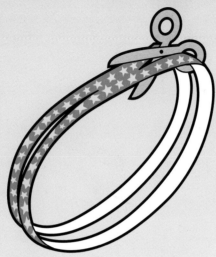

2. Cut the loop in half lengthways, like this. Hold up the two separate thin loops, to show the audience.

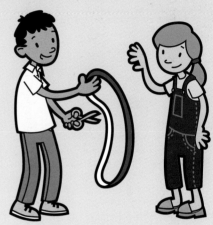

3. Put the two thin loops on one side and pick up the second loop you made. Ask for a volunteer from the audience.

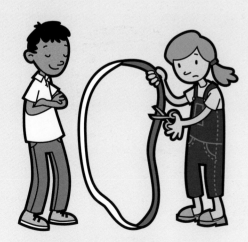

4. Challenge the volunteer to make two loops by cutting the loop in half. In fact, it will end up as one enormous loop.

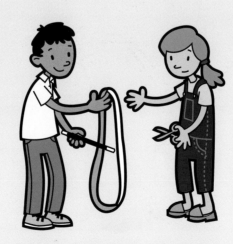

5. Now ask the volunteer to try again, using the third loop. Say that you will use your wand to help her.

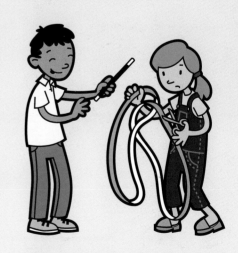

6. Wave your wand around over the loop. This time, your volunteer will end up with two loops joined together.

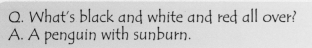
Q. What's black and white and red all over?
A. A penguin with sunburn.

Putting on a show

When putting on a show, it looks much better if you have a box to keep your tricks in. Make one by decorating a large cardboard box. Tape a piece of cardboard across the middle of it, to make two compartments.

Start your show by putting all of your tricks in one compartment.

When you've done a trick, put it into the other compartment.

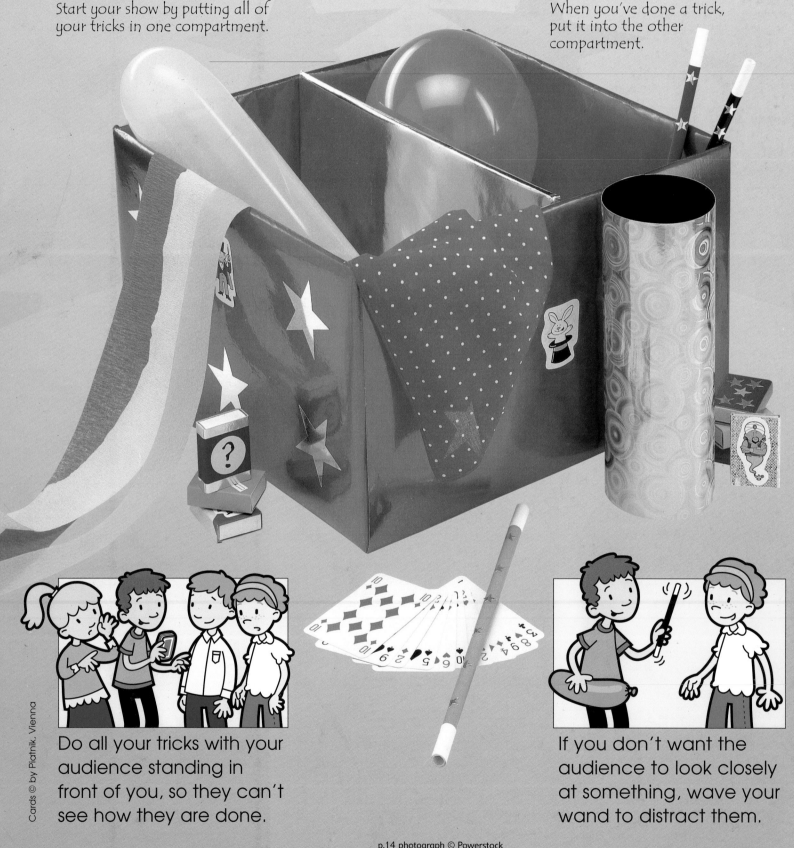

Do all your tricks with your audience standing in front of you, so they can't see how they are done.

If you don't want the audience to look closely at something, wave your wand to distract them.

p.14 photograph © Powerstock

First published in 2007 by Usborne Publishing Ltd. Usborne House, 83-85 Saffron Hill, London EC1N 8RT, England. www.usborne.com
Copyright © 2007, 2003 Usborne Publishing Ltd. The name Usborne and the devices ♀ ⊕ are Trade Marks of Usborne Publishing Ltd. All rights reserved. No part of this publication may be reproduced, stored in a retrieval system, or transmitted in any form or by any means, electronic, mechanical, photocopying, recording or otherwise, without prior permission of the publisher. UE. Printed in Malaysia. First published Tan America in 2007.